TECHNIQUES IN LIVER SURGERY

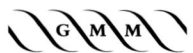

© 1997

GREENWICH MEDICAL MEDIA
219 The Linen Hall
162-168 Regent Street
London
W1R 5TB

ISBN 1 900151 251

First Published 1997

Apart from any fair dealing for the purposes of research or private study, or criticism or review, as permitted under the UK Copyright Designs and Patents Act, 1988, this publication may not be reproduced, stored, or transmitted, in any form or by any means, without the prior permission in writing of the publishers, or in the case of reprographic reproduction only in accordance with the terms of the licences issued by the Copyright Licensing Agency in the UK, or in accordance with the terms of the licences issued by the appropriate Reproduction Rights Organization outside the UK. Enquiries concerning reproduction outside the terms stated here should be sent to the publishers at the London address printed above.

The rights of Alighieri Mazziotti and Antonino Cavallari to be identified as editors of this work has been asserted by them in accordance with the Copyright, Designs and Patents Acts 1988.

The publisher makes no representation, express or implied, with regard to the accuracy of the information contained in this book and cannot accept any legal responsibility or liability for any errors or omissions that may be made.

British Library Cataloguing in Publication Data
A catalogue record for this book is available from the British Library

Distributed worldwide by
Oxford University Press

Designed and Produced by
Derek Virtue, DataNet

Printed in Hong Kong by
Dah Hua

TECHNIQUES IN LIVER SURGERY

Edited by

Alighieri Mazziotti
and
Antonino Cavallari

With the contribution of
J. Belghiti
E. Moreno González
L. Hannoun
M. Makuuchi
A.G. Tzakis

Foreword by
C. Broelsch

Greenwich Medical Media

This book is devoted to the memory of
Professor Giuseppe Gozzetti

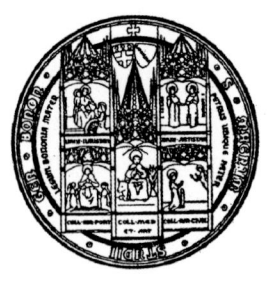

Alma Mater Studiorum

Under the auspices of the
University of Bologna

"E tu, che dici esser meglio il veder fare l'anatomia che vedere tali disegni, diresti bene se fosse possibile vedere tutte queste cose che in tali disegni si dimostrano in una sola figura, nella quale con tutto il tuo ingegno non verdrai e non avrai la notizia se non di alquante poche vene, delle quali io per averne vera e piena notizia ho disfatto più di dieci corpi umani distruggendo ogni altro membro... e un sol corpo non bastava a tanto tempo, che bisognava procedere in tanti corpi affinchè si finisse l'intera cognizione, la quale replicai due volte per vedere le differenze. ...E se tu avrai il disegno... egli non ti servirà se ti mancherà l'ordine... o se ti mancherà la pazienza... o se tu non sarai diligente".

"And you, who say that it is better to study anatomy by dissection rather than through these drawings, would be absolutely right if it were possible to see all those things which in these drawings can be shown in a single figure. However skilful you are, you will not see or be aware of more than just a few veins, whereas I, to understand them to the full, have had to dissect more than ten human corpses, destroying every other member... and the time available with one single corpse was not enough, so that I had to proceed gradually with many corpses until my knowledge was complete. This I repeated twice to see the differences. ...And if you have the drawing... this will be no help to you... if you lack the order... or you have no patience... or you are not diligent."

LEONARDO DA VINCI,
Quaderni di Anatomia,
vol 1, folio 13

TECHNIQUES IN LIVER SURGERY

CONTENTS

Contributors xi
Foreword xiii
Preface xv

SECTION ONE: BASIC ANATOMY 1

1. Surgical Anatomy of the Liver and
   Classification of Hepatectomies 3
2. Approaches in Liver Surgery 9

**SECTION TWO: STANDARD TECHNIQUES
OF LIVER RESECTION** 15

3. Right Hepatectomy 17
4. Left Hepatectomy 33
5. Left Lobectomy 43
6. Liver Segmentectomies 47
7. Liver Surgery in the Cirrhotic Patient 69
8. Extended Right Hepatectomy 79
9. Extended Left Hepatectomy 85

**SECTION THREE: COMPLEX TECHNIQUES OF
LIVER RESECTION** 91

10. 'Central Liver' Resection 93
11. Surgery of the Caudate Lobe 101

**SECTION FOUR: TECHNIQUES WITH
VASCULAR INVOLVEMENT** 117

12. Total Vascular Exclusion of the Liver 119
13. Liver Rescections with Involvement of
    the Retrohepatic Vena Cava 125

**SECTION FIVE: GENERAL ASPECTS OF
LIVER RESECTION** 133

14. Resection Technique 135
15. Evaluation of the Hepatic Functional Reserve 141

16. Tolerance of Liver Ischemia 145
17. Intra-operative Ultrasonography 149
18. Indications for Liver Resection 157
19. Pre-operative Portal Embolization 163

**SECTION SIX: SURGERY FOR LIVER
CYSTS AND TRAUMA** 169

20. Surgery for Non-Parasitic Liver Cysts 171
21. Surgery for Liver Hydatidosis 177
22. Liver Trauma 191

SECTION SEVEN: INTRA-ARTERIAL CHEMOTHERAPY 201

23. Intra-arterial Infusion for Locoregional Chemotherapy 203

SECTION EIGHT: BILIARY TUMORS 213

24. Resection of the Hilar Cholangiocarcinoma 215

SECTION NINE: INNOVATIVE TECHNIQUES 237

25. Major Liver Resections Using Hypothermic Perfusion 239

**SECTION TEN: STANDARD TECHNIQUES OF
LIVER TRANSPLANTATION** 249

26. Liver Procurement for Transplantation 251
27. Conventional Transplantation Technique 261
28. The 'Piggy-Back' Technique 275
29. Technical Problems and Complications of
    Liver Transplantation 287

**SECTION ELEVEN: ADVANCED TECHNIQUES OF
LIVER TRANSPLANTATION** 305

30. Reduced Grafts and Split Liver Transplantation 307
31. Transplantation from Living Related Donors 317
32. Auxiliary Liver Transplantation 325
33. Intestinal and Multiorgan Transplantation 337

APPENDIX 349
A Delayed Revolution: A History of Liver Surgery 351

INDEX 363

TECHNIQUES IN LIVER SURGERY
CONTRIBUTORS

Jacques Belghiti
PROFESSOR AND CHAIRMAN
Department of Digestive Surgery
Hôpital Beaujoin - Paris
France

Dominique C. Borie
FELLOW
Department of Digestive Surgery
Hôpital Saint Antoine - Paris
France

Christoph E. Broelsch
PROFESSOR OF SURGERY AND CHAIRMAN
Department of Surgery
University of Hamburg
Germany

Patricia Byers
ASSOCIATE PROFESSOR OF
CLINICAL SURGERY
Division of Trauma Services
Department of Surgery
University of Miami - USA

A. González Chamozzo
FELLOW
Department of Digestive Surgery
Hospital '12 de Octubre' - Madrid
Spain

Antonino Cavallari
PROFESSOR AND CHAIRMAN
Department of Surgery and Transplantation
University of Bologna
S. Orsola Hospital - Bologna
Italy

Giorgio Ercolani
RESIDENT
Department of Surgery and Transplantation
University of Bologna
S. Orsola Hospital - Bologna
Italy

Olivier Farges
ASSOCIATE PROFESSOR OF SURGERY
Department of Digestive Surgery
Hôpital Beaujoin - Paris
France

Georgios P. Fragulidis
ASSISTANT PROFESSOR OF SURGERY
Division of Liver/GI Transplantation
Department of Surgery
University of Miami - USA

I. García García
ASSOCIATE PROFESSOR OF SURGERY
Department of Digestive Surgery
Hospital '12 de Octubre' - Madrid
Spain

Enrique Moreno González
PROFESSOR AND CHAIRMAN
Division of General and
Transplantation Surgery
Hospital '12 de Octubre' - Madrid
Spain

Gian Luca Grazi
ASSISTANT PROFESSOR OF SURGERY
Department of Surgery and Transplantation
University of Bologna
S. Orsola Hospital - Bologna
Italy

Antony Gyampi
ASSOCIATE PROFESSOR OF
CLINICAL ANAESTHESIOLOGY
Department of Anaesthesiology
University of Miami - USA

Laurent Hannoun
PROFESSOR OF SURGERY
Department of Digestive Surgery
Hôpital Saint Antoine - Paris
France

xi

Elio Jovine
ASSISTANT PROFESSOR OF SURGERY
Department of Surgery and Transplantation
University of Bologna
S. Orsola Hospital - Bologna
Italy

Theodore Karatzas
VISITING ASSISTANT PROFESSOR
Division of Liver/GI Transplantation
Department of Surgery
University of Miami - USA

Tomoaki Kato
VISITING DOCTOR
Division of Liver/GI Transplantation
Department of Surgery
University of Miami - USA

Seiji Kawasaki
1st Department of Surgery
Shinshu University School of Medicine
Matsumoto
Japan

Farrukh A. Khan
ASSISTANT PROFESSOR OF CLINICAL SURGERY
Division of Liver/GI Transplantation
Department of Surgery
University of Miami - USA

Masatoshi Makuuchi
PROFESSOR AND CHAIRMAN
2nd Department of Surgery
University of Tokyo
Japan

Alighieri Mazziotti
PROFESSOR OF SURGERY
Department of Surgery and Transplantation
University of Bologna
S. Orsola Hospital - Bologna
Italy

J.C. Meneu Diaz
RESIDENT OF SURGERY
Department of Digestive Surgery
Hospital '12 de Octubre' - Madrid
Spain

José R. Nery
ASSOCIATE PROFESSOR OF CLINICAL SURGERY
Division of Liver/GI Transplantation
Department of Surgery
University of Miami - USA

Les Olson
DIRECTOR
Organ Procurement Organization
University of Miami - USA

M. Hildago Pasqual
PROFESSOR OF SURGERY
Department of Digestive Surgery
Hospital '12 de Octubre' - Madrid
Spain

Filippo Pierangeli
RESIDENT
Department of Surgery and Transplantation
University of Bologna
S. Orsola Hospital - Bologna
Italy

Camillo Ricordi
PROFESSOR AND CHAIRMAN
Division of Cellular Transplantation
University of Miami - USA

Philip Ruiz
ASSOCIATE PROFESSOR OF
CLINICAL IMMUNOLOGY
Department of Pathology
University of Miami - USA

Alain Sauvanet
ASSOCIATE PROFESSOR OF SURGERY
Department of Digestive Surgery
Hôpital Beaujoin – Paris
France

Tadatoshi Takayama
2nd Department of Surgery
University of Tokyo
Japan

Andreas G. Tzakis
PROFESSOR AND CHAIRMAN
Department of Surgery
Division of Transplantation
University of Miami - USA

Marc G. Webb
ASSISTANT PROFESSOR OF
CLINICAL SURGERY
Division of Liver/GI Transplantation
Department of Surgery
University of Miami - USA

Debbie Weppler
CLINICAL SPECIALIST
Division of Liver/GI Transplantation
University of Miami - USA

TECHNIQUES IN LIVER SURGERY

FOREWORD

Liver surgery has developed in the last 30 years from a prohibitive and highly risky endeavor performed by few surgeons to a rather standardized and calculable treatment modality. This area of surgery has been growing at a spectacular rate, extending its benefits into liver transplantation.

Clearly the entire achievements of reduced size and living related liver transplantation derive from the advances in conventional liver surgery. Despite the large number of publications in this field, *Techniques in Liver Surgery* presents a most suitable update of this fast developing branch of surgery still posing formidable challenges and problems.

It is a great honor for me to introduce this book conceived and mastered by Giuseppe Gozzetti, an admired friend and respected colleague, who, unfortunately prematurely deceased, is being deeply missed by all those who had the privilege to meet him closely. This remarkable work, which could not be finished by him personally, has been nevertheless completed and perfected by his associates and heirs Alighieri Mazziotti and Antonino Cavallari. Professor Gozzetti has evolved a s a pioneer in this field and continued to keep at the forefront with important contributions and with the creation of a surgical school in Bologna.

The book embodies the essence of liver surgery as conceived by Gozzetti: the liver surgeon as an expert in all aspects and facets of liver problems, where the knowledge of liver diseases, anatomy, physiology, pathology condense and blend in the practice of liver resection and transplantation.

The book is a contribution both for the neophyte liver surgeon with basic, detailed description of standard surgical techniques, as well as for the mature and expert liver surgeon who will be satisfied by the more advanced procedures, the newest techniques and updates in the field. The Editors managed to successfully integrate a major core of knowledge from the Bolognese School of Gozzetti with the newest developments as described by the very same experts who developed them. The structure of this work touches all of liver surgery, with major emphasis on technical aspects, but with insight on strategy and indications. The brief description of potential pitfalls and complications demonstrates the experience of the Authors and gives a particular interest and value to the publication. The illustrations from the Bologna school of Medical Drawing are of the greatest quality and very helpful in clarifying the essential and eloquent text.

Liver Surgery rises and stands strong and independent in this book as an enduring materialization of the ideas of Giuseppe Gozzetti, promoter and supporter Hepato-Biliary-Pancreatic Association throughout his career.

The book may contribute to honoring a surgeon who moved a particular field of surgery into a new dimension, thus serving many patients to receive a better treatment.

Christoph E. Broelsch MD PhD FACS
Professor and Chairman
HAMBURG, FEBRUARY 14, 1997

TECHNIQUES IN LIVER SURGERY

PREFACE

At the beginning of 1995, Professor Giuseppe Gozzetti began planning a book on liver surgery, describing the main techniques used in Bologna over 15 years of intensive work in the field of liver resection and transplantation. Unfortunately, these and other plans were curtailed by a long illness which Professor Gozzetti bore with a dignity and courage equal to the force of his spirit, well-known to all who had met him. We felt under an obligation to continue this work, certain that this was the best way to honor the memory of this great man and master of surgery.

The work of Professor Gozzetti marked an important step forward in the development of liver surgery worldwide. He lived through the great transformation in this branch of surgery in the early 1980s, from pioneer surgery oriented towards massive lesions, with inconsistent and in the long-term disappointing results, towards current hepatic surgery, perfectly programmed and safe. This was brought about in part by the progress of diagnostic radiology, and, above all the introduction of ultrasound which could detect small asymptomatic lesions that are more susceptible to radical surgery, with better immediate and long term results. In parallel, the development of liver transplantation from the end of the 1980s has greatly enhanced the experience of surgeons and anesthesiologists. This experience has enabled surgical indications to be extended to more extensive resections and right up to surgery defined as 'extreme' in view of the extent of the resection or the complexity of the procedure adopted. Interventional radiology techniques have encouraged this development with arterial chemoembolization reducing the volume of tumors which would otherwise not be resectable, and with portal embolization for the hypertrophy of remaining sections of the liver, thus enabling previously impossible resection surgery to be carried out successfully.

The complexity of problems associated with liver surgery, the growing body of literature increasing the number of clinical case studies, and the need for close collaboration with anesthesiologists, radiologists, oncologists and other specialists in liver disease and immunology, have led to the birth of a new specialty, Hepato-Bilio-Pancreatic surgery, of which Professor Gozzetti was one of the pioneers.

This book describes the main surgical techniques used in Bologna and elsewhere in the field of liver resection and transplantation. These include standard hepatectomies, anatomical segmentectomies, extended resection techniques and techniques associated with liver transplantation, taking into account indications and possible complications, their prevention and treatment. We have invited a number of highly regarded specialists to deal with subjects not directly undertaken in Bologna. Jacques Belghiti, in Paris, where the procedure for 'reglée' hepatectomy was developed by Lortat Jacob, describes heterotopic transplants and resection in cirrhotic livers. Laurent Hannoun, also from Paris, deals with "extreme" surgery with *ex vivo* and *ex situ* procedures. Masatoshi Makuuchi has given great impetus to modern resection liver surgery and contributes the chapter on liver transplantation from living donors. Andreas Tzakis, who trained alongside Professor Starzl in Pittsburgh, deals with multi-organ transplants, a subject in which he is a leading expert at international level. Finally, Professor Enrique Moreno Gonzalez takes an in-depth look at the treatment of hepatic hilar cholangiocarcinoma. Professor Moreno Gonzalez was one of Professor Gozzetti's closest friends, having trained together and shared a passion for surgery.

Two years of work have gone into this book. Considerable space has been dedicated to drawings illustrating anatomy and techniques. For these, we took advantage of the presence in Bologna of a long-established School of Artistic Anatomy and relied on the expertise of Patrizia Frascari, who combines technical precision in line with the traditions of Italian artistic anatomy. Thanks must go to our colleagues Gian Luca Grazi and Elio Jovine, who have written some of the chapters on liver transplantation; to Giorgio Ercolani, Marinella Morganti, Filippo Pierangeli, Michele Masetti and Salvo Gruttadauria, for their help in collecting the radiological and photographic illustrations and, last but by no means least, to Susan West, for her dedication in translating and revising this book.

We hope this book will be useful to surgeons training in liver surgery, and provide more experienced surgeons with an opportunity to review and reassess their techniques.

Alighieri Mazziotti
Antonino Cavallari
MARCH 1997

TECHNIQUES IN LIVER SURGERY

SECTION I

Basic Anatomy

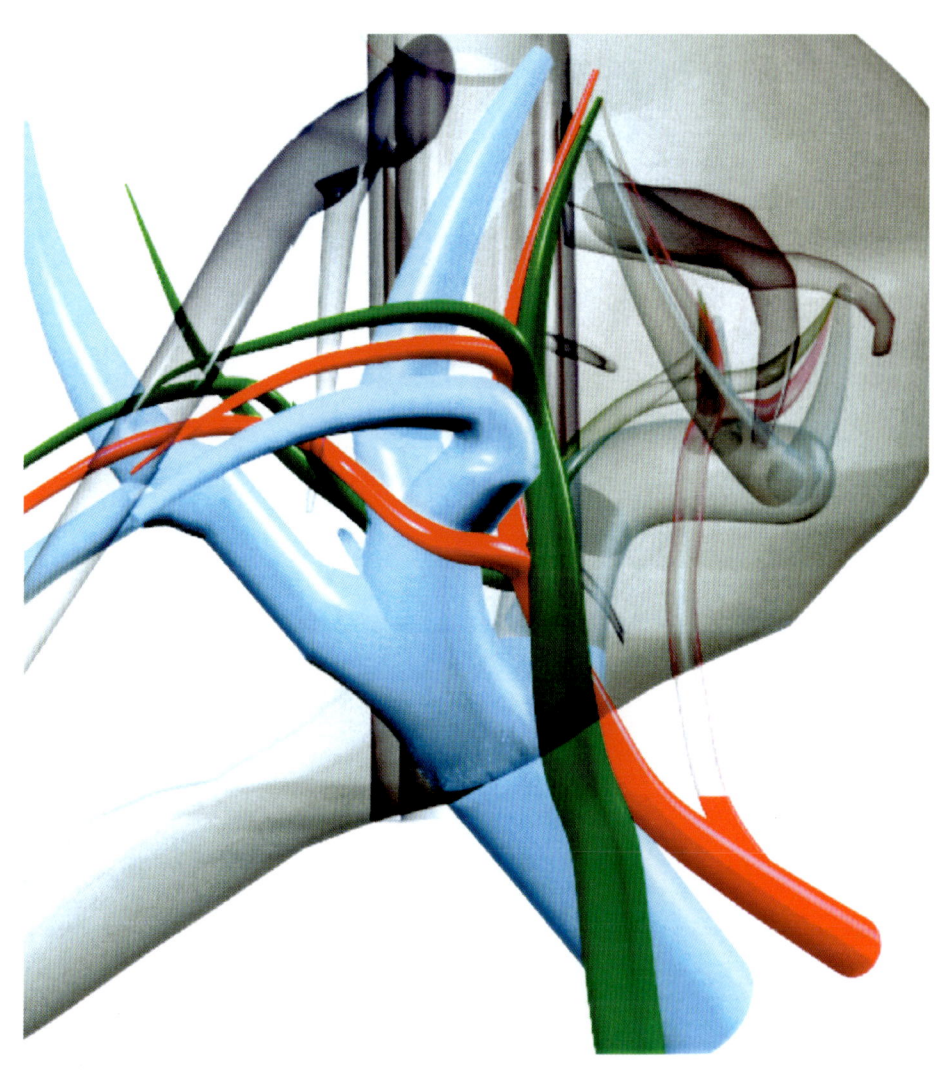

1

Surgical Anatomy of the Liver and Classification of Hepatectomies

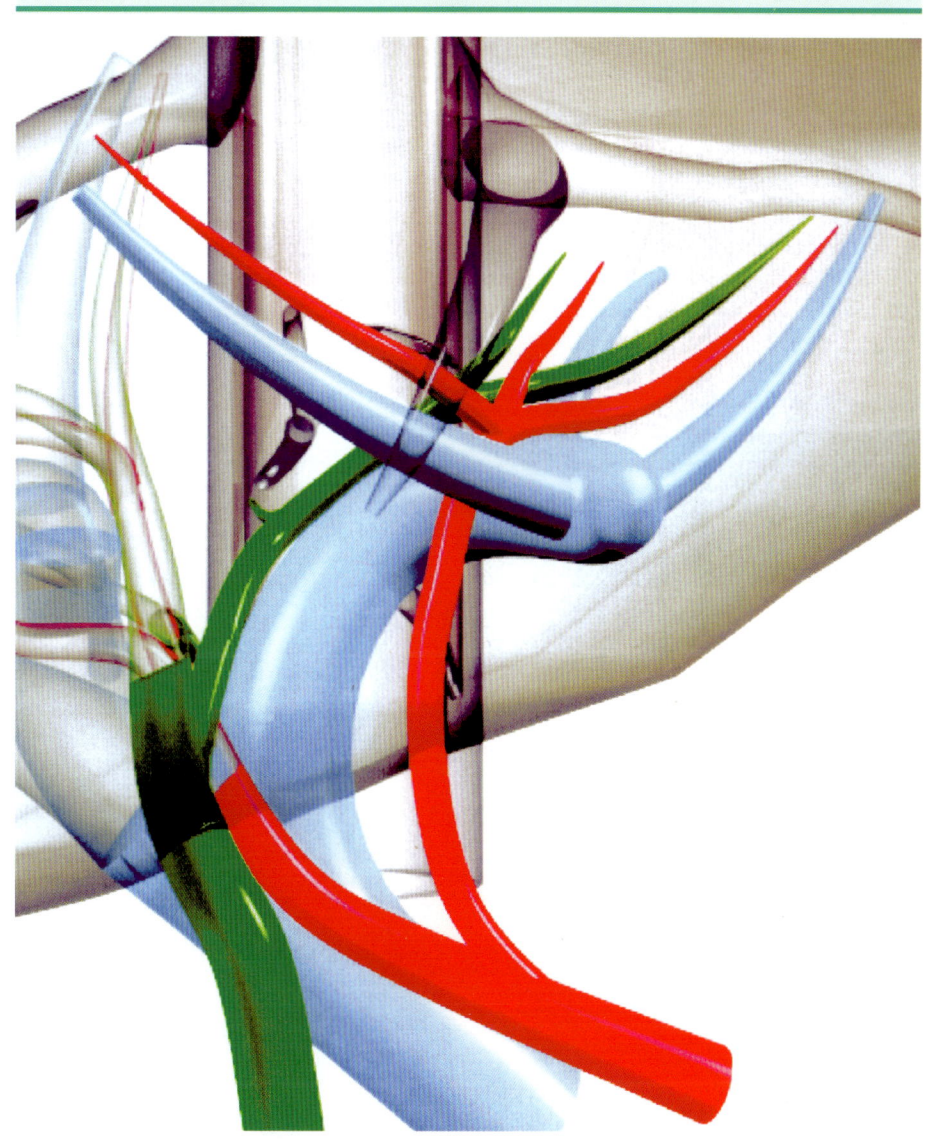

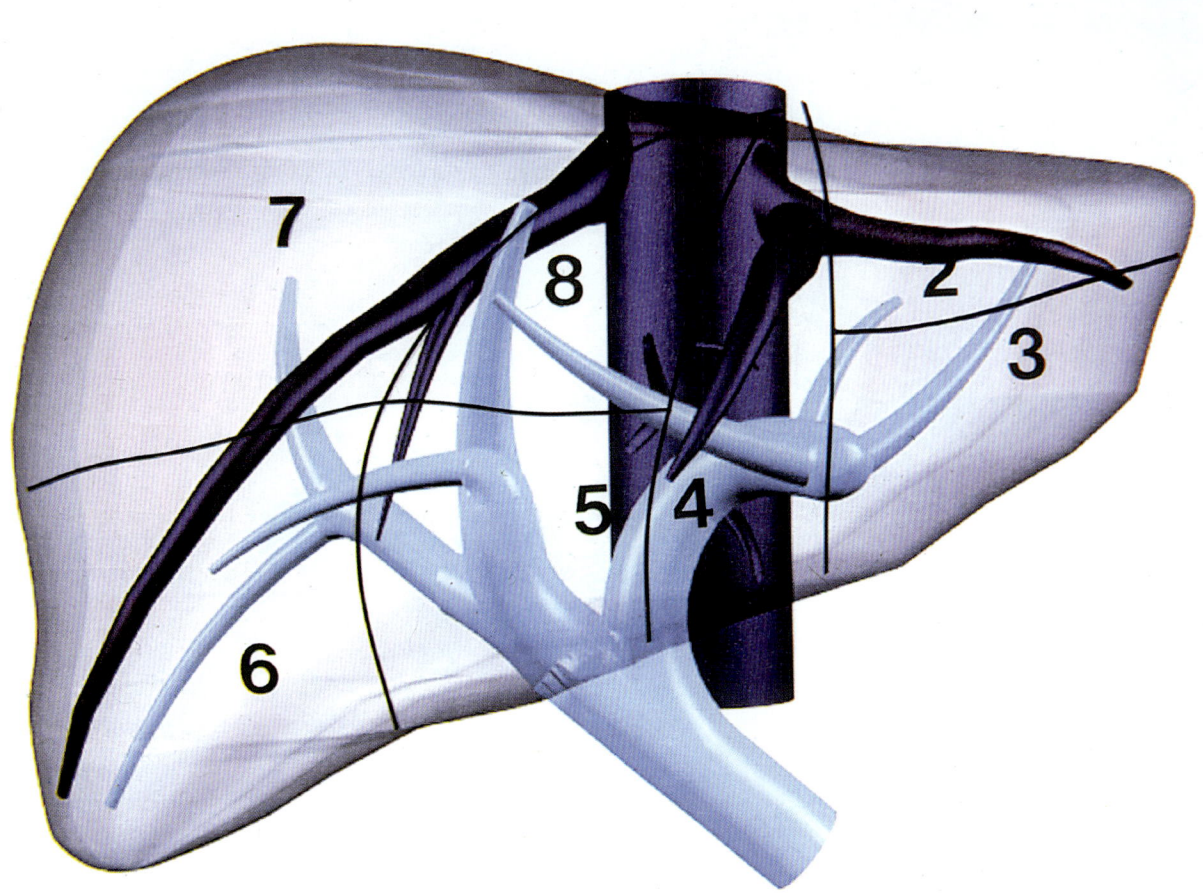

Figure 1.1 – *"Portal" segmentation according to Couinaud.*

The intrahepatic vascular distribution and segmentary anatomy of the liver are clearly defined.[1-4] In spite of this, different terms are still used which can lead to confusion. The segmentation described by Couinaud is used mainly by European surgeons and the terminology based on this definition will be used in this volume. Couinaud distinguishes eight segments which are numbered clockwise from the caudate lobe (segment 1) to the right. In the United States and in Japan, the terms used follow the subdivision into four hepatic segments described by Healey & Schroy. In practice, the two classifications overlap and are both based on the intrahepatic portal distribution (*Figure 1.1*).

At the hilum, the portal pedicles - accompanied by arterial branches and bile ducts - split into the right and left branches of the corresponding hemiliver which are divided by a sagittal plane, slightly oblique towards the left, known as the sagittal fissure or Cantlie line of the liver (*Figure. 1.2*). The division runs from the gallbladder fossa to the vena cava and corresponds to the ischemic demarcation line when a right or left Glissonian branch is ligated. This plane is followed when dividing the liver in routine right or left hepatectomy. The division into two 'hemilivers', therefore differs clearly from the classic anatomical division between left and right 'lobe', separated by the falciform ligament.

The right Glissonian pedicle (the name given to the combination of the portal, arterial and biliary pedicles which run together, joined inside the parenchyma and enclosed by a fibrous sheath which is an extension of the

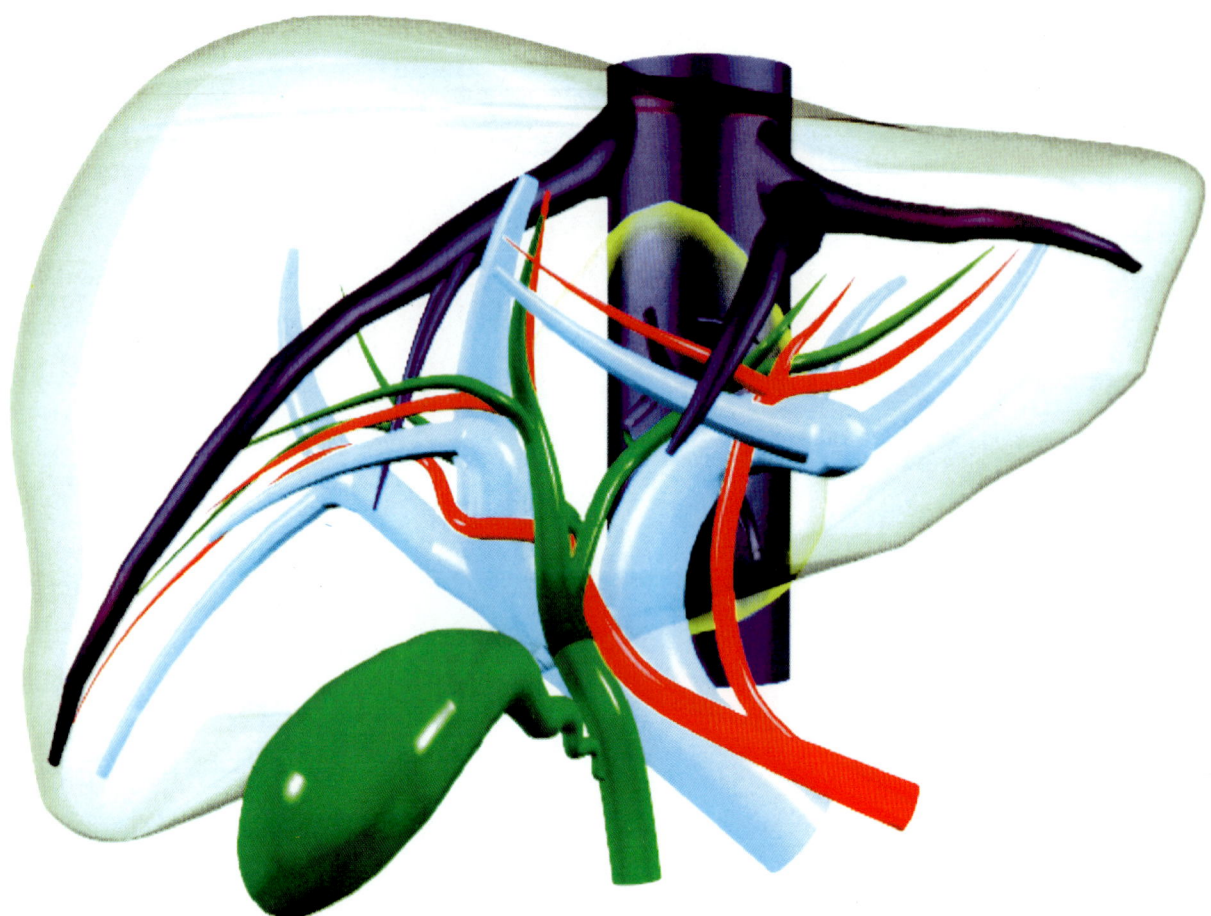

Figure 1.2 – *Hepatic vascular and ductal anatomy.*

hilar plate) is very short, 1-2 cm in length, and forks into an anterior or paramedian branch and a posterior or lateral branch (**Figure 1.3**). After turning forwards and upwards, the first separates into two pedicles, one anteroinferior and one posterosuperior respectively for the two right paramedian segments, segment 5 and segment 8 (also defined as the right paramedian sector). The posterior branch is longer, running laterally and dividing into two pedicles, one anterior and one posterosuperior, respectively, for the right lateral segments, 6 and 7 (or right lateral sector). On the left, the portal pedicle is longer, running first transversely and then anteriorly, as far as the insertion of the umbilical ligament (**Figure 1.4**). From the transverse part of the left Glissonian branch a small branch arises for the part of parenchyma situated behind the hilum, segment 1, corresponding to the Spigel lobe in the classic anatomical description. The vertical section of the left branch divides into a posterolateral branch for segment 2, an anterolateral branch for segment 3 (both these segments make up the left lateral sector in Couinaud's classification) and a medial branch for segment 4 (or left paramedian sector).

The hepatic veins run transversely in the direction of the Glissonian pedicles and delineate the edges of the segments; the right hepatic vein divides the lateral segments from the right paramedian segments, while the sagittal hepatic vein separates the right and left paramedian segments. The dividing line between the paramedian segment and the left lateral segments corresponds to the insertion line of the falciform ligament and not to the left hepatic vein which runs more laterally with respect to the left lobe.

Healey & Schroy's classification[5] differs only in terms of nomenclature from the segmentary description given above: the liver is divided into four segments, the left lateral, the left medial, the right medial and the right lateral, which correspond to Couinaud's "sectors".

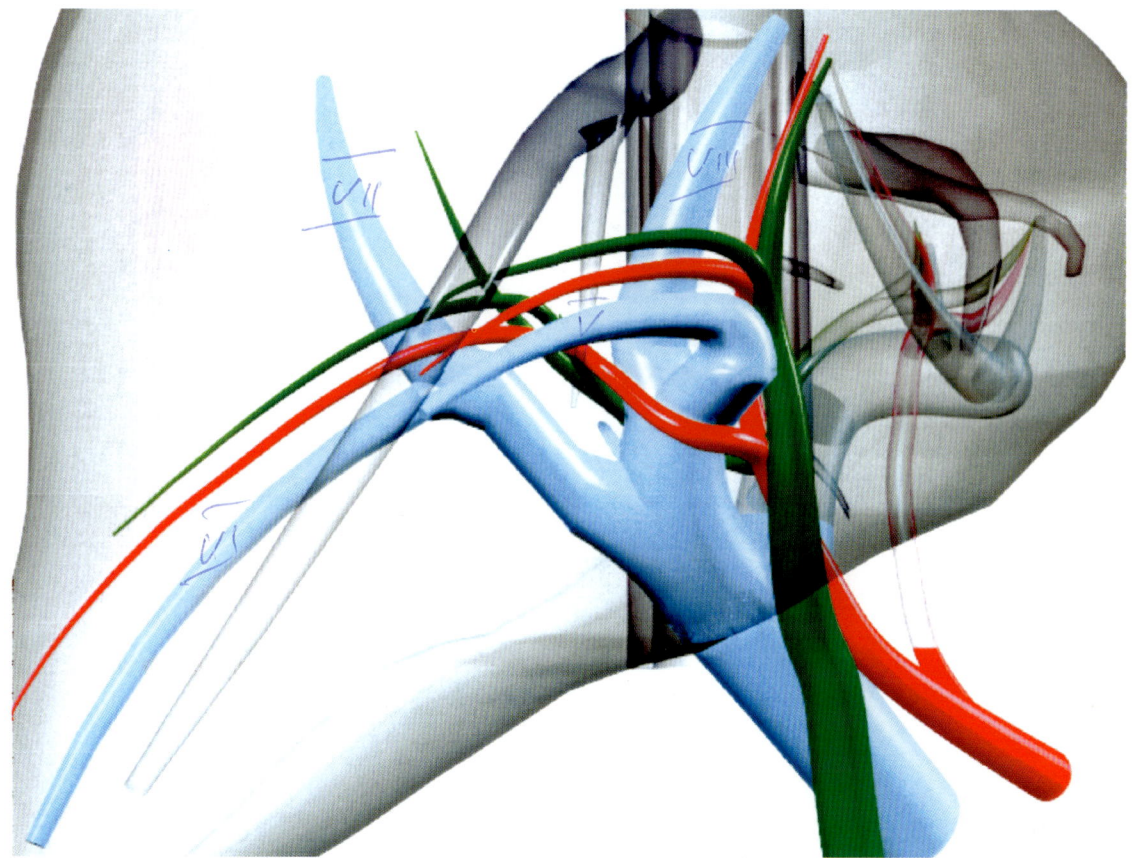

Figure 1.3 – *Right Glissonian pedicles*

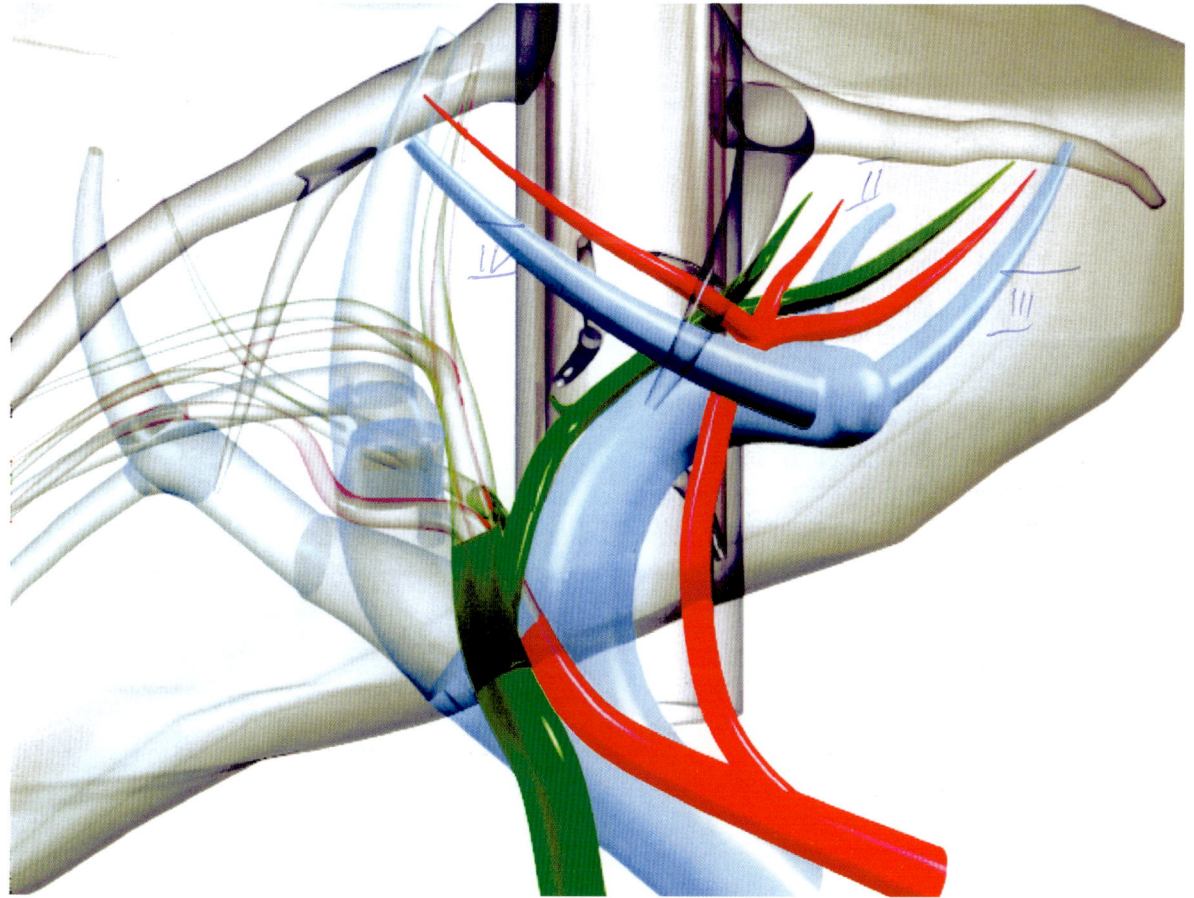

Figure 1.4 – *Left Glissonian pedicles*

SEGMENTS	COUINAUD'S CLASSIFICATION	HEALEY'S CLASSIFICATION
2, 3	Left lobe	Left lateral segment
4	Left paramedian sector	Left medial segment
2, 3, 4	Left hemiliver	Left lobe
5, 8	Right paramedian sector	Right anterior segment
6, 7	Right lateral sector	Right posterior segment
5, 6, 7, 8	Right hemiliver	Right lobe
1	Caudate (Spigel) lobe	Caudate lobe

Table 1.1 – *Liver anatomy classification.*

Each of these segments, except for the left medial, is divided into two subsegments, one anterior and one posterior, which correspond to Couinaud's segments: the left lateral (postero) superior (S2), the left lateral (antero) inferior (S3), the right medial (postero) superior (S8), the right medial (antero) inferior (S5), the right lateral (postero) superior (S7) and the right lateral (antero) inferior (S6). The left medial segment (S4) corresponds to Couinaud's segment 4. In both classifications the caudate or Spigel lobe is considered an independent unit (S1) (**Table 1.1**).

It must be emphasized that, on the basis of intrahepatic vascular anatomy, the term right or left 'lobe', which refers to an element of macroscopic anatomy, i.e. to the portions of parenchyma divided by the falciform ligament and the round ligament disappears. The term 'lobectomy' is nevertheless still sometimes used today to indicate the removal of a 'hemiliver'. In effect the removal of the right or left part of the liver along the plane of the sagittal fissure must be defined as a right or left (hemi) hepatectomy. Left lobectomy corresponds to the resection of the left anatomical lobe, i.e. to Couinaud's segments 2 and 3 or to Healey's left lateral sector. The term right 'lobectomy' leads to confusion since it is often used inappropriately to indicate a right hepatectomy and not the removal of the entire right anatomical lobe. This latter operation should be defined more precisely as a right hepatectomy extended to segment 4.

Resections along an anatomical fissure, and which take vascular anatomy into account, are defined as typical or anatomical resections. Extra-anatomical resections are known as wedge resections which correspond to exeresis carried out 'à la demande' without taking into account the segmentary anatomy within a segment, or even with respect to two adjacent segments. Segmentectomies, as they are defined in this book, refer to Couinaud's segments. Hepatectomies which include more than three segments are defined as major hepatectomies.

REFERENCES

1. Couinaud C. Le foie. Etudes anatomiques et chirurgicales. Masson, Paris, 1957.
2. Couinaud C. Hépatectomie droite, hépatectomie droite étendue ou trisegmentectomie? Considerations sur l'anatomie intra-hépatique et ses applications en chirurgie. *Ann Chir* 1979; **33**: 385-390.
4. Couinaud C. Controlled hepatectomies and exposure of intrahepatic bile ducts. Anatomical and technical study. C. Couinaud, Paris, 1981.
5. Bismuth H. Surgical anatomy and anatomical surgery of the liver. *World J Surg* 1982; 6: 3-9.
6. Healey JE Jr, Schroy PC. Anatomy of the biliary ducts within the human liver; analysis of the prevailing pattern of branching of the major variations of the biliary ducts. *Arch Surg* 1953; **66**: 599-616.

2
Approaches in Liver Surgery

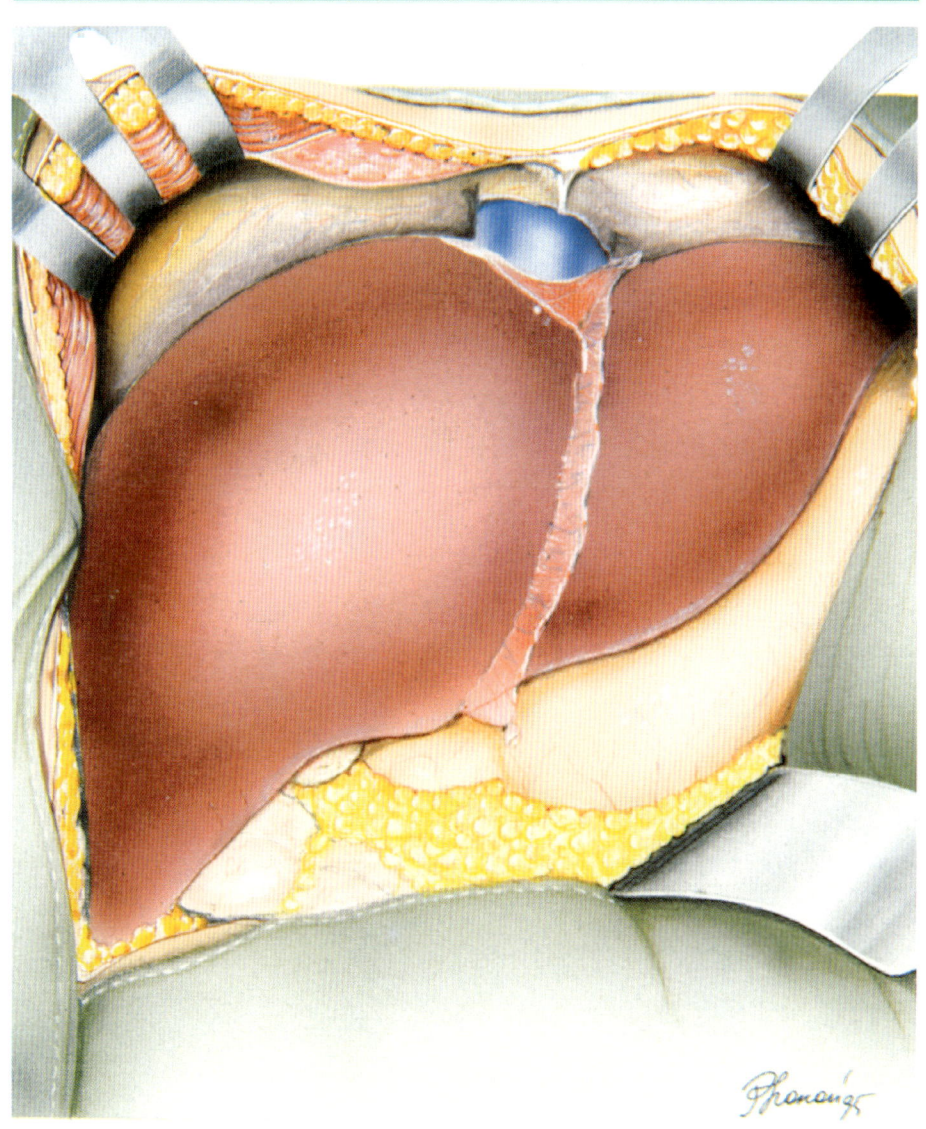

APPROACHES IN LIVER SURGERY

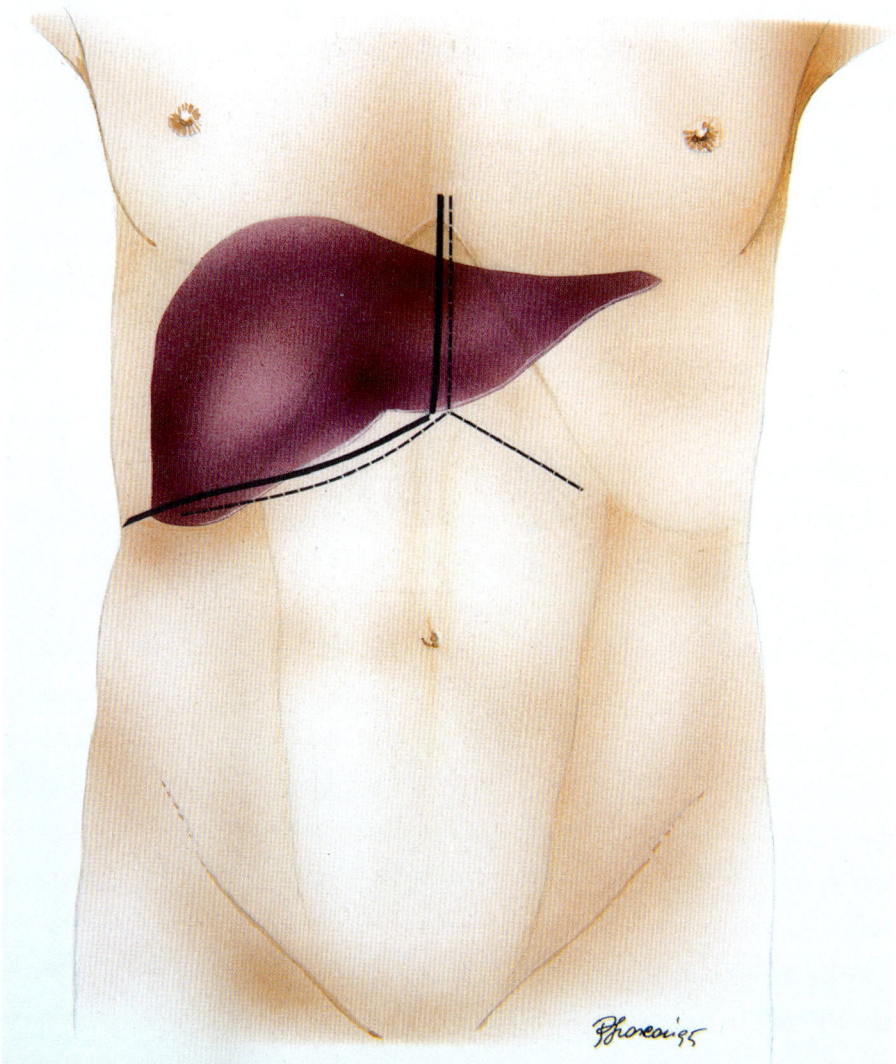

Figure 2.1 – *Incisions for liver surgery. The J incision (continuous line) is the routine access route in hepatectomies and the majority of liver transplants. The Mercedes incision (dotted line) is currently used in less than 5% of the liver resections (voluminous tumors extending towards the left) and transplants in our department*

All the hepatic resections performed in our department over the last 10 years have used the abdominal approach.

The bilateral subcostal approach, extended to the right as far as the midaxillary line, to the left as far as the lateral end of the rectus muscle, and medially upwards as far as the xiphoid process of the sternum *(Mercedes incision)* is the classic approach for major hepatectomies and for liver transplants (**Figure 2.1**). In reality, the extension to the left of the median line is generally not strictly necessary if there are no large tumors involving the left lobe. The central area of the incision, where three lines of perpendicular sections meet, represents the weakest point of the abdominal wall and may lead to post-operative eventration (5% in our series) or to ascitic fistulas in cirrhotic patients. The subcostal incision extended bilaterally also affects respiratory dynamics and is responsible for atelectasis and pleural effusions.

In the last 3 years, our most favored approach has been the so-called *J incision* (**Figure 2.2**), which involves a median laparotomy from the xiphoid cartilage, curving towards the right to the middle of the xipho-umbilical line and extending laterally to the right as far as the posterior axillary line below the 10th rib. A retractor holds back the right rib margin and another retractor is positioned on the median incision, opening the abdominal wall towards the left. We use the Kent retractor which is fixed to the operating table, above the shoulders, and allows retraction to be modified by the surgeon during the operation. This type of incision provides exposure equal to that of a bilateral subcostal approach, also in cases of left hepatectomy, with a reduced incidence of

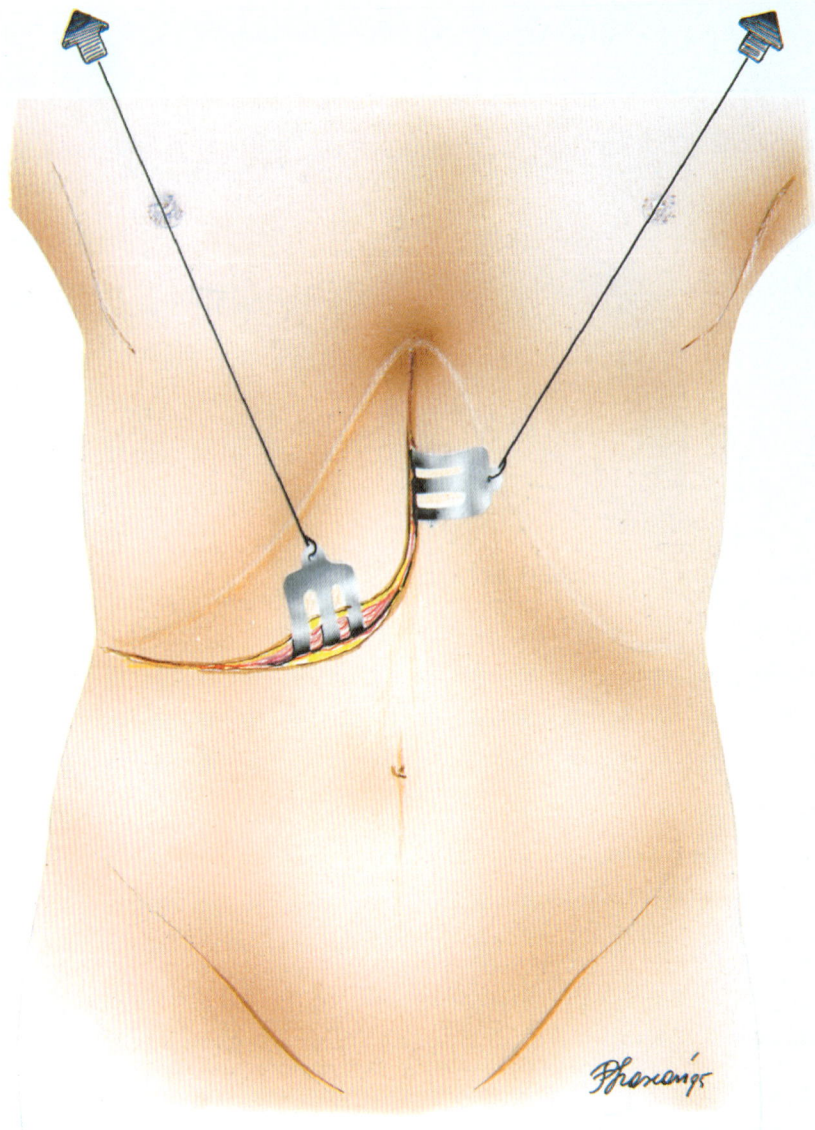

Figure 2.2 – *Position of the Kent retractors for exposure of the liver.*

abdominal wall complications and respiratory problems (*Figure 2.3*). The J incision represents the routine access route used for hepatic resections, while the classic Mercedes incision has been reserved for cases of large tumors of the left lobe. This access route is also commonly used in liver transplants.

Median laparotomy may be adequate when a left lobectomy is planned, if enlargement is not excessive and when the right side of the liver is known to be unaffected.

Thoracophrenolaparotomy was used in less than 1% of our series of 800 hepatectomies. This approach has been suggested for large posterior tumors involving the outlet of the right hepatic vein when access to the right atrium is necessary, or in hydatid cysts involving the right lung base. Complete exposure of the posterior hepatic segments and vena cava control can be easily achieved, without having to open the thorax, if complete division of the hepatic ligaments is undertaken, with exposure of the adrenal loggia and division of the dorsal ligament of the vena cava exposing the most

APPROACHES IN LIVER SURGERY

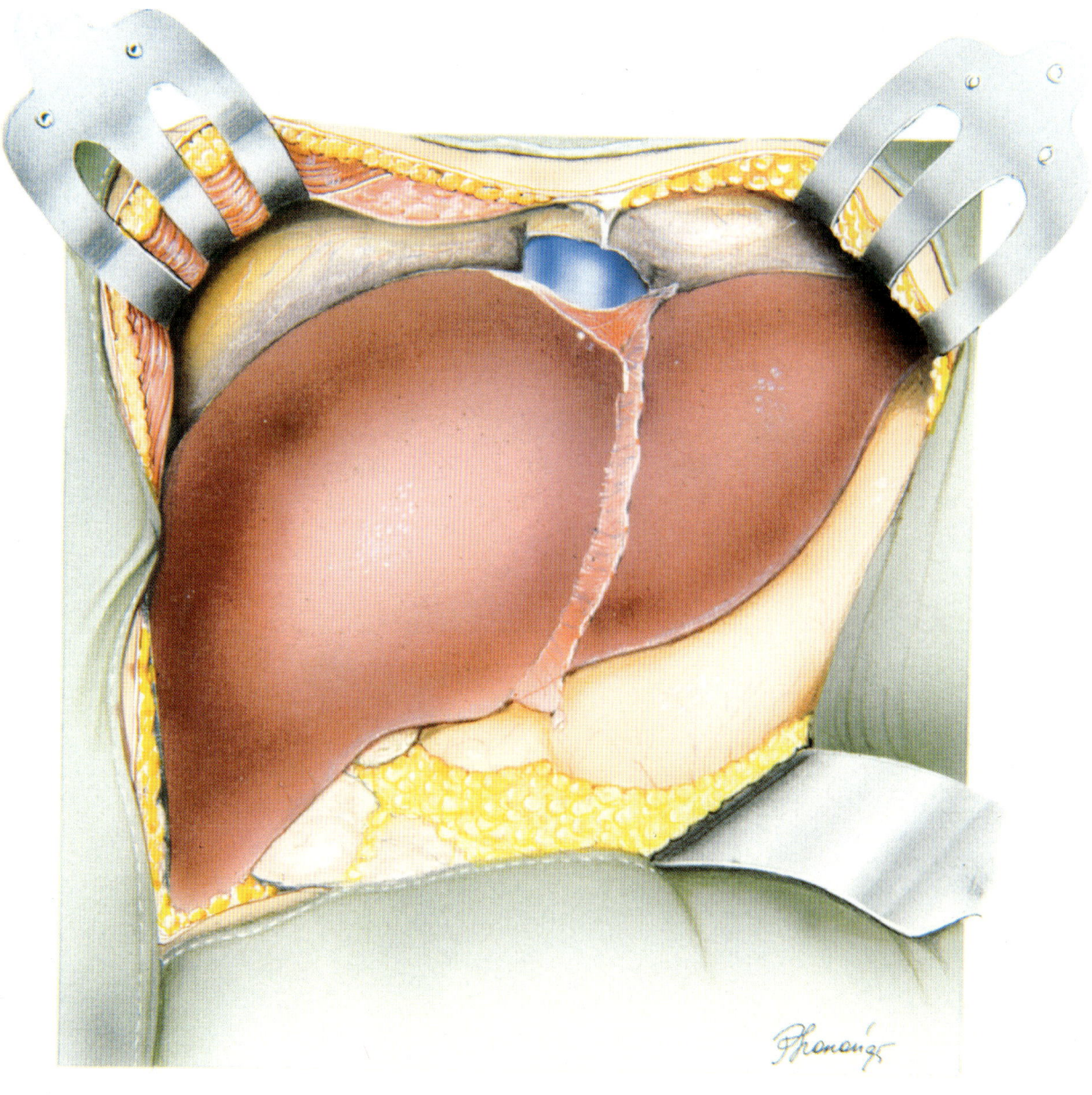

Figure 2.3 – *Abdominal exposure for liver surgery by means of the J incision.*

cranial portions of the vena cava and the outlet of the right hepatic vein. The latter can easily be controlled by the abdominal approach, after dissecting the anterior aspect and the right edge of the vena cava with progressive ligation of the hepatic vein branches of segment 7. The pleura was opened accidentally in 2% of our cases, especially in surgery for hydatid cysts when the diaphragm firmly adheres to the capsule and is weakened due to the progressive stretching of its fibers.

When a tumor infiltrates a limited area of the diaphragm, diaphragmatic resection can be performed without opening the pleura, closing the diaphragm to be resected with a large Satinsky clamp underneath which Vicryl® 0 (Polyclacin 910, Ethicon) sutures are applied to prevent air passing into the pleural cavity. For more extensive involvement, the diaphragm should be incised and the infiltrated portion removed *en bloc* with the tumor (**Figure 2.4**). The diaphragm is then sutured with Vicryl® 0 stitches when possible or with the interposition of a Gore-Tex® Patch

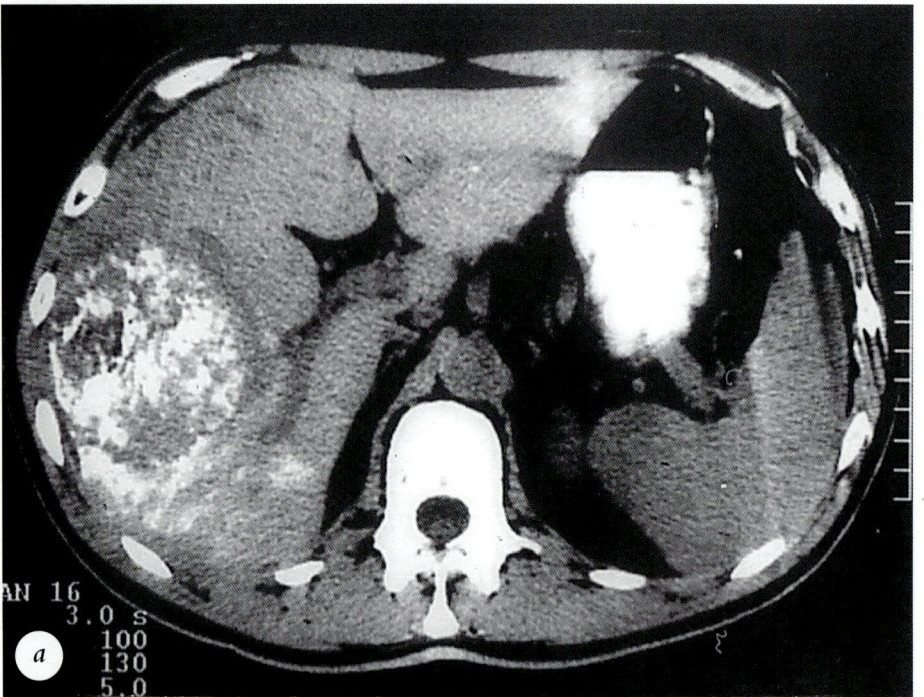

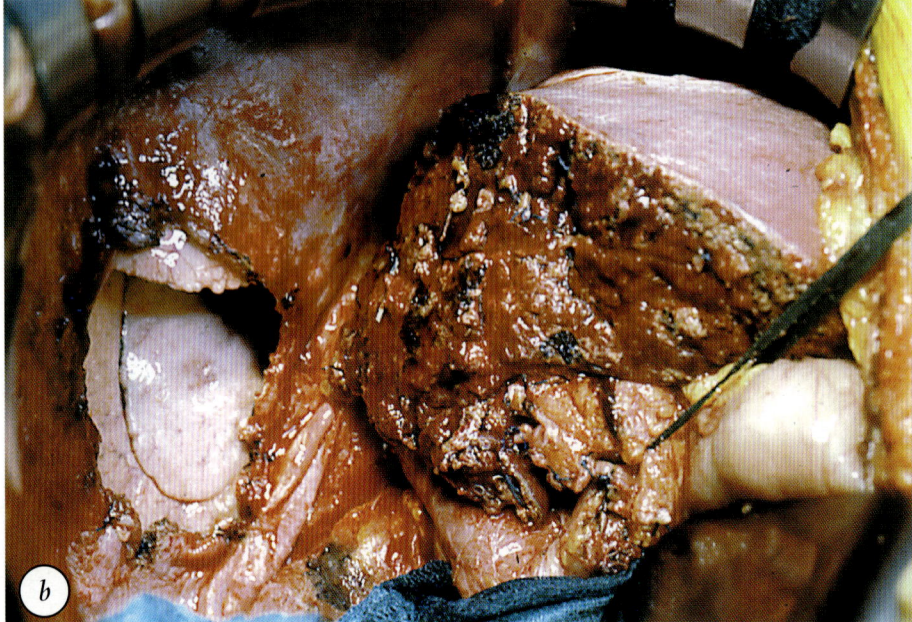

Figure 2.4 – *Right hepatectomy with resection of a portion of diaphragm for hepatocarcinoma. The patient underwent pre-operative chemoembolization which reduced the size of the tumor.*
a) *Pre-operative CT scan*
b) *The intra-operative field at the end of the resection. The diaphragm was simply sutured with Vicryl stitches after positioning of a pleural drainage.*

(Expanded PTFE, Surgical Membrane 0.1 mm, WL Gore and Associates Inc. Delaware, USA). In these cases a pleural drainage tube should be systematically positioned.

In *emergency surgery* for liver trauma, the median laparotomy approach is preferable, making it possible to examine and assess the entire abdominal cavity. This approach is adequate for capsular lacerations or for rupture of the left lobe. In the presence of more complex hepatic lesions, the incision must be extended to the right with a transverse inverted T section, penetrating laterally as far as the latissimus dorsi muscle.

TECHNIQUES IN LIVER SURGERY

SECTION II

Standard Techniques of Liver Resection

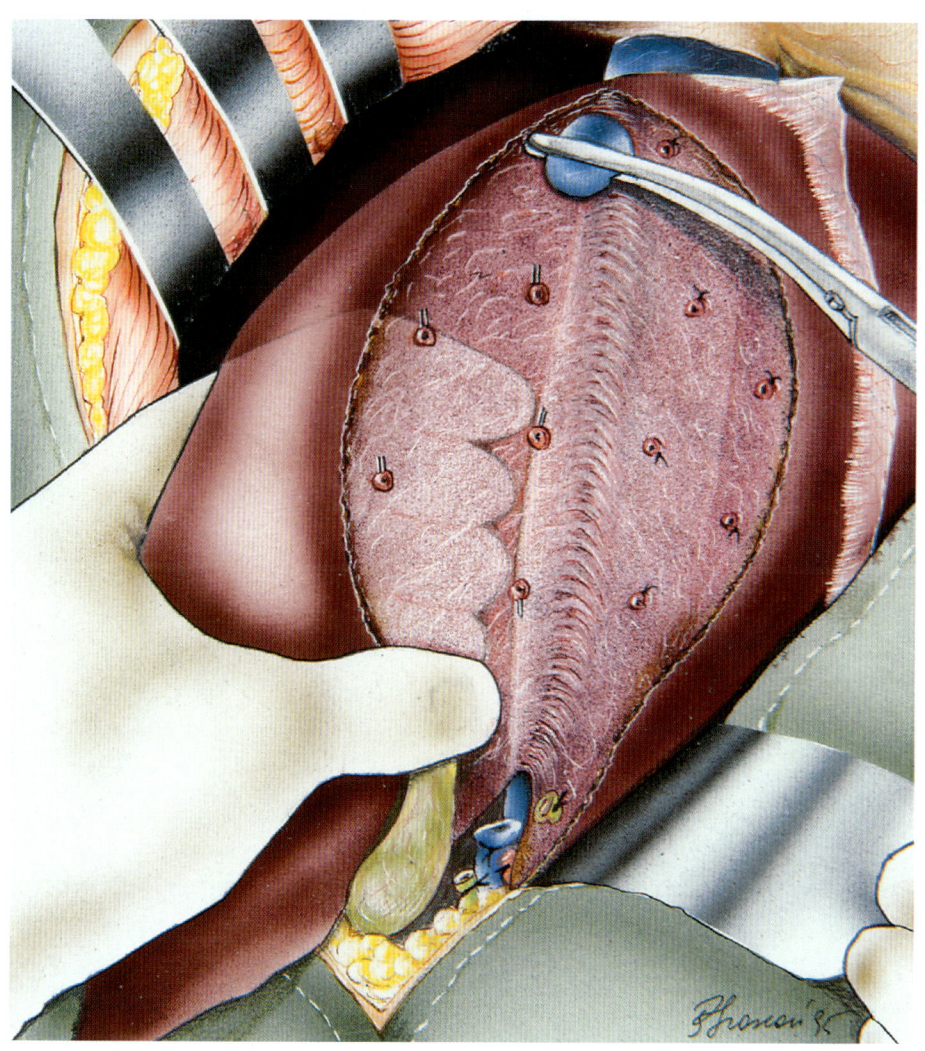

3

Right Hepatectomy

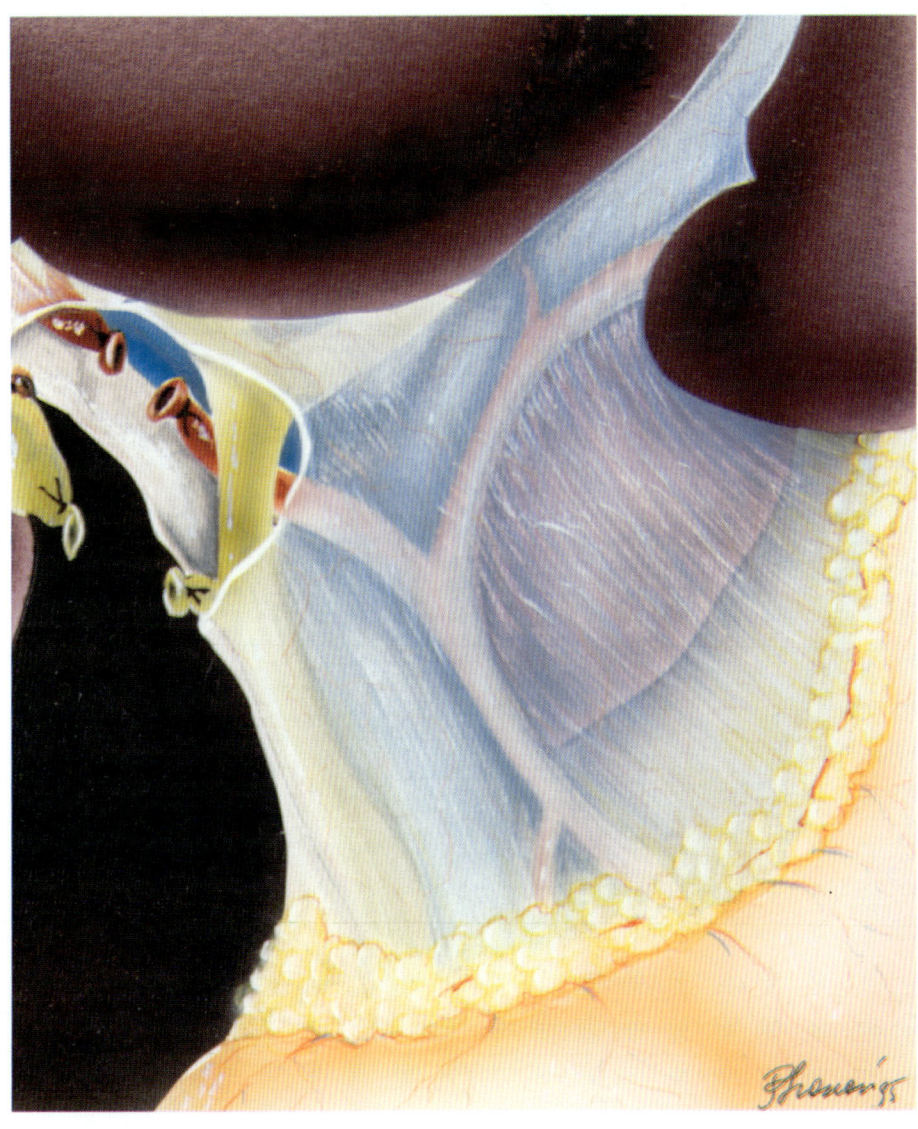

RIGHT HEPATECTOMY

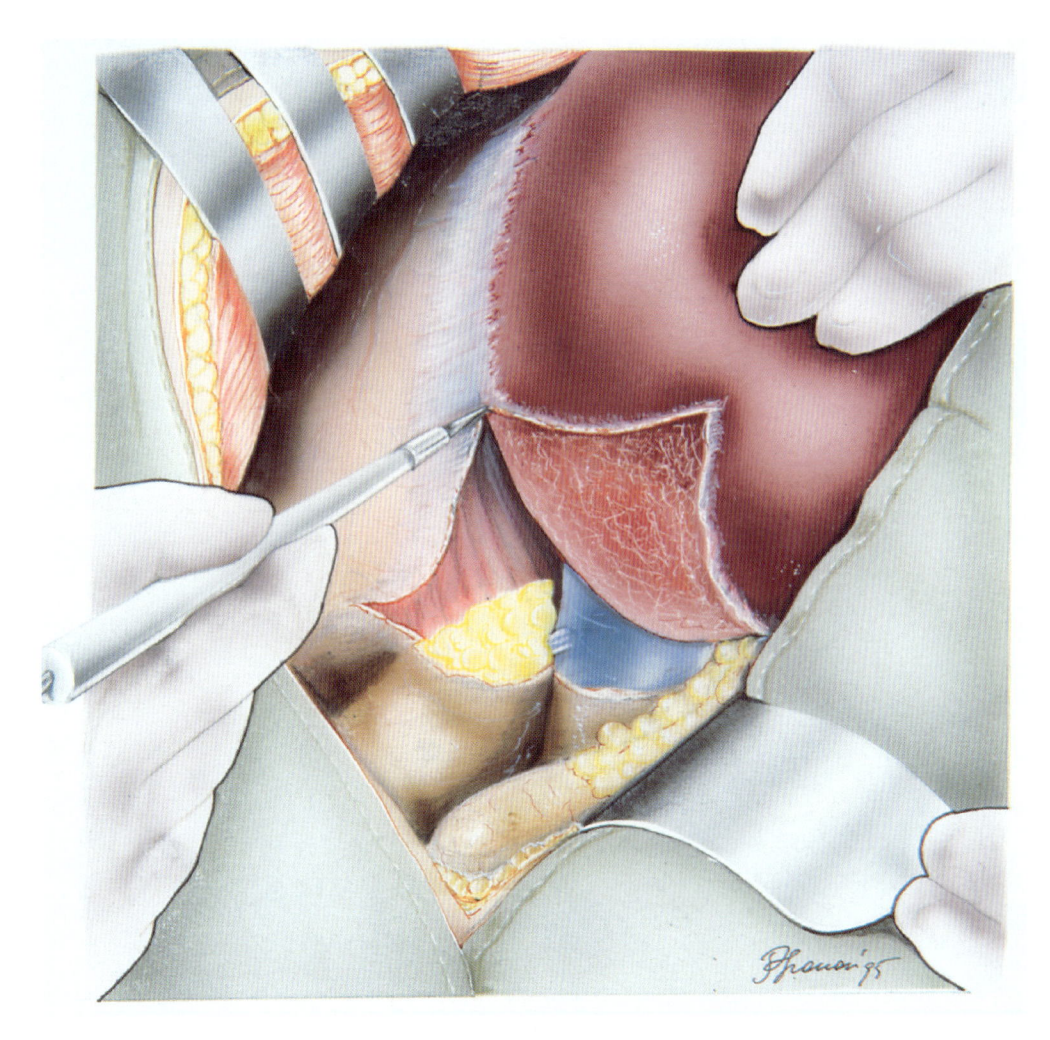

Figure 3.1 – *Division of the right triangular ligament.*

Right hepatectomy consists of resection of the right hemiliver, i.e. that part of the parenchyma vascularized by the right branch of the hepatic artery and the portal vein, and situated to the right of the plane passing between the gallbladder fissure and the right edge of the vena cava (segments 5, 6, 7, and 8 in Couinaud's classification). This is one of the most common hepatectomies, with a well standardized technique, albeit with some variations.[1,3,4,10,11]

A right subcostal incision extended along the median line is usually made. Surgical and ultrasound exploration is performed as soon as the subcostal part of the incision is made. Palpation assesses the extent of the neoplasm, any infiltration of the diaphragm, the presence of peritoneal nodules, and of lymph node involvement of the hepatic pedicle, in addition to any anatomical abnormalities of the hepatic artery. Intra-operative ultrasound does not necessitate division of the hepatic ligaments. The neoplasm must be identified and the relation with the hepatic veins and with the Glissonian pedicles must be assessed correctly to define the resection margins. The other hepatic segments must be examined for satellite nodules or portal thrombosis. Ultrasound investigation should not take more than 5-10 minutes.

The first stage of the hepatectomy consists of mobilizing the right part of the liver and dividing the hepatic ligaments. The round ligament is divided between ligatures. The falciform ligament is divided by cautery as far as its separation into the two lateral layers which continue in the right and left triangular ligaments. It is not necessary to divide the left triangular ligament. The right triangular ligament is exposed by applying traction to the right lobe upwards and towards the left. The assistant surgeon plays an important role at this stage in applying the correct tension to the liver and the progressive rotation of the organ as the ligament is divided (*Figure 3.1*). The lower layer of the triangular ligament is then divided,

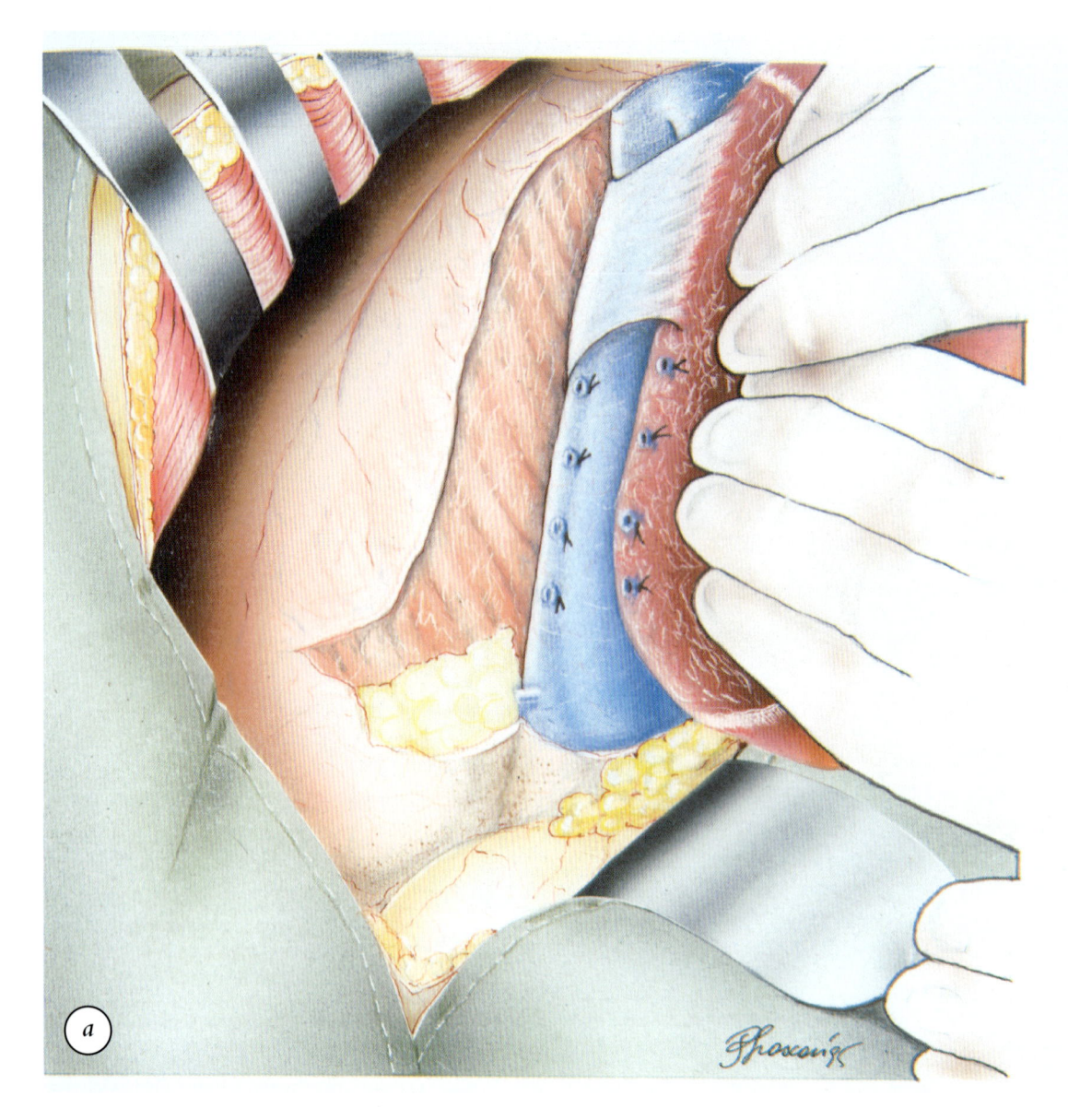

Figure 3.2 – *Detachment of the bare area of the right lobe and exposure of the lateral border of the vena cava. Note that the outlet of the right hepatic vein is covered by the dorsal ligament of the vena cava,* **a)**. *The ligament is shown by the clamp,* **b)**. *Only after the ligament has been divided can the right hepatic vein be safely exposed,* **c)**.

elevating the liver upwards. Division proceeds until the subhepatic vena cava is exposed, the constant landmark being the caudate process. The triangular ligament contains only small vessels and lymphatics and can be divided with cautery. In cirrhotic patients the ligaments contain dilated vessels and lymphatics which may have to be ligated. Superiorly the division of the triangular ligament must be continued as far as the posterior insertion of the falciform ligament. Keeping the liver elevated and turned towards the left, the detachment of the retroperitoneal part ('bare area') of the right lobe is continued. Care must be taken to respect the adrenal gland, potentially the site of major hemorrhage, particularly in the presence of cirrhosis. The adrenal gland must be detached from the hepatic capsule. Dissection continues until the right lateral edge of the vena cava is exposed. The right suprarenal vein is not ligated for a conventional right hepatectomy. This stage is simplified by turning the operating table towards the left and progressively increasing traction on the rib arch. The Kent retractor is particularly useful at this stage.

Complete mobilization of the right lobe is essential for a correctly performed operation and to establish whether the lesion can be resected. Partial infiltration of the diaphragm is not a contraindication to hepatic resection. The portion of infiltrated diaphragm must be removed *en bloc* together with the tumor. If the infiltration is limited to an area of a few centimeters, the diaphragm can be resected without opening the pleura, clamping the affected portion with a large Satinsky clamp below which Vicryl® sutures are applied.

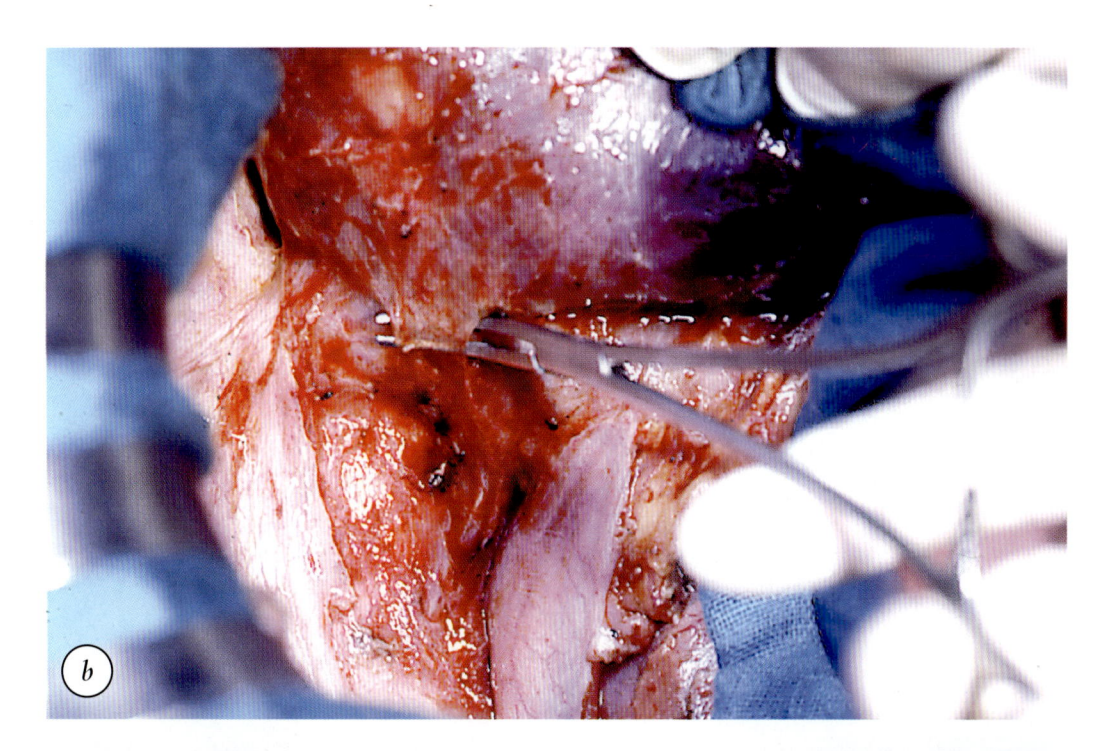

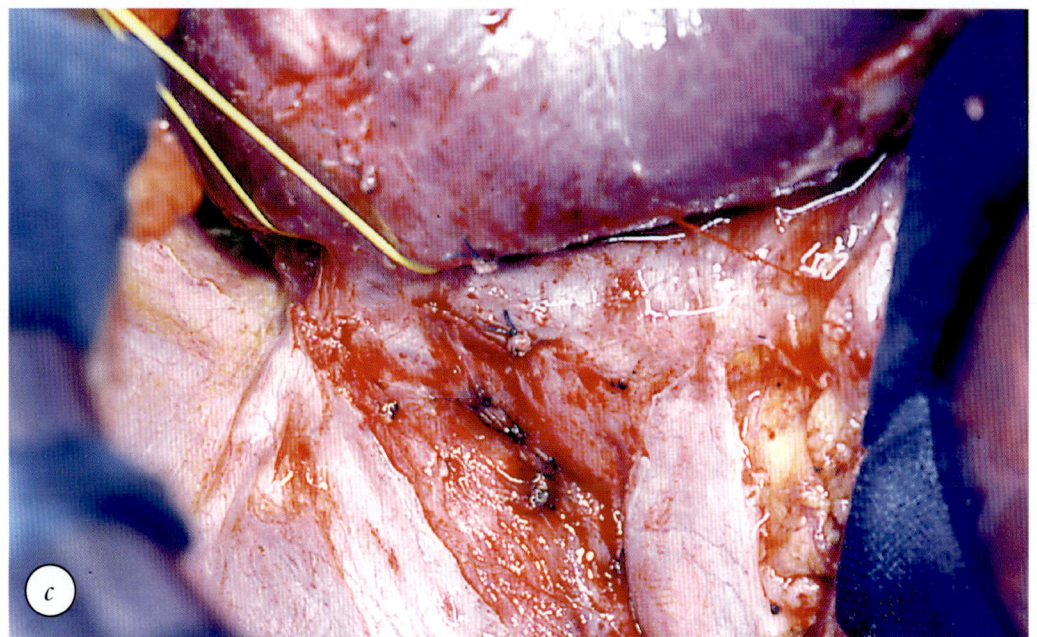

Dissection of the right edge of the vena cava is an important stage of the operation: the freer the vena cava, the easier and safer the last stage of resection. Lifting the liver upwards exposes the small secondary hepatic veins of segments 6 and 7. These veins are only a few millimeters in length but are surrounded by slack connective tissue which facilitates dissection; the caval side of these veins should be ligated and sutured to prevent hemorrhage if one of the ligatures should slip during the subsequent stages of the operation due to movement of the vena cava. The hepatic side of these veins can be closed with metal clips.

Proceeding cranially towards the right hepatic vein, the dorsal ligament of the vena cava is exposed (**Figure 3.2**). This ligament is an avascular connective thickening situated at the rear

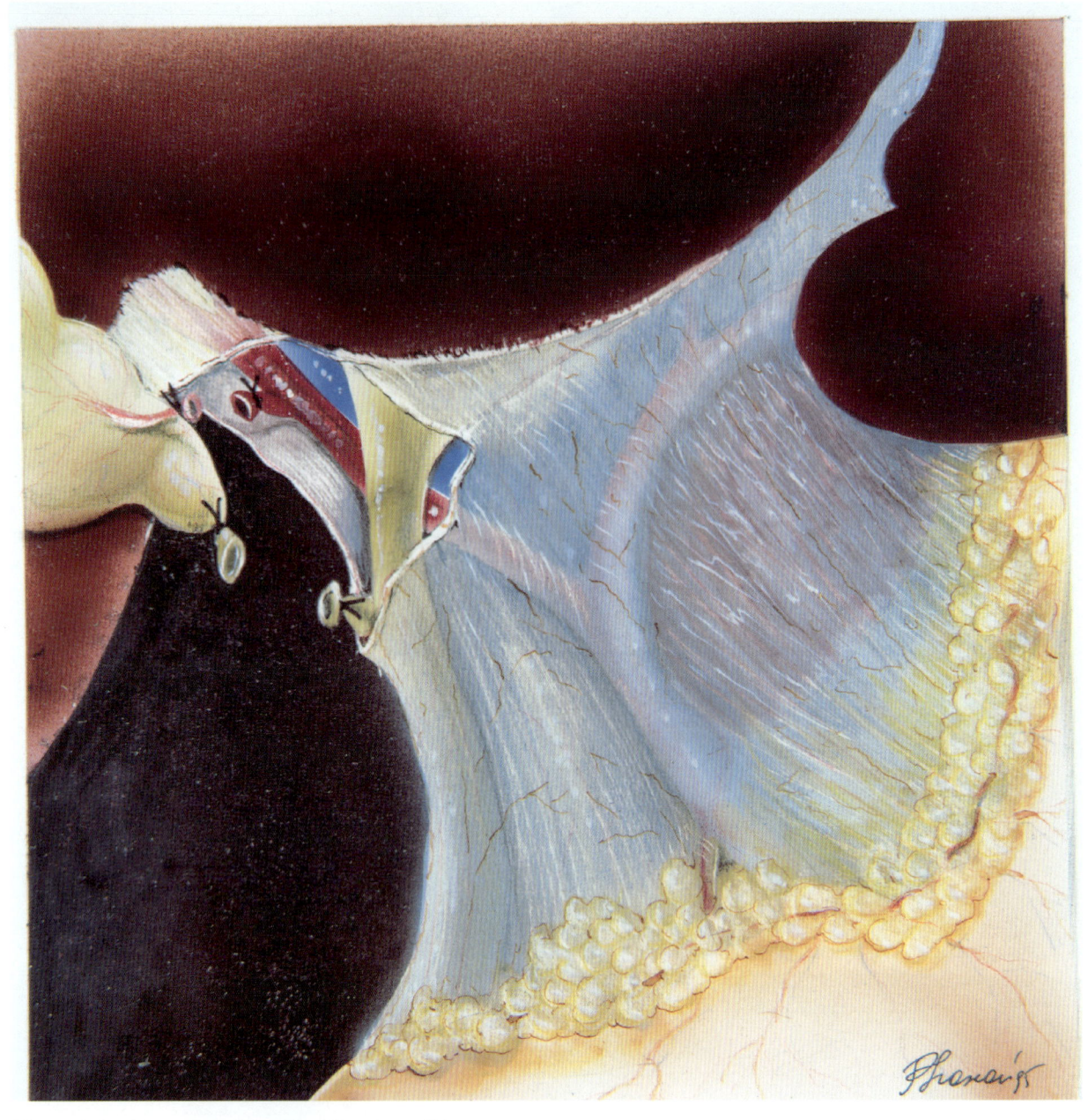

Figure 3.3 – *Preparation of the right Glissonian pedicle. Division of the cystic duct and the cystic artery.*

of the vena cava between segment 7, immediately below the parenchymal fossa where the right hepatic vein penetrates, and the left part of the caudate lobe. Division of the dorsal ligament exposes the more cranial part of the vena cava and the outlet of the right hepatic vein.

After complete mobilization of the right lobe, the Glissonian pedicles at the hilum are isolated. The first stage is the dissection of Calot's triangle. The cystic duct and artery are ligated and divided, and the infundibulum and the left portion of the gallbladder bed are detached (*Figure 3.3*). The plane which divides the gallbladder fissure represents the lower plane of the parenchymal division. Dissecting along the right border of the biliary tract, the right branch of the hepatic artery can be identified. This usually crosses the hepatic duct posteriorly, and is surrounded by neural and lymphatic tissue. More rarely, the artery may be situated in front of the biliary tract or may run vertically, behind the common bile duct, originating from the superior mesenteric artery. The artery is encircled with rubber tape and before ligation the left arterial branch should be exposed and palpated. The right branch of the hepatic

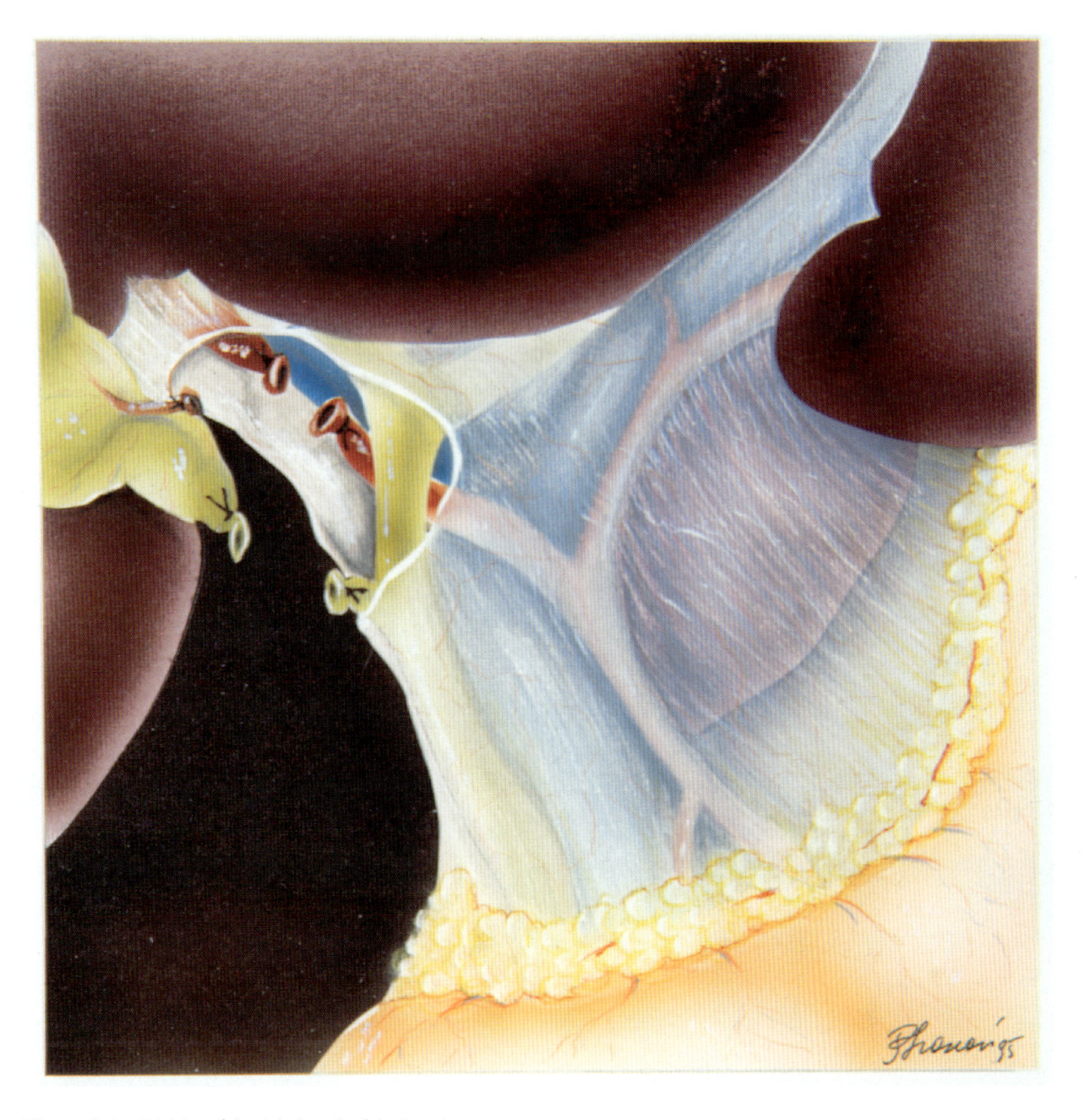

Figure 3.4 – *Division of the right branch of the hepatic artery.*

artery may sometimes already be divided at this point into the right anterior and posterior branches. The artery should be divided distally to prevent devascularization of the common bile duct or the blocking of other collaterals for segment 4 (**Figure 3.4**).

After dividing the artery, the right branch of the portal vein is exposed, contained in loose connective tissue which makes dissection easier. The extrahepatic section of the right branch may sometimes be very short (about 1 cm in length); exposure in these cases may be made easier by mobilizing the portal vein distally with division of the posterior layer on the hepatoduodenal ligament and continuing the dissection upwards, to the right of the hilum, after displacing the common hepatic duct to the left. The portal branch must be clamped both proximally and distally. The proximal stump must always be ligated with a Prolene® (Polypropylene, Ethicon) 4-0 transfixed suture or with a whipstitch (**Figure 3.5**).

We never identify the right hepatic duct for extraparenchymal ligation. The walls of the hepatic duct are delicate and can be easily damaged. There are also frequent anatomical

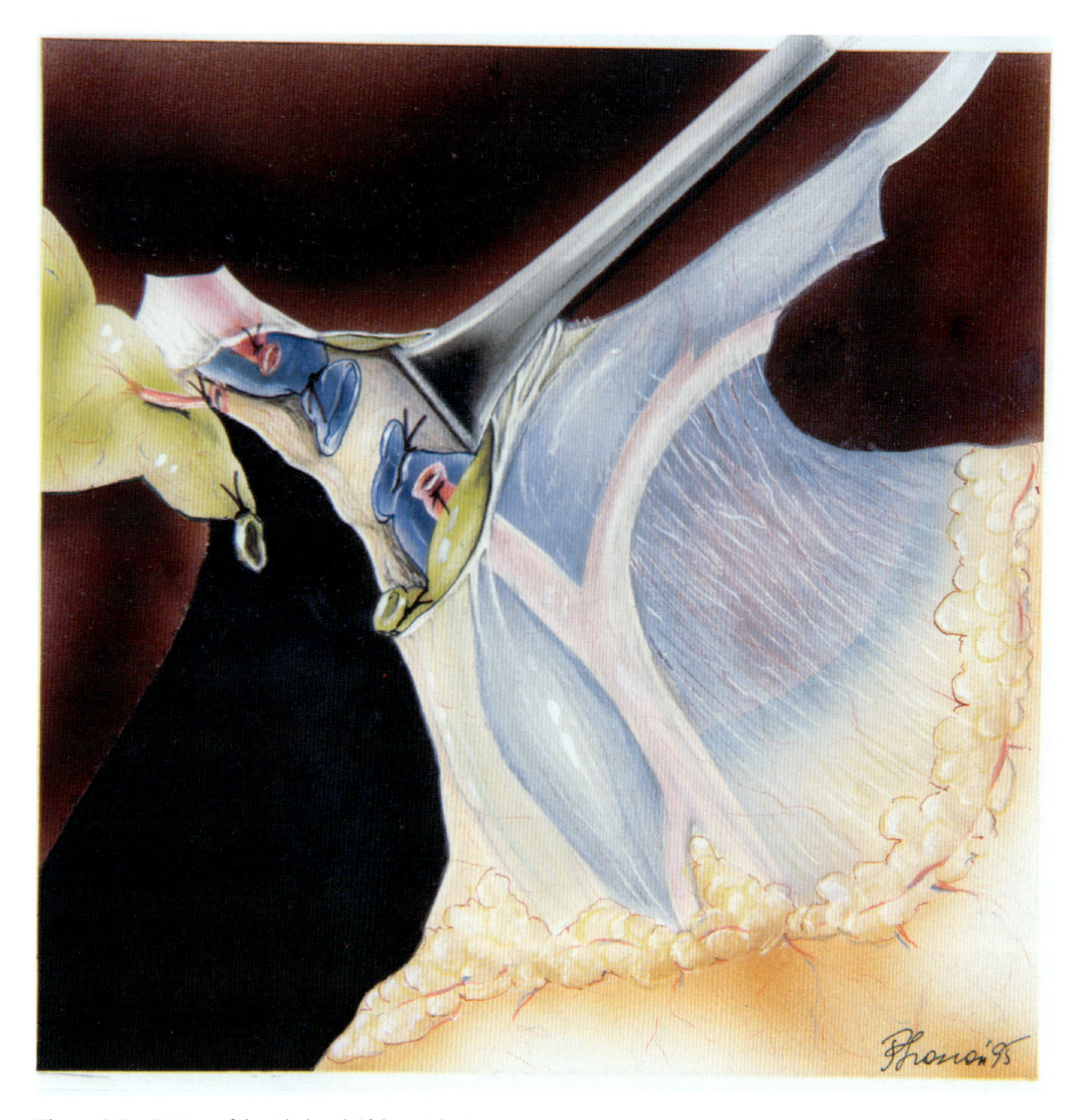

Figure 3.5 – *Division of the right branch of the portal vein.*

RIGHT HEPATECTOMY

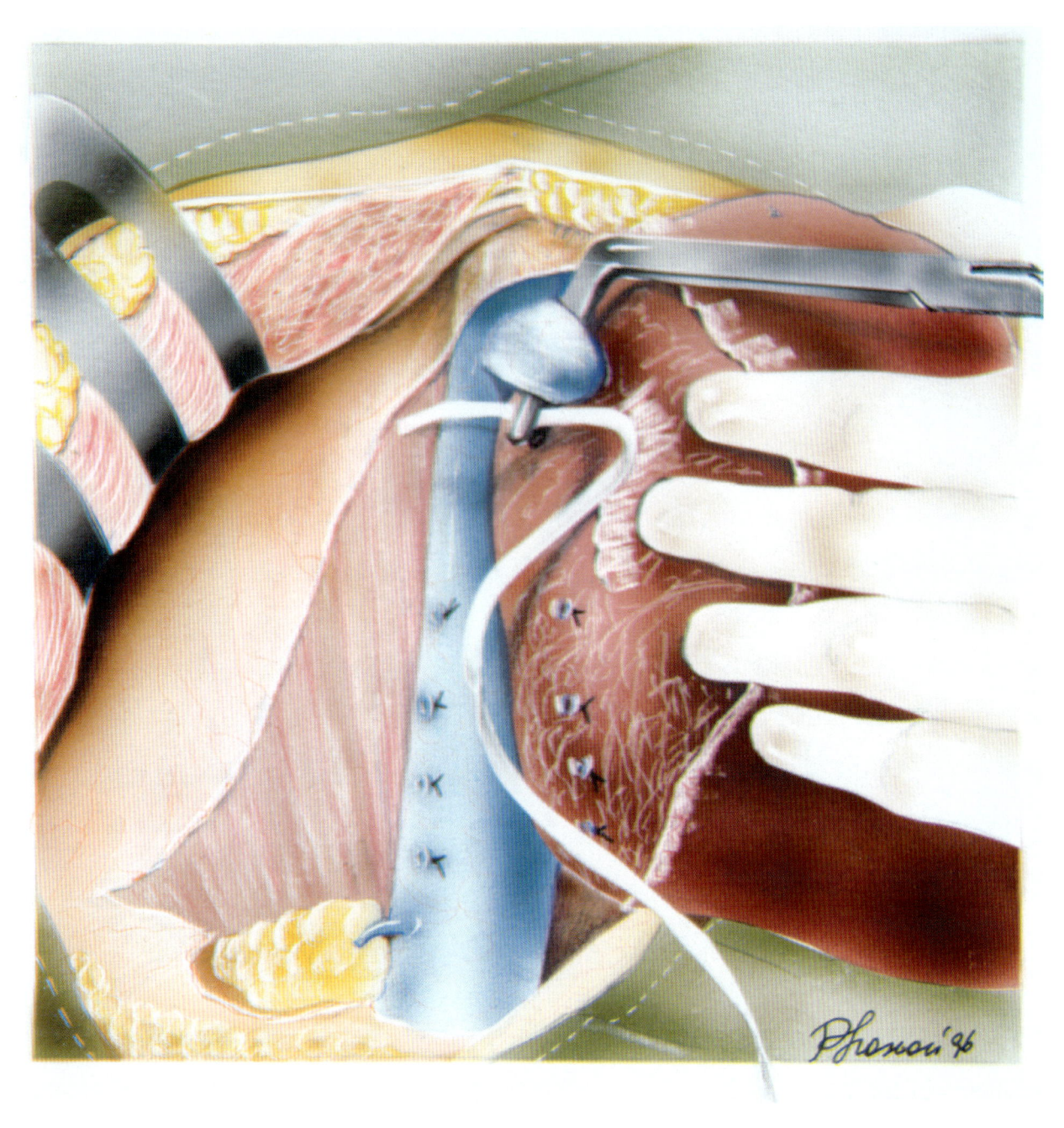

Figure 3.6 – *Preparation of the right hepatic vein*

variations at the outlet of the paramedian and right lateral bile ducts, in the paramedian duct and in the small canaliculi of the caudate lobe, making extraparenchymal ligation of the right hepatic duct inadvisable during the hilar stage of resection. We systematically perform ligation of the right hepatic duct during parenchymal dissection, ensuring that the bifurcation is avoided, without the risk of encountering anatomical variations or of damaging the wall of the biliary tract in its more delicate extraparenchymal part.

Once the artery and the portal branch have been ligated, the right hemiliver darkens in color, clearly distinguishing it from the remaining parenchyma (***Figure 3.6***). When the hilar stage is complete, the right hepatic vein is divided. In our more recent experience, extrahepatic ligature of the right hepatic vein is routinely performed in conventional right hepatectomies. When the dorsal ligament of the vena cava has been completely divided, the convergence of the vena cava and the hepatic vein is fully exposed and the vein can be easily

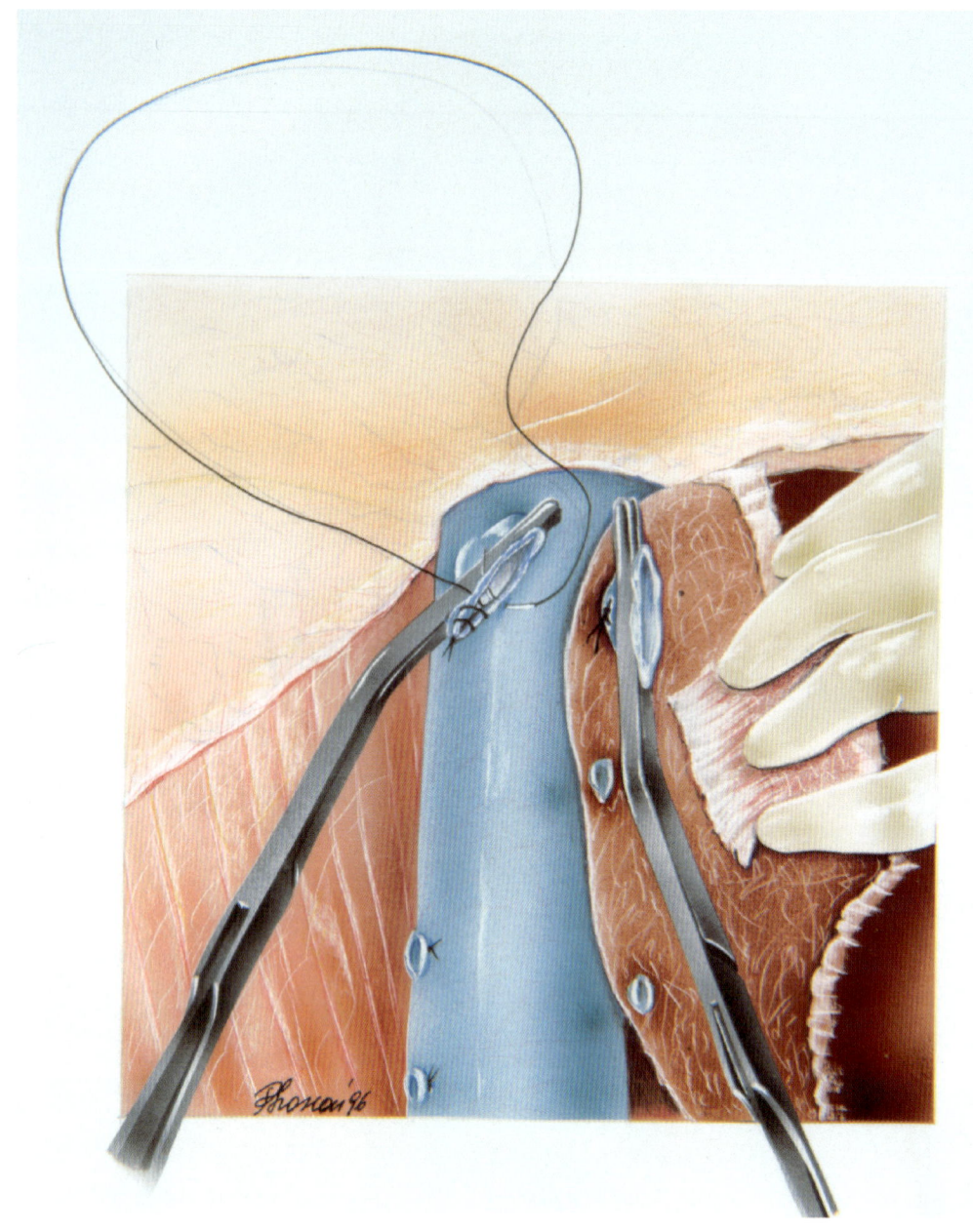

Figure 3.7 – *Division of the right hepatic vein.*

encircled, clamped and divided (*Figure 3.7*). The caval edge of the vein should be sutured with Prolene® 3-0 whipstitches, while the hepatic end can be ligated with a transfixed stitch. Extraparenchymal ligation of the right hepatic vein, which must follow division of the right Glissonian pedicle, allows complete mobilization of the part of the liver to be removed and reduces blood loss during resection.[8] Complete exposure of the vena cava behind the liver may, however, be difficult in cases of large posterior tumors. In such cases extraparenchymal ligature of the right hepatic vein can be particularly risky and it is preferable to postpone this stage until completion of the parenchymal division, when the right hemiliver is almost completely detached. This only happens in less than 10% of our current practice.

Glisson's capsule must be divided along this ischemic demarcation line by cautery, proceeding upwards beyond the V insertion of the falciform ligament. On the inferior aspect of the liver, the incision should be made to the midpoint of the gallbladder bed. Dissection of the parenchyma proceeds from the anterior margin of the liver, pinching small portions of the parenchyma with Kelly forceps so that the intrahepatic vessels are displayed. The smallest vessels are simply coagulated while the larger

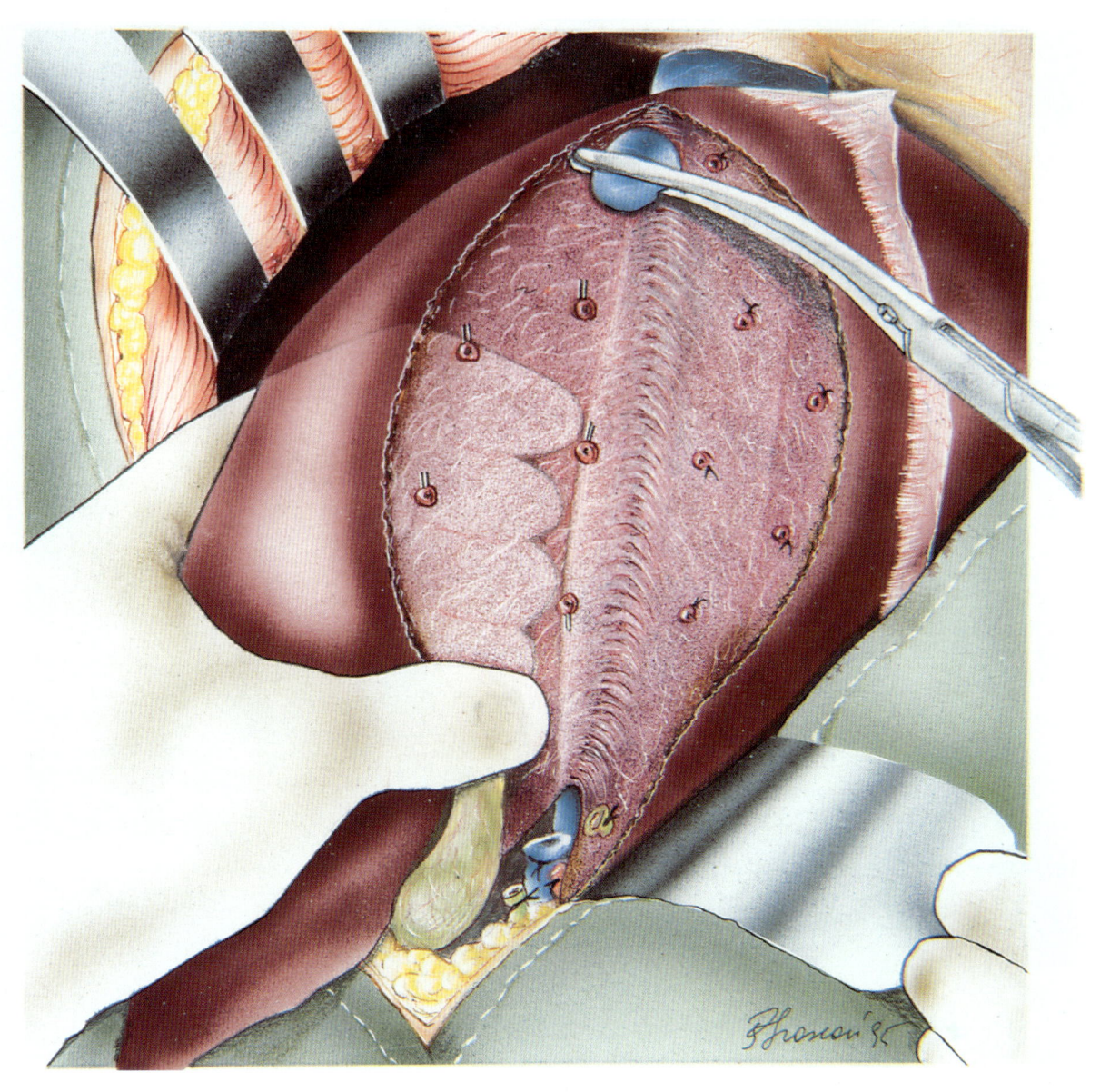

Figure 3.8 – *Division of the right hepatic vein.*

pedicles are closed with metal clips (Premium Surgclip M-11-5, AutoSuture) or ligated and divided. When dividing the parenchyma, care should be taken not to cut too far to the left, close to the middle hepatic vein: the walls of this vein are delicate with numerous small branches which are easily lacerated, leading to hemorrhage. Hemostasis is elective, with ligation or Vicryl® 3 or 4-0 sutures. Larger sutures over the entire thickness, ("mattress" suturing) ,or with stronger threads should be avoided at all costs, since these can lead to parenchymal necrosis and sequestration. It is preferable to ligate progressively and to avoid using numerous forceps which would inevitably tear some vessels from the vein; these would then retract into the parenchyma making hemostasis more difficult. Noting these precautions and following a clear resection plan limits hemorrhage during parenchymal dissection to a minimum. Over 50% of the hepatectomies carried out in our department are currently performed without the need for transfusions.[6] Hemorrhage can, however, sometimes become abundant as the deeper layers of the parenchyma are divided. In these cases it is advisable to clamp the hepatic pedicle at the hilum. Having passed the plane of the hilum, the right liver is only attached to the parenchyma of segment 8. At this point it is advisable for the surgeon to hold

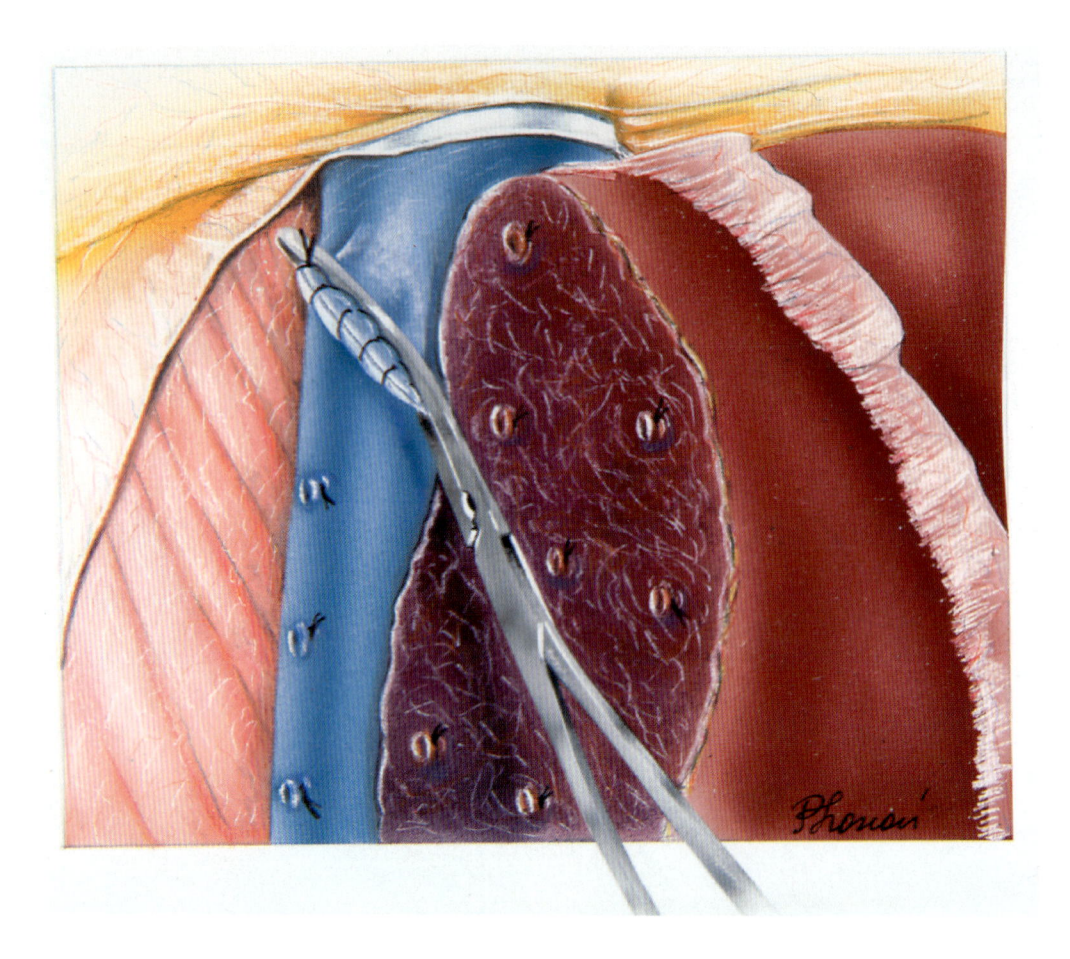

Figure 3.9 – *Suturing of the right hepatic vein.*

the portion to be removed in his left hand, touching the edge of the vena cava with his index finger as a reference point. Once the right hepatic vein has been ligated, the last portion of parenchyma can be divided before reaching the posterior aspect of Glisson's capsule. If, on the other hand, the right hepatic vein was not ligated previously outside the parenchyma, it can be identified in this last stage of the resection and clamped intraparenchymally close to the confluence with the vena cava, and then divided and sutured with Prolene® 3-0 whipstitches (**Figures 3.8 and 3.9**)

If a meticulous parenchymal division technique is followed, further hemostasis sutures are not generally necessary. Minor bleeding of the parenchyma can be coagulated with cautery or, even better, with an Argon beam coagulator. Particular attention should be paid to biliostasis. If there are traces of bile from the incision, methylene blue should be injected through the cystic duct. Cholangiography should be performed in particular cases of large biliary fistulas or when the anatomy is unclear.

Two drains are systematically positioned. The right colon and the omentum are maneuvered to the empty hepatic compartment. If the patient has had an anterior laparotomy (e.g. a colectomy for carcinoma) colonic adhesions and the omentum must be mobilized to fill the hepatic compartment.

Complications

Right hepatectomy is a well-defined procedure. It is, however, a major operation involving a series of technical principles that must be carefully observed. Intra- and post-operative complications must be recognized so they can be dealt with correctly.

Hemorrhagic complications

HEMORRHAGE FROM THE RESECTED SURFACE

Preliminary ligature of the right Glissonian pedicles, step-by-step resection, and careful surgical hemostasis are the best means of preventing hemorrhage of the resected surface. Clamping of the hepatic pedicle during standard right hepatectomy is not a routine procedure and is only performed in the event of major hemorrhage during resection. 32% of right hepatectomies in our unit have been carried out without clamping of the hepatic pedicle. Hemorrhage usually originates from the hepatic vein side. In addition to surgical hemostasis, an effective means of preventing this type of hemorrhage is to maintain a low central venous pressure during the operation.[7]

LESIONS OF THE PORTAL BIFURCATION

These lesions are caused when attempting to encircle the right branch of the portal vein in order to ligate it, either when the surgeon causes a direct lesion, or when a posterior branch for the caudate lobe is damaged. Careful dissection, proceeding from the anterior to the posterior aspect of the vessel, and mobilization of a portion of the portal trunk in order to create sufficient space before encircling the right branch with the ligature carriers, help prevent this type of incident. In the event of hemorrhage, the portal trunk must be clamped and the lesion sutured with Prolene® 5-0. Hepatectomy can only proceed if patency and the absence of stenosis of the portal trunk and the left branch are confirmed.

LESIONS OF THE VENA CAVA

The most common lesions are the tearing of an accessory hepatic vein or of the vena cava during mobilization of the liver either due to excessive traction or during the detachment of large posterior tumors. Hemorrhagic lesions must be sutured with Prolene® 3-0 or 4-0, starting from the caval side while pressure is applied to the parenchymal laceration which will be sutured subsequently. More extensive tearing of the vena cava is less frequent and more complex. Before attempting to suture, it is important to pack the hemorrhage site to allow the anesthesiology team to stabilize the patient and compensate for blood loss. Once the lesion is packed, it is advisable to complete the mobilization of the liver in order to expose the vena cava and be able to position a lateral clamp or two transverse clamps above and below the laceration which must be sutured electively. Complete clamping of the vena cava is only advisable if hemodynamic stability has been achieved.

LACERATION OF THE RIGHT HEPATIC VEIN

This is a dramatic event due to the resultant massive hemorrhage and the risk of air embolism. Laceration occurs when attempting to encircle the hepatic vein for extraparenchymal ligature. It is advisable to remember that exposure of the right hepatic vein is much easier if the dorsal ligament of the vena cava is divided. The importance of this structure in hepatectomy has been stressed by Makuuchi: the dorsal ligament is stretched between the left portion of the caudate lobe and segment 7 and surrounds the vena cava posteriorly. Division of this ligament frees the more cranial portion of the retrohepatic vena cava and allows complete exposure of the right hepatic vein which can thus be safely encircled with a clamp, ligated and sutured.

If the hepatic vein is torn, Positive End Expiratory Pressure (PEEP) should be applied to reduce the risk of air embolism: this however increases venous hemorrhage and accentuates hypotension. The hemorrhage should first be stopped by digital pressure, so that the vena cava can be freed and then clamped laterally for elective hemostasis. If the situation is so extreme that the vena cava cannot be clamped laterally, it is necessary to clamp the hepatic pedicle and the vena cava above and below the liver in order to achieve hemostasis in a bloodless field.

Biliary complications

BILIARY FISTULAE

Assessment for biliary leaks in the resection area is a very important stage of hepatectomies: biliary leakage is the main cause of post-operative subphrenic abscesses. If there are traces of bile in the cut surface, methylene blue must be injected to display the fistula which must be electively sutured with Vicryl® 4-0 stitches. A post-operative biliary fistula revealed by abdominal drainage generally tends to close spontaneously, if the ducts involved are small and there are no obstructions in the main biliary tract. Persistent post-operative fistulae require retrograde cholangiography with placement of a nasobiliary tube or endoprosthesis;[2] if this is unsuccessful a re-operation is necessary.

BILIARY TRACT DAMAGE

This is a rare complication. In our unit we have had 2 cases, one during a right hepatectomy for a large angioma and one for a hydatid cyst. Damage to the biliary tract may occur during preparation of the hilum due to accidental ligation of the hepatic duct during dissection, or due to accidental coagulation or ischemia from excessive devascularization. More complex lesions may occur during difficult hepatectomies, e.g. for hydatidosis, when the anatomy of the hepatic ducts is altered by the presence of the intrahepatic mass. Damage to the biliary tract must be suspected if bilirubin values are high after the first 4 post-operative days and there are no other signs of hepatic insufficiency. Ultrasound will confirm the dilatation of the biliary tract in the remaining liver. Retrograde cholangiography is essential to establish the site and type of obstruction. Complete obstruction or transection of the biliary tract should be treated with a hepaticojejunostomy with Roux loop: the operation must be performed without delay, before regeneration of the left lobe hinders exposure of the hepatic hilum. Endoscopic dilatation (dilatation with balloon and stent positioning) may be attempted for incomplete stenosis or in particular situations with impaired hepatic function.

Hepatic insufficiency

Right hepatectomy involves removal of 60% of the hepatic parenchyma. This amount increases in inverse proportion to the size of the mass to be removed. The operation requires careful post-operative care with infusion of fluids and albumin for 4-5 days. Oral feeding should start as early as possible. In spite of the importance of parenchymal reduction, right hepatectomies are generally very well tolerated by a normal liver. Even hepatectomies performed for trauma, when all the removed parenchyma is healthy, are not complicated by signs of hepatic insufficiency if there is no prolonged liver ischemia, hypotension or portal thrombosis. There is a risk of hepatic insufficiency if the liver is cholestatic or there is chronic liver disease, particularly cirrhosis. Prolonged clamping of the hepatic pedicle and intra-operative hypotension can cause postoperative hepatic insufficiency. If signs of hepatic insufficiency appear in the post-operative stage, the presence of sepsis, portal thrombosis, or thrombosis of the hepatic veins must be excluded. Doppler investigation of the portal vein and the hepatic veins make it easy to evaluate these last two conditions. CT and scintigraphy with marked leukocytes are indispensable in the detection of intrahepatic abscesses. The lidocaine test[5,9] is particularly useful in evaluating the extent of the hepatic insufficiency in these circumstances. The test is not affected by the simultaneous infusion of fresh plasma or coagulation factors which could falsify common laboratory parameters. In our experience, a dramatic reduction in MEGX - the primary metabolite of lidocaine - below 10% suggests severe hepatic insufficiency. Liver transplantation can be considered in end-stage hepatic insufficiency after major hepatectomies, which is fortunately a rare occurrence.

REFERENCES

1. Bismuth H. Les hépatectomies. Technique de l'hépatectomie droite. *Encyclop Méd Chir*, Paris, Techniques chirurgicales. 4/2/07, 40762-40763.
2. Born P, Bruhl K, Rosh T, Ungeheuer A, Neuhaus H, Classen M. Long term follow-up of endoscopic therapy in patients with post-surgical biliary leakage. *Hepato-Gastroenterol.* 1996; **43:** 477-487.
3. Broelsh C. *Atlas of Liver Surgery*. Churchill Livingstone, New York, 1993. pp. 8-29.
4. Couinaud C. Principes directeurs des hépatectomies réglées. *Chirurgie* 1980; **106:**103-106.
5. Ercolani G, Mazziotti A, Grazi GL, Jovine E, Callivà R, Morganti M, Masetti M, Pierangeli F, Cavallari A. Evaluation of liver function with lidocaine (MEGX) test. Proceedings 2nd World IHPBA

Congress, Bologna 1996. Monduzzi, Bologna, 1996. Vol. I, pp. 143-148.
6. Gozzetti G, Mazziotti A, Grazi GL, Jovine E. Liver resections without blood transfusions. *Br J Surg* 1995; **82:**1105-1110.
7. Hanna SS, Proctor J, Hanna TP. A low central venous pressure reduces blood loss during liver surgery. Proceedings 2nd World IHBPA Congress, Bologna 1996. Monduzzi, Bologna, 1996. Vol. I, pp. 411-415.
8. Makuuchi M, Yamamoto J, Takayama Y, Kosuge T, Gunven P, Yamazaki S, Hasegawa H. Extrahepatic division of the right hepatic vein in hepatectomy. *Hepato-Gastroenterol* 1991; **38:** 176-179.
9. Oellerich M, Raude E, Burdelski M, Shulz M, Schmidt F, Ringe B, Lamesch P, Pichlmayr R, Raith H, Scheruhn M, Wrenger M. Wittekid C. Monoethylglycinexylidide formation kinetics: a novel approach to assessment of liver function. *J Clin Chem Clin Biochem* 1987; **25:** 845-853.
10. Possati L, Cavallari A, Gozzetti G, Mazziotti A. Chirurgia del Fegato. Masson It., Milano, 1982, pp. 83-93.
11. Tôn Thât Tùng. Les Résections Majeures et Mineurs du Foie. Masson, Paris, 1979.

4

Left Hepatectomy

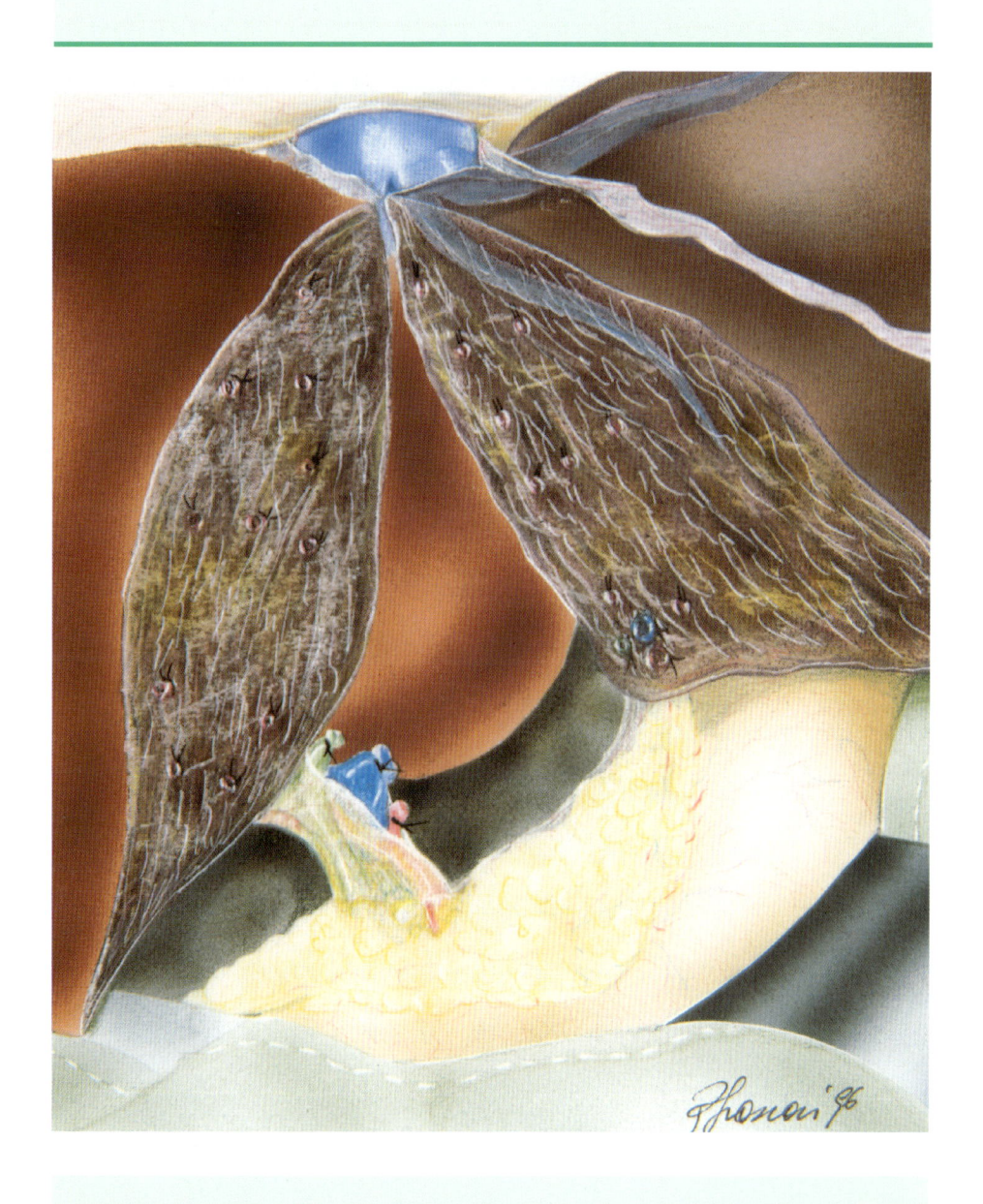

LEFT HEPATECTOMY

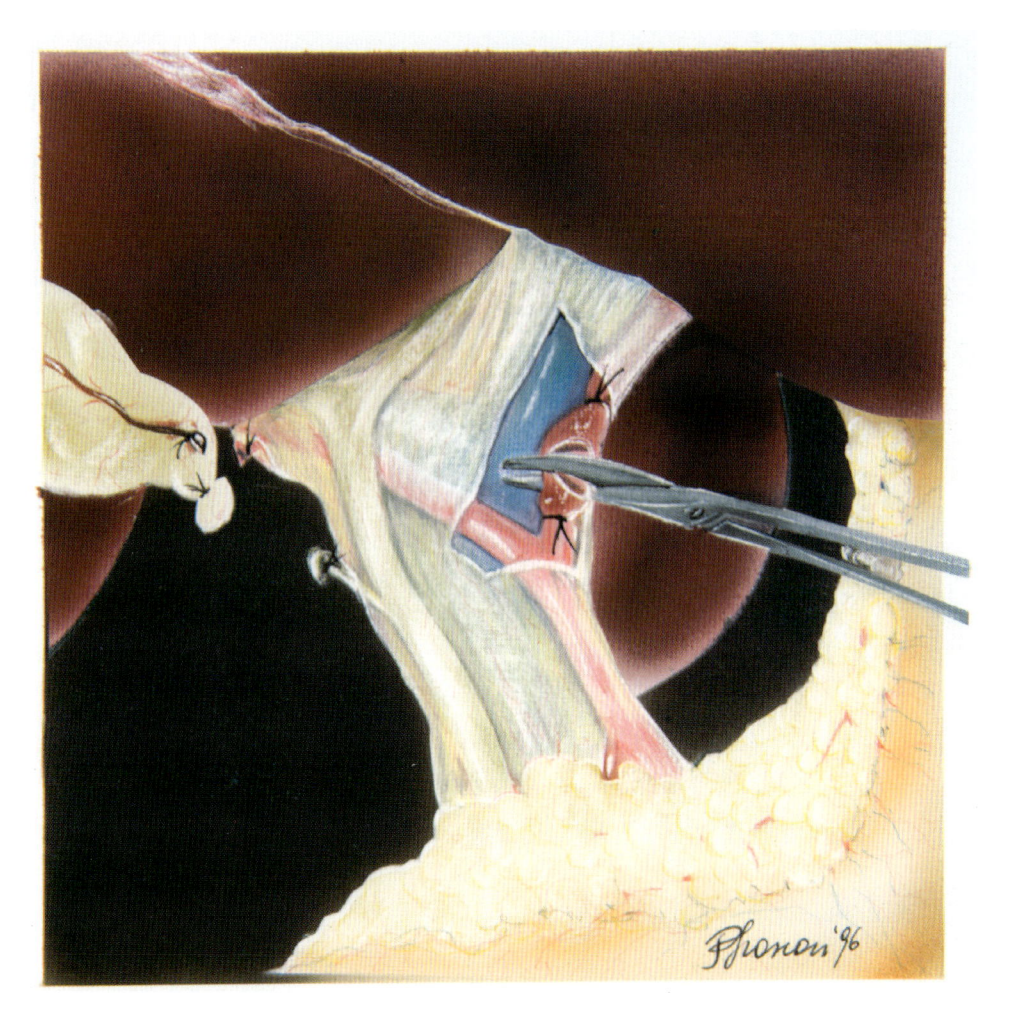

Figure 4.1 – *Left hepatectomy. Division of the left branch of the hepatic artery.*

Left hepatectomy consists of the removal of the left hemi-liver, i.e. the portion of parenchyma which receives its blood supply from the left branch of the portal vein and from the left branch of the hepatic artery (anatomical left lobe and left paramedian segment; segments 2, 3 and 4). This portion is demarcated by the sagittal-Cantlie plane and is drained by the left and middle hepatic veins. The caudate lobe is left in place in a conventional left hepatectomy. The abdominal incision is the same as the one used for right hepatectomy: a J incision extended to the right as far as the median axillary line and medially to the xiphoid cartilage which is removed; for particularly large tumors, a bilateral subcostal incision extended along the midline is advisable. Mobilization of the left hemiliver requires division of the umbilical ligament, the falciform ligament and the left triangular ligament by cautery. The left lobe may extend laterally as far as the splenic loggia. In this case, there may be a risk of damaging the upper pole of the spleen if excessive traction is exerted on the liver to stretch the end of the triangular ligament. In such cases we prefer to start the division of the triangular ligament closer to the vena cava and then to proceed towards the left. The left diaphragmatic vein runs along the diaphragmatic insertion of the ligament and sometimes crosses the triangular ligament before draining into the left hepatic vein. In this case, the diaphragmatic vein must be ligated, sutured and divided, completing the division of the ligament up to the vena cava. The lesser omentum must be divided close to the liver, taking care to identify a left hepatic artery in the upper part, originating from the left gastric artery and present in 15-20% of cases.

When mobilization of the left lobe is complete, the hilar stage is carried out. We systematically remove the gallbladder. Parenchymal division on the anterior face of the liver is carried out along the intermediate plane of the gallbladder bed as far as the vena cava. Division of the anterior peritoneum of the hepatoduodenal ligament is performed medially with respect to the common bile duct. The arterial bifurcation is exposed and the left branch of the artery (or the left branches leading respectively to the left lobe and the left paramedian segment) is divided between two ligatures (***Figure 4.1***). Below

TECHNIQUES IN LIVER SURGERY

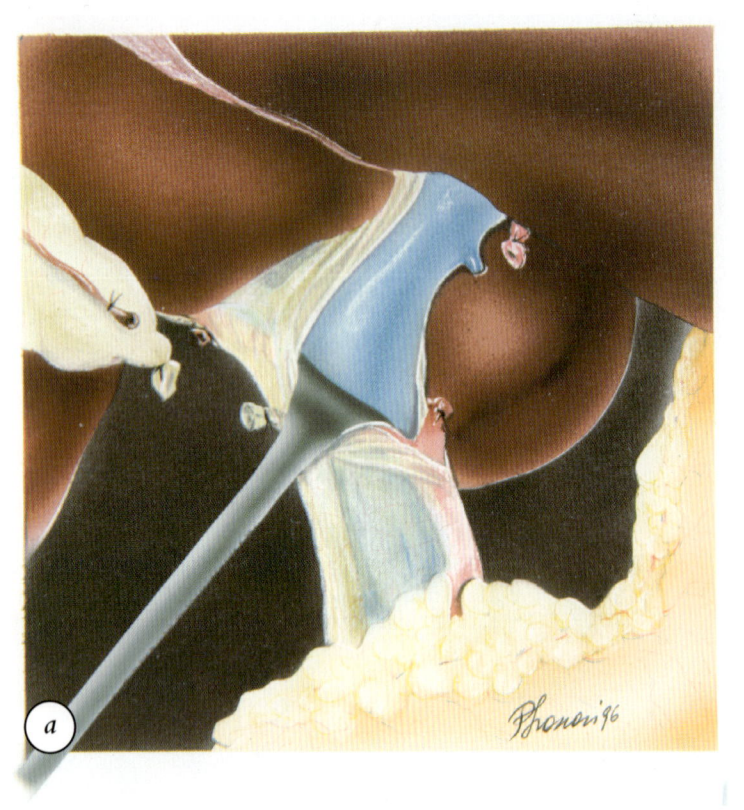

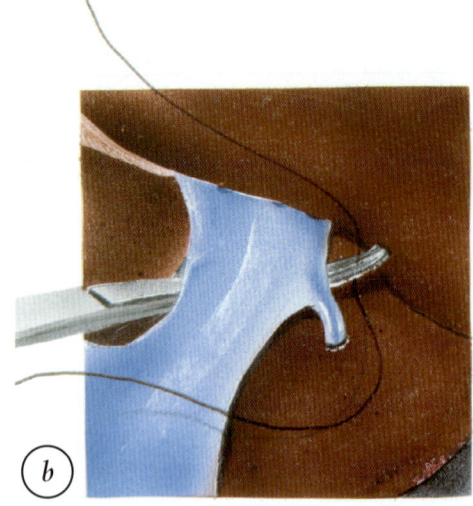

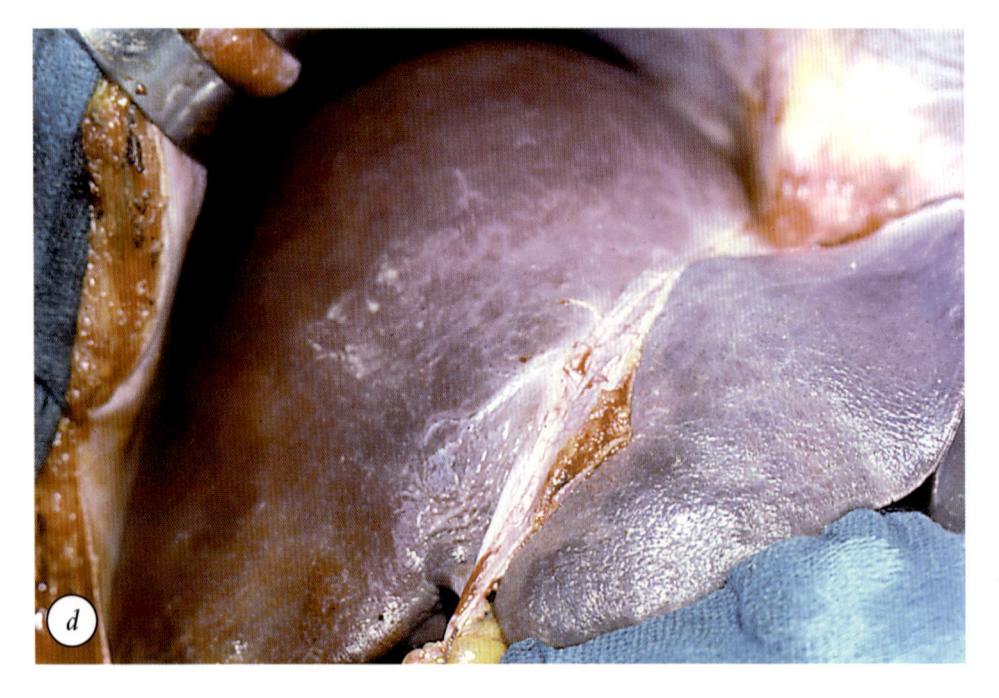

Figure 4.2 – *Exposure of the left branch of the portal vein, **a**). When the vein is ligated, the pedicle for the caudate lobe must be preserved, **b**). Ischemic demarcation of the left hemiliver, **c**).*

the artery, surrounded by very loose connective tissue, the left branch of the portal vein can be identified on a more cranial plane; this vein should be followed for a few centimeters beyond the bifurcation, outside the parenchyma. On the posterior aspect of the portal vein, 1-2 cm from the bifurcation, is a branch running towards the caudate lobe; this must be identified and left intact. The portal ligature must always be distal to this Spigelian branch (**Figure 4.2**). The left hepatic duct is not identified extraparenchymally. In this type of surgery, even more so than in right hepatectomies, division of the hepatic duct is always performed distally, during resection of the parenchyma: at the level of the left hepatic duct, variations in biliary distribution are even more frequent.[1,4] Examples include the

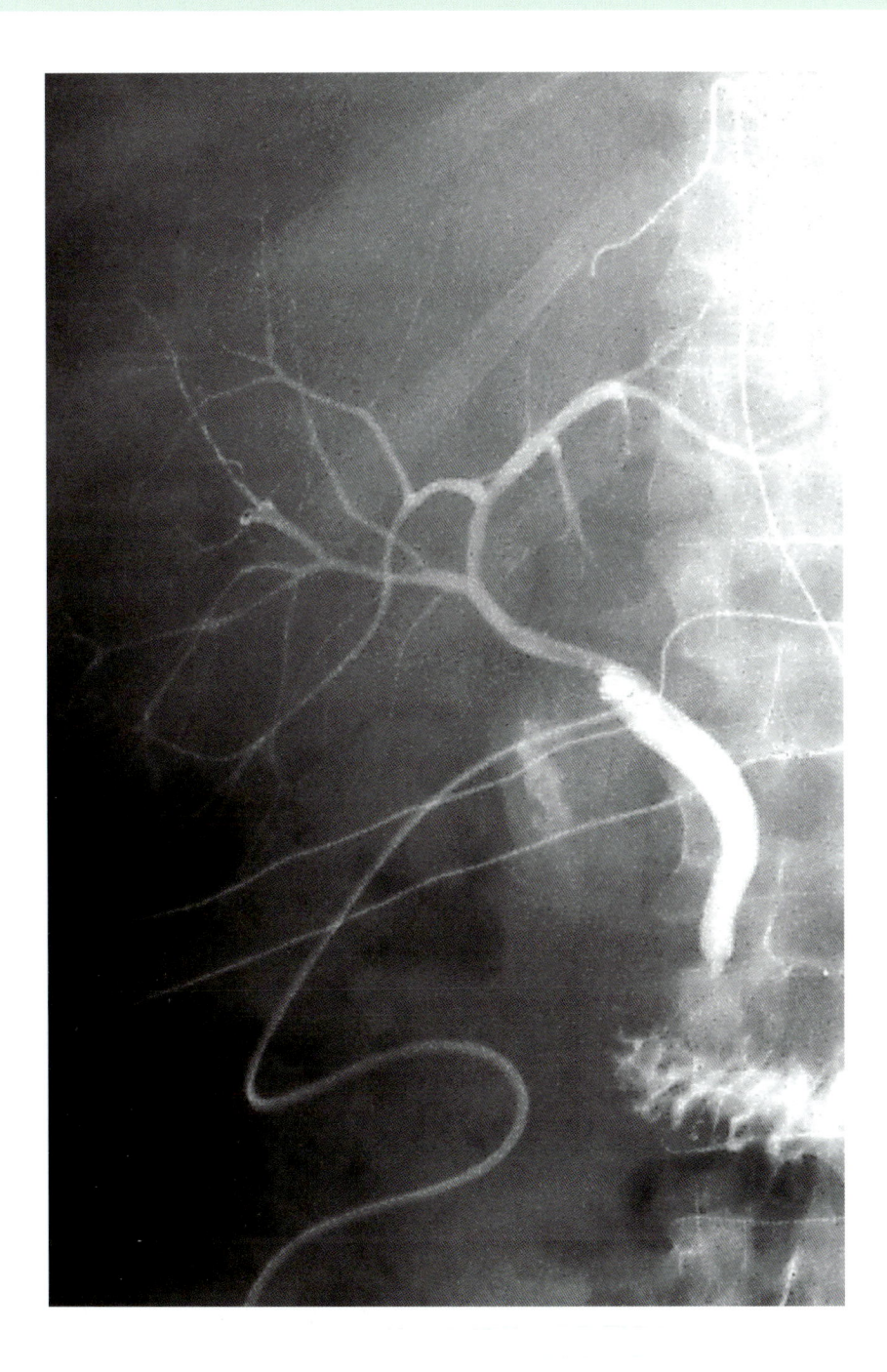

Figure 4.3 – *Right paramedian duct which runs into the left hepatic duct (trans-Kehr cholangiography in a liver transplant).*

presence of ducts for the caudate lobe and a right paramedian duct which may cross the portal bifurcation and drain into the left hepatic duct in 63 to 20% of cases (**Figure 4.3**).

After ligation of the portal branch, the left hemi-liver becomes ischemic with a demarcation line along the main sagittal plane of the liver (**Figure 4.4**). Division of the parenchyma is performed as for right hepatectomy. After incising Glisson's capsule with cautery, the parenchyma is divided with Kelly forceps, coagulating, ligating or using clips to close the small branches encountered during resection. Division proceeds to the right of the sagittal hepatic vein which is included in the resection. Continuing the division, and taking care to remain to the left of the hilar fissure, the left hepatic duct is encountered very distally,

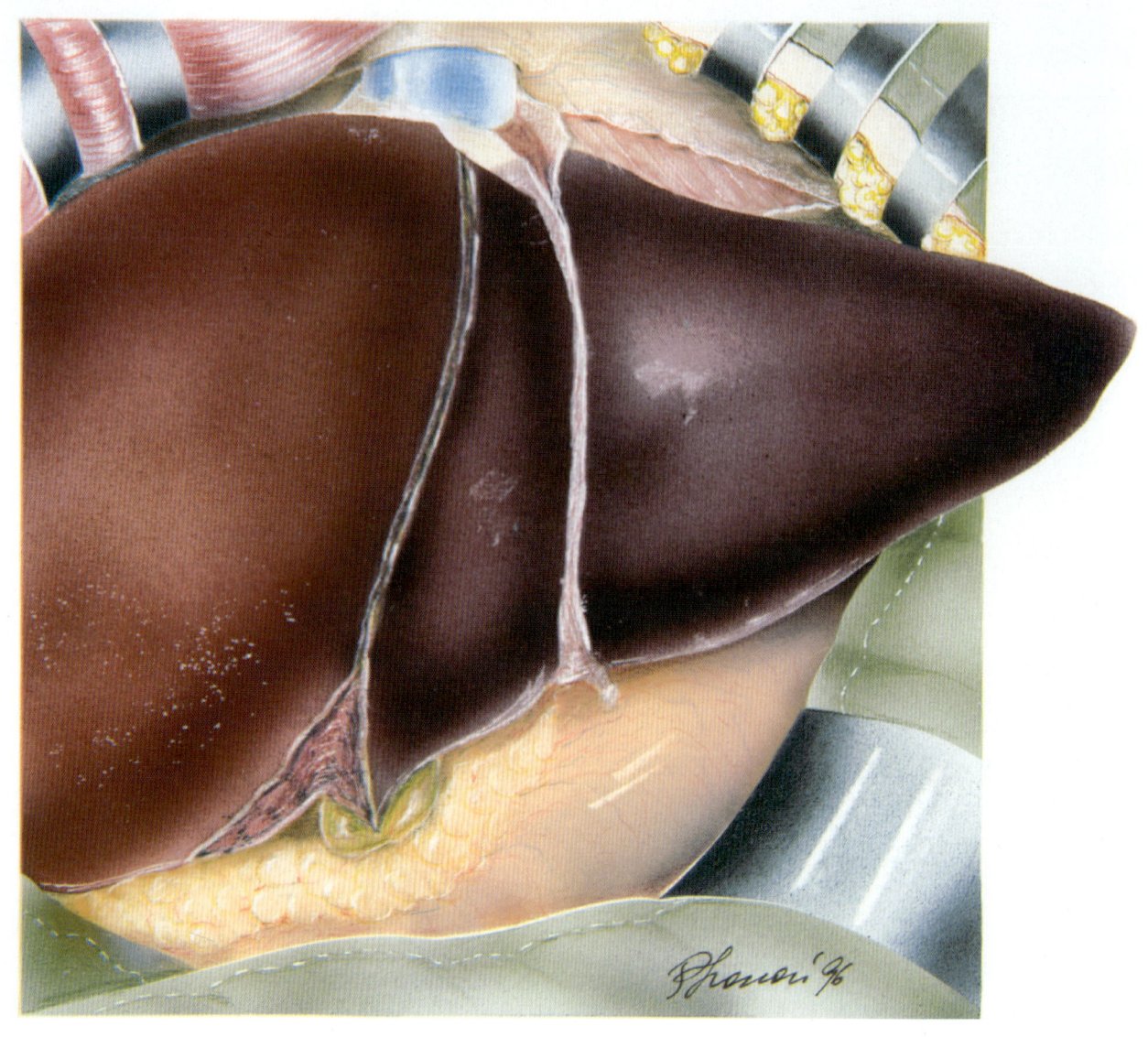

Figure 4.4 – *Division of the parenchyma along the Cantlie line.*

within the parenchyma. The hepatic duct is ligated *en bloc* with its Glissonian sheath, using two ligatures (**Figure 4.5**). This procedure prevents lesions to any anomalous bile duct originating from the right hemiliver. The left hemiliver thus remains attached by a thin bridge of parenchyma to the caudate lobe, which can be easily divided, and by a portion of parenchyma of the posterior part of segment 4, containing the sagittal and left hepatic veins. Continuing the division of the parenchyma with smooth forceps, the common trunk of the hepatic vein is identified, clamped, divided and sutured with a Prolene® 3-0 stitch (**Figure 4.6**).

LEFT HEPATECTOMY

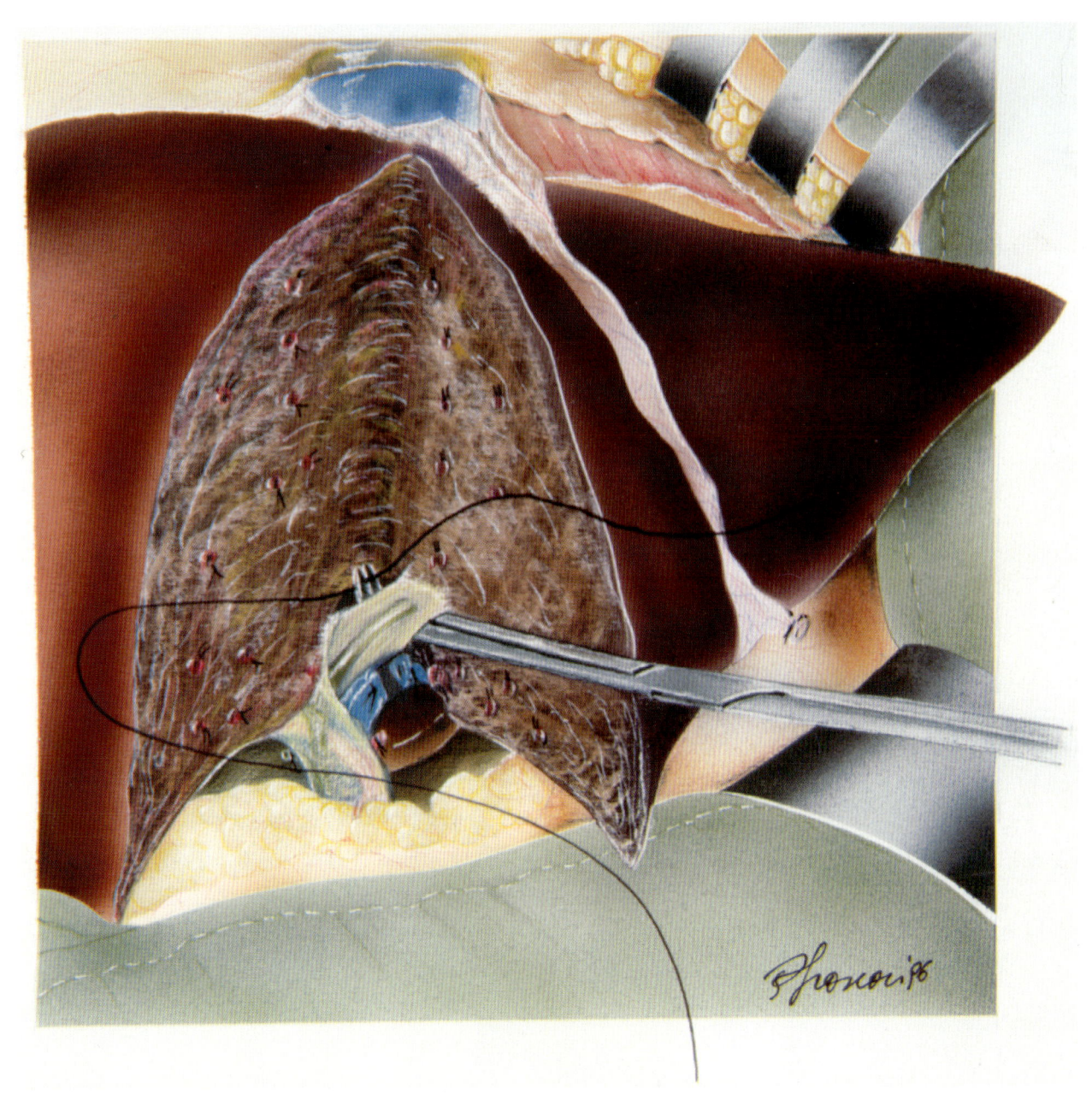

Figure 4.5 – *Intraparenchymal ligature of the left hepatic duct.*

Progressive and meticulous hemostasis makes it possible to perform the hepatectomy without blood loss. In the event of hemorrhage, temporary clamping of the hepatic pedicle may be necessary during the more advanced stages of the hepatectomy. The operation is concluded with the positioning of a gravity drain situated in the lesser sac and passed to the right through the hiatus of Wislow. The same considerations described for right hepatectomy should be given for the treatment of the resected surface.

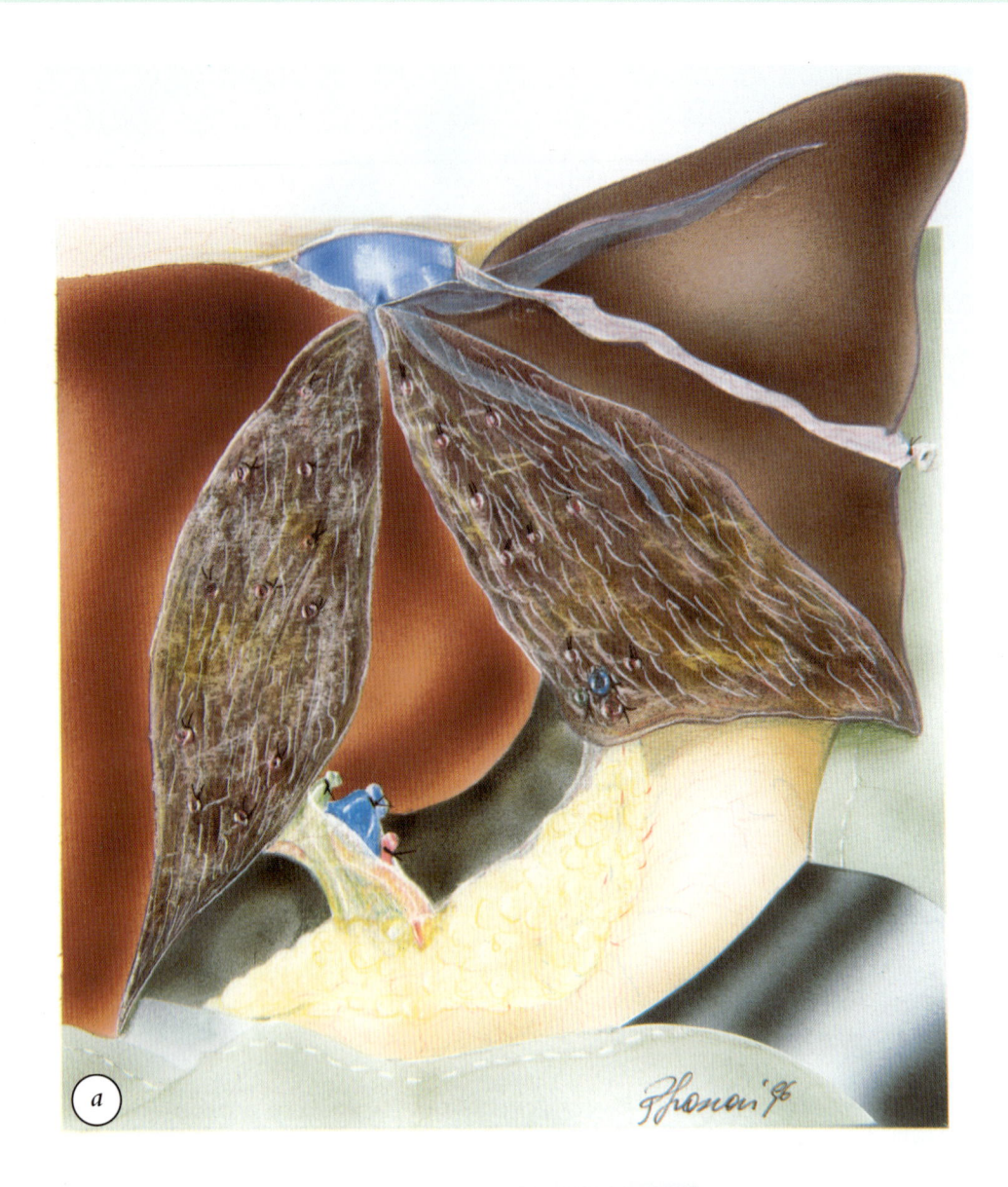

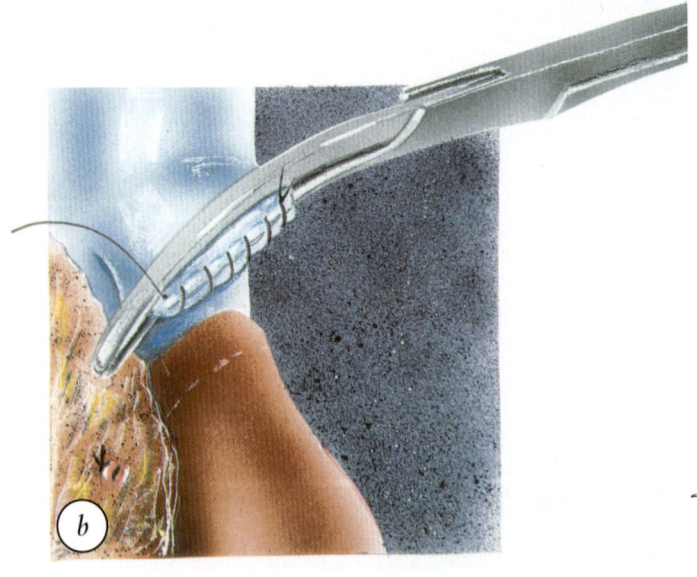

Figure 4.6 – *Exposure of the common trunk of the middle and left hepatic veins at the end of parenchymal division, a). The stump of the vein is clamped and sutured, b).*

Complications

Lesions of the left hepatic vein

The end of the left hepatic vein runs immediately below Glisson's capsule before reaching the vena cava in the loose tissue at the posterior insertion of the triangular ligament. This section of the vein has a thin wall and it is usually difficult to identify its confluence with the sagittal hepatic vein. We, therefore, prefer to divide the vein transparenchymally, after the liver has been dissected. Hemorrhage may also occur due to damage to a left diaphragmatic vein which may cross the triangular ligament and drain into the left hepatic vein a few centimeters from its convergence with the vena cava. Hemorrhage from this vein should be treated by suturing first the diaphragmatic aspect and then the liver.

Biliary damage

Biliary damage may occur due to the division of small bile ducts in the caudate lobe or accidental section of an anomalous duct originating from the right hemiliver. In the first case it is advisable to remove the caudate lobe in order to prevent biliary fistulae or cholangitis. If damage to an anomalous right duct draining into the left hepatic duct is suspected, transcystic cholangiography must be performed to determine intrahepatic biliary anatomy. The biliary branch must be sutured with PDS® (Polydioxanone, Ethicon) 6.0 stitches over a Silastic stent which can be passed through the cystic duct or directly from the main bile duct below the convergence.

REFERENCES

1. Couinaud C. Exposure of the left hepatic duct: anatomical limitations. *Surgery* 1989; **105**: 21-27.
2. Linder RM, Cady B. Hepatic resection. *Surg Clin N Am* 1980; **60**: 349-367.
3. Mizumoto R, Sutuki H. Surgical anatomy of the hepatic hilum with special reference to the caudate lobe. *World J Surg* 1988; **12**: 2-10.
4. Russel E, Yrizzary JM, Montalvo BM, Guerra JJ, Al Refa F. Left hepatic duct anatomy. Implications. *Radiology* 1974; **174**: 353-356.

5

Left Lobectomy

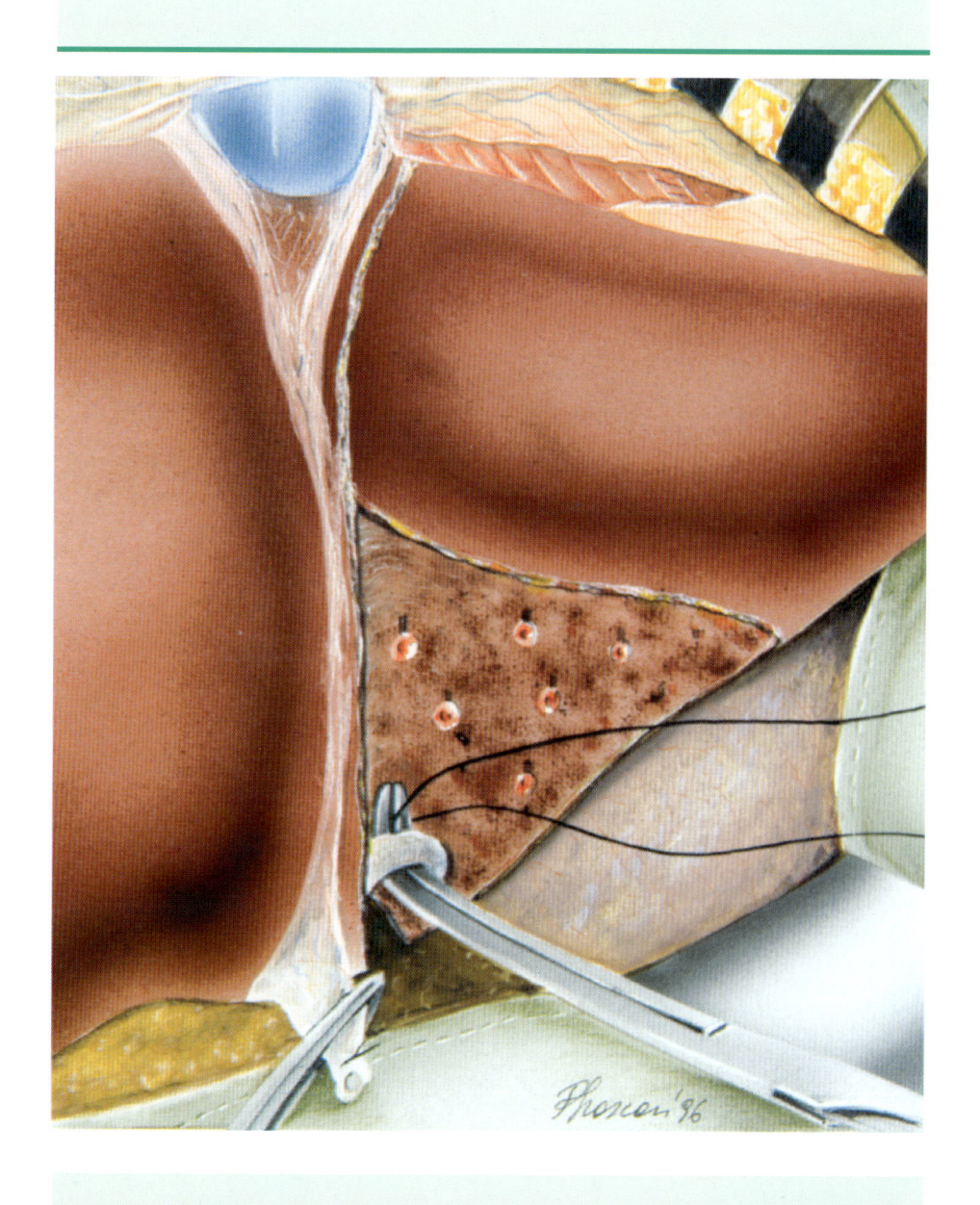

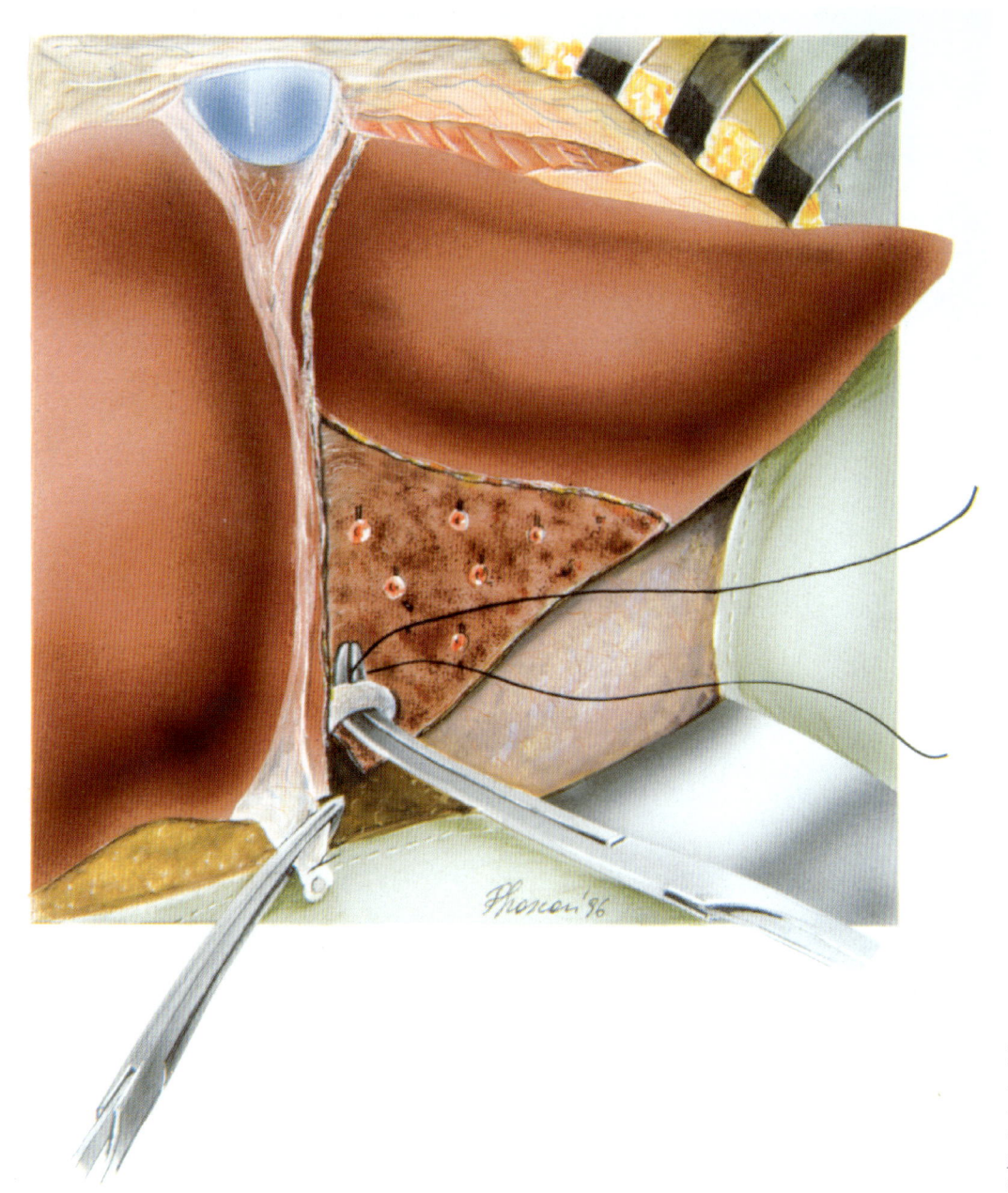

Figure 5.1 – *Left lobectomy. Ligation of the Glissonian pedicle for segment 3.*

Left lobectomy consists of the resection of the left anatomical lobe, i.e. the portion of the parenchyma situated to the left of the falciform ligament (segments 2 and 3 in Couinaud's classification, left lateral sector in Healey's classification). It is the simplest and most common of the typical hepatectomies, and is indicated for tumors localized in the left lobe, direct infiltration from a gastric tumor, hydatid cysts or traumatic lesions involving the left lobe of the liver.

The usual approach is a xiphoumbilical median incision. The bilateral subcostal approach, extended along the midline, is used for particularly large tumors.

The most commonly used procedure in left lobectomy is the transparenchymal technique. The liver is mobilized by dividing the falciform ligament, the left triangular ligament and the lesser omentum. Incision of Glisson's capsule is performed immediately to the left of the insertion of the falciform ligament. Parenchymal division proceeds from the anterior edge of the liver. The Glissonian pedicle of segment 3 is situated at the level of the insertion of the umbilical ligament, on its left side, immediately above Glisson's capsule on the inferior surface of the liver. The arterial, biliary and portal branches run together enclosed by a thickening of Glisson's capsule and are ligated en bloc (**Figure 5.1**). About 2 cm to the rear, on a plane that extends to the left part of the

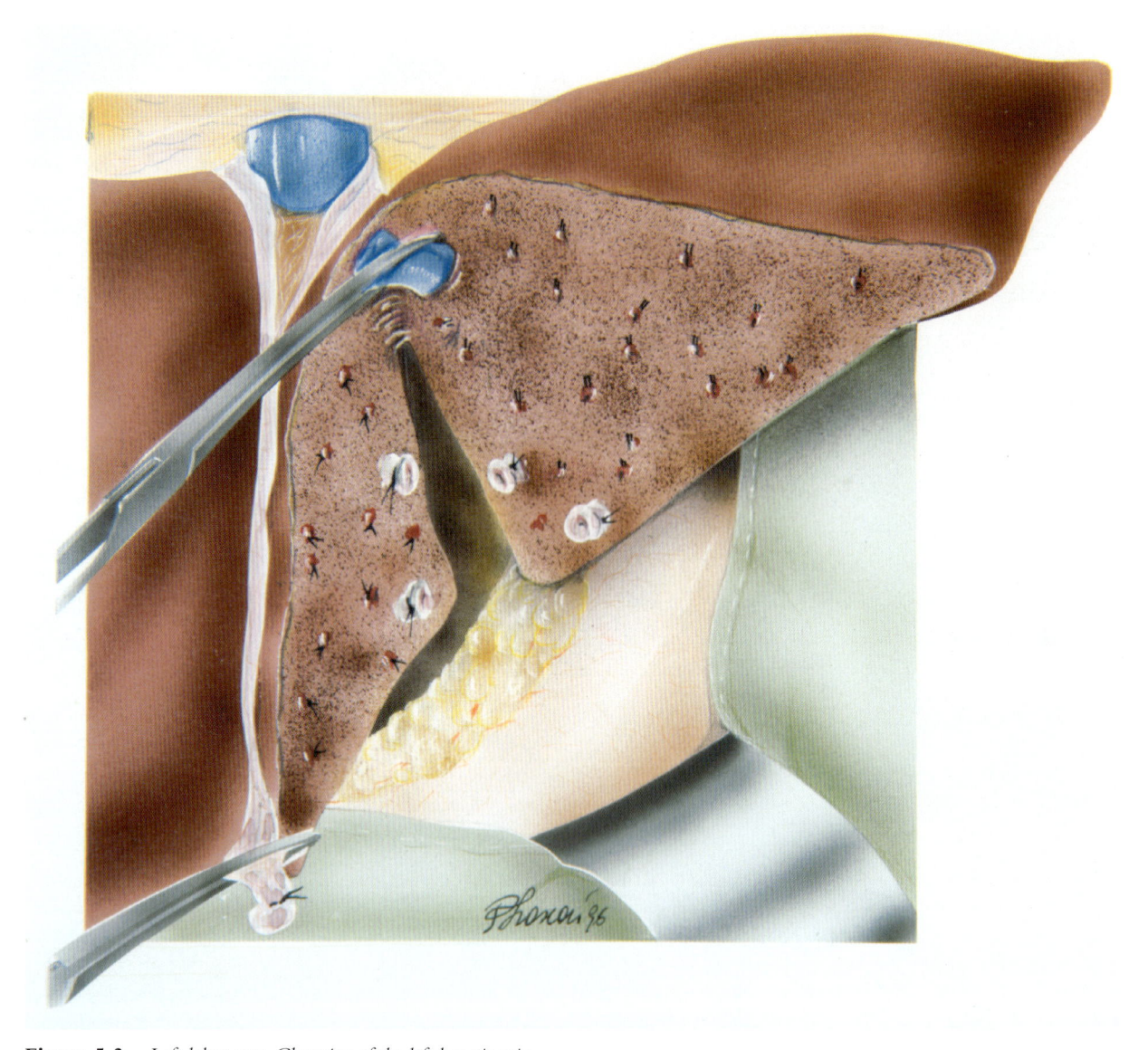

Figure 5.2 – *Left lobectomy. Clamping of the left hepatic vein.*

hilum, the Glissonian pedicles of segment 2 are encountered. The pedicles are clamped and divided with two ligatures. Dissection proceeds posteriorly as far as the trunk of the left hepatic vein which is clamped, divided and sutured with a Prolene® 3-0 transfixed stitch (**Figure 5.2**).

At times, especially in thin subjects and in non-cirrhotic livers, the Glissonian pedicles can be easily isolated on the inferior surface of the liver, to the left of the umbilical ligament fissure, and ligated extraparencyhmally.

6

Liver Segmentectomies

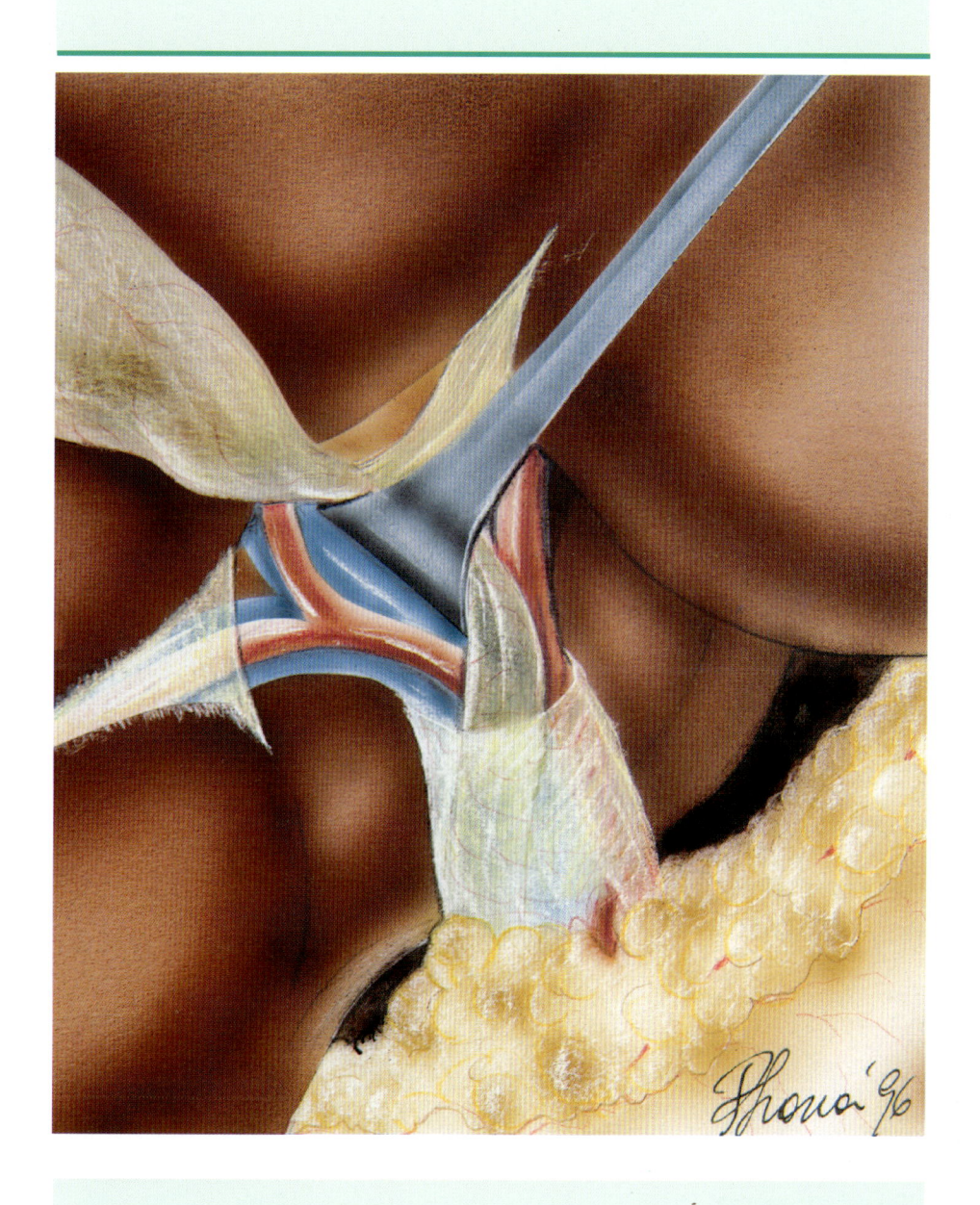

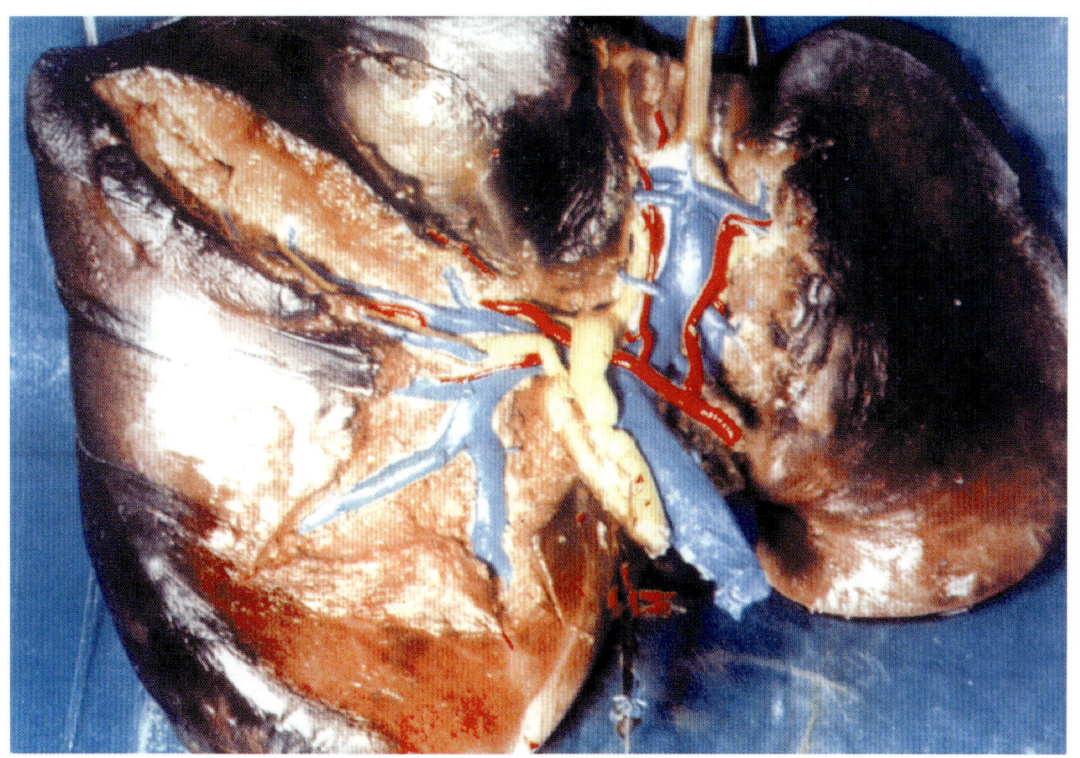

Figure 6.1 – *Anatomy of the hepatic hilum in a liver cast. The biliary duct is colored yellow (the gallbladder has been removed), the artery red and the portal vein blue.*

Resections of a single hepatic segment, or of two or more segments, can be performed anatomically, after assessing the vascular pedicles. The hepatic segments are anatomical entities based on the presence of afferent vascular pedicles which have a defined arrangement, despite possible anatomical variations. The terminology used in this volume follows the 'European' classification of the hepatic segments according to Couinaud.[3,4] Healey and Schroy's classification, more popular in the United States and Japan, includes four 'segments' - left lateral, left medial, right anterior and right posterior – (which correspond to the 'sectors' in Couinaud's classification) divided into 'subsegments' (which correspond to the 'segments' in Couinaud's classification[8]).

At the hepatic hilum it is possible to identify the arterial and portal branches of the left lateral segments, 2 and 3, (anatomical left lobe), of segment 4, of the right paramedian segments, 5 and 8, and of the right lateral sector segments, 6 and 7. By the left extraparenchymal route it is possible to also identify the individual segmentary branches of segments 2 and 3, which are enclosed by a sheath of connective tissue, to the left of the umbilical fissure. On the right side, the division of the main pedicles into individual segmentary branches lies within the parenchyma and elective ligation of the individual branches is only possible after dissection of the parenchyma (***Figure 6.1***). The portal pedicles of segment 1 can be identified and divided extraparenchymally.

Anatomical segmentectomies are based on the resection of a single hepatic segment or of several segments at the same time, after the identification and selective clamping of the vascular pedicles. While resection is a simple matter for anterior segments 5 and 6 and the anterior portion of segment 4 and segment 3, the situation is more complex for posterior segments 7 and 8 and all segment 4. This chapter describes anatomical single segmentectomies (apart from segment 1 which will be dealt with in chapter 11).

Other segmentectomy techniques described in the literature advise pre-operative elective injection of a dye into the segmentary portal pedicle, under the guidance of intra-operative ultrasound. The identification of the segment with the resultant staining indicates the limits of the resection.[10] This technique, however, requires skill and familiarity with intra-operative ultrasound. For segments 6 and 8, which often receive two or more afferent pedicles, elective injection is more difficult. Staining may also prove ineffective in the presence of an artero-portal shunt, a frequent occurrence in cirrhotic livers.

The technique described in this chapter, based on the elective clamping of the vascular pedicles, is in our opinion a rational approach to anatomical segmentectomy, in which resection is based on true intra-hepatic vascularization and not on arbitrary criteria. The method prevents devascularized zones remaining in the parenchyma, as these could become a possible source of parenchymal sequestration, abscess and biliary fistula.

Anatomical landmarks of liver segments

There are constant landmarks present on the outer surface of the liver which identify the intra-hepatic vascular structures. These landmarks make it possible to identify the margins of the segments and can be a useful guide in performing segmentary hepatectomies.

The most clearly visible landmark on the anterior surface of the liver is the fissure of the umbilical ligament. The termination of the left portal branch, Rex's recess, is situated at the end of this fissure, and the right horns for segment 4 and the left horn for segment 3 originate from here. These portal branches run together to the corresponding arterial and biliary branches, enclosed in connective tissue and visible on the left after detachment of Glisson's capsule and on the right after dissecting a small portion of parenchyma.

The plane passing between the gallbladder bed and the vena cava indicates the sagittal fissure of the liver, the Cantlie line, along which conventional right or left hepatectomy is carried out. The middle hepatic vein is just to the left of this plane and contains only small hepatic branches of segment 5 before reaching the large right Glissonian vascular pedicles. There are a further two landmarks in the right lobe consisting of two vascular pedicles. On the inferior surface of the liver, to the right of the gallbladder and running obliquely and posterior to the plane of the hilum, is Ganz's incisure[6] along which runs the posterior Glissonian pedicle for segments 6 and 7. On the lateral surface of the liver, clearly visible after dissecting the right triangular ligament, is a fissure in the parenchyma which corresponds to the trunk of the right hepatic vein. This indicates the upper limit between segments 7 and 8.

Indications for segmentectomy

Segmentectomies are indicated for small hepatic lesions, limited to a single segment, to adjacent lesions in 2 or 3 segments, or to multiple lesions situated at some distance from each other in the two lobes of the liver. The most typical conditions are benign tumors or small malignant lesions such as single or multiple metastases in several segments. One example is hepatocarcinoma associated with cirrhosis. This operation, required with increasing frequency as a result of ultrasound screening detecting small asymptomatic tumors, must preserve as much parenchyma as possible in cirrhotic patients while ensuring radical intervention.

The correct surgical management of hepatic malignancies should guarantee a radical intervention, ensuring a clear margin of at least 1cm, and should preserve as much non-involved liver parenchyma as possible. Segmentectomies can satisfy these requirements and offer several advantages compared with conventional hepatectomies. Most segmentectomies do not require blood transfusions. Additionally, surgical trauma is limited and the post-operative recovery period is shorter, without the need for administration of plasma derivatives. Segmentectomies are not usually followed by phenomena of hepatic anatomy alterations caused by compensatory hypertrophy, common after major hepatectomy. It is also much simpler to re-operate in the event of tumor recurrence. The main advantage of segmentectomies is, however, represented by patients with chronic hepatitis or with confirmed cirrhosis who cannot tolerate major hepatectomy. The selective clamping of the vascular pedicles of the hepatic sector adjacent to the segment to be removed, as described in our technique, limits damage to the parenchyma caused by the *en bloc* clamping of the hepatic pedicle at the hilum. This advantage appears even greater in livers affected by chronic diseases.

Resection of segment 4

Segment 4 consists of the most medial portion of the left hemiliver, bordered on the left margin by the insertion of the falciform ligament and by the umbilical fissure, and on the right by a plane passing from the gallbladder bed to the vena cava. The Glissonian

LIVER SEGMENTECTOMIES

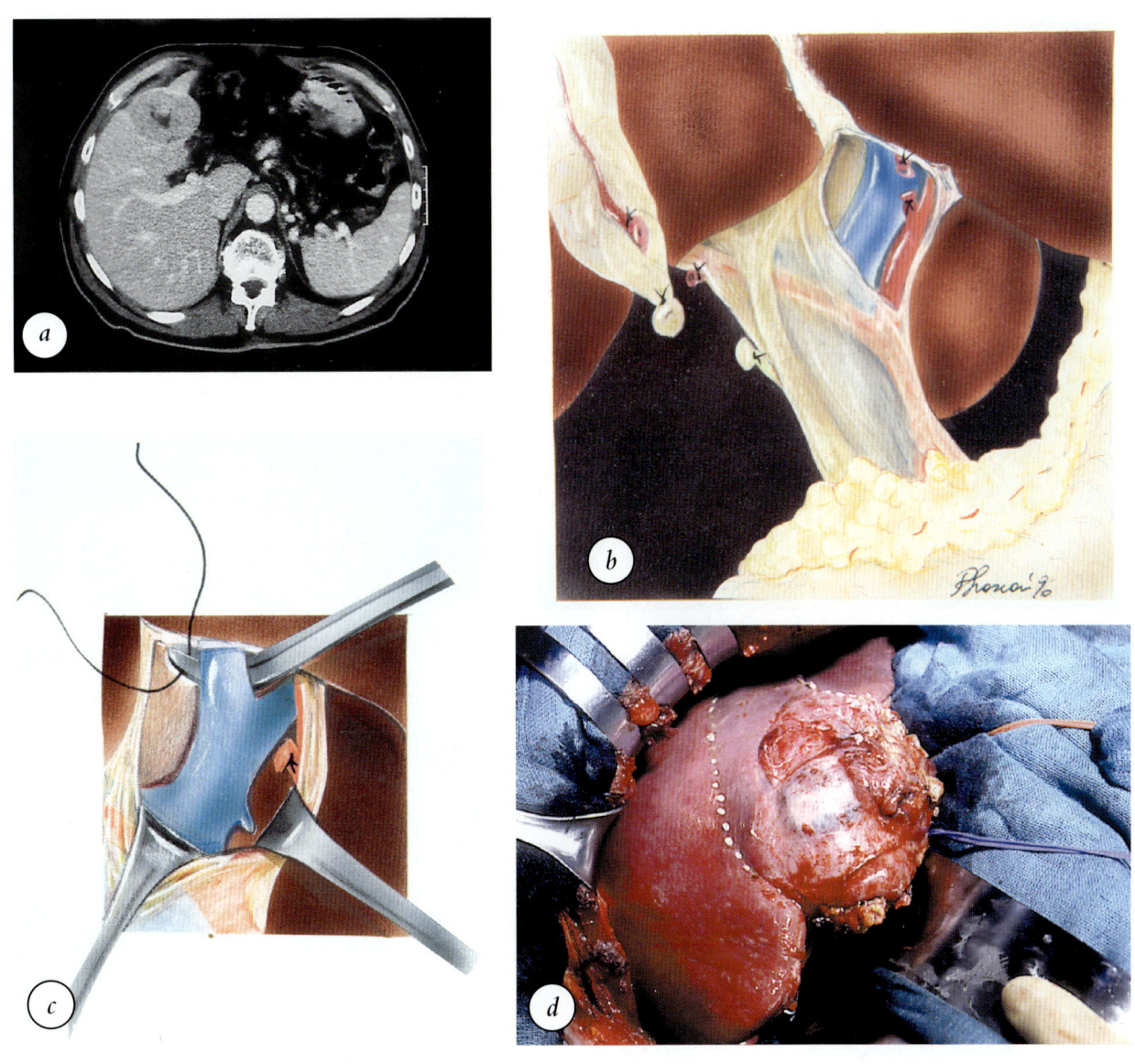

Figure 6.2 – *Resection of segment 4 for hepatocarcinoma. **a)** Preoperative CT scan. **b)** Ligature of the left paramedian arterial branch. **c)** Ligature of the left paramedian portal branch. **d)** Ischemic demarcation of segment 4.*

pedicles of segment 4 originate from the left portal branch and from the left branch of the hepatic artery or from a middle hepatic artery originating directly from the common hepatic artery. The biliary branch drains into the left hepatic duct, or distally adjacent to the right horn of Rex's recess or directly on the anterior aspect of the left hepatic duct. Venous drainage takes place through the middle hepatic vein which runs deep within the parenchyma and drains into the vena cava, generally with a common trunk with the right hepatic vein.

Anatomical resection of segment 4 is based on the extraparenchymal ligation of the afferent vessels. After dissecting the peritoneum of the hepato-duodenal ligament, the left branch of the hepatic artery is followed and the lateral branches (for the left lobe) and the medial branch (for segment 4), are identified: the latter is ligated and divided (**Figure 6.2b**). The right branch of the artery is also identified. Posterior to the artery, the portal bifurcation is dissected. The left branch is long and can be easily mobilized as far as its terminal branches. The medial branch corresponds to the pedicle of segment 4, which should be ligated (**Figure 6.2c**). The biliary branch is not identified at this stage. The convergence of the hepatic ducts is not divided and, during isolation of the vascular pedicles, remains on an anterior and superior plane. When the vascular pedicles have been ligated the ischemic demarcation line for parenchymal dissection appears on the surface of segment 4 (**Figure 6.2d**). Right dissection is carried out along the gallbladder-vena cava plane (**Figure 6.3a**). At this stage, selective clamping

TECHNIQUES IN LIVER SURGERY

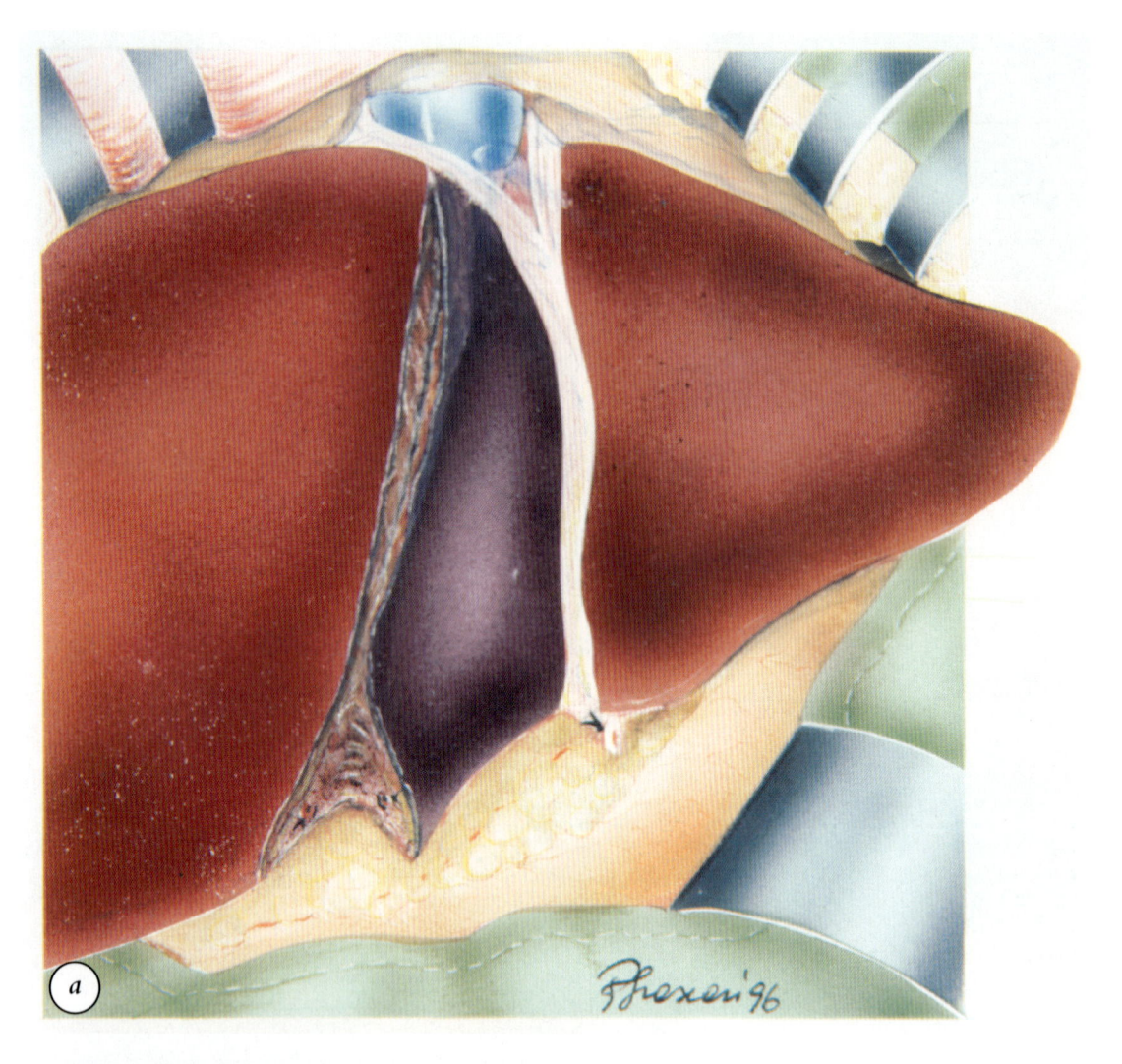

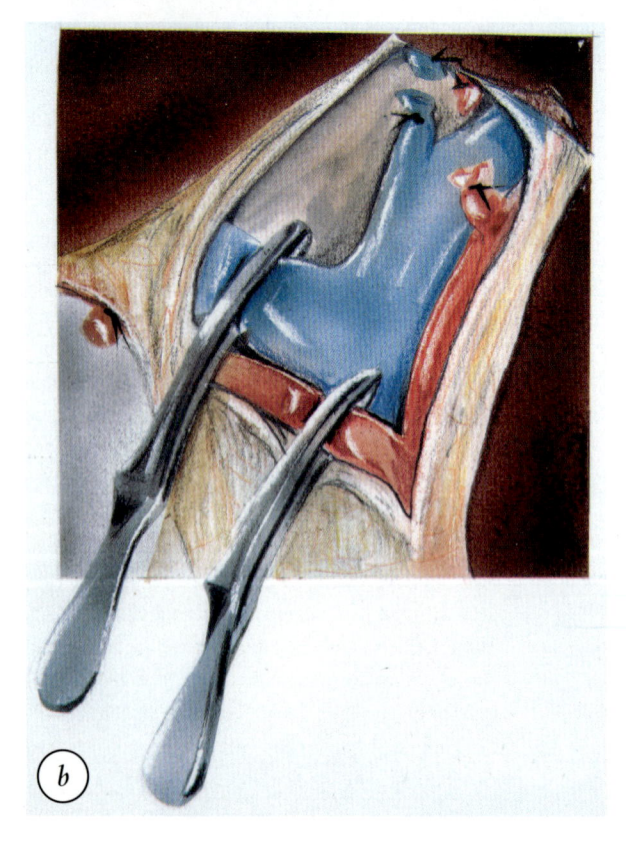

Figure 6.3 – *a) Parenchymal division along the gallbladder – vena cava plane. During resection, the right portal and arterial branches are clamped b).*

LIVER SEGMENTECTOMIES

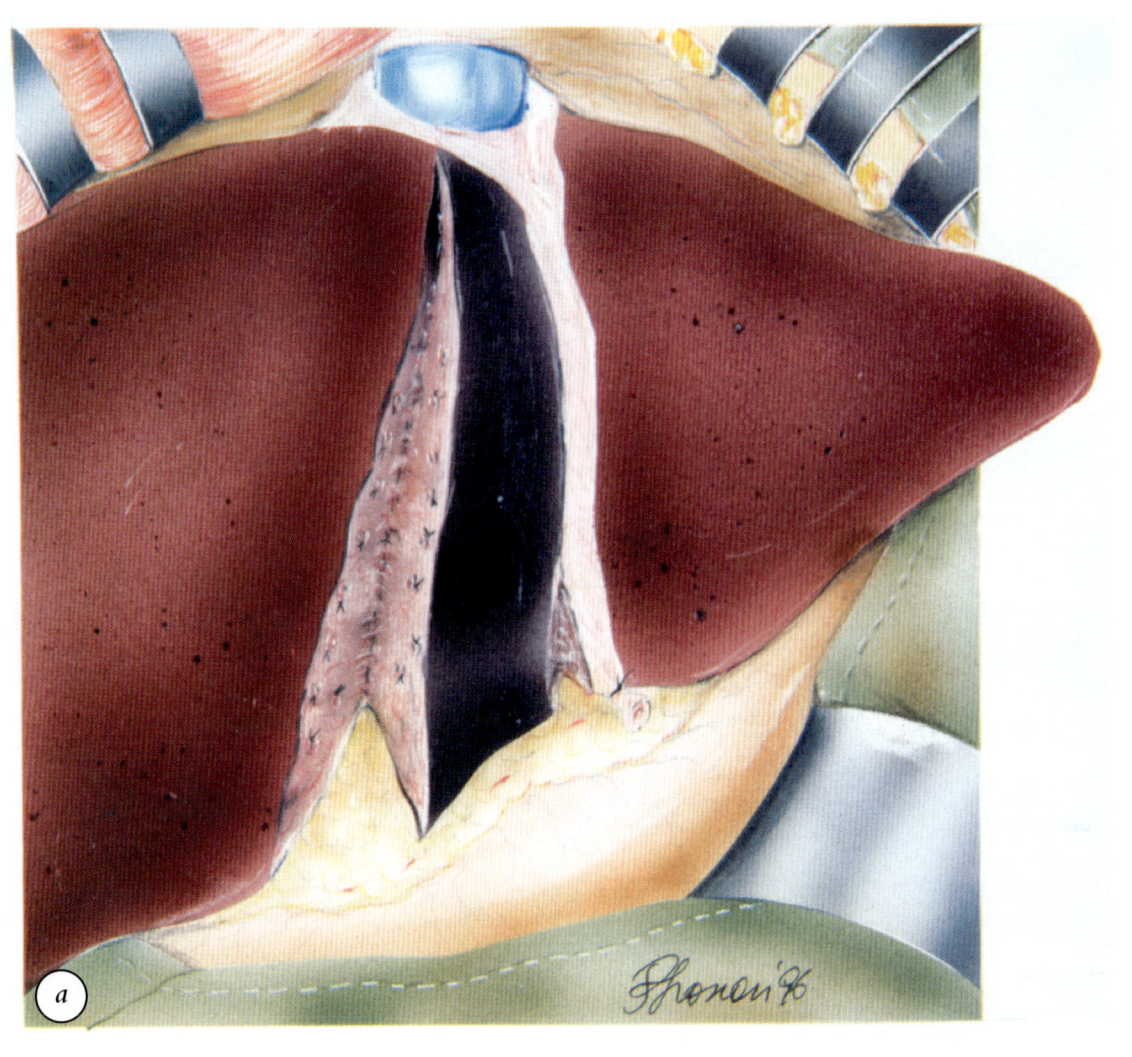

Figure 6.4 – *a) Left parenchymal division along the insertion plane of the falciform ligament. The left portal and arterial pedicles are clamped b).*

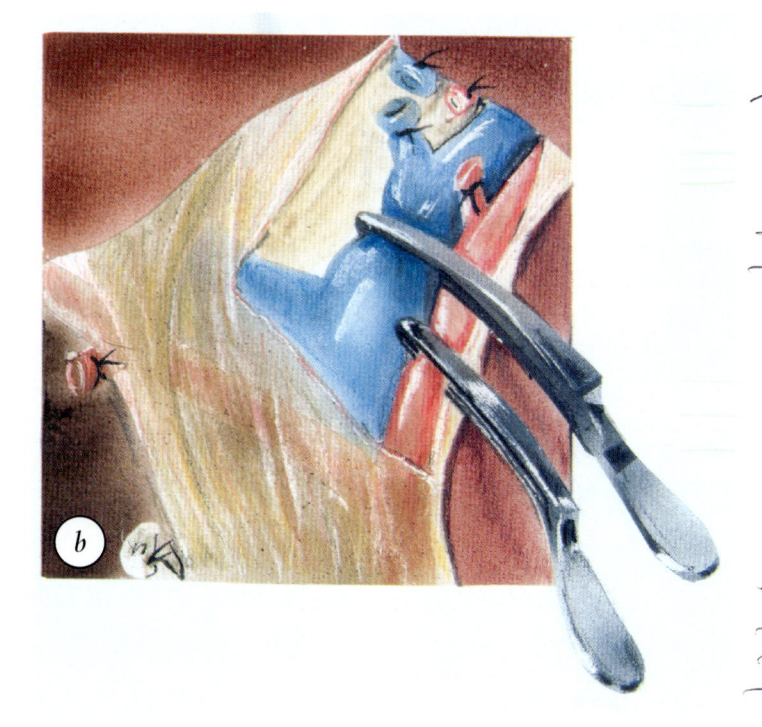

of the right Glissonian pedicle is advisable in order to limit blood loss (**Figure 6.3b**). The root of the middle hepatic vein appears early along the resection plane; the vein is followed along its right border to the point where it drains into the vena cava. Once dissection along the right margin is complete, the clamp can be removed from the right arterial and portal branch. Dissection continues on the left along the insertion plane of the falciform ligament (**Figure 6.4a**). During parenchymal dissection it is advisable to clamp the previously prepared left branch of the artery and of the portal vein to prevent bleeding during resection. A few centimeters posterior to the insertion of the round ligament, the Glissonian pedicle for the anterior portion of segment 4 is encountered on the right, and must be ligated with Vicryl® 3-0. Dissection proceeds posteriorly, where several small hepatic

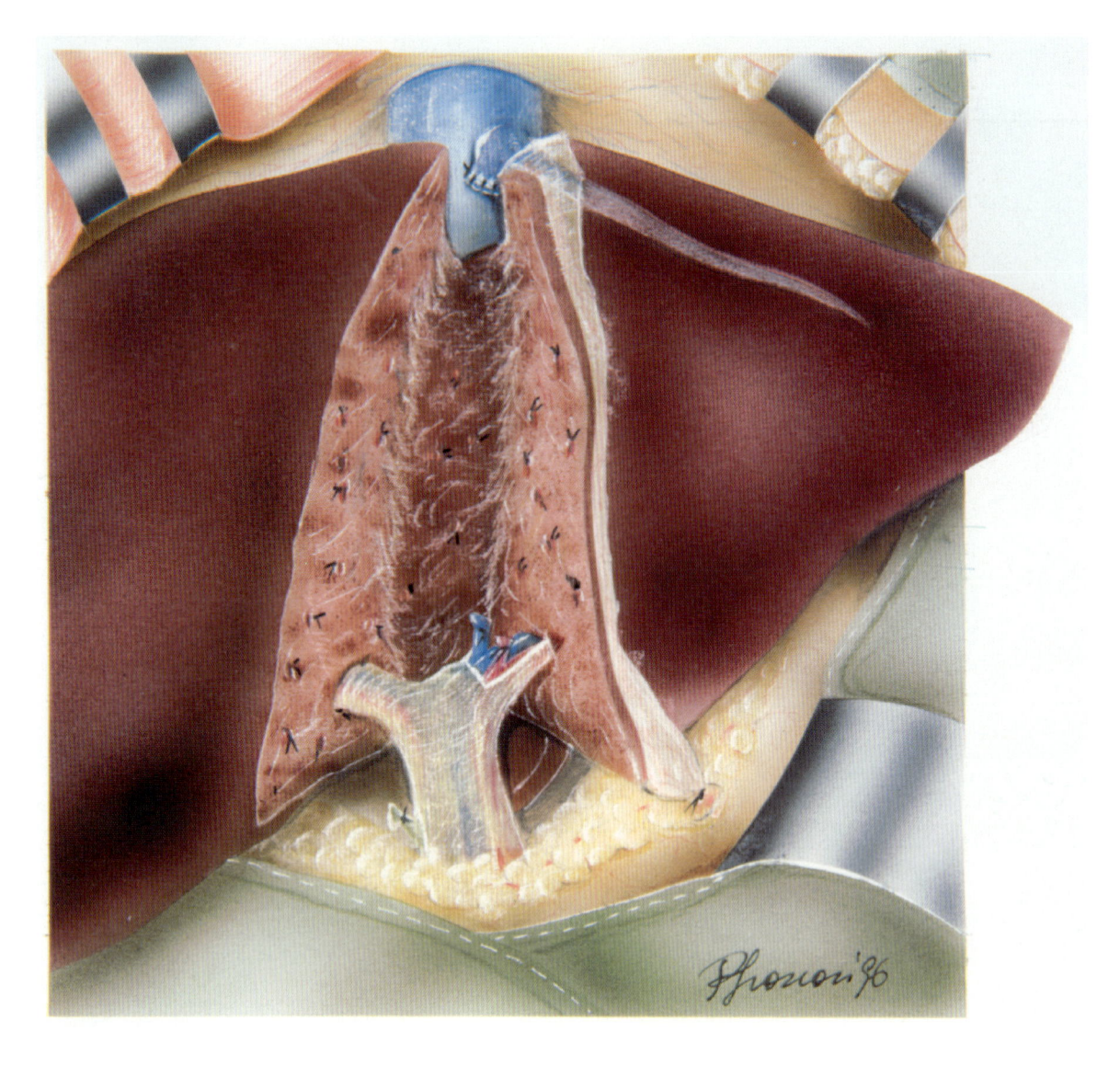

Figure 6.5 – *Division of the middle hepatic vein.*

branches and normally a further Glissonian branch originating from the main left pedicle are encountered. Once parenchymal dissection is complete, the left pedicle is unclamped. Immediately below the hilum, Glisson's capsule is divided above the hilar plate, taking care to identify a possible biliary branch of segment 4 which may drain more proximally into the anterior border of the left hepatic duct. This biliary duct must be sutured with Vicryl®. At this point the whole of segment 4 is attached only to the trunk of the middle hepatic vein which must be clamped, divided and sutured (*Figure 6.5*).

Resection of the anterior part of segment 4 is indicated for small lesions, situated between the gallbladder and the insertion plane of the falciform ligament (*Figure 6.6a*). The portal pedicle of this part of segment 4 always originates from the right horn of Rex's recess and runs along the bile duct and the anterior branch. These can easily be identified once the parenchyma to the right of the round ligament has been divided (*Figure. 6.6b and d*). Ligation of the pedicles is followed by the appearance of a demarcation line of the anterior sub-segment 4 (*Figure 6.6c*) which can thus be removed electively (*Figure 6.6d and e*).

Resection of segment 8

Isolated resection of segment 8 as proposed by Couinaud,[3] and described by Bismuth,[2] Franco,[5] Scheele,[14] Yu[16] and Makuuchi,[11] remains a technical challenge. The deep position of the afferent Glissonian pedicle

LIVER SEGMENTECTOMIES

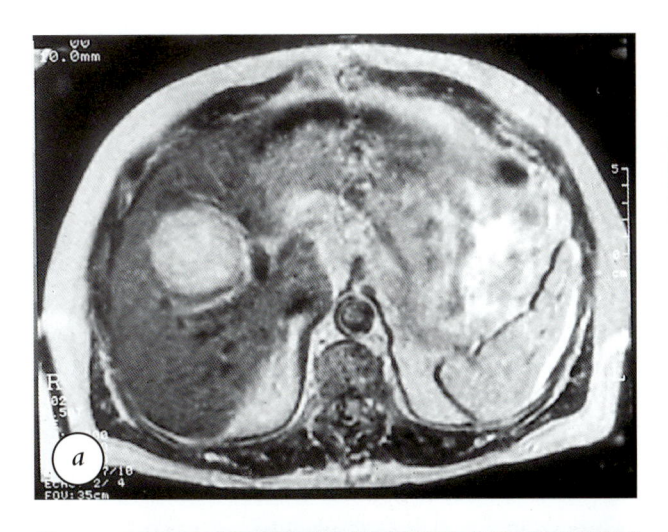

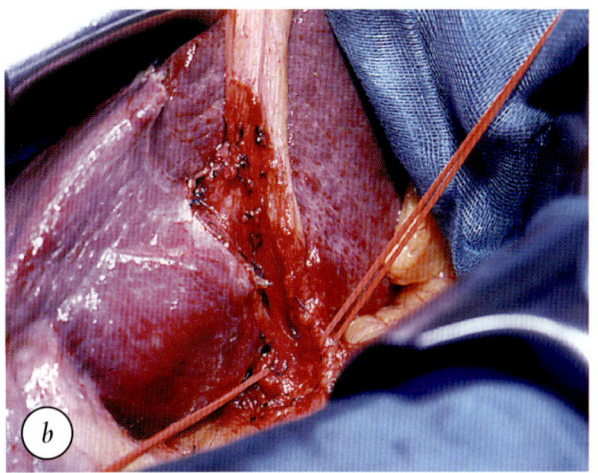

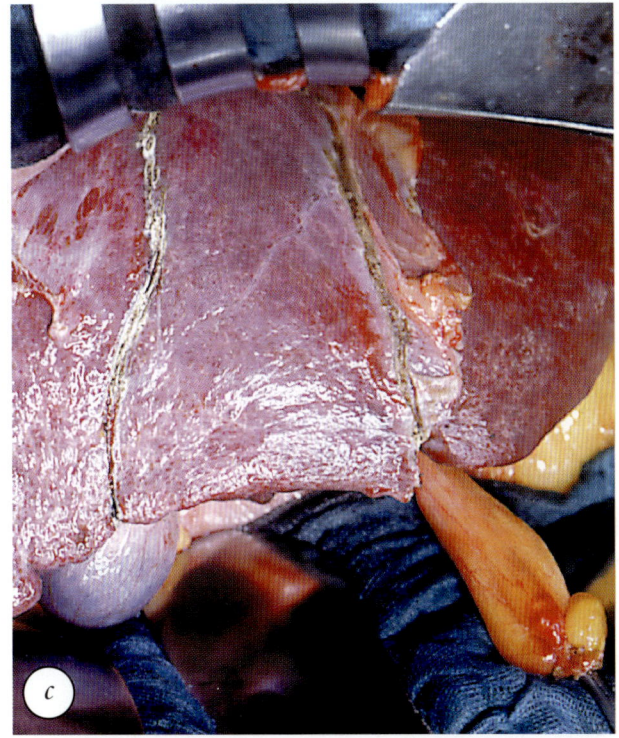

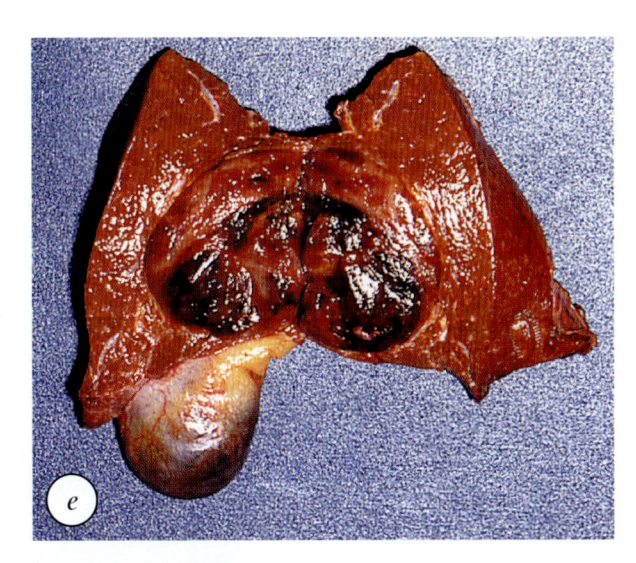

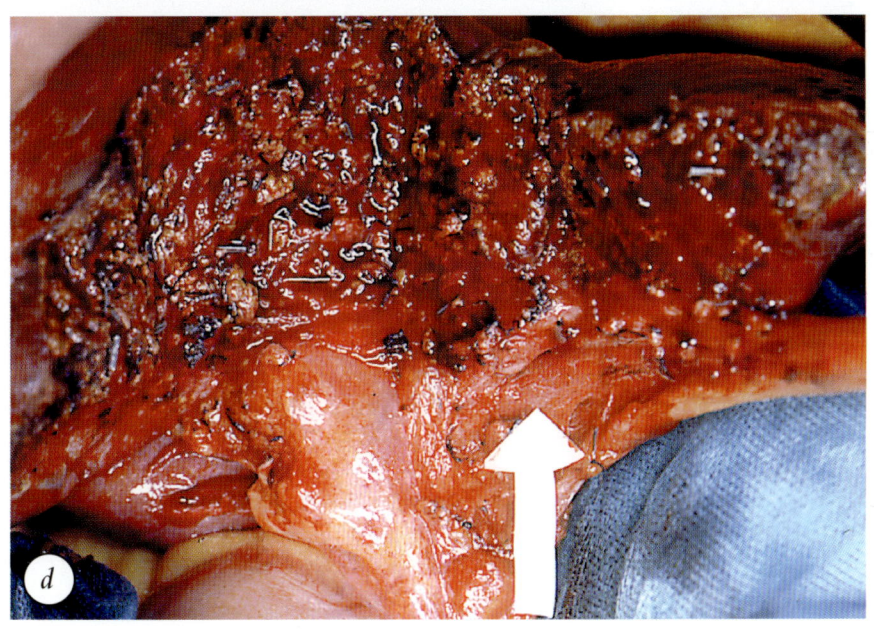

Figure 6.6 – *Resection of the anterior part of segment 4 for hepatocarcinoma.*
a) *Preoperative MRI.*
b) *Identification of the arterial and portal branches.*
c) *Ischemic demarcation of the anterior part of segment 4 following ligation of the vascular pedicles.*
d) *The arrow indicates ligation of the vascular pedicles along the left horn of Rex's recess.*
e) *Resection specimen, including the gallbladder.*

55

necessitates a wedge resection. This leaves a large resection plane that goes deep into the parenchyma at an acute angle, where it becomes very difficult to achieve hemostasis. The relation with the right and median hepatic veins, which delimit segment 8 laterally, and with the vena cava posteriorly, make dissection hazardous. Furthermore, the extremely variable dimensions of segment 8, especially in the presence of cirrhosis, make it very difficult to establish the extent of the resection. In the absence of anatomical surface landmarks on segment 8, the borders may be arbitrarily chosen. The difficulties are greater in the presence of large tumors, since it is necessary to ensure a safe margin of clearance of at least 1 cm from the tumor edge. This measure can be easily missed during an isolated resection of segment 8. Conventional resection of segment 8 has been shown to be statistically associated with a higher post-operative morbidity.[15] We have consistently encountered considerable problems in achieving hemostasis when removal of segment 8 alone was carried out transparenchymally. One cirrhotic patient died of a post-operative hemorrhage.[7]

To perform a more anatomical, safer and, from the oncological point of view, more complete operation, we suggest the anatomical removal of segment 8 by prior clamping of the right paramedian arterial and portal branches, and complete opening of the hepatic fissure. This procedure appears better in achieving hemostasis and decreases the risk of damaging the surrounding parenchyma and providing an adequate resection margin, which can be obtained once the liver has been widely dissected.

Anatomical premises

Segment 8 corresponds to the anterosuperior portion of the right paramedian sector, extending to the middle and right hepatic veins. Macroscopically the medial limit is represented by the plane of the sagittal fissure and the lateral limit of the oblique plane is marked by the fissure of the right hepatic vein. The inferior border of segment 8, adjacent to segment 5, has no apparent landmarks. The Glissonian pedicles of the entire paramedian sector can be isolated at the hilum extraparenchymally. The right branch of the portal vein is quite short and runs deep inside the parenchyma. It runs to the right end of the hilum and becomes visible after mobilization of the infundibulum of the gallbladder and dissection of the fibrous tissue of the hilar plate. After about 1 cm, the right paramedian branch originates from its superior edge and runs within the parenchyma on a sagittal plane, directed anteriorly and upwardly. The right paramedian artery is, usually, easily identified medial to the common hepatic duct, anterior to the portal branch. Within the parenchyma, the paramedian pedicle has a fairly consistent course, enclosed in a fibrous sheath together with the bile ducts, and turns to continue anteriorly[4] before dividing into the segmentary branches. These pedicles are related anteriorly to segment 5 and posteriorly to segment 8. There are always two segmentary branches for segment 8, one anterior branch and one which runs posteriorly. The venous drainage of segment 8 is by means of a series of small veins that run transversely. These small veins drain into the right and middle hepatic veins.

Operative technique

The technique of segment 8 resection first requires division of the cystic artery and duct. The gallbladder is removed. After dividing the anterior layer of the hepato-duodenal ligament, the arterial branches can be identified (*Figure 6.7b*). Two branches originate from the right branch of the hepatic artery, one running vertically, generally to the left of the common hepatic duct, and one obliquely in a lateral and posterior direction, passing behind the common bile duct and entering the parenchyma in correspondence with Ganz's incisure (*Figure 6.7c*). After lifting the right anterior branch of the artery, the portal bifurcation is mobilized. Dissection of the right portal branch is preferably carried out below the bile duct, after opening the lateral peritoneal layer. The right branch of the portal vein soon divides into an anterior medial branch and a lateral branch that turns posteriorly with respect to the plane of the hilum, parallel to the corresponding artery (*Figure 6.7d*). The two portal branches are lifted. The bile duct is not isolated at this stage: the sectorial biliary pedicles have many anatomical variations and are not easy to identify during extraparenchymal dissection. Consequently, we never dissect the biliary branches in the extraparenchymal stage of segmentectomies, but only after the parenchyma has been divided. The artery and the paramedian portal pedicle are clamped (*Figure 6.8a*), thus leading to demarcation of the entire paramedian sector, the limits of which can be traced on Glisson's capsule by cautery (*Figure 6.8b*). The liver is then opened along the sagittal fissure plane. Temporary clamping of the left pedicle at this stage prevents hemorrhage from the resected portion.

LIVER SEGMENTECTOMIES

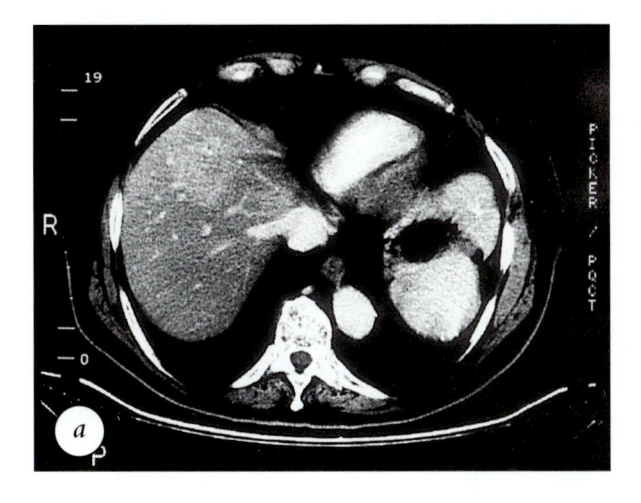

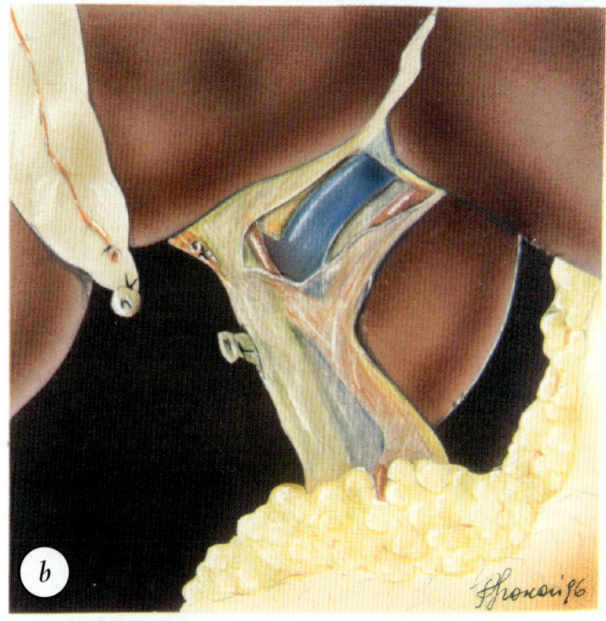

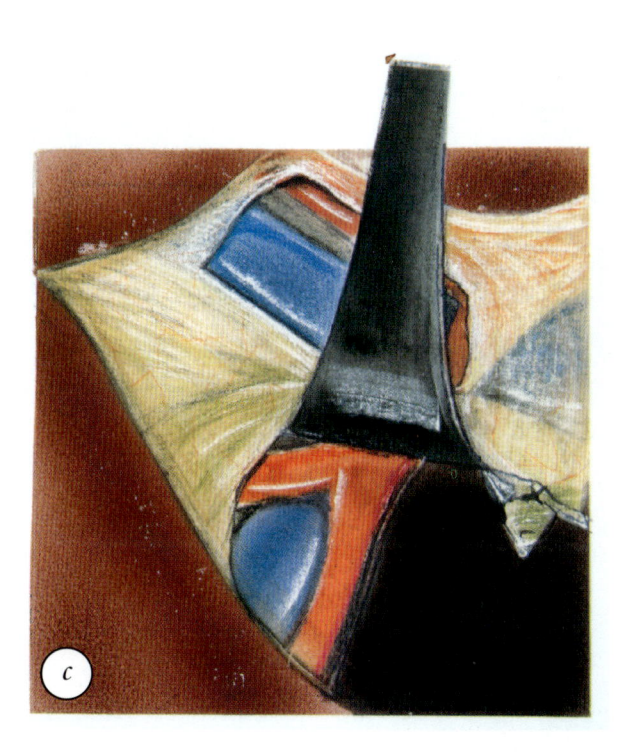

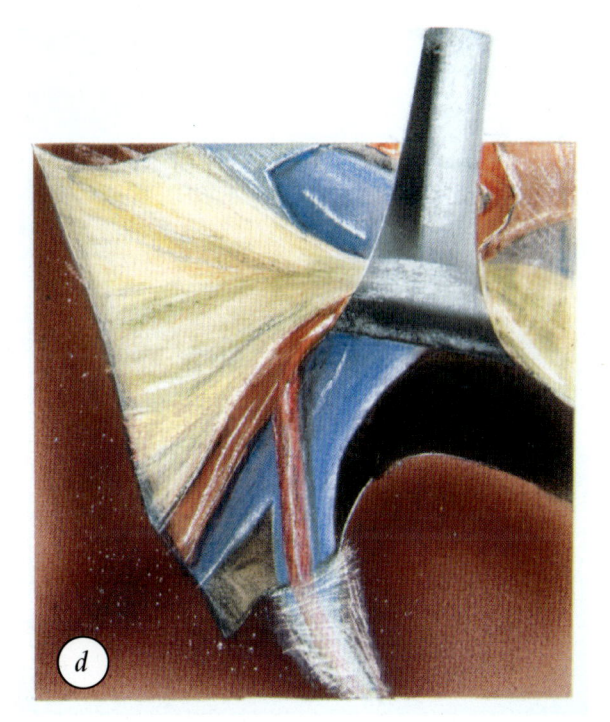

Figure 6.7 – *Resection of segment 8 for hepatocarcinoma. **a)** Pre-operative CT scan. **b)** Resection of the gallbladder pedicle and the anterior layer of the hepato-duodenal ligament. **c)** Identification of the right arterial branches. **d)** Identification of the right portal branches.*

57

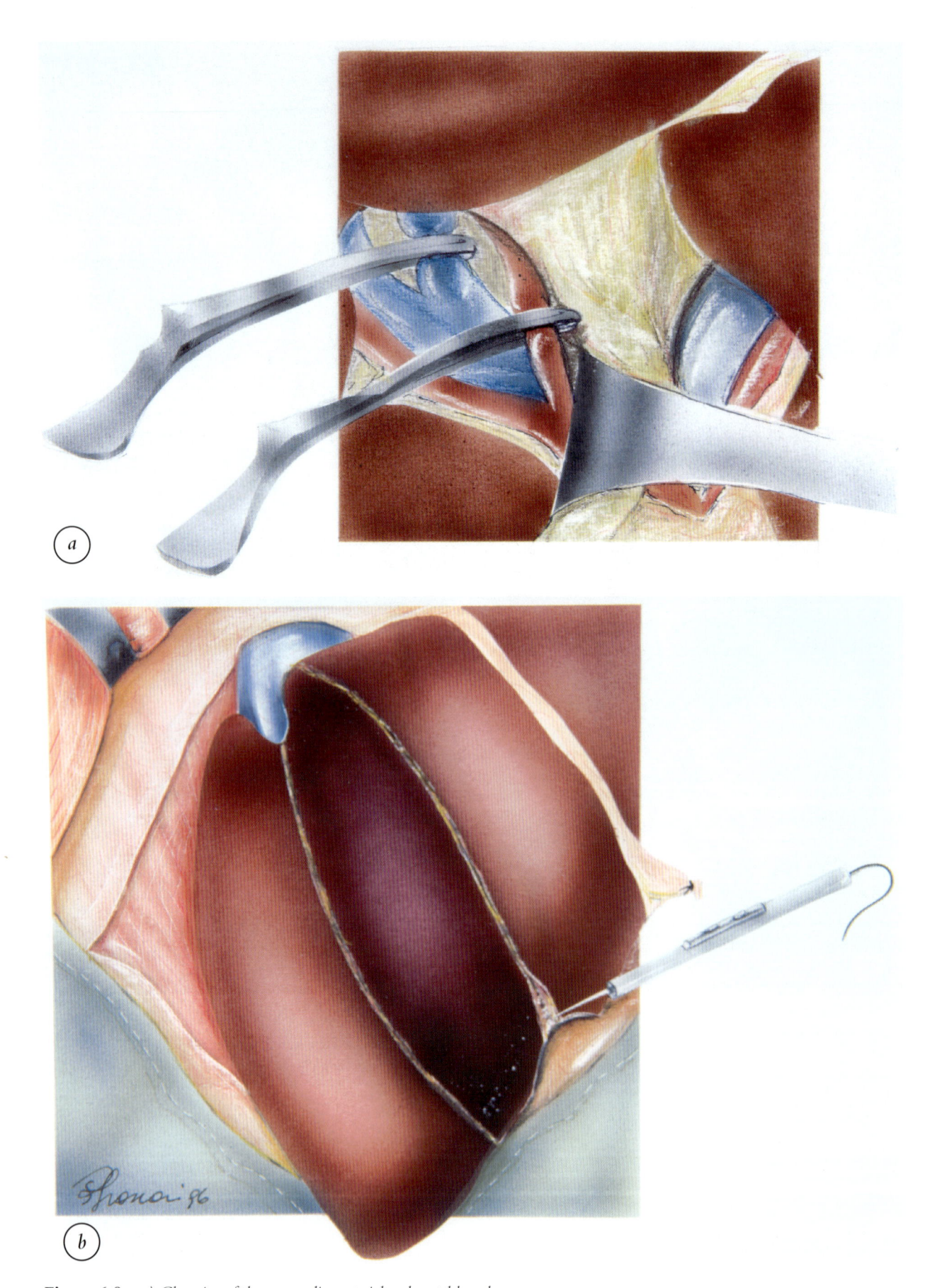

Figure 6.8 – **a)** *Clamping of the paramedian arterial and portal branches and ischemic demarcation of the right paramedian sector. Parenchymal dissection begins along the Cantile line,* **b).**

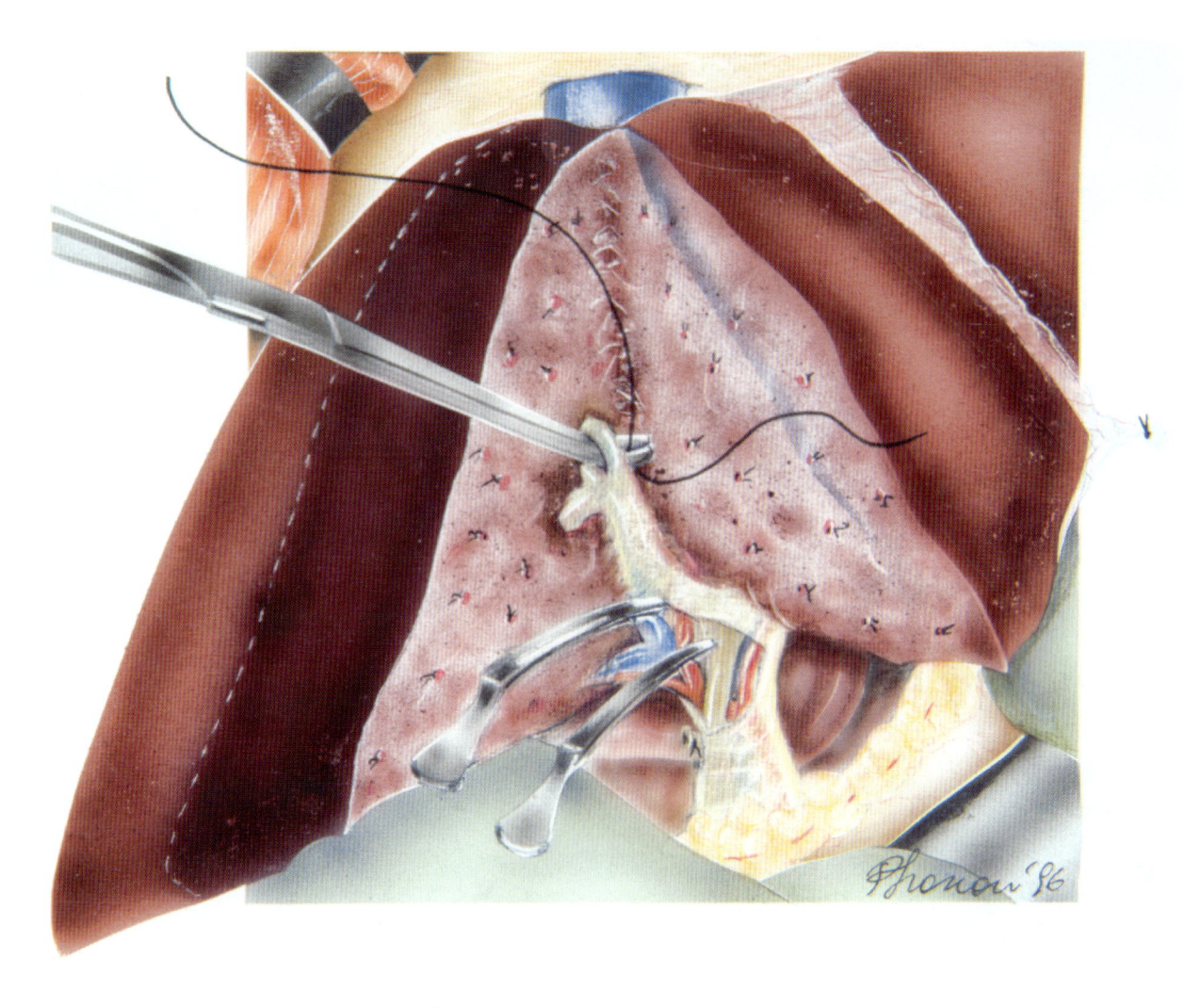

Figure 6.9 – *Ligation of the ventral and dorsal Glissonian pedicles of segment 8.*

Dissection of the parenchyma continues towards the plane of the hilum, remaining slightly more oblique to the right compared with conventional hepatectomy, until the paramedian Glissonian pedicle is encountered. This is followed along its anterior border as far as its upper dividing branches, dorsal and ventral for segment 8 (**Figure 6.9**). After ligation of the pedicles of segment 8, the clamps which closed the paramedian pedicles to the hilum are released. Segment 5 returns to its normal color and the demarcation line with segment 8 represents the plane for transverse dissection of the parenchyma (**Figure 6.10**). Lateral dissection also follows a second ischemic demarcation line, the fissure of the right hepatic vein acting as a landmark (**Figure 6.11**). At this stage of lateral resection, temporary clamping of the right lateral pedicle may help to limit blood loss. The resection plane exposes the trunk of the right hepatic veins as segment 8 is completely removed (**Figure 6.12**).

The technique described above allows anatomical resection of segment 8. The opening of the sagittal fissure plane enlarges the operating field, making hemostasis easier. None of the resections that we have done using this technique needed transfusions. No particular problems were encountered.

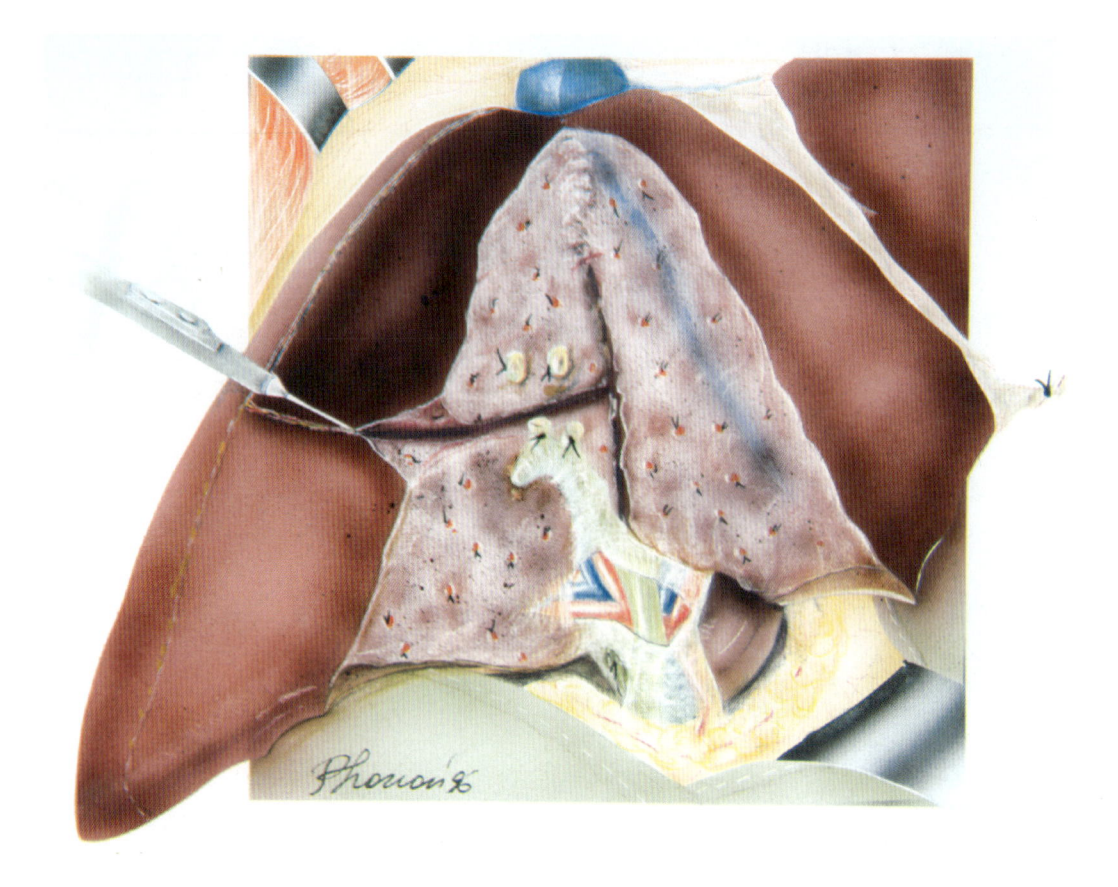

Figure 6.10 – *After removing the clamps on the paramedian pedicles, the parenchyma is divided between segments 5 and 8 following the ischemic demarcation line of segment 8.*

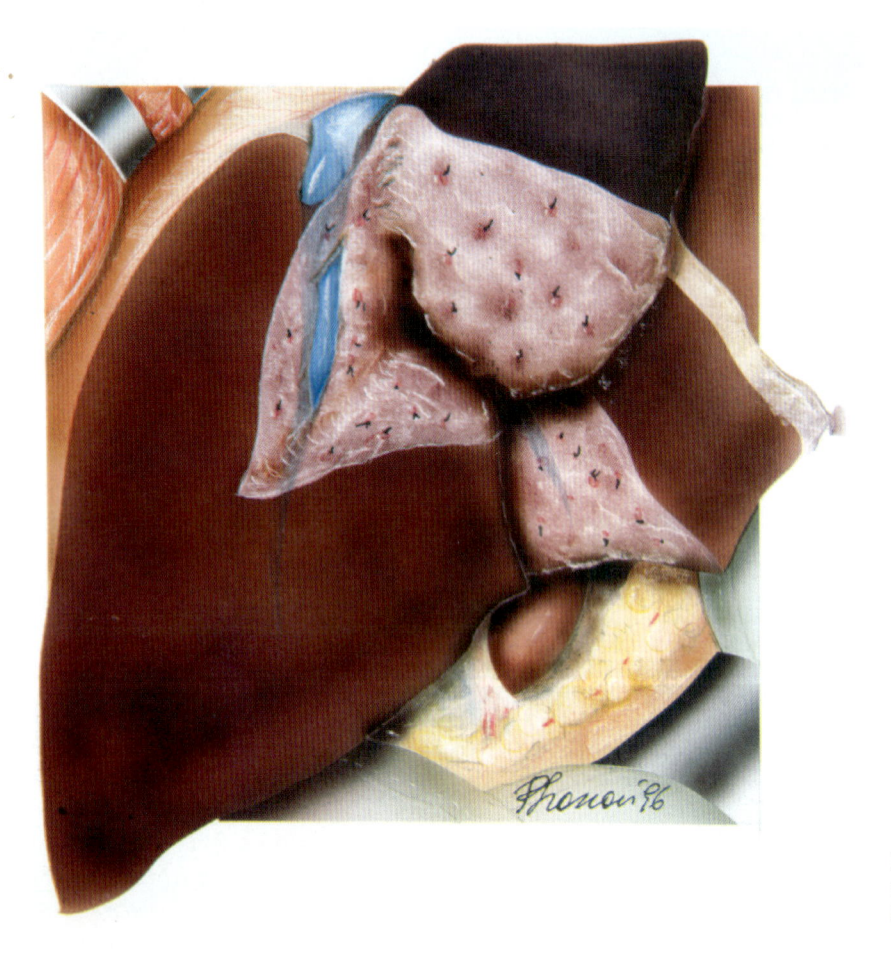

Figure 6.11 – *Lateral section with the fissure of the right hepatic vein as a landmark.*

LIVER SEGMENTECTOMIES

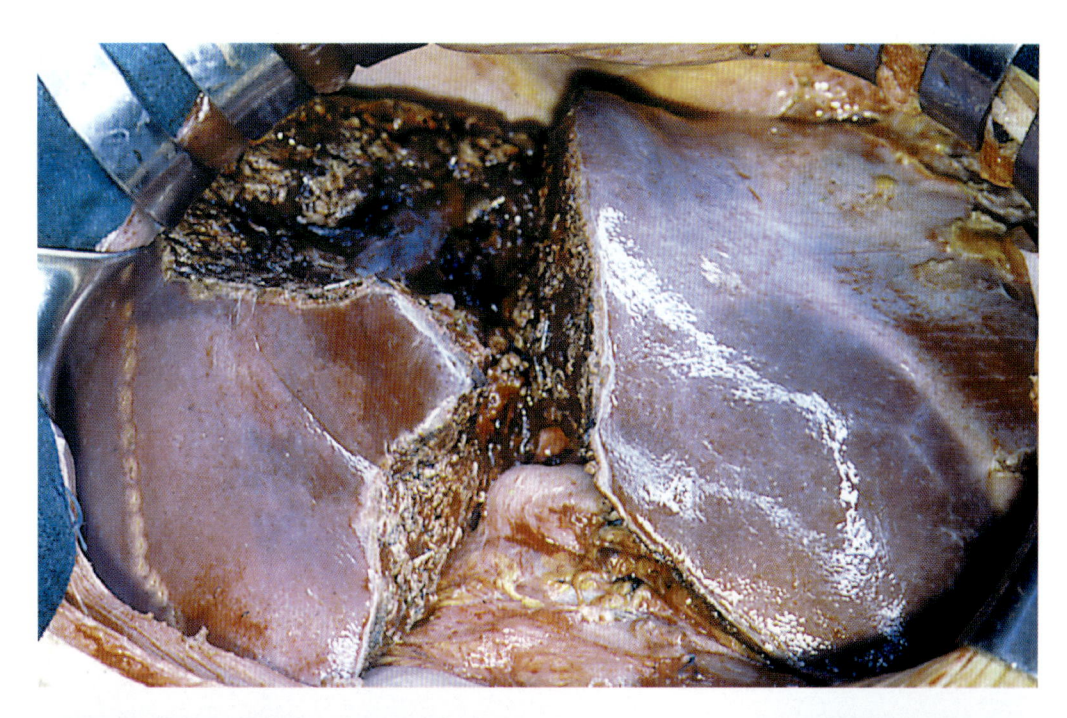

Figure 6.12 –
The operating field after removal of segment 8.

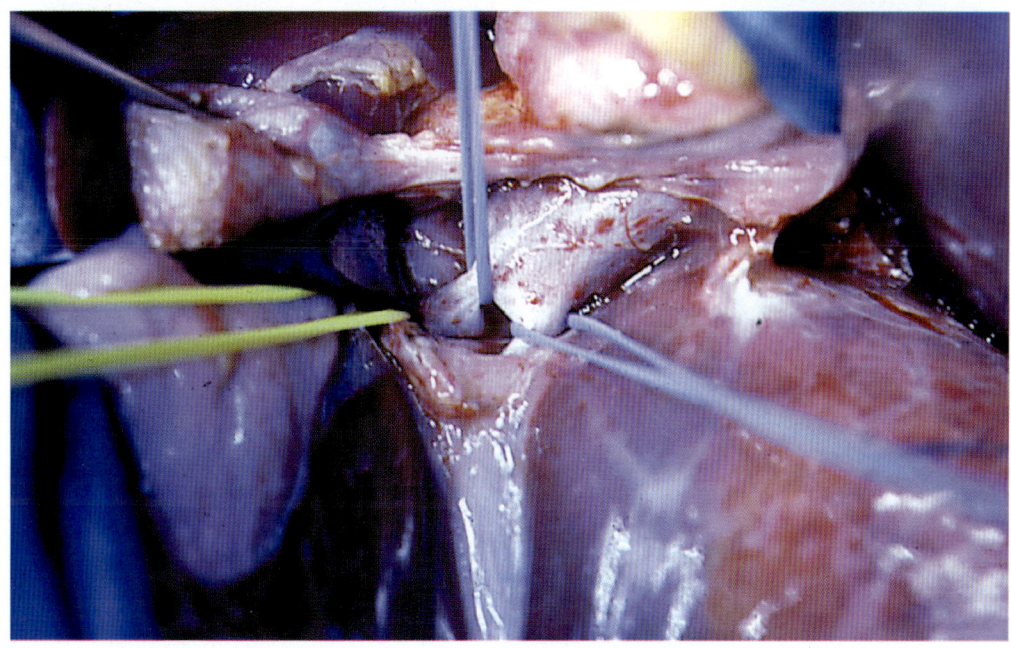

Figure 6.13 –
Lateral Glissonian pedicles for segments 6 and 7, which enter the parenchyma in correspondence with Ganz's incisure.

Resection of segment 7

Segment 7 corresponds to the superior and dorsal portion of the right lobe of the liver. Dissection of the right triangular ligament is necessary to completely expose it. The vascular pedicles of segment 7 originate from the right lateral Glissonian pedicle and enter the parenchyma in a common trunk at segment 6, in correspondence with Ganz's incisure (**Figure 6.13**). This right lateral Glissonian pedicle runs deep into the parenchyma, almost transversely, and subsequently divides into two segmentary branches, the anterior one to segment 6, and the posterior one running upwards to segment 7.

The lateral pedicle can be easily freed outside the parenchyma; after mobilizing the infundibulum of the gallbladder and dividing the lateral peritoneum of the hepato-duodenal ligament, the artery can be identified (**Figure 6.14a**). Once this has been mobilized together with the bile duct, the right branch of the portal vein is then freed, and dissection continues towards the parenchyma until the secondary division branches are identified (**Figure 6.14c**). Here too, the bile ducts are never sought outside the parenchyma, but only

61

TECHNIQUES IN LIVER SURGERY

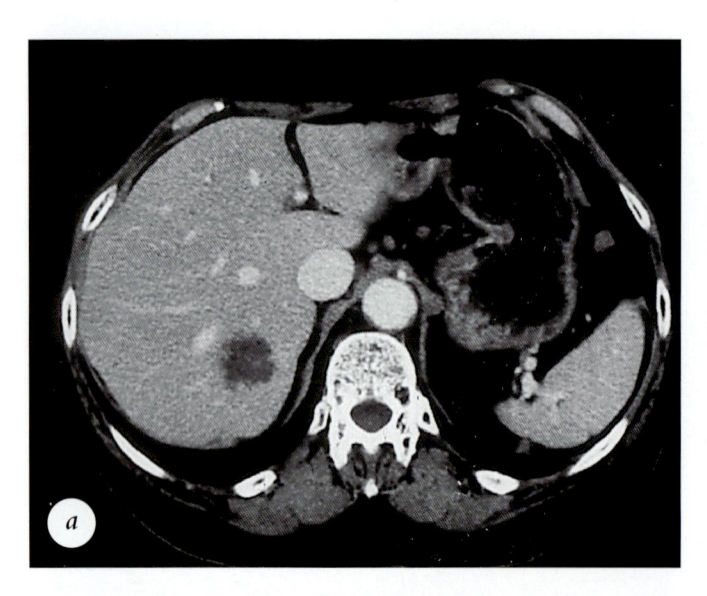

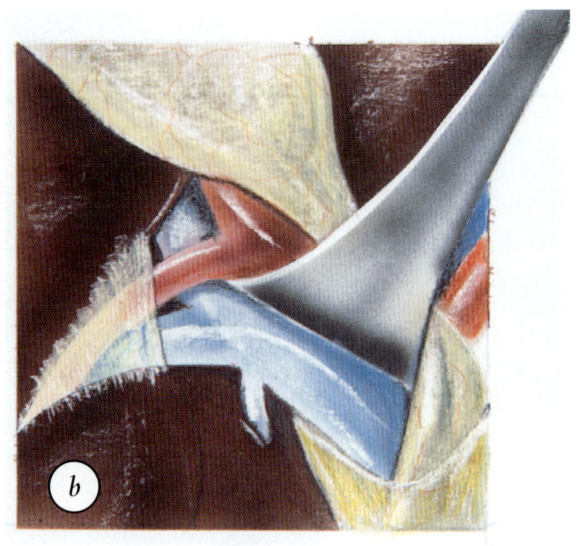

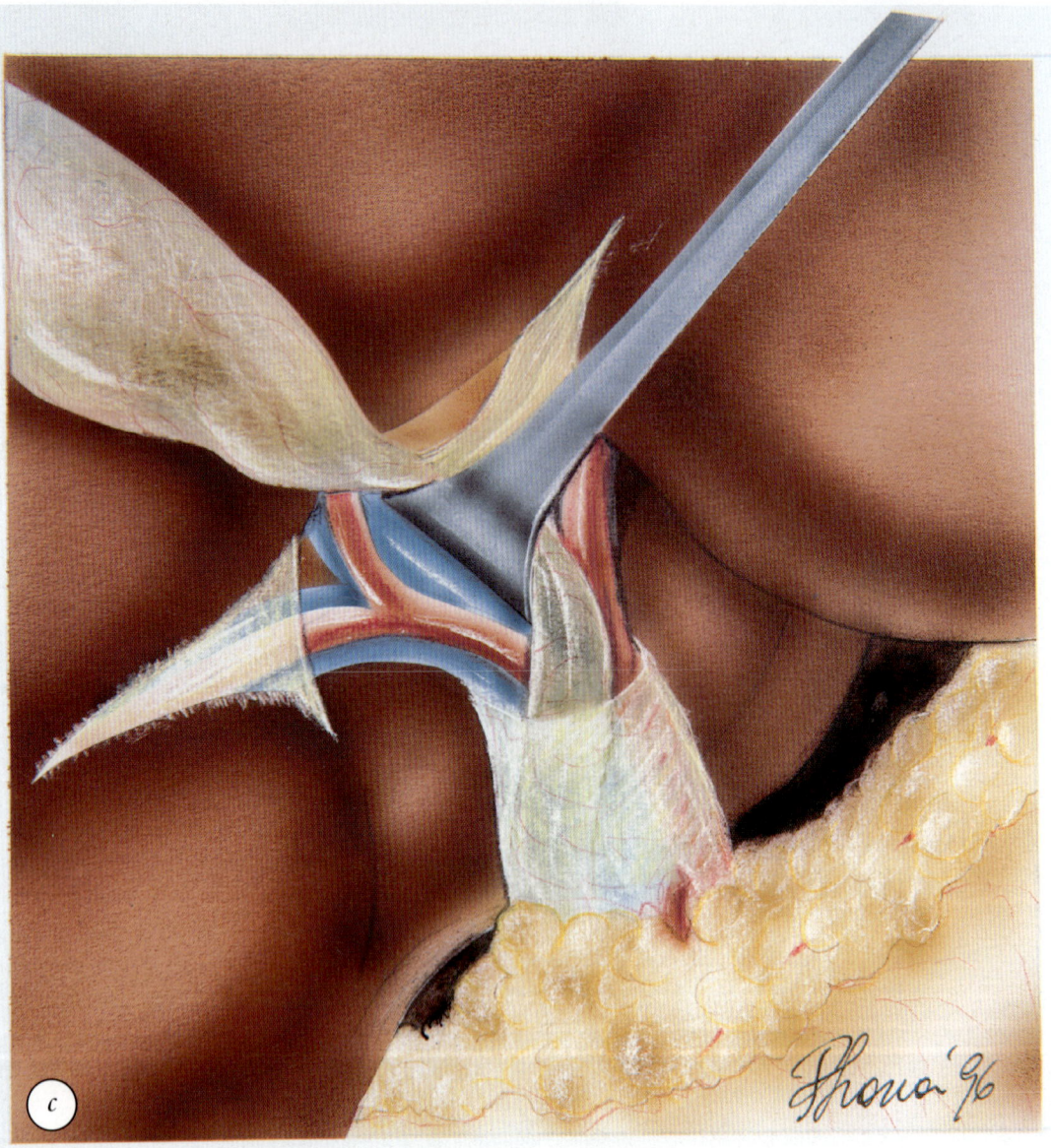

Figure 6.14 – *Resection of segment 7 for metastases from colonic carcinoma.* ***a)*** *Pre-operative CT scan.* ***b)*** *Isolation of the right arterial branches after division of the posterior peritoneal layer of the hepato-duodenal ligament.* ***c)*** *Isolation of the right portal branches.*

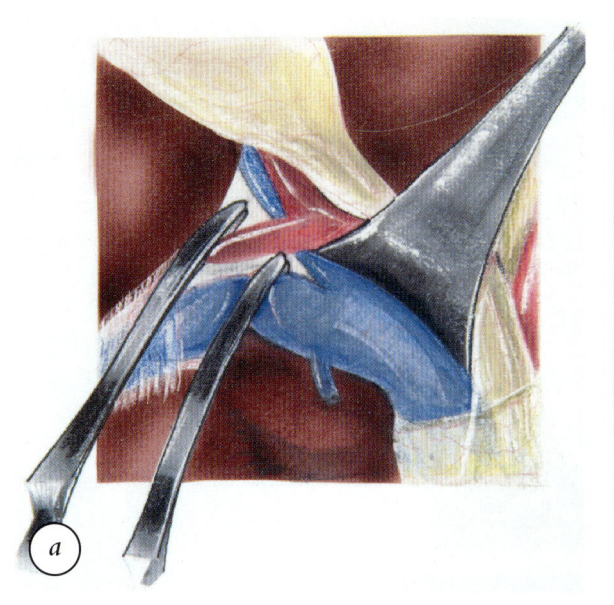

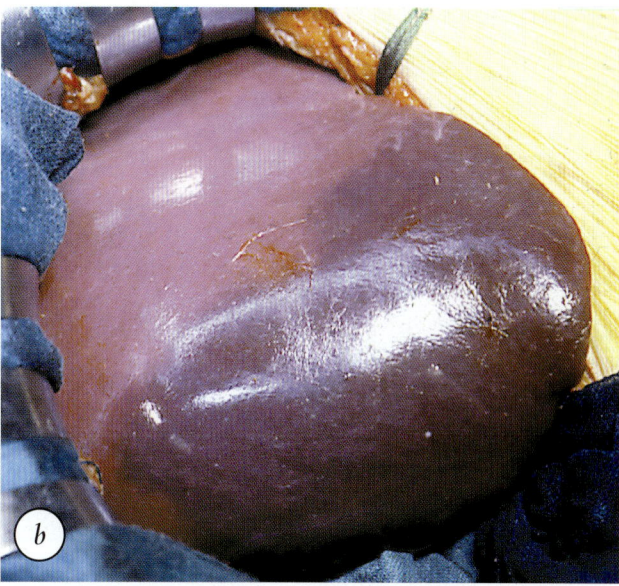

Figure 6.15 – **a)** *Selective clamping of the lateral arterial and portal pedicles, followed by ischemic demarcation of the lateral sector,* **b)**.

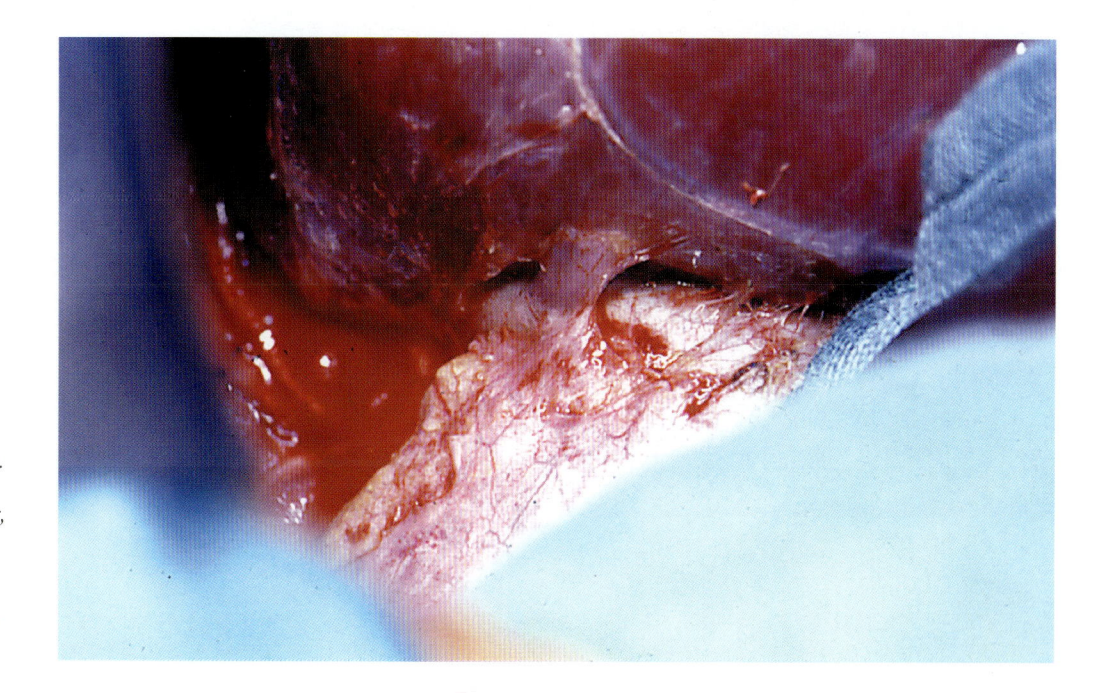

Figure 6.16 – *Lower hepatic vein. The vein is clearly visible in the center, after detachment of the bare area of the liver as far as the right margin of the vena cava.*

divided trans-parenchymally, at the end of the resection, to prevent accidental damage to the adjacent hepatic ducts in the presence of anatomical variations. Clamping of the arterial branch and lateral portal branches leads to blanching of the entire right lateral sector (**Figure 6.15**). The fissure of the right hepatic vein indicates the upper resection margin. The right hepatic vein can be left in place or may be removed if the neoplastic lesion is adjacent to the vein or has infiltrated the vein (**Figure 6.14a**). Isolated resection of segment 7 with ligation of the right hepatic vein can be safely performed.[1] However, ligation of the right hepatic vein leaving segment 6 in place leads to a transitory venous congestion of this segment with hemorrhage of the resected margin which may be difficult to control. Venous outflow of segment 6 should be ensured by preserving the accessory hepatic veins and in particular the right inferior hepatic vein (**Figure 6.16**). This vein is present in

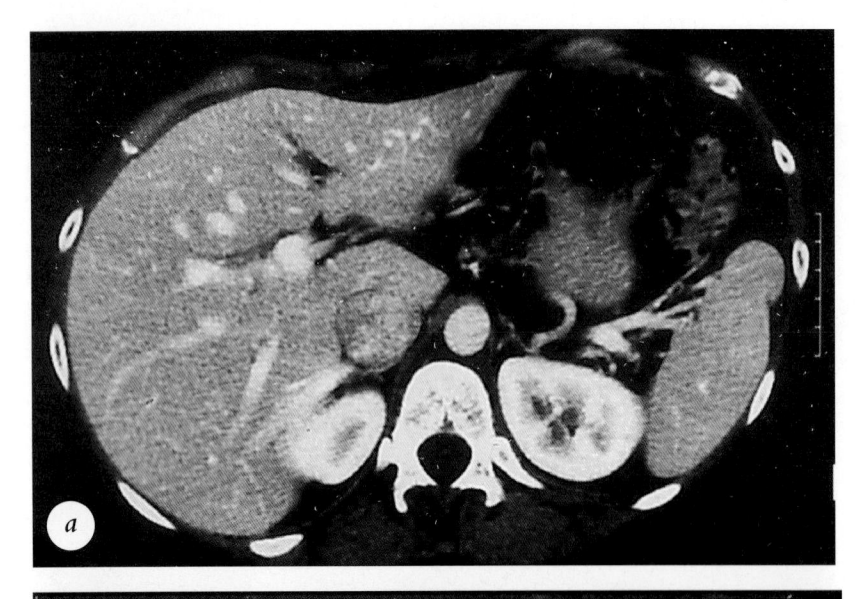

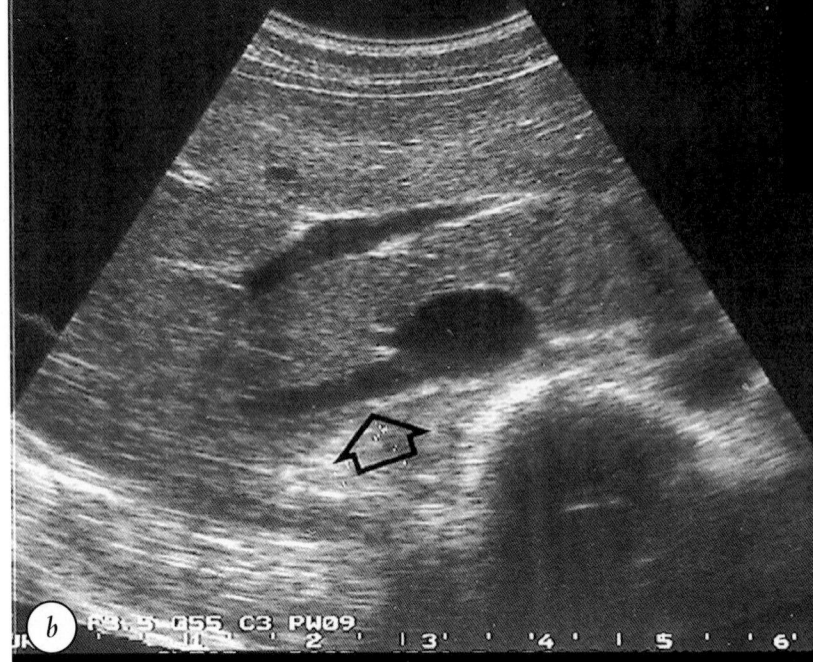

Figure 6.17 – *Lower hepatic vein. a) CT liver scan. The vein is visible in a scan that passes immediately above the upper tip of the right kidney. b) Transverse section of a US liver scan: the lower hepatic vein (arrow) is visible at its outlet into the vena cava.*

about 25% of cases (9-12) and will be visible on the pre-operative CT scan (**Figure 6.17a**) and even on the US scan (**Figure 6.17b**). The trunk of the hepatic vein is surrounded after division of the right triangular ligament. After clamping the lateral Glissonian pedicles, the trunk of the right hepatic vein is clamped (**Figure 6.18a**) and divided, and the two stumps are sutured (**Figure 6.18b**). The parenchymal dissection line follows the ischemic demarcation plane.

Dissection begins at the top, proceeding downwards between segments 7 and 8. During dissection, it is advisable to clamp the pedicles of the paramedian sector to limit blood loss. The pedicle of segment 7 lies deep within the parenchyma and is exposed during dissection, clamped and sutured together with all the vascular and biliary branches. Once the Glissonian pedicle of segment 7 has been divided, the arterial and portal branches at the

LIVER SEGMENTECTOMIES

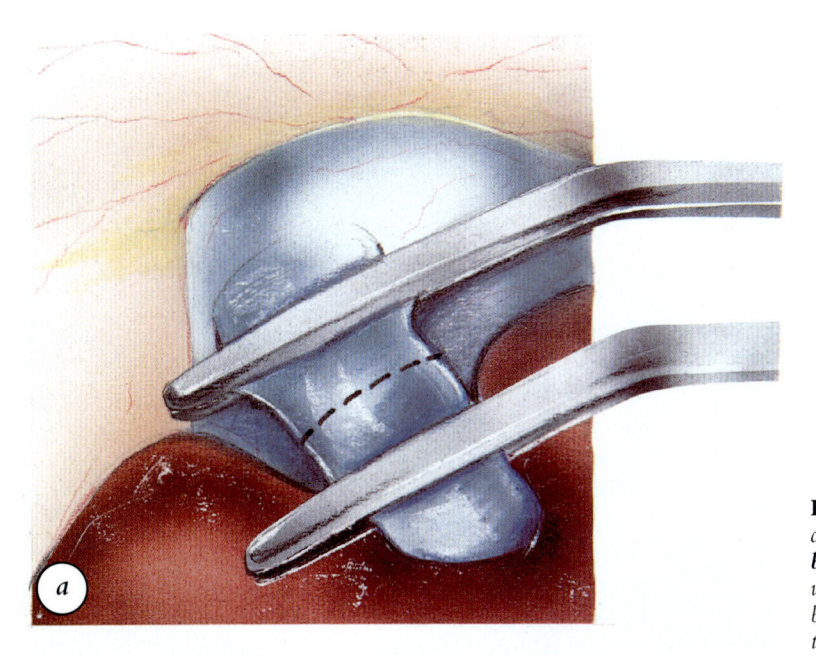

Figure 6.18 – *a)* *Extraparenchymal clamping of the right hepatic vein.*
b) *After division of the right hepatic vein, the parenchyma is dissected between segments 7 and 8, following the demarcation line.*

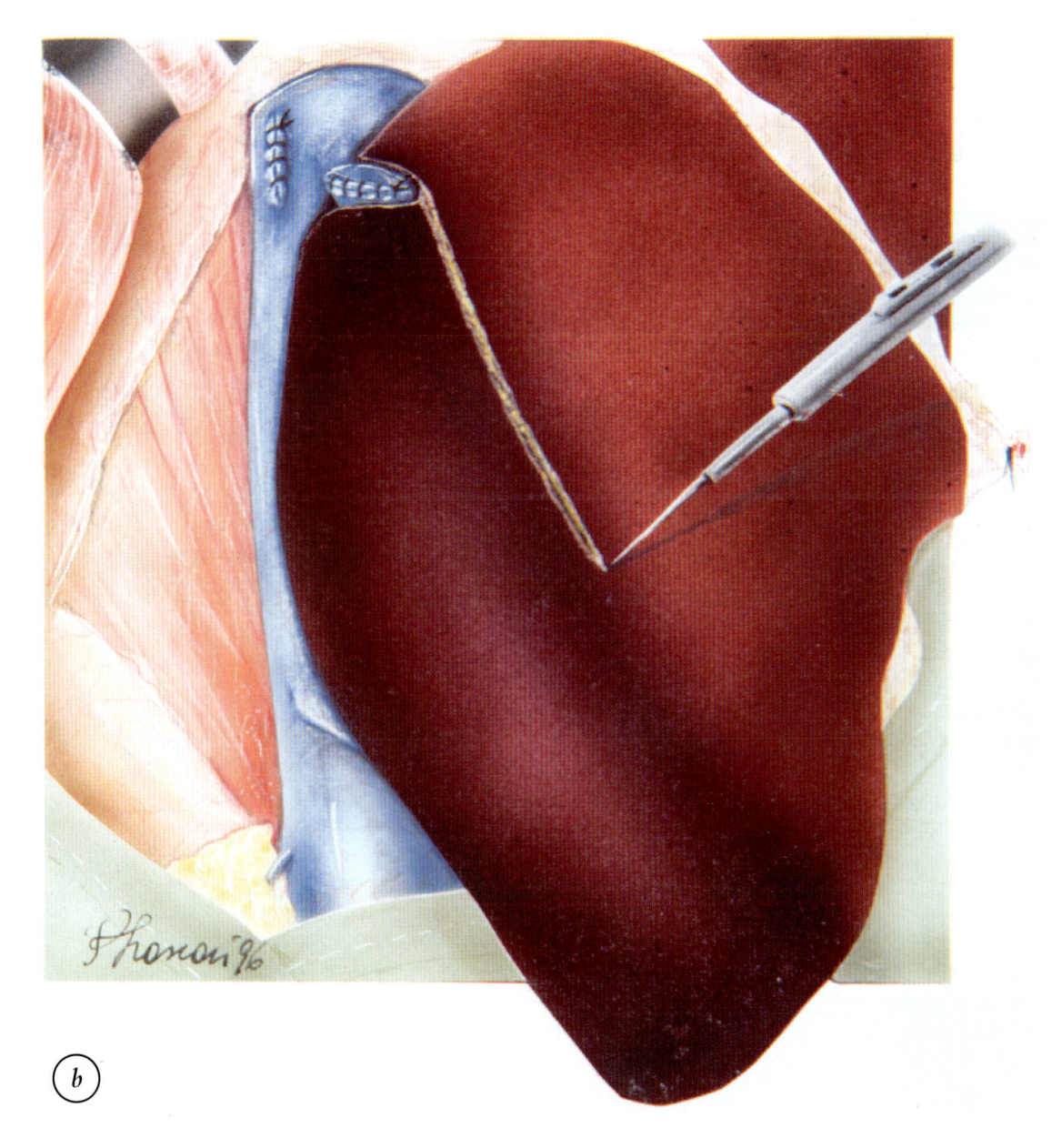

hilum can be unclamped; segment 6 returns to its normal color and the ischemic demarcation line marks the inferior dissection plane between segments 6 and 7 (**Figure 6.19**).

Resection of segments 6 and 5

The basic stages for the exeresis of segments 6 and 5 are the same as those described for the resection of segments 7 and 8, respectively.

For segment 6, the right lobe of the liver is mobilized by dividing the triangular ligament and freeing the right margin of the vena cava as far as the distal ligament. If present, the inferior accessory suprahepatic vein is ligated. Clamping of the arterial and portal lateral Glissonian pedicles produces ischemic demarcation of the entire right lateral sector. The parenchyma is divided starting from the lower margin of the liver, proceeding along an oblique plane from right to left and from the front towards the back. Deep inside the parenchyma, the lateral pedicles are encountered (generally two), which are ligated and sutured *en bloc* with the connective tissue which surrounds them. The Glissonian pedicles are then unclamped at the hilum and segment 7 thus returns to its normal color. The upper dissection margin follows the ischemic demarcation line between segments 6 and 7.

For segment 5 the cystic duct and the cystic artery are divided and the lateral margins of the incision are indicated by the ischemic demarcation line after clamping of the paramedian Glissonian pedicles. Dissection starts on the medial face, corresponding to the gallbladder-vena cava plane, and follows a slightly oblique direction towards the right. Dissection stops at the plane of the hilum, then follows the lateral margin between segments 5 and 6, remaining in front of Ganz's incisure, so as not to encounter the posterior Glissonian pedicle. The pedicle for segment 5, generally only one, is identified inside the parenchyma when, branching off from the paramedian sectorial pedicle, it runs forward. After clamping and dividing the pedicle of segment 5, the paramedian artery and portal branch can be unclamped. Segment 8 returns to its normal color and the ischemic demarcation line indicates the dissection line between segments 5 and 8.

Complications

Hemorrhage

Most segmentectomies can be performed without blood transfusions. Ischemia of the segment to be removed and the temporary occlusion of the adjacent sectorial branches prevent blood loss during dissection of the parenchyma. Nevertheless, resection of the right posterior segments 7 and 8 involves a risk of hemorrhage, due to the relationship with the right and middle hepatic veins. It should be remembered that the walls of the hepatic veins are thin and tearing of the small collaterals is a potential source of hemorrhage. Dissection along the main hepatic veins must be performed with great care. Small defects must be closed with sutures (Prolene® 5 or 6-0). Maintaining low central venous pressure reduces the risk of hemorrhage. To prevent damage to the vein walls, it is advisable to leave a thin layer of parenchyma above the veins.

Biliary damage

Damage to the biliary convergence is a risk in resections of segment 4 and to a lesser extent of segments 5 and 8. Anatomical variations in intrahepatic biliary distribution are also frequent. We recommend that the bile duct should not be ligated extra-parenchymally but at the end of the resection and *en bloc* with the connective tissue that surrounds the Glissonian elements. Injection of methylene blue and air through the cystic duct is required to recognize biliary leakage. Transcystic cholangiography should be performed when a biliary lesion is suspected. Defects in biliary ducts must be sutured with Vicryl® 6-0. It is advisable to drain the biliary tract upstream of the suture with a fine silicone catheter which can be passed through the cystic duct or the biliary duct of the removed segment.[11]

Abscesses

Infectious complications after segmentectomy are mainly caused by collections of bile which become infected, or by ischemic necrosis of a portion of the parenchyma. In our opinion, the segmentectomy technique described here, performed after clamping of the afferent vascular pedicle, seems to reduce the risk of the devascularization of the remaining portions of parenchyma. Percutaneous drainage is the treatment of choice for abscesses and postoperative biliary collections.

LIVER SEGMENTECTOMIES

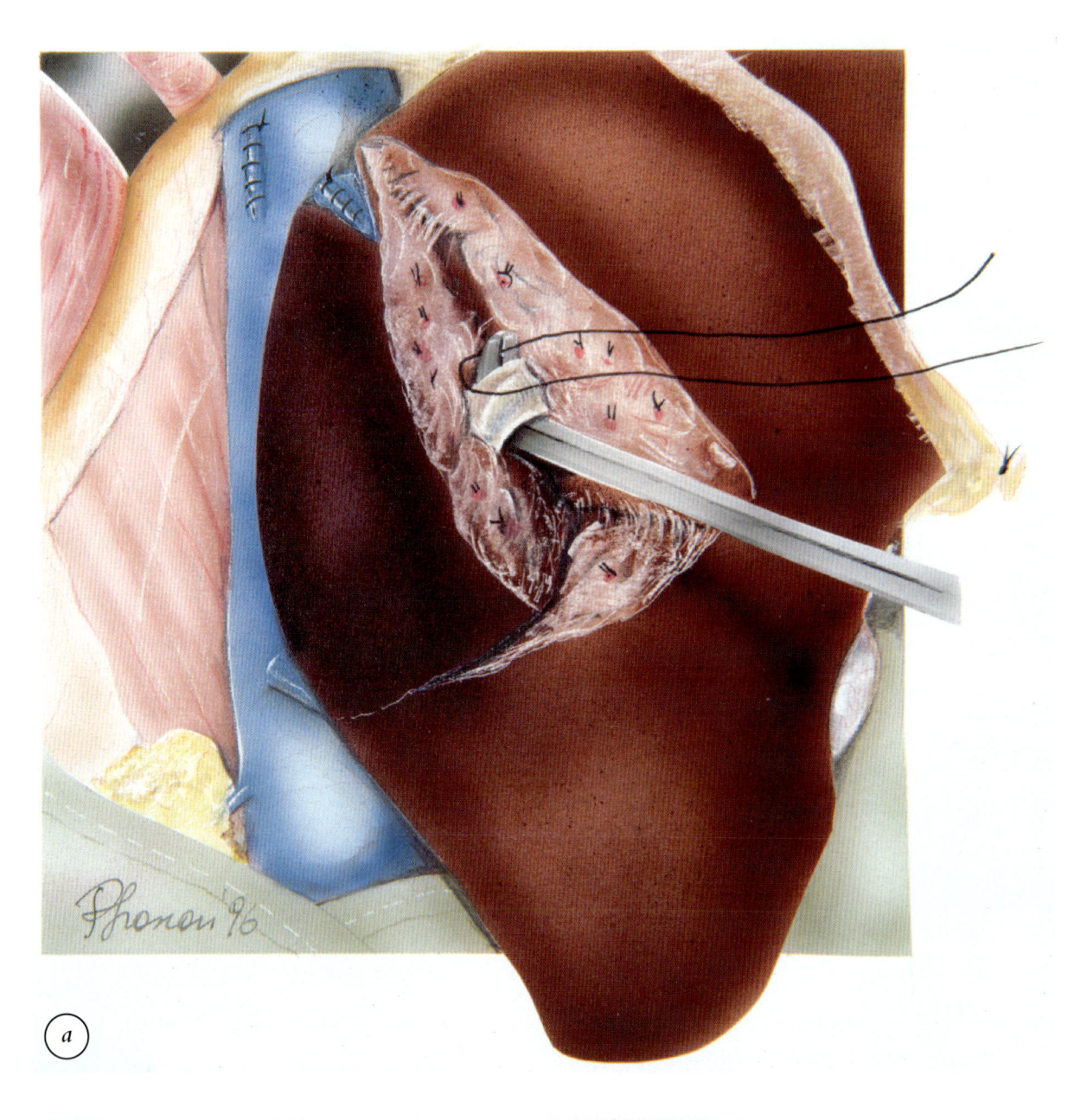

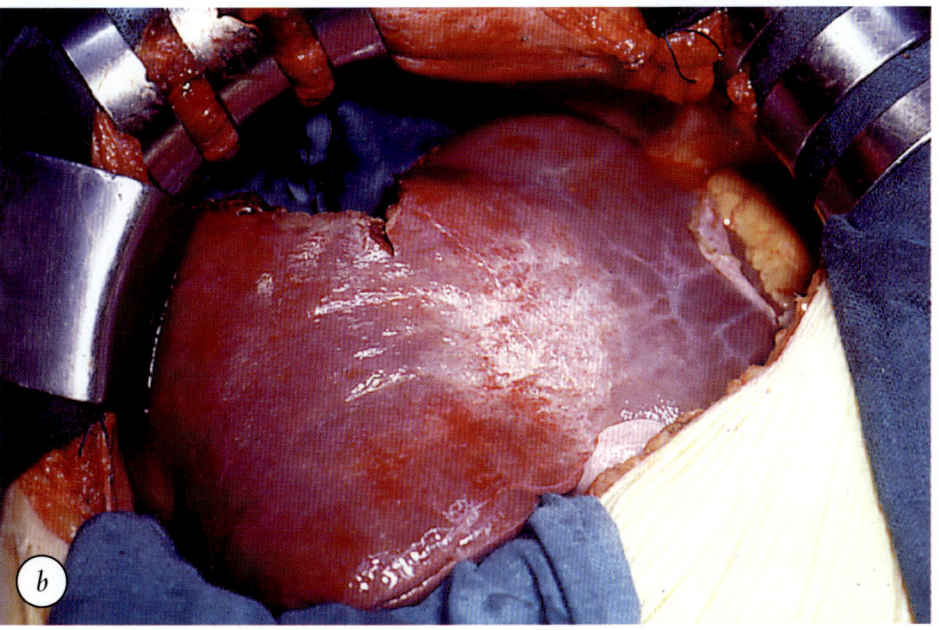

Figure 6.19 – *a) Intraparenchymal division of the Glissonian pedicle of segment 7. b) Operating field after resection of segment 7.*

REFERENCES

1. Beppu M, Fukuzaki T, Mitani K, Fujimoto K, Tariguchi S. Hepatic subsegmentectomy with segmental hepatic vein sacrifice. *Arch Surg* 1990; **125:** 1170-1176.
2. Couinaud C. Controlled hepatectomies and exposure of intrahepatic bile ducts. In: *Anatomical and technical study*. Couinaud C, Paris, 1981.
3. Couinaud C. *Surgical anatomy of the liver revisited*. Couinaud C, Paris, 1989.
4. Bismuth H, Houssin D, Castaing D. Major and minor segmentectomies "reglées" in liver surgery. *World J Surg* 1982; **6:** 10-24.
5. Franco D, Bonnet P, Smadja C, Grange G. Surgical resection of segment VII (antero-superior subsegment of the right lobe) in patients with liver cirrhosis and hepatocellular carcinoma. *Surgery* 1985; **98:** 949-954.
6. Ganz H. *Introduction to hepatic surgery*. Elsevier, Amsterdam, 1995.
7. Gozzetti G, Mazziotti A, *et al*. Esperienza su 400 resezioni epatiche. *Chirurgia* 1992; **5:** 398-408.
8. Healey JE Jr., Schroy PC. Anatomy of the biliary ducts within the human liver: analysis of the prevailing pattern of branching and the major variation of the biliary ducts. *Arch Surg* 1953; **66:** 599-616.
9. Makuuchi M, Hasegawa H, Yamasaki S et Al. The inferior right hepatic vein: ultrasonic demonstration. *Radiology* 1983; **148:** 213-217.
10. Makuuchi M, Hasegawa H, Yamasaki S. Ultrasonically guided subsegmentectomy. *Surg Gynecol Obstet* 1985; **161:** 346-350.
11. Makuuchi M. Segmentectomy and subsegmentectomy. In: Lygidakis NJ and Makuuchi M. *Pitfalls and Complications in the Diagnosis and Management of Hepatobiliary and Pancreatic Diseases*, Thieme, New York, 1993, pp.133-145.
12. Nakamura S, Tsuzuki T. Surgical anatomy of hepatic veins and the inferior vena cava. *Surg Gynecol Obstet* 1981; **152:** 43-50.
13. Scheele J. Segment oriented resection of the liver: rationale and technique. In: Lygidakis N and Tytgat G *Hepatobiliary and Pancreatic Malignancies*. Thieme, Stuttgart, 1989, pp. 219-247.
14. Scheele J. Die segmentorientierte Leberresektion: Grundlagen, Technik, Stellenwert. *Chirurg* 1989; **60:** 251-165.
15. Shimada M, Matsumaat T, Akasawa K, Kamakura T, Itasaka H, Sugimaki K, Nose Y. Estimation of risk of major complications after hepatic resections. *Am J Surg* 1994; **167:** 399-403.
16. Yu Ye-Quin, Tang ZY, Zhon XD, Mack P. Resection of segment VIII of the liver for treatment of primary liver cancer. *Arch Surg* 1993; **128:** 224-227.
17. Takayama T, Makuuchi M, Watanabe K *et al*. A new method for mapping hepatic segments: counter staging identification technique. *Surgery* 1991; **109:** 226-9.

7

Liver Surgery in the Cirrhotic Patient

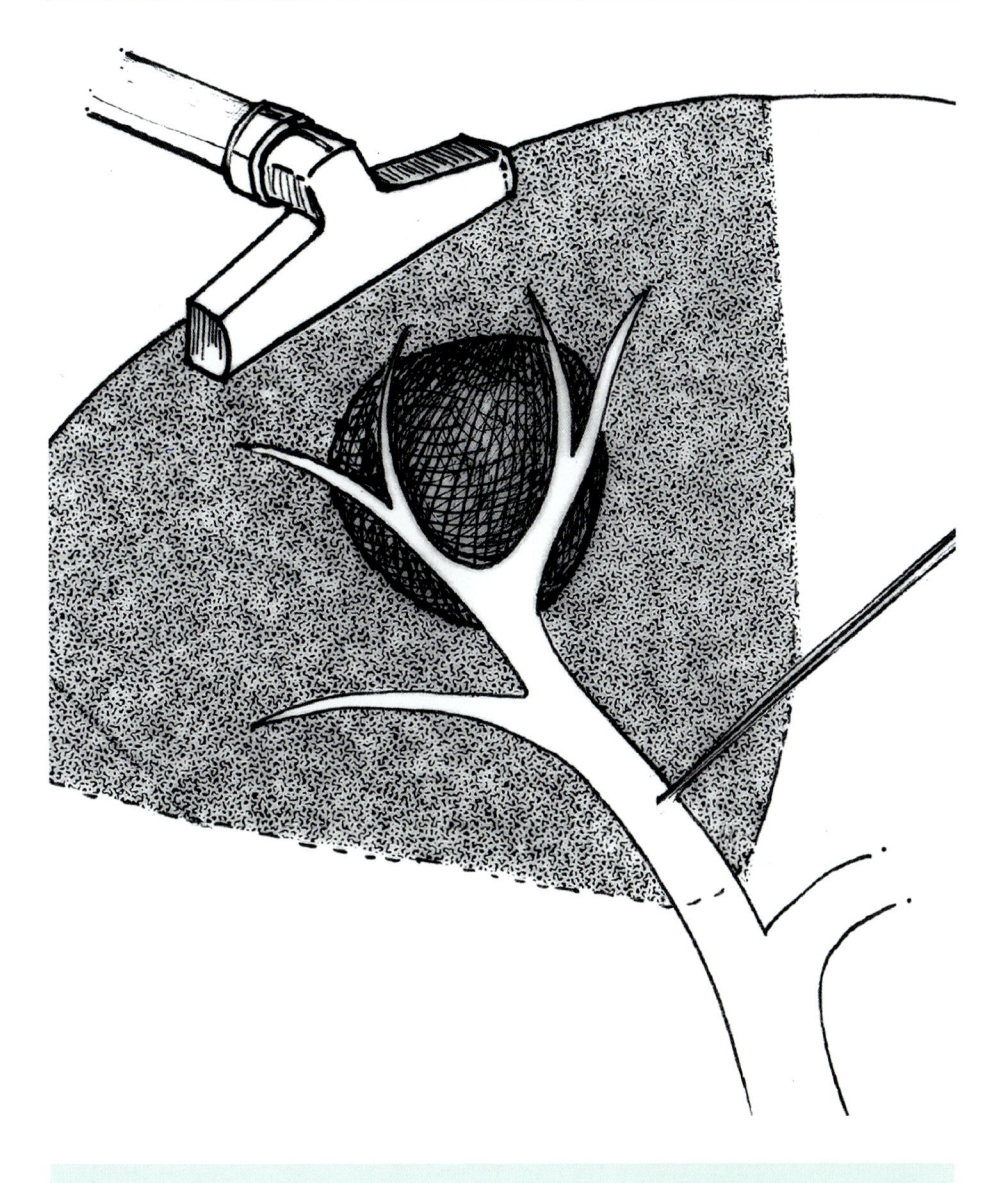

J. Belghiti, O. Farges

Hepatocellular carcinoma (HCC) is the most common primary malignant tumor of the liver. This tumor develops in 80 to 90% of the patients with a history of cirrhosis. The precise nature of the relationship between cirrhosis and HCC is still unclear. One mechanism may relate to hepatocyte regeneration and increased cell proliferation associated with cirrhosis, acting to promote carcinogenesis through DNA damage by environmental mutagens. This, in turn, may be promoted by a lower activity of enzymes involved in DNA repairing. There is, in addition, evidence that both HBV and HCV infections are independent risk factors for hepatocarcinogenesis for the following reasons. Firstly, the very high rate of serological markers of HBV and/or HCV infection amongst HCC patients in high endemic area, and secondly, the possible development of HCC in non-cirrhotic HBV or HCV-positive patients. Initially, most HCCs were thought to be HBV related. Over the past 2 decades, however, the importance of HCV has become predominant. The reasons for this are, firstly, a better knowledge of the mode of transmission of HBV infection and the development of effective vaccination plans, these having been associated with a reduction in the proportion of HBV carriers and of HBV related HCC. Secondly the identification of the HCV as the principal cause of non-A, non-B hepatitis, the recognition of the high prevalence of HCV-infection (HCV-carrier rate of 1% world wide, including Europe, as compared to an HBV-carrier rate of 0.1% in Europe) and the lack of vaccination against the HCV. Thirdly, the high proportion of HCV positive patients who progress to cirrhosis (20 to 30% over a 20 years follow-up). And, finally, the comparable or even greater (up to 2.7 times) carcinologic potential of the HCV as compared with the HBV. Over 60 to 75% of HCC patients in Japan, Italy, Spain, France (and presumably other countries) are HCV positive and this trend is expected to become even more pronounced in the near future. The incidence of HCC in patients with cirrhosis has been calculated to range between 3 and 7% per year. In patients with chronic active hepatitis, i.e. at a pre-cirrhotic stage, the incidence of HCC is lower, but figures as high as 0.5 to 1% have been reported. Hence, HCCs are anticipated to become a significant health problem in the next decade.

Although alcohol injection, transcatheter arterial embolization and liver transplantation have greatly extended the range of therapeutic options available for the treatment of HCC complicating cirrhosis, hepatic resection remains the treatment of choice. Liver resection in cirrhotic patients however has additional requirements to those needed in non-cirrhotic patients. Indeed, cirrhotic patients tend to have coagulation disorders and portal hypertension, both of which will increase the risk of intraoperative bleeding. These patients are at risk of post-operative liver failure, because they have a decreased functional volume of liver, and because their liver has an impaired ability to regenerate. Finally, they are particularly vulnerable to sepsis and post-operative electrolyte imbalances. Considerable improvements in the safety of liver resection in cirrhotic patients over the last decade has resulted from the better identification of these features and the development of better surgical techniques.

Pre-operative considerations

The pre-operative evaluation of the cirrhotic patient undergoing surgical resection should focus on the patient, the liver and the tumor.

Evaluation of the patient

Careful pre-operative assessment and optimisation of the patient's status will reduce the operative risk. Nutritional status is evaluated and malnutrition is treated. Adequate renal, pulmonary and cardiac function are essential to withstand the enhanced post-operative hyperdynamic state. Fluid and electrolyte disorders have to be corrected. Abnormal coagulation may be transiently overcome by fresh frozen plasma or platelet transfusion if thrombocytopenia, due to portal hypertension, is present. Esophageal varices are looked for and their risk of bleeding assessed by endoscopy. If this risk is high, or if the patient has previously bled, it is probably wise to pre-operatively treat these varices by ligation or sclerotherapy. Diabetes mellitus should be identified, as it increases the risk of post-operative complications and may, besides cirrhosis, be associated with impaired hepatic regeneration.

Evaluation of the functional reserve of the liver

The risk of post-operative liver failure depends both upon the quantity and the quality of the liver parenchyma spared by the resection. It is generally agreed that in the normal liver the paramedian sector, the posterolateral sector, segments I and IV and the left lateral segment account for 30%, 35%, 20% and 15% of the entire organ respectively. However, these estimations do not take into account the tumor mass, nor the frequent dystrophy of the cirrhotic liver. An accurate measurement can nowadays be obtained by CT assisted image analysis.

Assessment of the functional reserve of the cirrhotic liver is more difficult to achieve. The most common relies on the Child-Pugh classification that includes clinical (ascites and encephalopathy) and laboratory (serum bilirubin, albumin and prothrombin time) parameters. It has been demonstrated that the incidence of post-operative mortality and liver failure correlates closely to this classification.[1,2] Therefore, resection is contraindicated in patients who are grade C at the time of surgery, while only limited resection should be allowed in patients who are grade B. In grade A cirrhotic patients, several models have, retrospectively, been developed to assess the extent of a safe resection as a function of bromosulphalein or indocyanine green clearance, glucose tolerance test, redox tolerance index or a combination of these. Yet these tests are not always easily available and may be influenced by functional hepatic blood flow (i.e. the hepatic blood supply and the intrahepatic/extrahepatic shunt) or minor degrees of biliary obstruction so that their influence on the post-operative course has not always been confirmed. Superimposed acute alcoholic hepatitis, as well as chronic active viral hepatitis, identified by raised pre-operative transaminase levels, are also associated with increased risk and should be considered, at least transiently as operative contraindications.[3]

Assessment of the tumor

Hepatic resection may be considered if the tumor is solitary, and if there is no associated portal vein thrombosis or extrahepatic metastases. The pre-operative assessment of the number of tumors is based on ultrasound, CT performed 2 to 4 weeks after intraarterial injection of lipiodol, or on spiral CT scan. It has however been recognised, based on the pathological analysis of the explant liver of liver transplant recipients, that all these radiological procedures lack accuracy in detecting multiple small tumors. Overall, US, CT and angiography fail to demonstrate multiple tumors in 50 to 80% of the patients.[4] An increasing problem, related to the ability of these imaging techniques to identify very small focal lesions, is the differentiation of HCC from macroregenerative nodules or borderline nodules within a cirrhotic liver. This may, to some extent be achieved by MRI and arteriography.

Operating technique
Anesthesia

The anesthesiologist should be informed of the severity of the underlying liver disease and should plan anesthetic requirements accordingly. Intravascular volume is maintained by colloid or fresh frozen plasma, rather than crystalloid. In cases of extensive resection, cardiovascular indices are monitored by the placement of a Swan Ganz catheter and a radial arterial line. A Foley catheter is required to follow urine output. Continuous monitoring of oxygen saturation is helpful, as are frequent electrolytes and coagulative profiles. Blood and blood products should be available, but with technical advances are often not required. In any case, undue transfusions should be avoided to prevent immunisation. In addition, a hematocrit level greater than 30-35% is associated with increased blood viscosity and may favor vascular thrombosis. Prophylactic antibiotics and histamine H_2 blockers should be given.

Position of the patient

The position of the patient is important and can make the difference between an easy and a difficult operation. The patient should be positioned supine with the right arm extended along the body. The rib margin is positioned

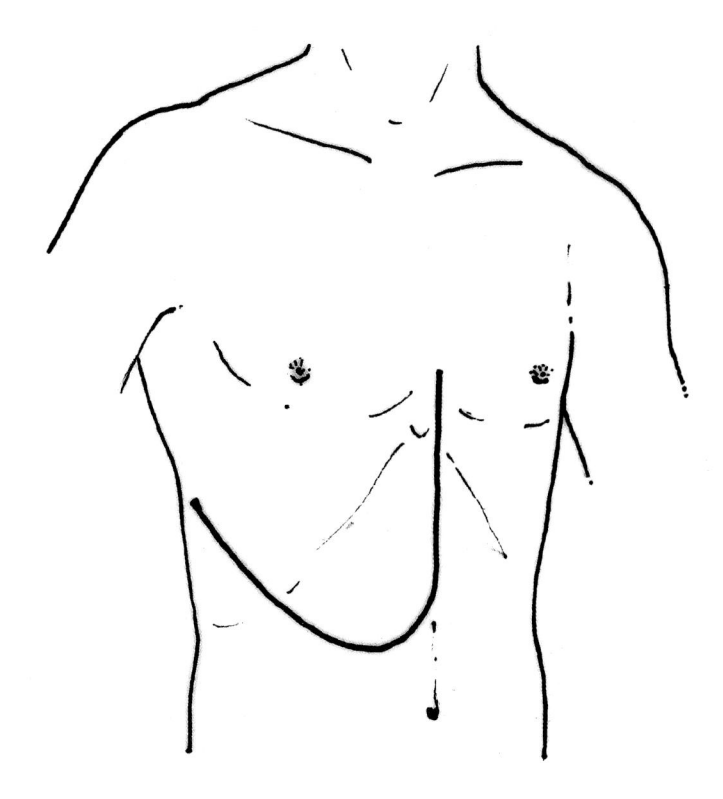

Figure 7.1 – *J-shaped incision consisting of an upper midline incision extended to the right at the level of the umbilicus to the mid axillary line.*

over a rolled blanket to facilitate exposure of the liver. The hips are taped in the supine position to allow subsequent rotation of the table to either side.

The incision

The choice of the incision is influenced by several goals. It should give a good access to all parts of the liver, should be easily extended if required, and should prevent leakage of ascitic fluid in the post-operative period. Liver surgery is usually performed through a bilateral subcostal incision. This incision should follow the coastal margin exactly, 1 cm below it, especially along the right flank, to give good access to the retrohepatic IVC. If a closer access to the suprahepatic IVC is required, this incision may be easily extended by a median incision along the xyphoid process. An alternative is the J-shaped incision, that starts medially along the xyphoid process down to approximately 5 cm above the umbilicus, before curving laterally along the right ninth intercostal space to end at the posterior axillary line. The J incision is indicated for surgery of the right lobe and provides particularly good access to the area around the junction between the inferior vena cava and the right hepatic vein (***Figure 7.1***). The costal arches on both sides are retracted cranially and laterally.

Intraoperative tumor staging

ABDOMINAL INVESTIGATION

Abdominal investigations detect intrahepatic or extrahepatic spread. Needle biopsy is helpful in the evaluation of a suspect nodule, but it is often difficult to distinguish on frozen section between a cancerous nodule and a nodule of regeneration. Satellite nodules can be resected at the time of operation if the area concerned does not involve massive resection of the liver. Abdominal investigation in 5% of operable tumors may reveal, pedicular node extension, which precludes further hepatic resection.

INTRAOPERATIVE ULTRASONOGRAPHY

This procedure is essential in surgery of the cirrhotic liver, which may reveal otherwise invisible or non-palpable tumors. Intraoperative ultrasonography localises the tumor accurately and determines its relationship to vascular structures. It may detect tumor thrombus or intrahepatic occult lesions not apparent in the pre-operative radiological work-up or on palpation, and which will affect the intended surgical procedure.

This technique is also useful to guide pre-operative biopsies, allow transportal methylene blue staining, permit selective portal clamping by intraportal balloon catheter, and provide guidance during parenchymal transection (see below).

Vascular occlusion

Intraoperative blood loss is traditionally considered a significant risk factor for postoperative complications in cirrhotic patients. This assumption is derived from several uni- and multivariate analyses, but it is still unclear whether hemorrhage *per se* is the risk factor or whether it simply reflects the difficulty of the resection, hemostatic disorders, portal hypertension, or the hyperkinetic state associated with superimposed chronic active hepatitis. In addition, it is still somewhat unclear whether any transfusion or only massive transfusions (above 5 units of packed red blood cells) increase this risk. Nevertheless, it is agreed that every effort should be made to avoid intraoperative blood loss.

Several techniques of inflow, with or without outflow occlusion, are available to reduce intraoperative blood loss. Inflow occlusion may be achieved by preliminary extrahepatic control of the arterial and venous branch of the segments to be removed. This is easily achieved in formal right or left hepatectomies, left lateral segmentectomies or segment IV resections are contemplated. The arterial and portal pedicle to the right anterior or posterior segments may also be controlled in patients with a proximal division of the right arterial and portal branches. Alternatively, possible to achieve selective occlusion of the segmental portal branches of the right liver using a balloon catheter, introduced transparenchymally using intraoperative ultrasound.

In addition to these techniques which devascularize the liver segment(s) to be removed, it is also possible to minimize bleeding at the time of liver transection by clamping the hepatic pedicle. This clamping may be either continuous or intermittent. Continuous vascular occlusion of up to 60 minutes is well tolerated by non-cirrhotic livers, especially if it associated with a complete vascular occlusion of the liver (see below). We have, however, recently shown in a controlled study that cirrhotic livers tolerated continuous clamping poorly and, in these patients intermittent clamping (of 15 minutes separated by periods of 5 minutes during which the clamps are released) was safer.

Inflow occlusion is very effective in preventing bleeding of arterial or portal origin but will not prevent bleeding from the hepatic veins. The latter may first be minimized by reducing the central venous pressure below 8 - 10 cm H_2O. Division of the hepatic veins draining the segments to be removed (after having divided the afferent portal vein and arterial branches) will also help reduce bleeding. Alternatively, it is possible to perform the hepatectomy under total vascular occlusion. This technique involves clamping of the hepatic pedicle and the vena cava below and above the liver, after having ligated the right adrenal vein. Total vascular occlusion seems, however, poorly tolerated by cirrhotic livers.

Vascular occlusion techniques are very useful in preventing intraoperative blood loss. One should, however, be aware that these occlusions will inevitably result in some ischemia (and/or reperfusion) injury. In patients with cirrhotic livers who are particularly sensitive to these injuries it is important to find a good compromise between the benefits (prevention of transfusion) and drawbacks (liver injury) of these occlusions. A cautious step by step division of the liver parenchyma with selective coagulation or ligation of all the vascular branches crossed, is essential to prevent blood loss.

Margin of safety and choice of resection

There is, currently, no absolute consensus on the extent of a safe margin during resection of HCC in cirrhotic livers. Obviously, the larger the resection, the more likely that the tumor and potentially adjacent satellite nodules, are removed. If this approach is followed, then the entire segment in which the tumor is located should be removed (***Figure 7.2***). HCC, indeed, tends to spread through the portal vein, potentially both in the hepatopetal and the hepatofugal direction. Segmentectomies will, therefore, ensure that tumor cells that might have spread in this segment are also removed. However, as indicated above, large resections are not always feasible in cirrhotic patients. On the other hand, a "minimal" approach is to perform only a tumorectomy. This is usually made feasible by the presence of a tumor capsule which facilitates enucleation from the surrounding parenchyma, provided the tumor is superficial. These resections may be very well tolerated, even in patients with impaired liver function tests. There is, however, a risk that they are incomplete, in particular if the capsule is invaded by tumor cells (a frequent situation), if satellites nodules are present, or if there is a thrombosis of the portal branch adjacent to the tumor. An intermediate approach is to excise the tumor with at least a 1 cm thick margin of non-affected parenchyma around it. This is probably a safe

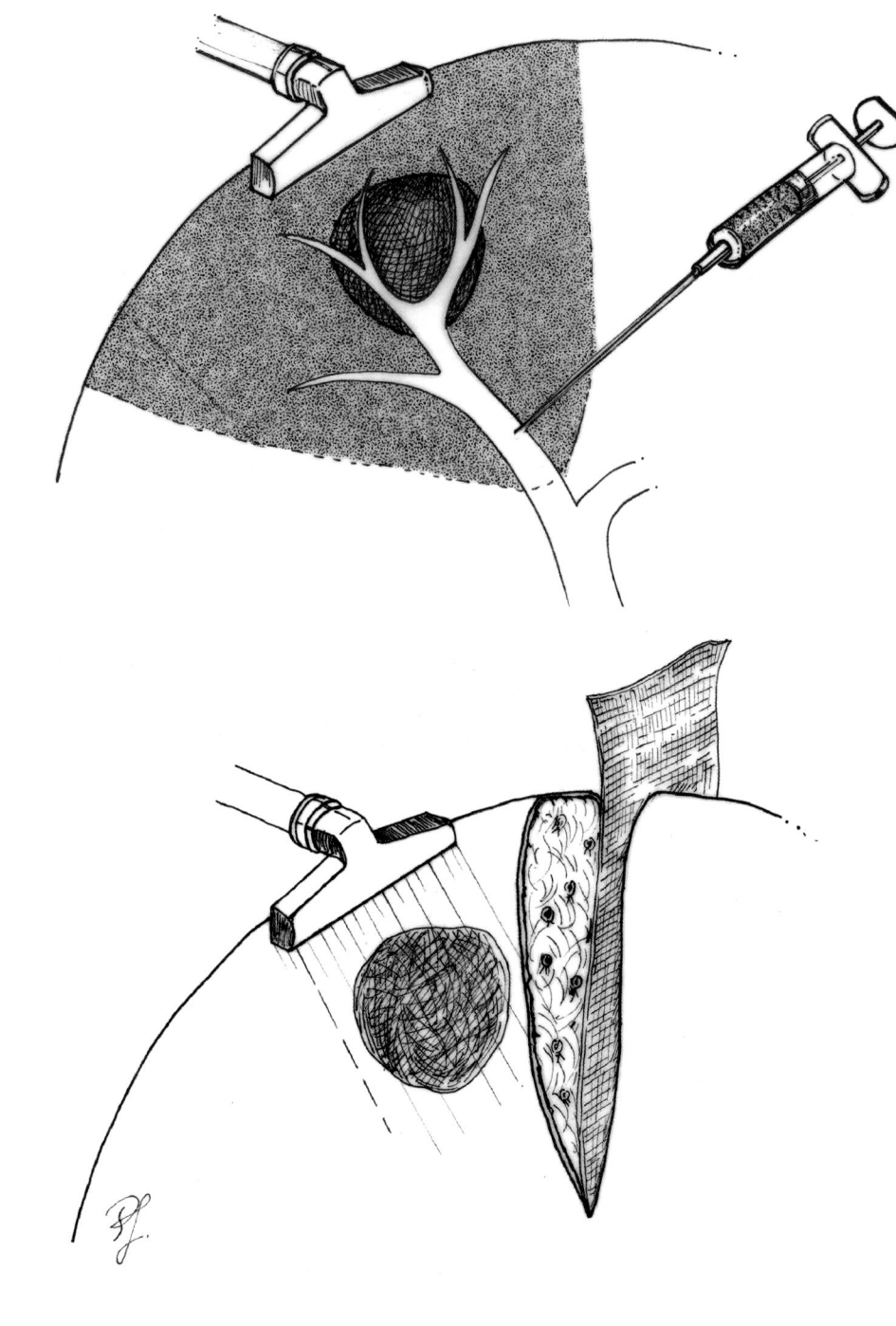

Figure 7.2 – *Procedure for identification of the intersegmental plane in the liver. Due to the extension of HCC through the portal vein, the main branch should ideally be removed. Methylene blue is injected under ultrasound control; this stains the capsula of the liver corresponding to the segment.*

Figure 7.3 – *Technique of parenchymal transection. The distance between the tumor and the transection plane can be controlled by intraoperative ultrasound, placing a mersylene mesh in the cut-section to amplify interference with air. All vascular and biliary radicles are ligated at the transection margin.*

procedure if segmentectomies are considered too large at resection as 80 % of intrahepatic recurrence occurs away from the resected zone.

Parenchymal transection

Liver transection in cirrhotic patients does not markedly differ from that used in non-cirrhotic patients and should follow the following steps: (a) the tumor is localized by intraoperative ultrasonography; (b) the portal unit to be resected is identified. It may be useful at this stage to inject methylene blue in the portal branch under intraoperative ultrasound to clearly identify the boundaries of the segment, or the subsegment, vascularised (c) the incision is traced on Glisson's capsule with a cautery; (d) the parenchymal transection is guided by ultrasound, and the appropriate safety margin is estimated by measuring the distance between the tumor and a mersylene mesh introduced into the cut section; (e) all vascular and biliary pedicles are ligated at the transection margin (*Figure 7.3*). Transection of the parenchyma is best achieved by kellyclasia; because the cirrhotic liver has a hard consistency, the ultrasound dissector proves less useful than when used for the division of normal liver.

Treatment of the raw surface

After the specimen is removed, the clamps are released and the cut surface is packed for 5 minutes. The gauze packs are placed over a plastic drape laying against the raw surface. This non-adherent material prevents the gauze packs from sticking to the exposed parenchyma, and bleeding at the time of stops removal. Bleeding vessels are secured with fine Prolene® 5/0 sutures. Biliary leakage is best located by injecting methylene blue through the cystic duct. Finally, sealing of the raw surface with fibrin glue is probably useful to prevent collection of bile or blood, especially in cirrhotic patients who are at risk of impaired coagulation due to liver failure and/or hypersplenism related thrombopenia, and in whom post-operative ascites may preclude the natural sealing of the cut surface by neighbouring organs and omentum.

Drainage

Liver resections in cirrhotic patients are associated with a high risk of post-operative ascites. This is caused by the extent of the dissection, which will invariably open lymphatics. These are particularly developed in cirrhotics, because of liver failure and portal hypertension, as well as a potentially impaired ability of the peritoneum of cirrhotic patients to clear ascites. Post-operative ascites may be associated with two complications. One is leakage through the abdominal incision that will prevent wound healing. The second is ascites superinfection. Ascites superinfection may result from leakage of ascites through the abdominal wall, from a biliary leakage from the raw surface of the liver, or from an ascending infection from abdominal drainage.

Whether abdominal drainage should be used after liver resection in cirrhotic patients is controversial. It will prevent accumulation of ascites in the peritoneal cavity, and hence encourage the abdominal wound healing. However, it is associated with a risk of ascending bacterial infection of the peritoneal cavity. Furthermore, ascites may persist for several weeks or months. Two options are, therefore, available. One is to insert a one-way (suction) drain that is removed after a few days ; the orifice left by the drain should be closed once the drain has been removed. The other option, (that we usually favor) is to close all abdominal wall layers as tightly as possible without drainage and to perform repeated paracenthesis should ascites occur.

Post-operative ascitis may, to some extent, be prevented by reducing the administration of sodium-containing intravenous fluids and by using diuretics, if there is an adequate renal function. Intravascular volume expanders, such as albumin, may be used if the patient is hypotensive, oliguric, or has a rising serum creatinine. One week prophylactic antibiotics may be used to prevent ascites superinfection.

Post-operative care and management

Cirrhotic patients undergoing liver resection are at increased risk of post-operative liver failure and sepsis. It is of the utmost importance to achieve optimal oxygenation of the liver remnant by establishing an adequate cardiopulmonary status. Monitoring should rely on; peripheral blood level, pulse rate and oxygen saturation, although these may not parallel intrahepatic hemodynamics, hematocrit levels maintained around 30-35% (greater levels may put the patient at risk of vascular thrombosis) and on serial blood gas levels. Liver function tests, including serum bilirubin, transaminases, alkaline phosphatase and gamma glutamyl transferase, as well as prothrombin and factor V plasma levels should be monitored daily or every other day in the initial post-operative period. Similarly, kidney function should be monitored and maintained by adequate fluid and electrolytes balance based on the daily record of fluid input and output, the patient's weight, as well as on serum and urine electrolyte concentrations and serum creatinine level.

The normal kinetics of liver function tests in cirrhotic patients are characterised by an early drop in prothrombin activity on post-operative day 1, and a progressive increase in serum bilirubin levels up to day 3. Both parameters should, however, start to progressively normalize from post-operative day 5 onwards.

Abnormal recovery (or secondary deterioration) of liver function tests should prompt the rapid investigation for complications. The most feared complication in this setting is sepsis. One should be aware that fever and increased white blood cell count may be absent. Blood and ascites, if present, should be sampled for bacterial culture. Perihepatic fluid collections should be looked for and aspirated, or drained, percutaneously. Failure to treat these infections promptly will inevitably result in the progressive development of irreversible multiorgan failure. Another possible complication, although rare, is portal vein thrombosis, that should be detected by Doppler ultrasound.

Segmental or partial thrombosis may reverse with anticoagulation. Complete thrombosis is almost always fatal. Rupture of esophageal varices is another complications specific to cirrhotic patients.

Conclusion

Over the past decade, there has been considerable improvement in liver surgery. These are associated with more accurate pre-operative assessment of liver volumes and functional reserve, thus allowing a better selection of patients, improved knowledge of the anatomy of the liver, the development of segment-oriented resections more selective use of clamping techniques (thus allowing as much functional parenchyma as possible to be spared), the availability of surgical tools such as intraoperative and better post-operative management. This has allowed resections, and, if required, repeated resections to be performed in cirrhotic patients with an in-hospital mortality rate of 5 to 10%.

REFERENCES

1. Franco D, Capussoti L, Smadja C et al. Resection of hepatocellular carcinomas: results in 72 European patients with cirrhosis. *Gastroenterology* 1990 ; **98:** 733 -738.

2. Nagao T, Inoue S, Goto S. et al. Hepatic resection for hepatocellular carcinoma: clinical features and long term prognosis. *Ann Surg* 1987 ;**205:**33-40.

3. Noun R, Jagot P, Farges O, Sauvanet A, Belghiti J. High pre-operative serum alanine transferase levels increases the risk of liver resection in Child grade A cirrhotic patients. *World J Surg* (in press).

4. Rizzi PM, Kane PA, Ryder SD. *et al.* Accuracy of radiology in detection of hepatocellular carcinoma before liver transplantation. *Gastroenterology* 1994; **107:** 1425-1429.

8

Extended Right Hepatectomy

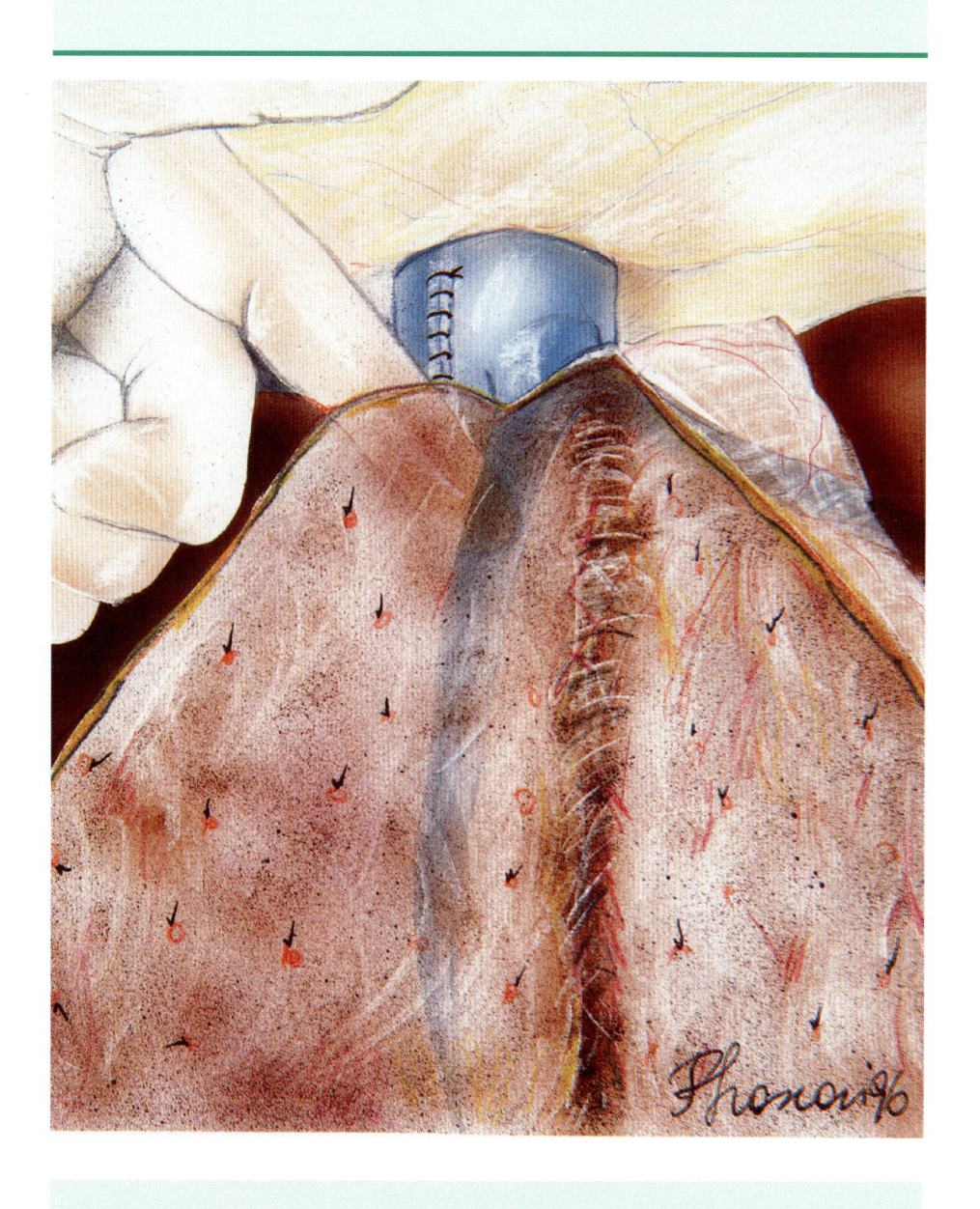

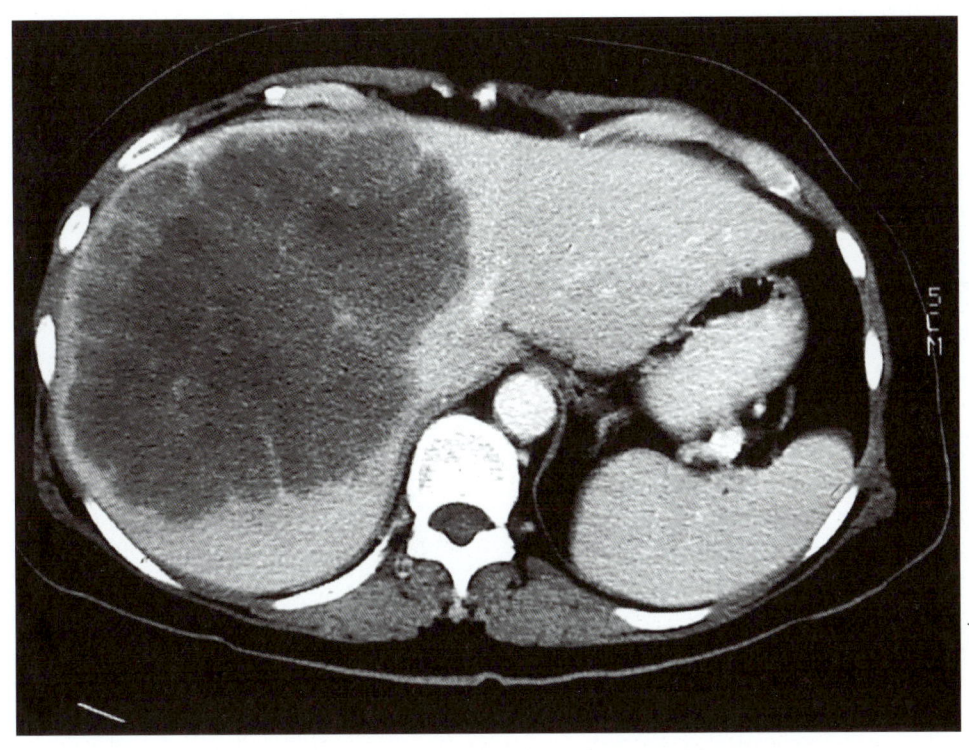

Figure 8.1 – *Huge metastases from colonic carcinoma of the right hemiliver extending towards segment 4. Preoperative CT.*

Extended right hepatectomy consists of the removal of the right anatomical lobe (segments 5, 6, 7, 8 and 4). The operation is indicated for large tumors which extend from the right hemiliver beyond the sagittal incisure plane towards segment 4 (***Figure 8.1***). This is a major operation and requires functional and anatomical integrity of the remaining left lobe. The operation is well tolerated in patients with extensive tumor masses which replace a large portion of the parenchyma of the right lobe. If a large part of the liver to be removed is healthy and if the left lobe is relatively small, there is a risk of postoperative hepatic insufficiency. When planning an extended hepatectomy it is therefore advisable to consider pre-operative embolization of the right portal branch in order to produce compensatory hypertrophy of the left lobe (see Chapter 19).

The initial stages of the operation are identical to conventional right hepatectomy: after dividing the right triangular ligament and the falciform ligament, the gallbladder pedicle and the right branch of the hepatic artery and of the portal vein are divided, without isolating the right hepatic duct (***Figure 8.2a***). Extrahepatic ligature and division of the right hepatic vein is particularly advisable (***Figure 8.2b***). Once the right hepatic vein has been divided, a space is created between the vena cava and the parenchyma where it is easier to identify the middle hepatic vein during resection. In Starzl's original description, the right hepatic vein is divided transparenchymally during the resection.[2,3] Glisson's capsule is divided to the right of the insertion of the falciform ligament on the anterior surface of the liver. On the inferior surface the parenchymal bridge is divided below the umbilical ligament. Division

TECHNIQUES IN LIVER SURGERY

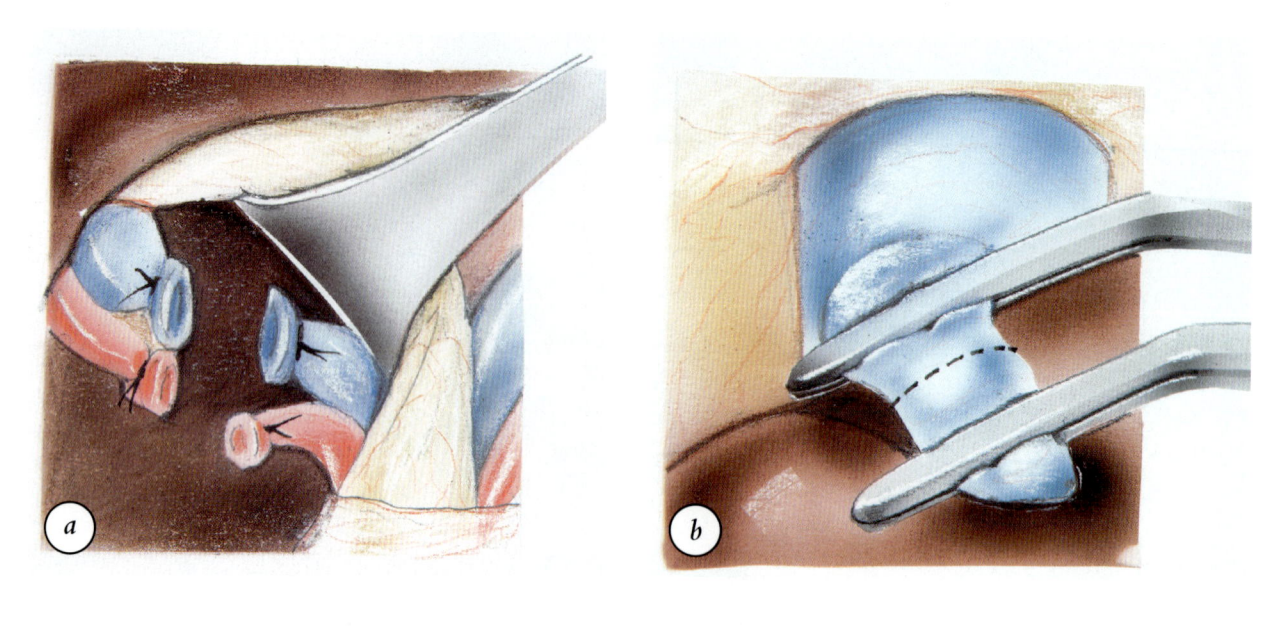

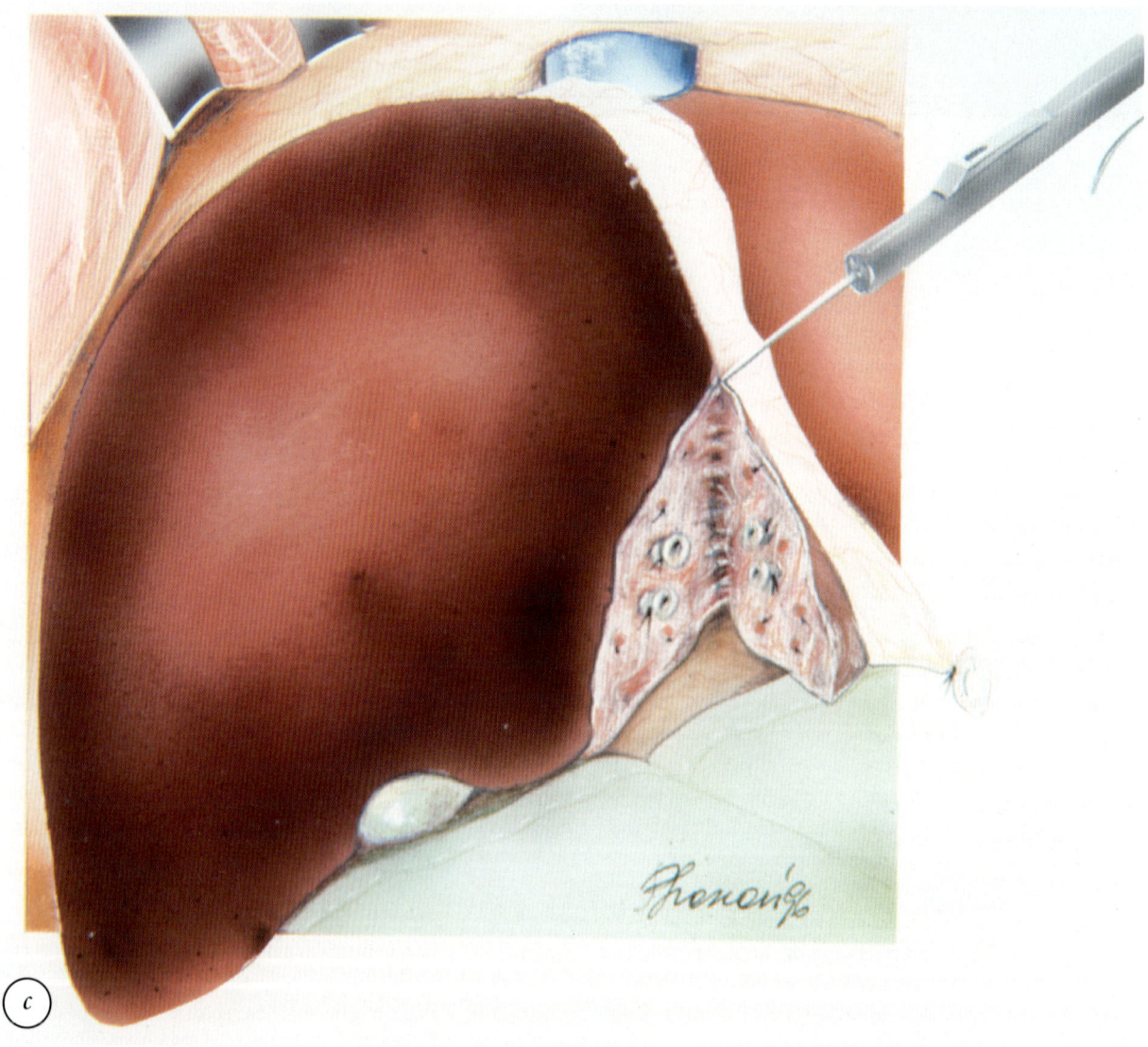

Figure 8.2 – *Extended right hepatectomy. **a)** Ligature of the right branches of the hepatic artery and portal vein. **b)** Clamping and division of the right hepatic vein. **c)** Division of the parenchyma to the right of the insertion of the falciform ligament.*

EXTENDED RIGHT HEPATECTOMY

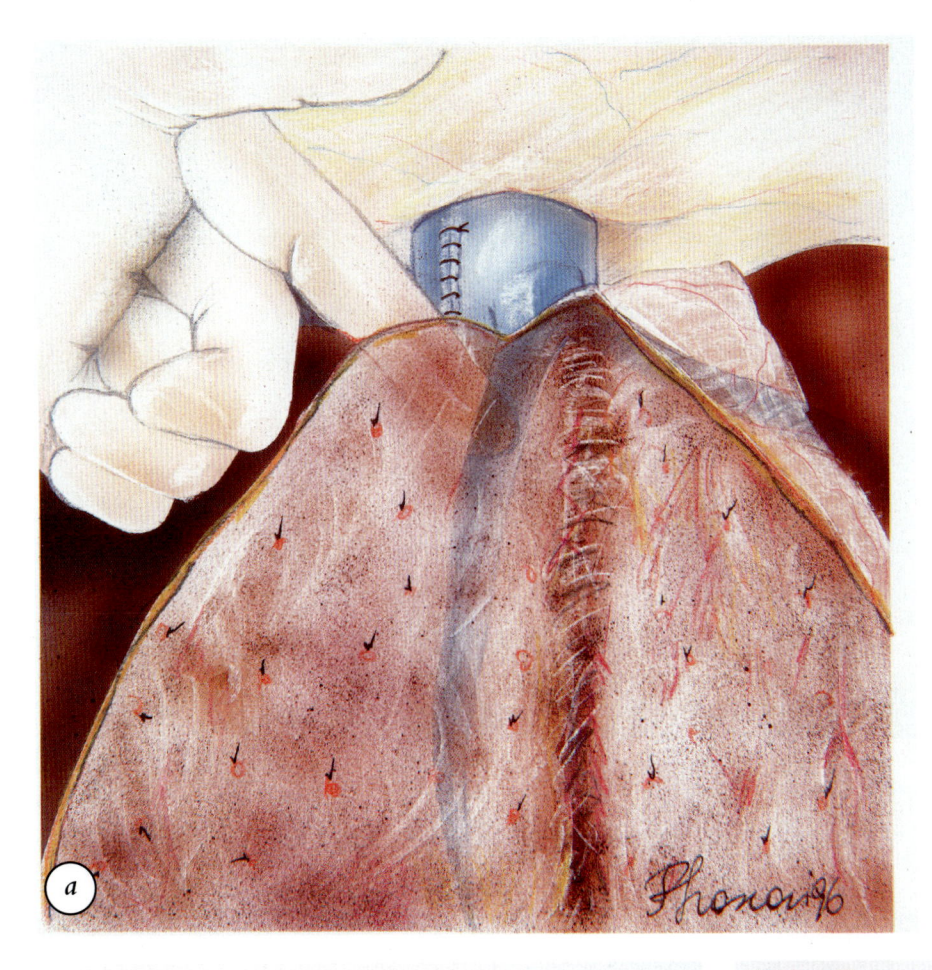

Figure 8.3 – *Extended right hepatectomy. Division of the parenchyma is completed with isolation **a)** and clamping of the middle hepatic vein **b)**. The right hepatic duct is the last structure to be interrupted **c)**.*

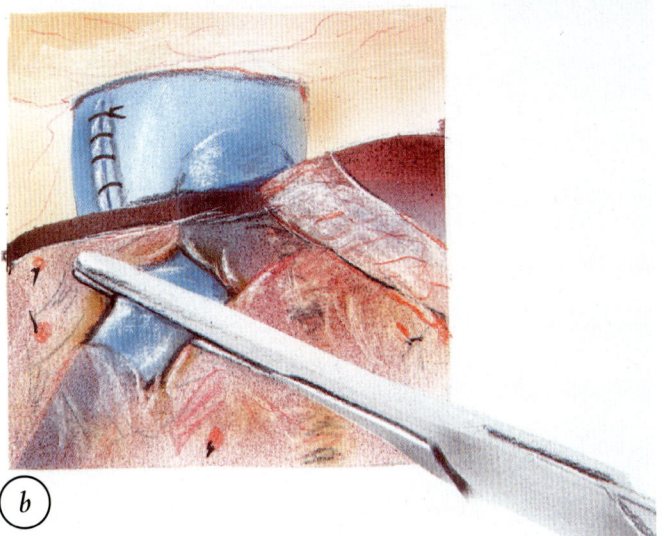

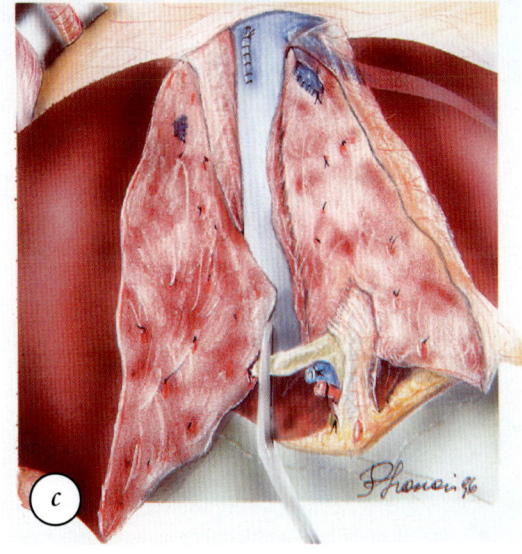

of the parenchyma proceeds from the front towards the back, maintaining the umbilical ligament in traction. A few centimeters from the anterior aspect of the liver, the Glissonian pedicles of segment 4 are encountered; they are clamped and sutured (***Figure 8.2c***). Glisson's capsule is then divided on the inferior face of segment 4, immediately above the insertion of the hilar plate, taking care to avoid any accessory bile duct of segment 4 which may drain directly into the horizontal portion of the left hepatic duct. Division of segment 4 proceeds progressively deeper into the parenchyma as far as the trunk of the middle hepatic vein. At this stage it is advisable to insert a finger in the space created in front of the retrohepatic vena cava so that the layer of parenchyma surrounding the middle hepatic vein can be detached more easily, without damaging the wall of this vein or the vena cava (***Figure 8.3a***). The hepatic vein is clamped, divided and sutured just before it drains into the left hepatic vein (***Figure 8.3b***). The right lobe of the liver is now only connected by the

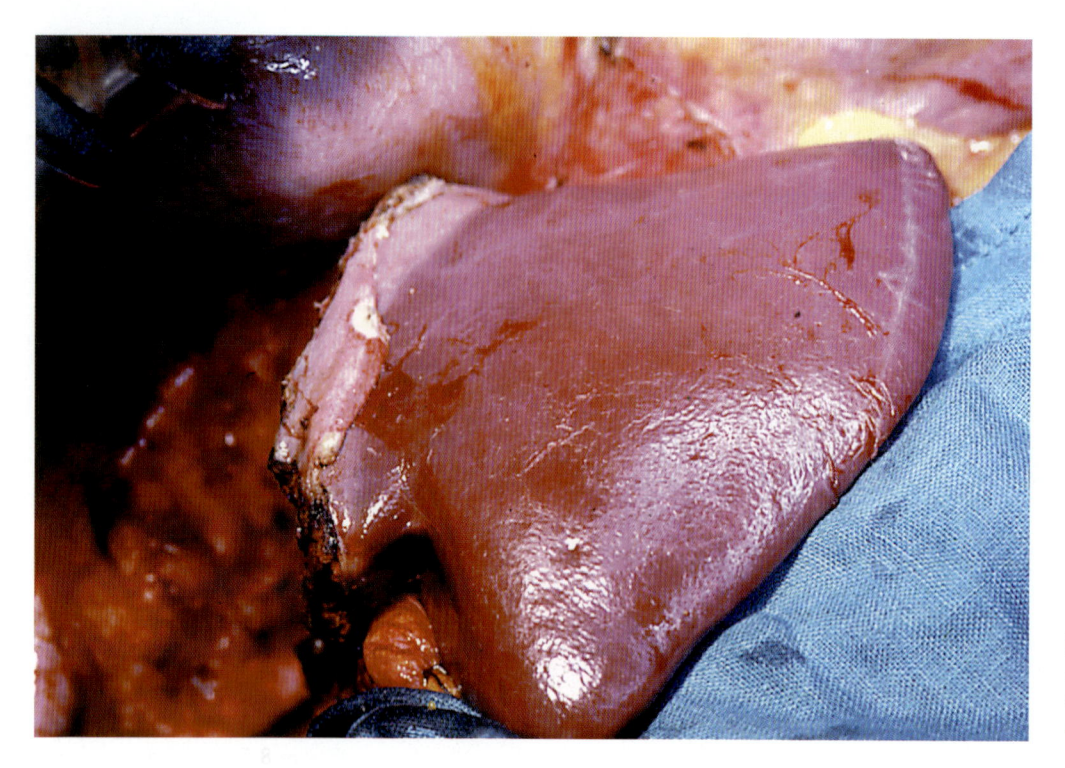

Figure 8.4 – *Extended right hepatectomy. Resection field.*

right Glissonian pedicle where the right hepatic duct must now be clamped at some distance from the bifurcation, at a safe point at the level of the secondary bifurcation (**Figure 8.3c**). By following this technique it may not be necessary to clamp the hepatic pedicle at the hilum. The use of methylene blue and transcystic cholangiography is advisable, in order to identify any biliary leakage from the left hepatic duct due to accidental division of a duct originating from segment 4.[1] The resected surface is left open and the left lobe free (**Figure 8.4**). There is no risk of torsion of the remaining lobe if the left triangular ligament is left intact.

REFERENCES

1. Brower ST, Miller C, McElhinney AJ. Avoidance of injury to the left hepatic duct during parenchymal dissection for hepatic trisegmentectomy. *Surg Gynecol Obstetr* 1989; **168:** 457-458.
2. Starzl TE, Bell RH, Beart RW, Putnam CW. Hepatic trisegmentectomy and other liver resections. *Surg Gynecol Obstetr* 1975; **141:** 429-437.
3. Starzl TE, Koep LJ, West R *et al*. Right trisegmentectomy for hepatic neoplasms. *Surg Gynecol Obstetr* 1980; **150:** 208-214.

9

Extended Left Hepatectomy

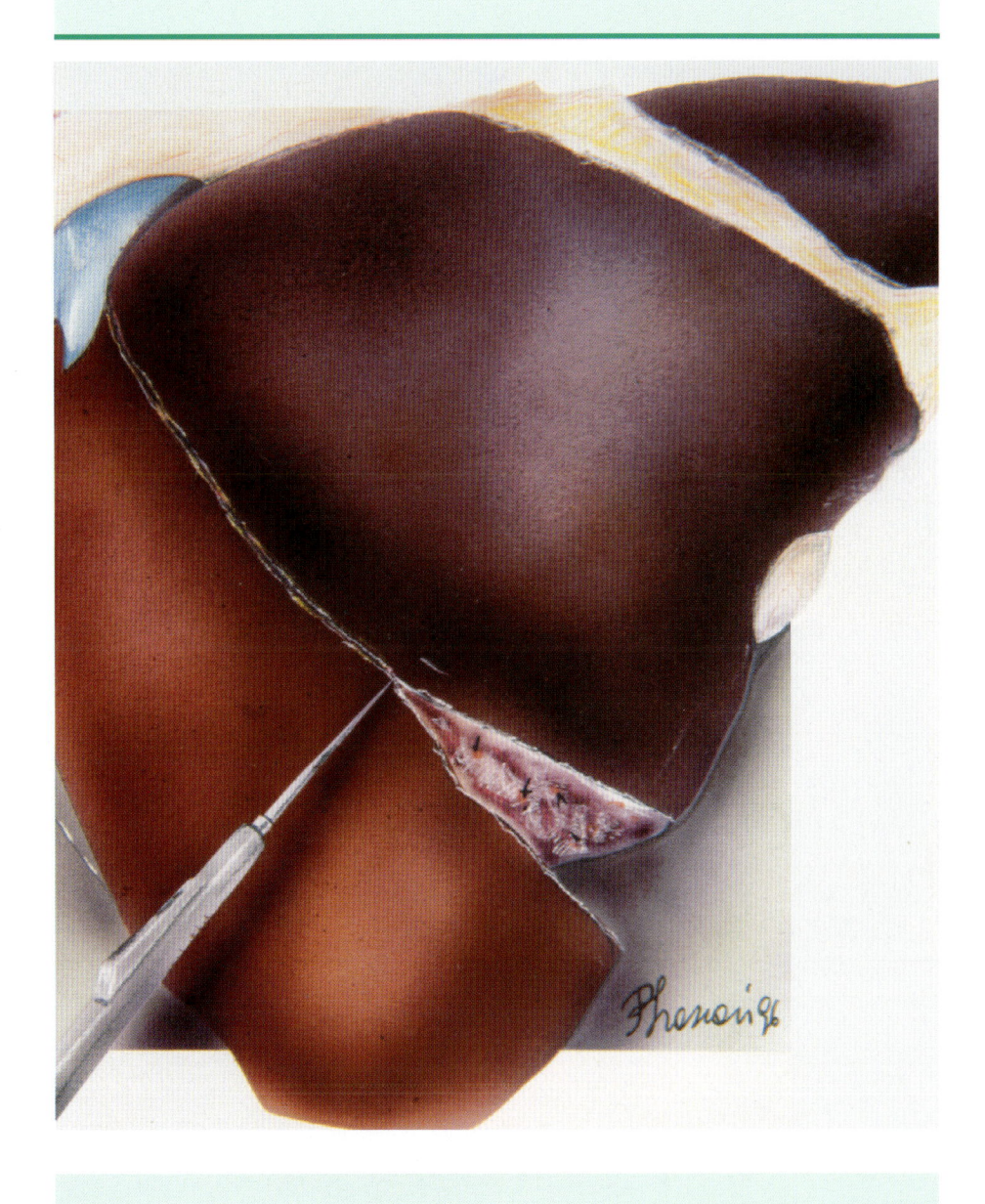

Extended left hepatectomy consists of removal of the left hemiliver and the right paramedian segments (segments 2, 3, 4, 5 and 8). From a functional point of view this hepatectomy involves approximately 70% of the parenchyma, and should be limited to patients with completely healthy residual parenchyma without fibrosis or cholestasis. Indications for this operation are tumors which extend from the left hemiliver beyond the main hepatic fissure towards segments 5 and 8. It may also be indicated for tumors localized in the posterior segments, close to the middle hepatic vein, which protrude into the posterior portion of segments 4 and 8. Resection in this case may consist of left hepatectomy extended to segment 8, leaving segment 5 in place.

The technique for extended left hepatectomy was defined by Starzl[2] and has more recently been described, with some variations, by Kawasaki & Makuuchi.[1] We describe the technique used in our department.

Operative landmark

The key point of the technique for extended left hepatectomy is related to the right hand margin of resection, due to the anatomical relationships with the right hepatic vein and with the posterior Glissonian pedicle. These structures have landmarks on the external surface of the liver dictates guide the limit of the resection. The outlet of the right hepatic vein is always indicated by a fissure which can be identified on the surface of the hepatic dome, after having completely divided the right triangular ligament, the falciform ligament and its posterior layers. This fissure is easily recognizable and constitutes a reliable landmark of the right hepatic vein. The course of the posterior Glissonian pedicle can be identified on the inferior aspect of the liver by an obliquely posterior incisure (Ganz's incisure) which extends from the gallbladder bed, encircles the caudate process anteriorly and continues towards the right to around 3-5 cm from the edge of the liver. The posterior Glissonian pedicle is always found adjacent to this incisure, within the hepatic parenchyma.

Technique

The left hemiliver is completely mobilized, dividing the triangular ligament, the hepatogastric ligament and the falciform ligament as far as its posterior layers. After dividing the gallbladder pedicle, the left Glissonian pedicle structures are prepared. If the caudate lobe is to be preserved, ligature of the left portal branch must be more distal beyond the transverse part of the vein. Division of the left hepatic duct can be more distal, and we prefer to divide the bile tract during parenchymal resection, where there is less risk of anatomical variations (***Figure 9.1a***). Ligature of the left Glissonian pedicle produces ischemic demarcation of the hemiliver along the gallbladder-vena cava line. The arterial and portal right paramedian pedicles are identified extraparenchymally.

Proceeding along the right aspect of the common bile duct, underneath the bile tract, the two dividing branches of the right hepatic artery can be identified: the paramedian branch, which runs vertically, parallel to the common hepatic duct, and the lateral pedicle which runs towards Ganz's incisure. The arterial branches are lifted upwards and to the right to expose the right branch of the portal vein which is followed distally as far as its dividing branches, the paramedian branch for segments 5 and 8 and the lateral branch parallel to the lateral artery. The two paramedian vascular pedicles are clamped to produce ischemic demarcation of segments 5 and 8 and are then ligated (***Figure 9.1b***). The parenchymal resection line is indicated by the anatomical landmarks already described, approximately 1 cm in front of Ganz's incisure, and of the fissure of the right hepatic vein, following the ischemic demarcation line.

TECHNIQUES IN LIVER SURGERY

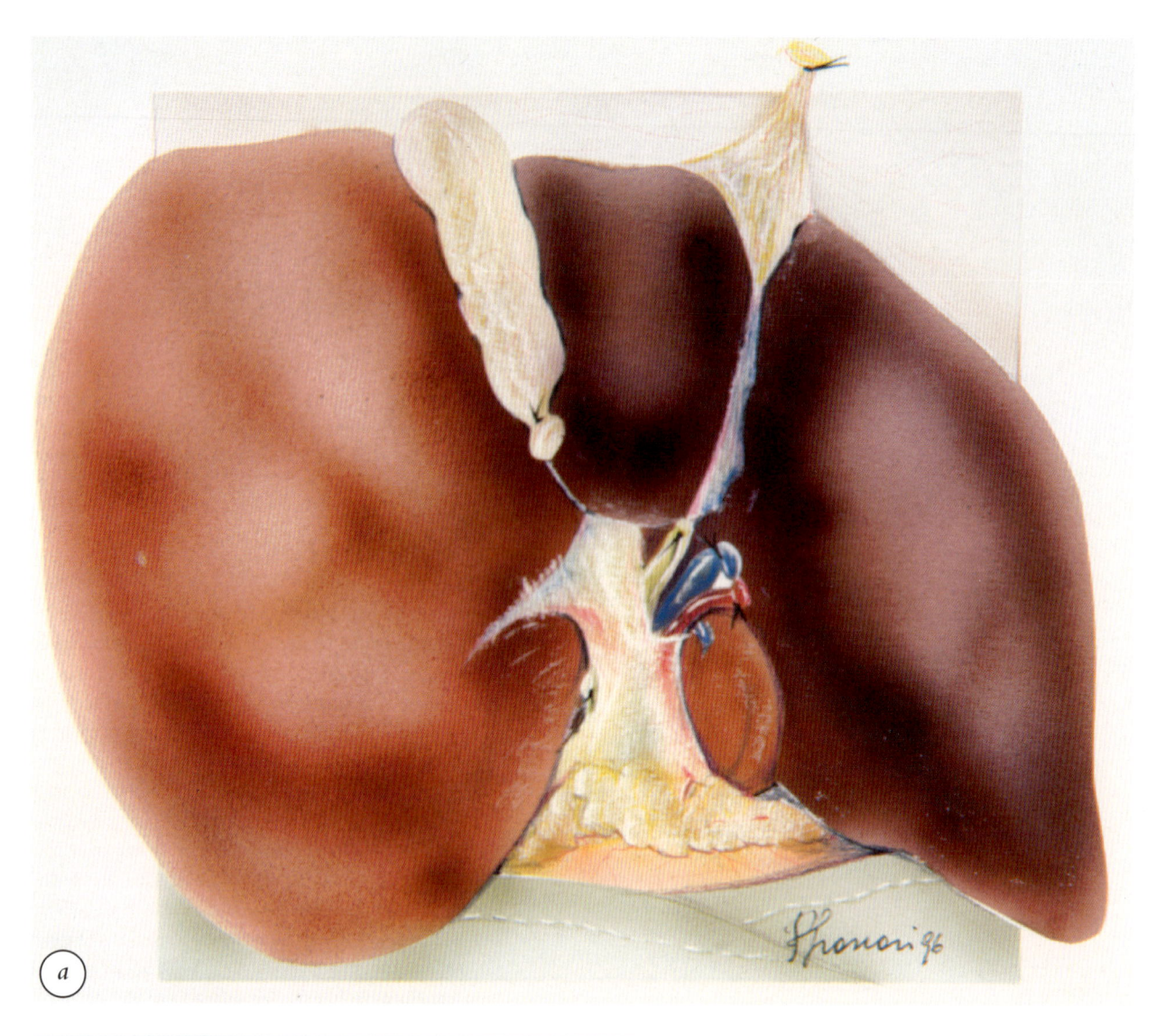

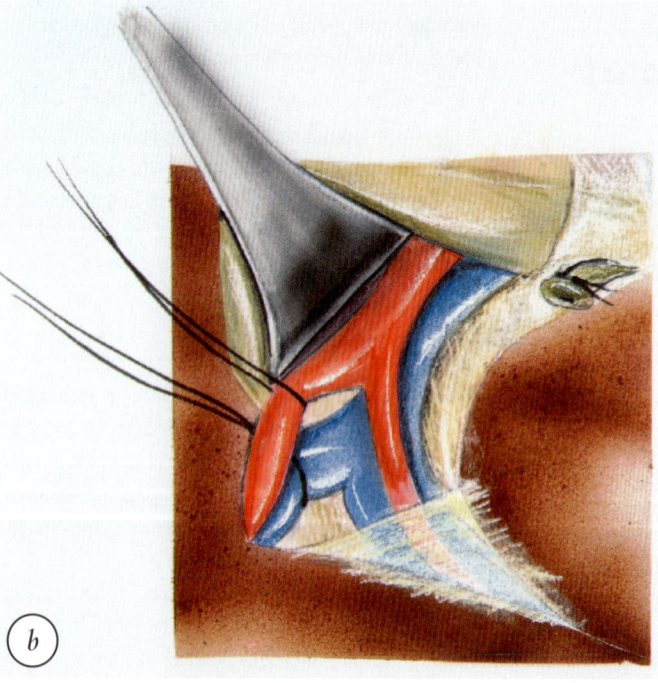

Figure 8.1 – *Extended left hepatectomy.* **a)** *Division of the left Glissonian pedicles.* **b)** *Ligature of the arterial and portal right paramedian branches.*

EXTENDED LEFT HEPATECTOMY

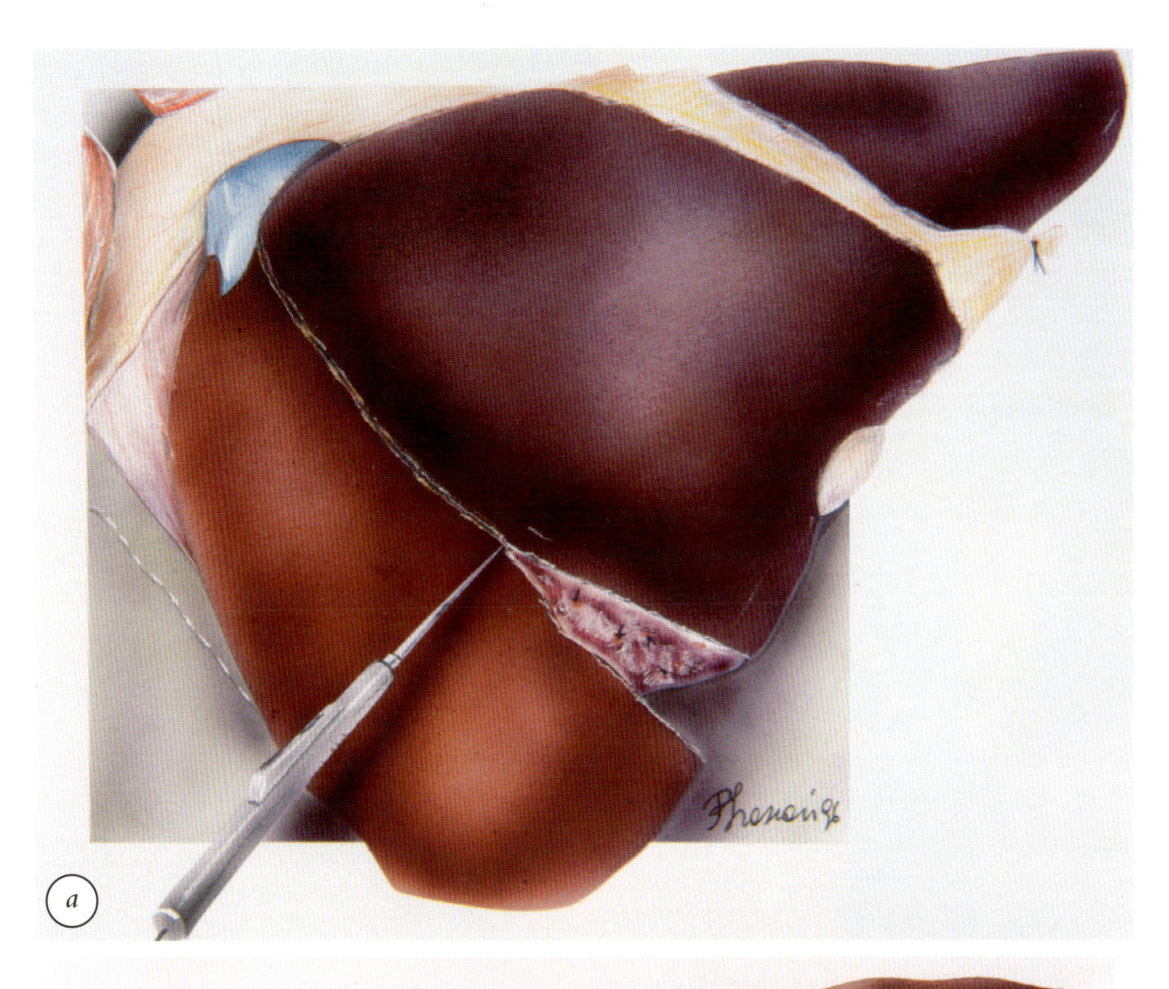

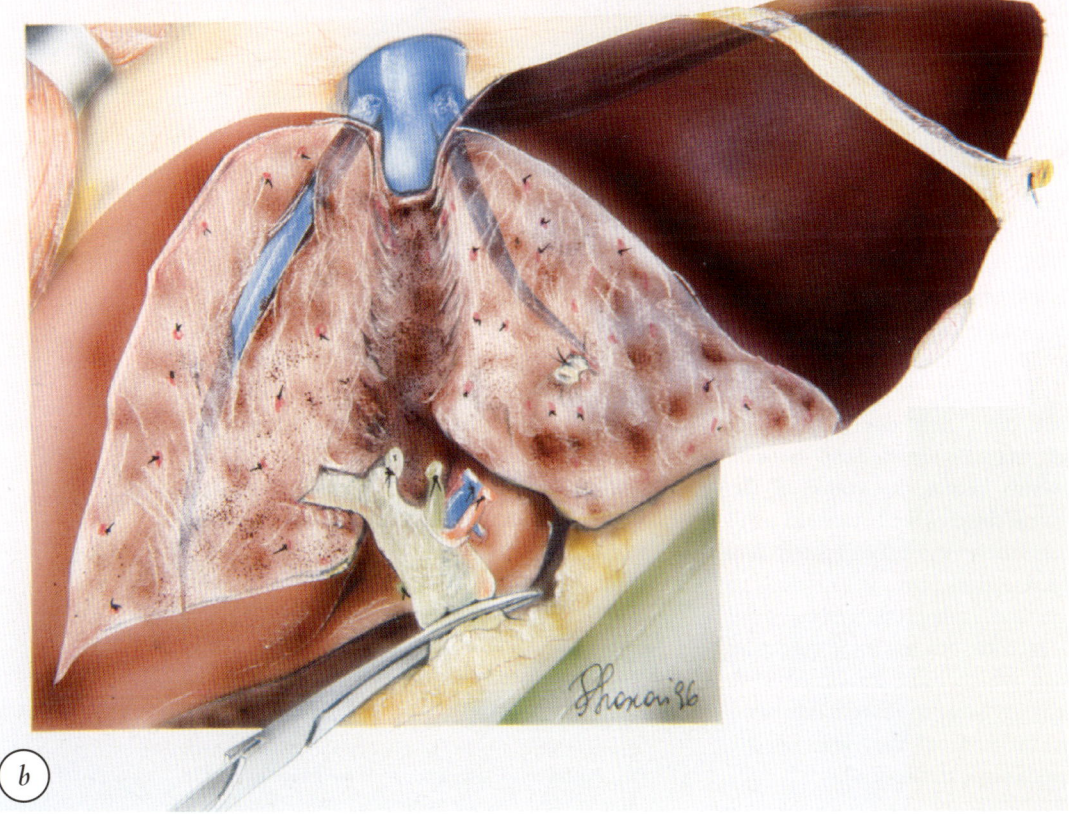

Figure 9.2 – *Extended left hepatectomy.* ***a–b)*** *Division of the parenchyma under intermittent clamping of the hepatic pedicle.* (***c.*** *over page*)

c) Division of the common trunk of the middle and left hepatic veins.

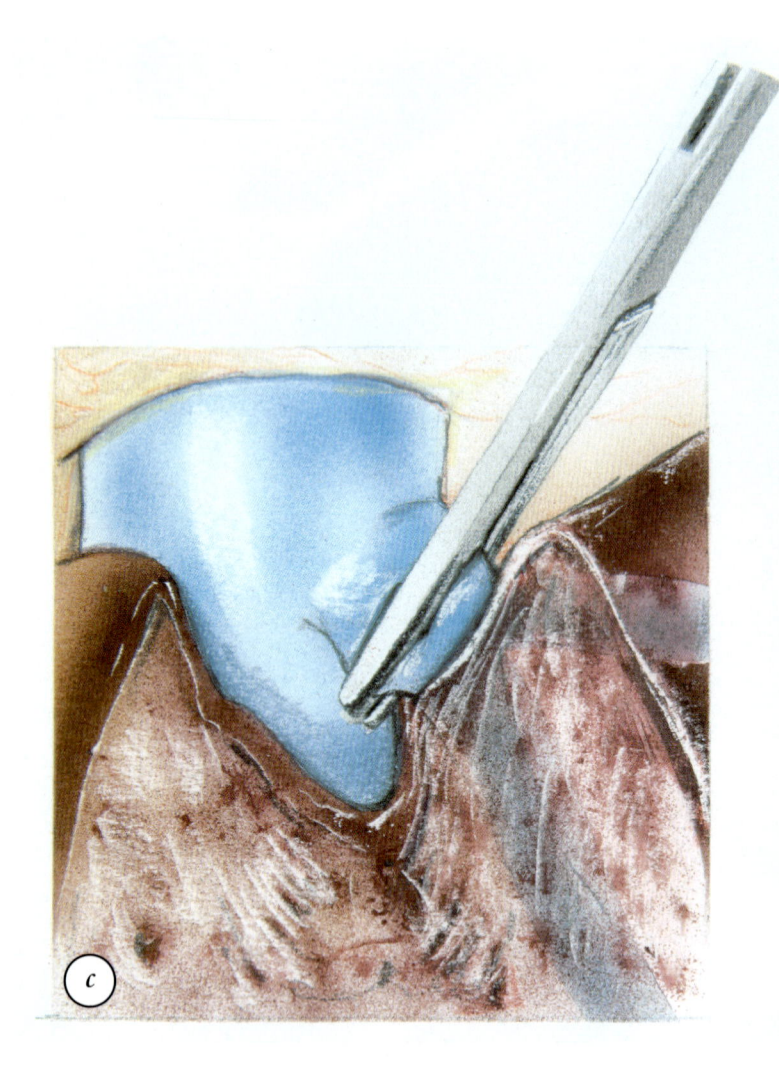

Division of the parenchyma is performed during intermittent clamping of the Glissonian pedicle at the hilum, on a very oblique plane, proceeding from right to left to reach the lateral fissure of the hilum. As dissection continues, the paramedian pedicle is encountered; this should be clamped *en bloc*, ligated and sutured (it is only at this point that the paramedian bile duct, not identified during the extrahepatic stage, is divided). Dissection continues upwards, along the trunk of the right hepatic vein into which various small collaterals flow; these must be ligated and sutured. If the resection plane is too close to the trunk of the vein, laying it bare, these small collaterals may be torn, causing small defects in the venous wall which must be closed with 5-0 sutures. It is advisable to leave a thin layer of parenchyma in front of the right hepatic vein to prevent damage to the wall.

Dissection continues beyond the confluence of the right hepatic vein into the vena cava, in front of the right portion of the caudate lobe (***Figure 9.2a***). The liver is, therefore, now attached to the vena cava by the trunk of the left vein and to the left wall of the caudate lobe by the fibrous cord which corresponds to Arantius' ligament. This fibrous cord must be divided to free the inferior aspect of the left hepatic vein and to completely detach the left hemiliver from the caudate lobe. The common trunk of the left hepatic vein can finally be clamped, divided and sutured with a Prolene® 3-0 whipstitch (***Figure 9.2b***). The resected surface is treated as usual. Transcystic cholangiography is advisable. The residual cavity is drained with two tubes and filled with omentum.

REFERENCES

1. Kawasaki S, Makuuchi M. Left hepatic trisegmentectomy. In: Lygidakis NJ and Makuuchi M, *Pitfalls and Complications in the Diagnosis and Management of Hepatobiliary and Pancreatic Disease*. Thieme, Stuttgart, 1993, pp. 146-149.
2. Starzl TE, Iwatsuki S, Shaw BW *et al*. Left hepatic trisegmentectomy. *Surg Gynecol Obstetr* 1982; **155:** 21-27.

TECHNIQUES IN LIVER SURGERY

SECTION III

Complex Techniques of Liver Resection

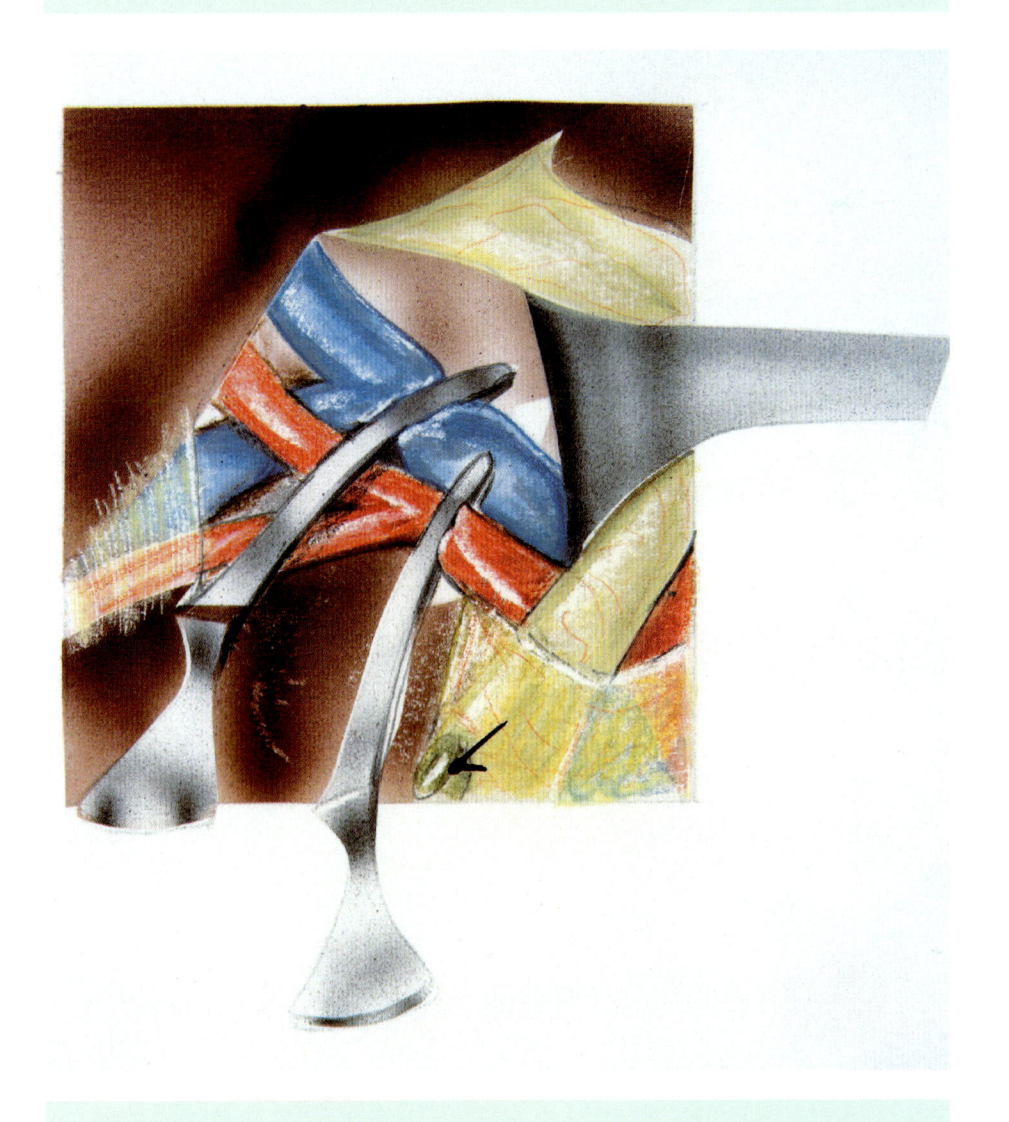

10

'Central' Liver Resection

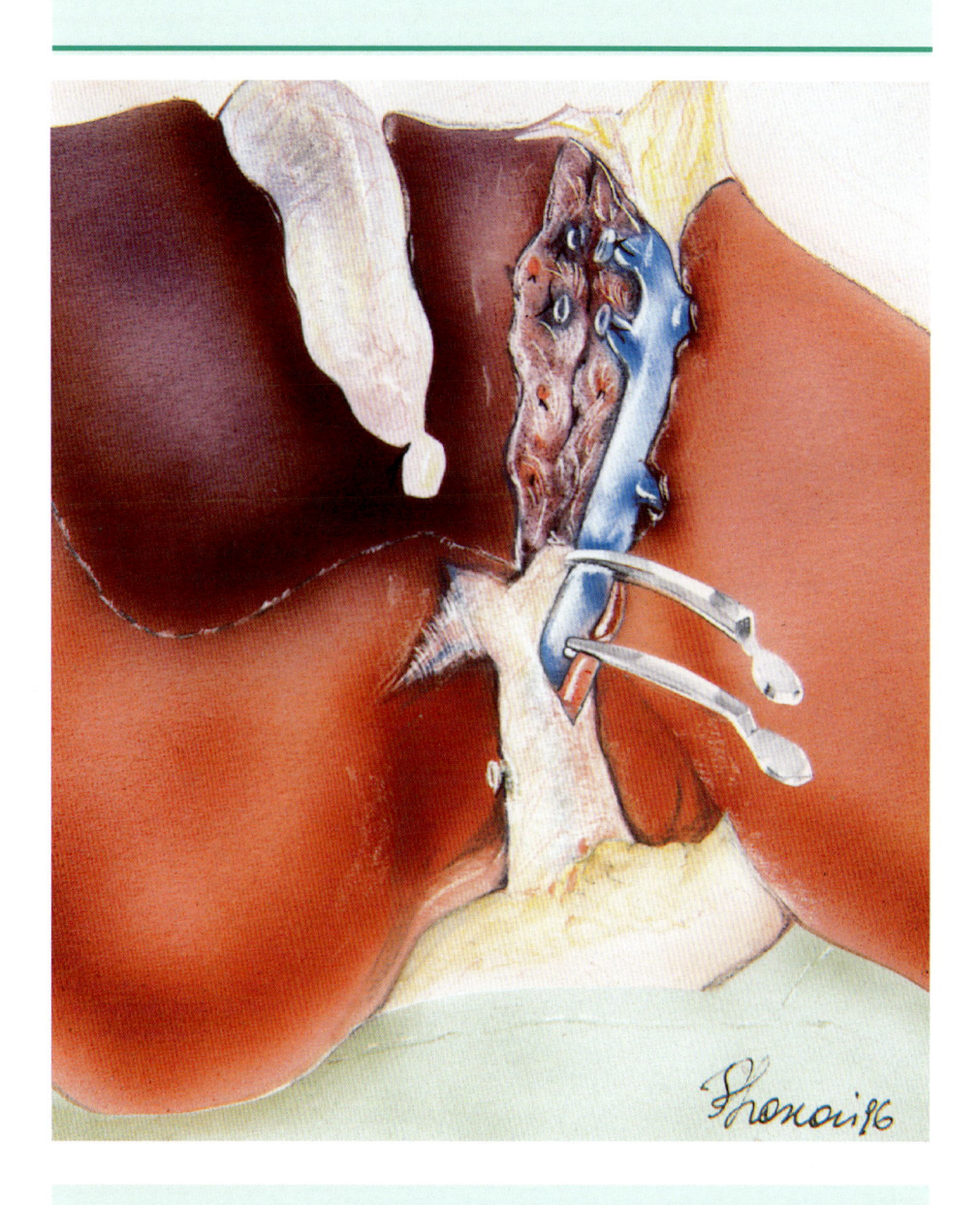

'CENTRAL' LIVER RESECTION

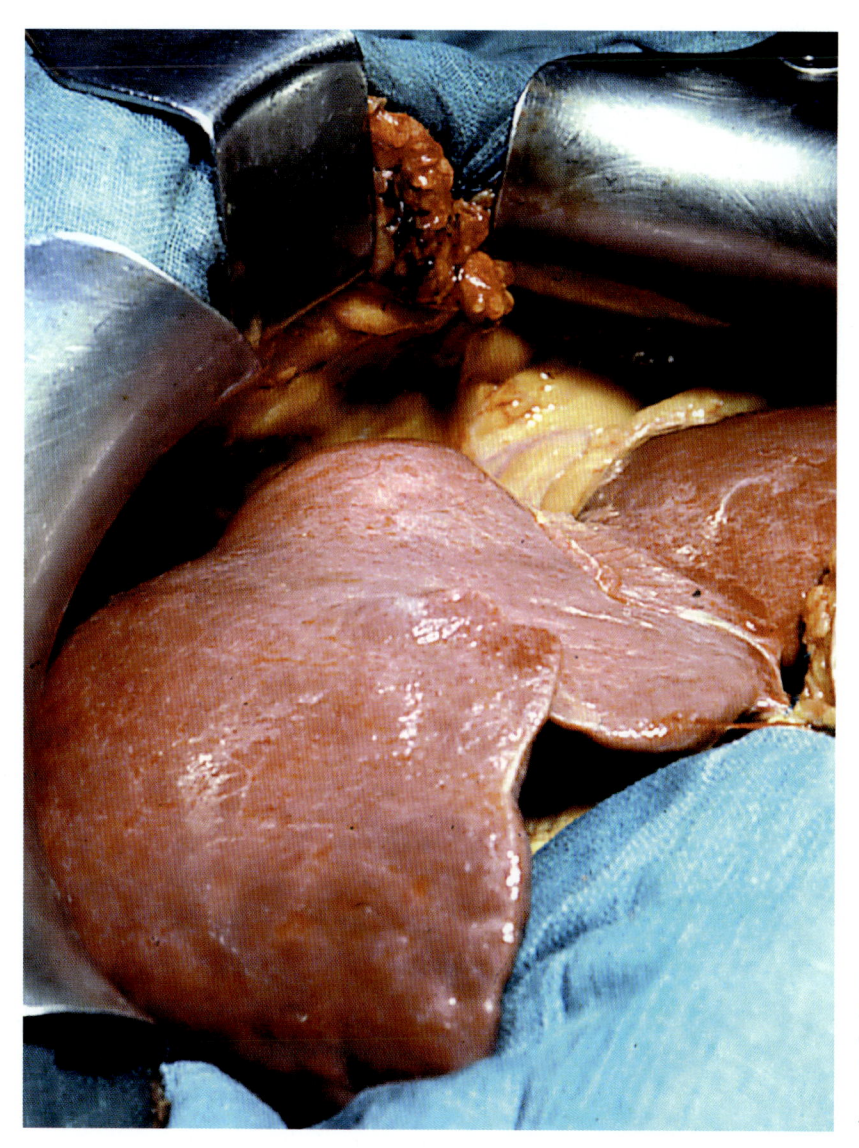

Figure 10.1 – *Hepatocellular carcinoma associated with cirrhotic liver developed between segments 4 and 8.*

Central liver resection or mesohepatectomy consists of the resection of the medial segments 4, 5 and 8. This operation is indicated for tumors which develop between segments 4 and 8 (**Figure 10.1**) and, occasionally, for tumors of the hepatic hilum or of the gallbladder. The basic stages of the operation are the same as those described for resection of segment 4 and 8 (see Chapter 6).

The hilar stage, after division of the cystic duct or the cystic artery, requires isolation and clamping of the right paramedian arterial and portal pedicles (**Figure 10.2a**). The ischemic demarcation line indicates the right lateral limit of the resection which is marked by cautery. The main right branch of the artery and the portal vein are encircled with tape and clamped during division of the right portion of the parenchyma. On the left the resection plane is defined by the insertion of the falciform ligament. The left arterial and portal pedicles are also encircled with tape and clamped during division of the left portion of the parenchyma, resulting in a hemi-hepatic vascular occlusion on both the left and the right during resection. This hemi-hepatic clamping limits ischemic damage and is particularly advisable in patients with cholestasis or cirrhosis.

Division of the parenchyma begins on the left. The umbilical ligament is held in traction and division proceeds from the front towards the back, to the right of the ligament, until the Glissonian pedicles of segment 4, corresponding to the right horn of Rex's recess, are encountered (**Figure 10.2b**). The arterial, biliary and portal pedicles are surrounded by a sheath of connective tissue and are clamped *en bloc*, sutured and divided. On the inferior aspect of the liver, Glisson's capsule is divided above the hilar plate and care should be taken to identify an occasional biliary branch of segment 4, which could drain into the horizontal section of the left hepatic duct. Division

TECHNIQUES IN LIVER SURGERY

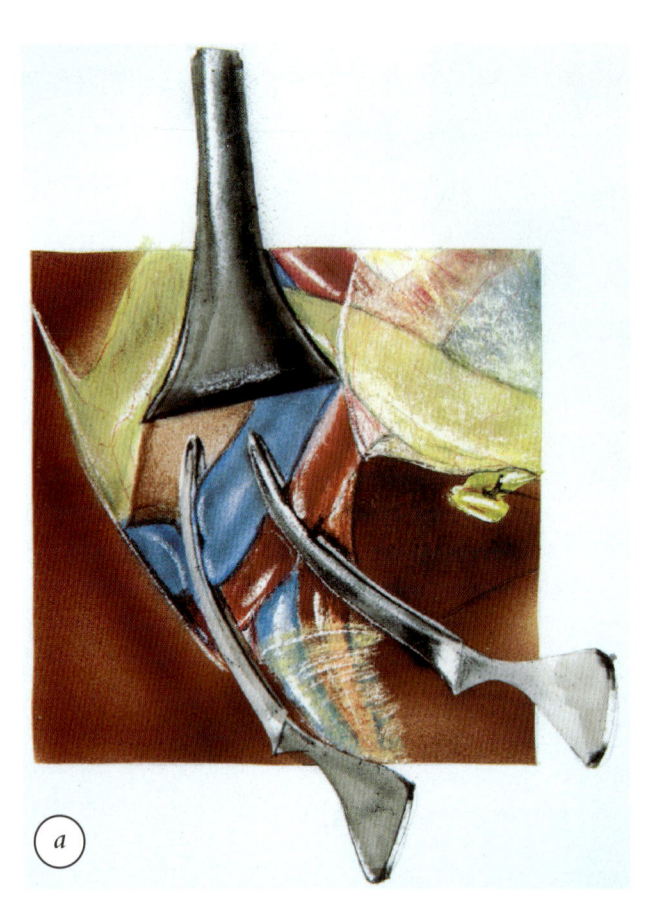

Figure 10.2 – *"Central" liver resection. **a)** Clamping of the right paramedian arterial and portal branches. **b)** Glisson's capsule is incised by cautery along the ischemic demarcation line on the right side. The left branch of the portal vein and of the hepatic artery are clamped, and the parenchyma divided along the insertion of the falciform ligament.*

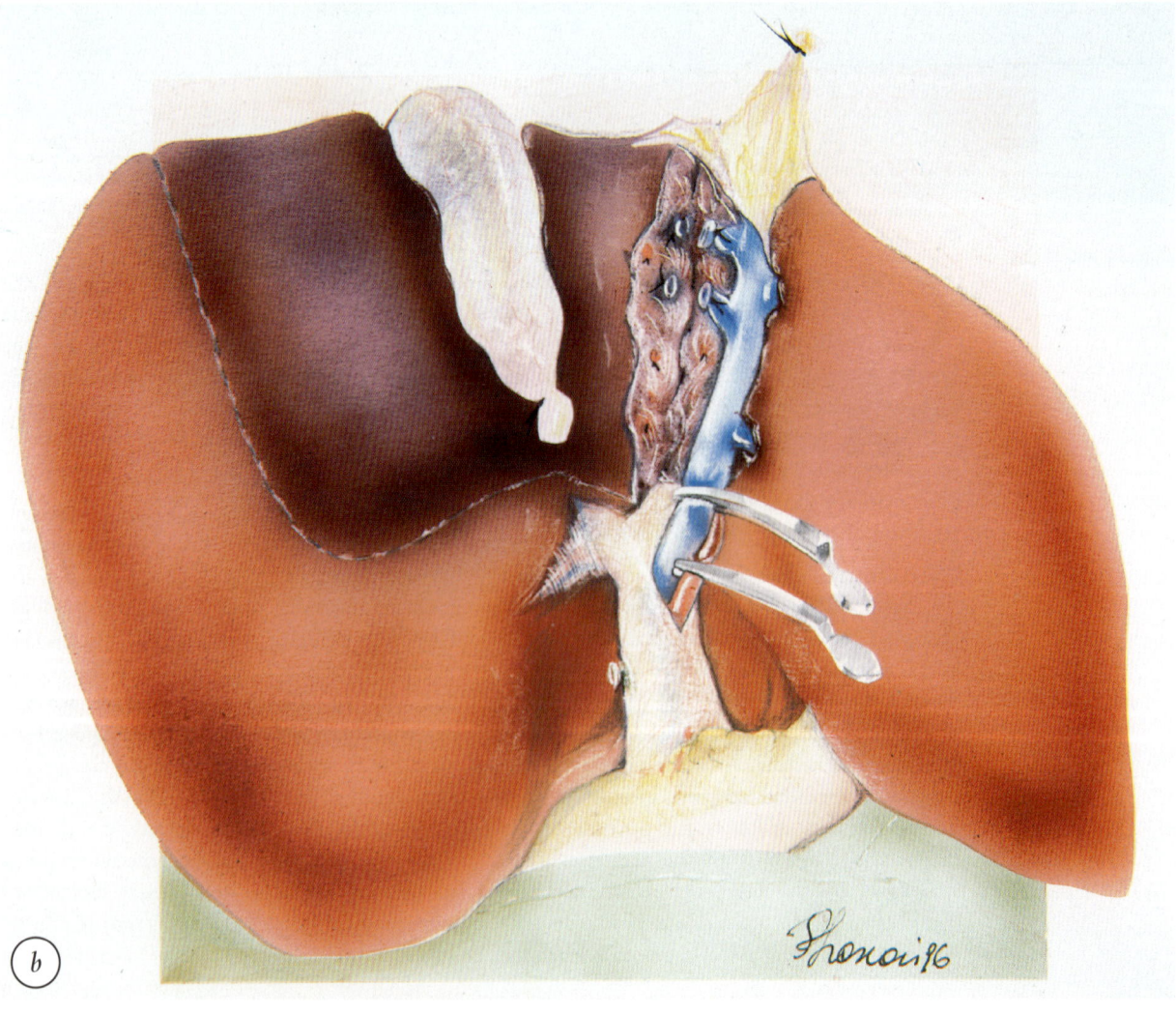

'CENTRAL' LIVER RESECTION

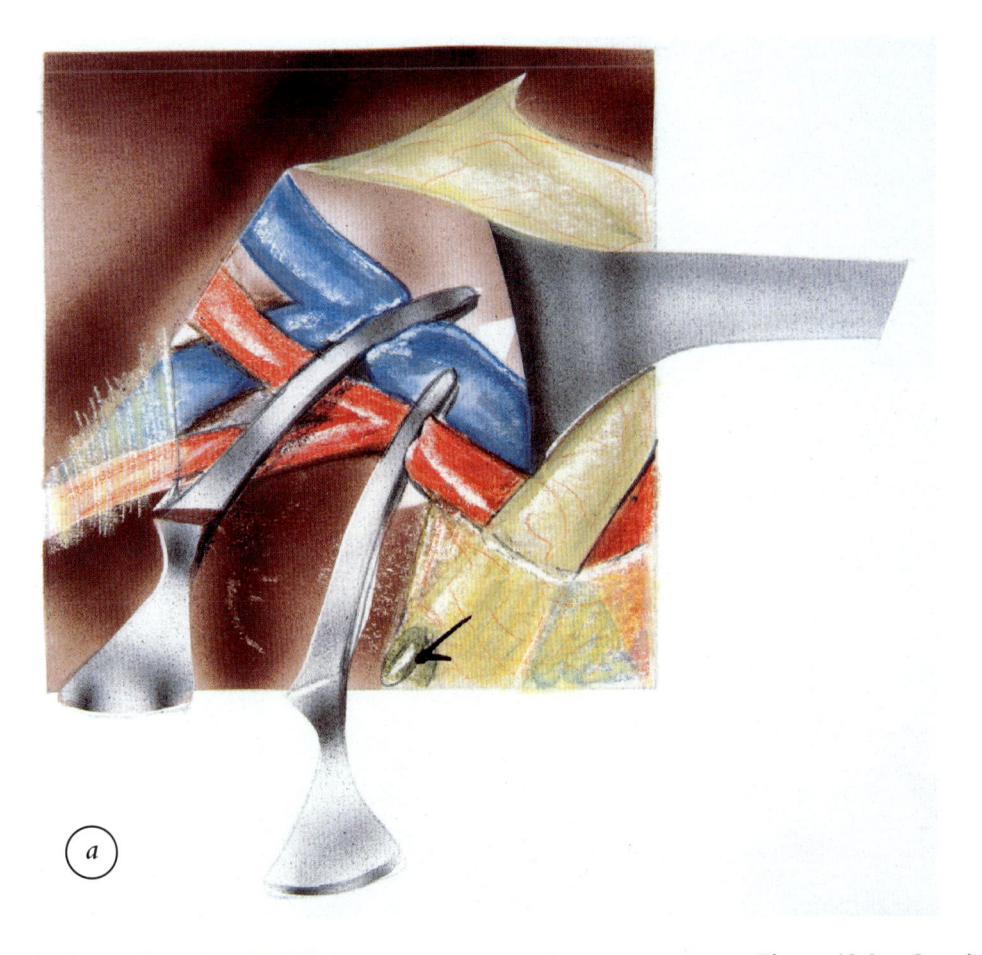

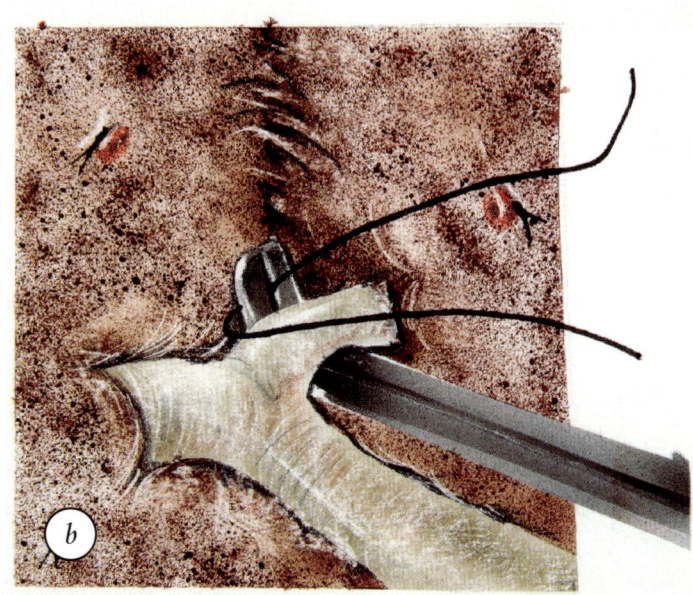

Figure 10.3 – *Once division of the parenchyma on the left side has been completed, the right branch of the hepatic artery and the portal vein are clamped **a)** followed by parenchymal division on the right side. Intraparenchymal ligation of the paramedian Glissonian pedicle **b)**.*
*(**c.** and **d.** over the page.)*

of the parenchyma continues upwards where no significant vessels are encountered, apart from some branches of the left hepatic vein. Division stops close to the middle hepatic vein and the left Glissonian pedicle and the hilum is unclamped to confirm hemostasis. On the right, division follows the ischemic demarcation line previously indicated. Also, at this stage of parenchymal division, the main right branch of the hepatic artery and of the portal vein are clamped to reduce blood loss (**Figure 10.3a**). Right parenchymal division is oblique from right to left and from anterior to posterior, proceeding in the direction of the fissure of the right hepatic vein, which represents the superior landmark of the resection plane.

TECHNIQUES IN LIVER SURGERY

d

e

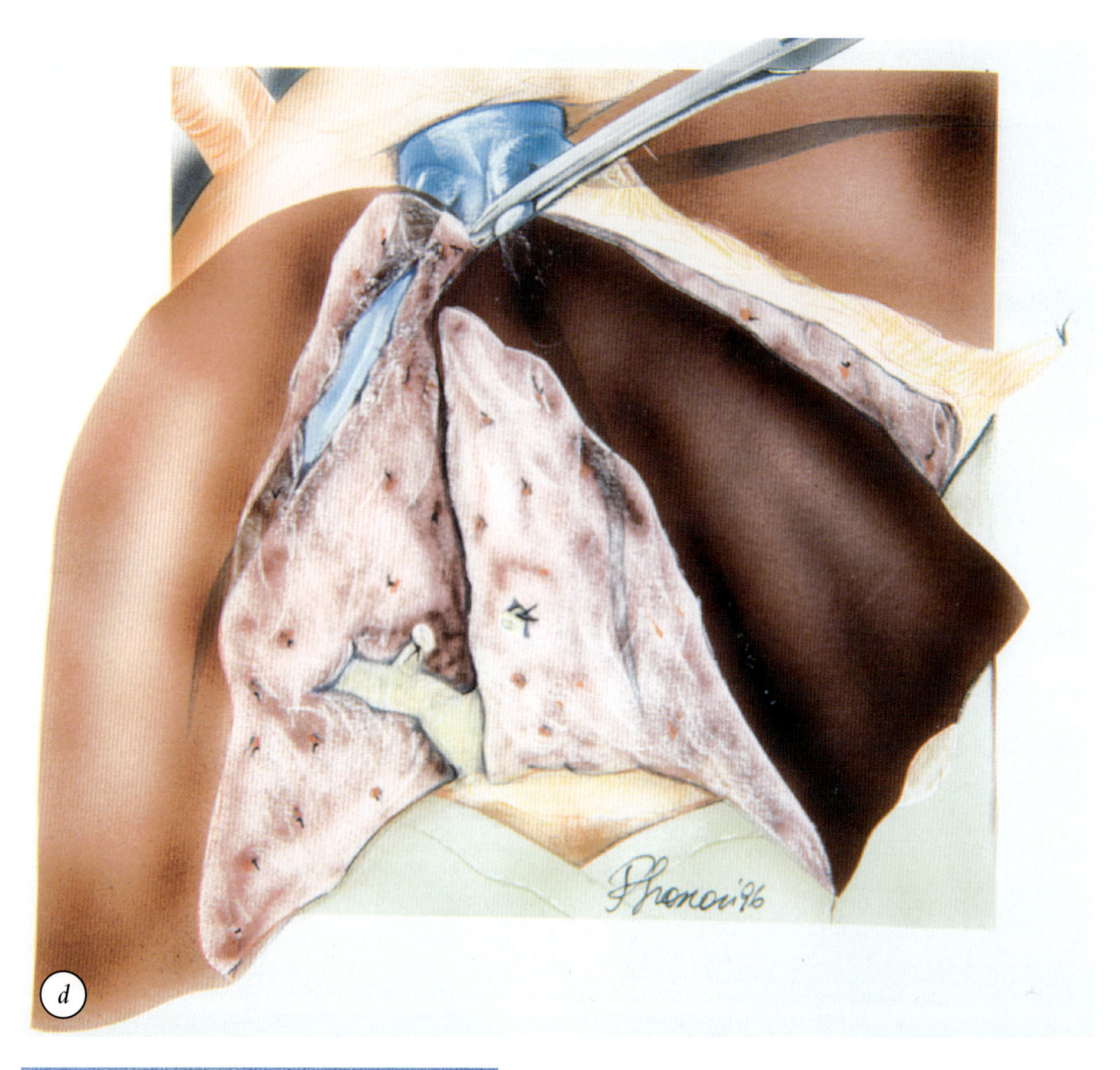

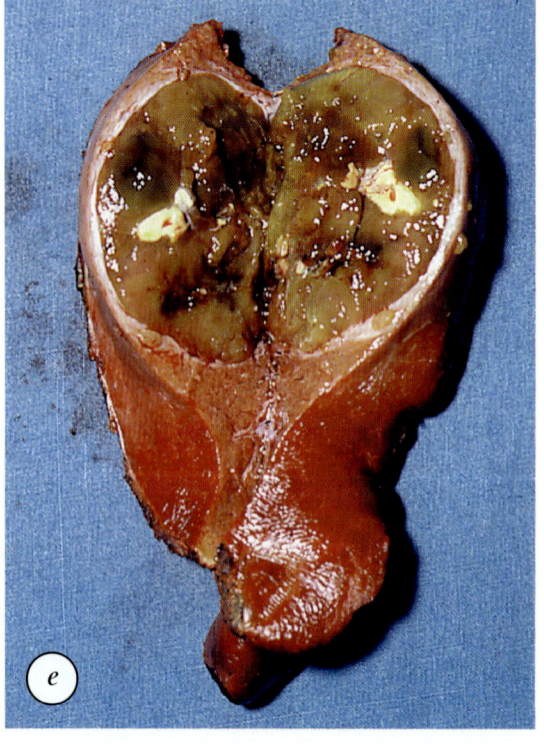

Figure 10.3 (continued) – *Clamping and division of the middle hepatic vein on completion of the parenchymal division **c)**. Operative specimen **d)**.*

98

'CENTRAL' LIVER RESECTION

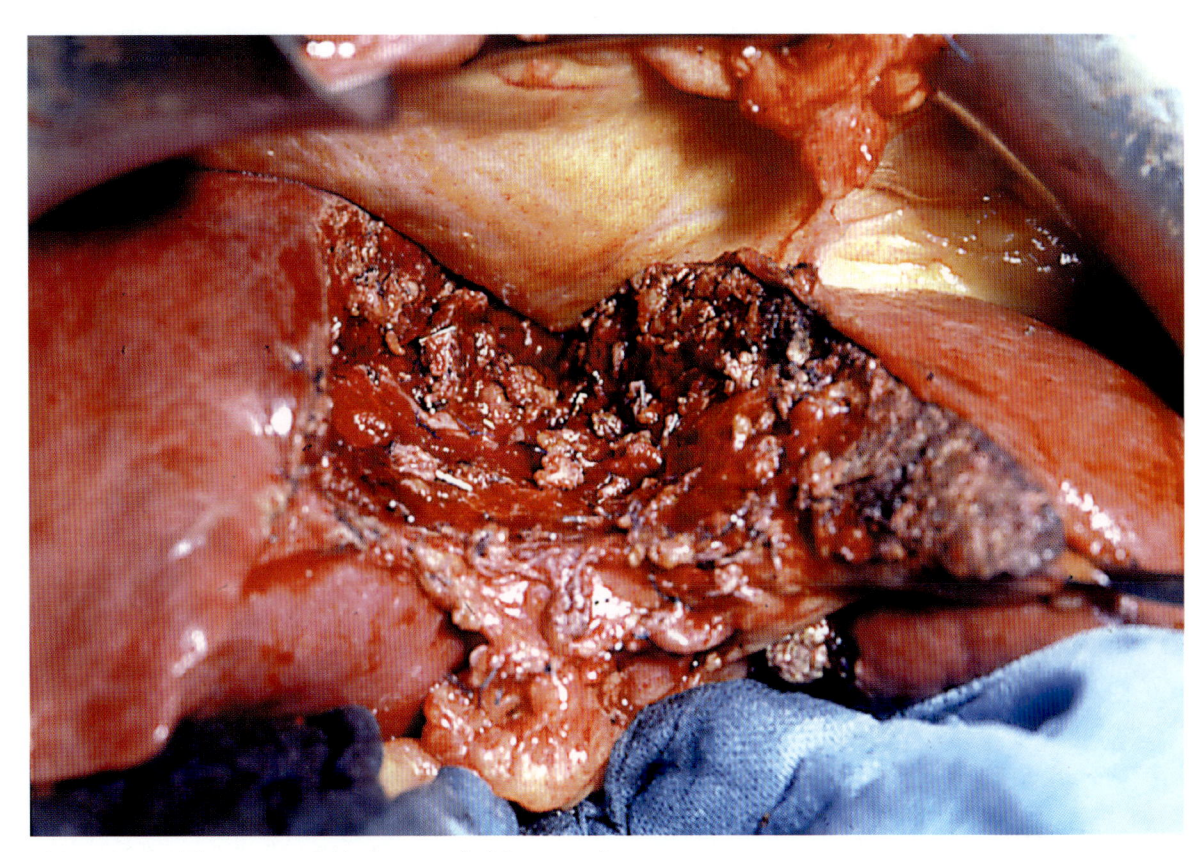

Figure 10.4 – *The operating field after removal of the paramedian segments.*

A series of tributary branches of the right hepatic vein are first encountered along the resection plane. To prevent tearing, it is advisable to retain some parenchyma anterior to the hepatic vein, which is particularly delicate and thin walled. Deeper within the parenchyma, at the level of the hilum, the right paramedian Glissonian pedicle is encountered, running anteriorly and branching off from the lateral pedicle, which has a more posterior course, and running towards Ganz's incisure. The anterior Glissonian pedicle is exposed and clamped *en bloc* with its connective sheath and sutured with Vicryl® (**Figure 10.3b**). Division continues posteriorly, with the fissure of the right hepatic vein as a constant landmark, until the left resection plane is reached. The remaining parenchymal bridge contains the middle hepatic vein which is isolated, clamped and sutured (**Figure 10.3c**). The resected portion is removed together with the gallbladder (**Figure 10.3d**).

Figure 10.4 shows the path of the resection planes, the left one sagittal and the right one oblique; the Glissonian hilum can be seen at the front while at the back the caudate lobe covers the retrohepatic vena cava. Considering the wide exposure of the left hepatic duct, where an additional biliary duct of segment 4 or an anomalous right paramedian duct may branch off, it is particularly advisable to check the integrity of the biliary system with transcystic cholangiography, and to check biliostasis with injection of methylene blue.

11

Surgery of the Caudate Lobe

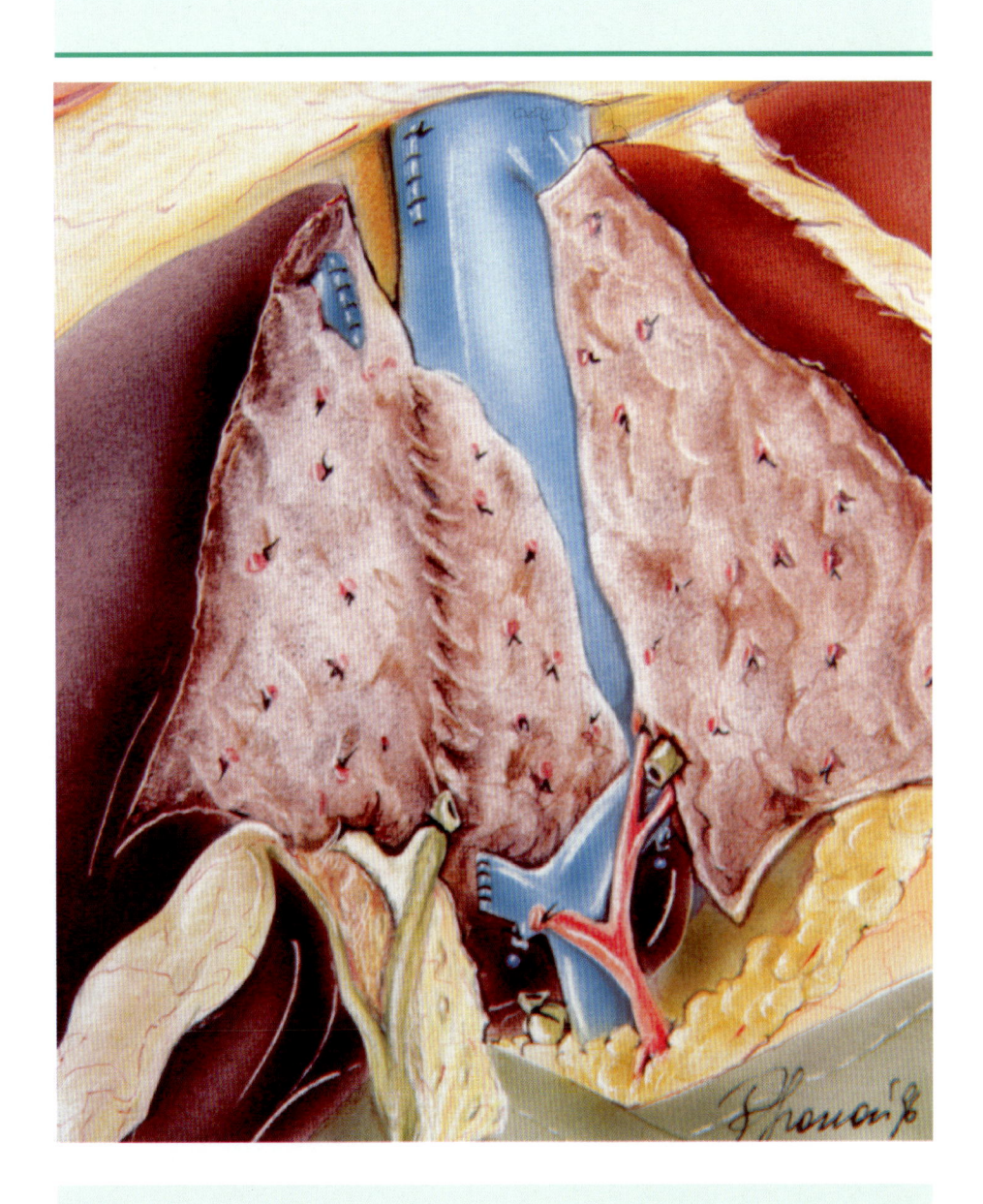

SURGERY OF THE CAUDATE LOBE

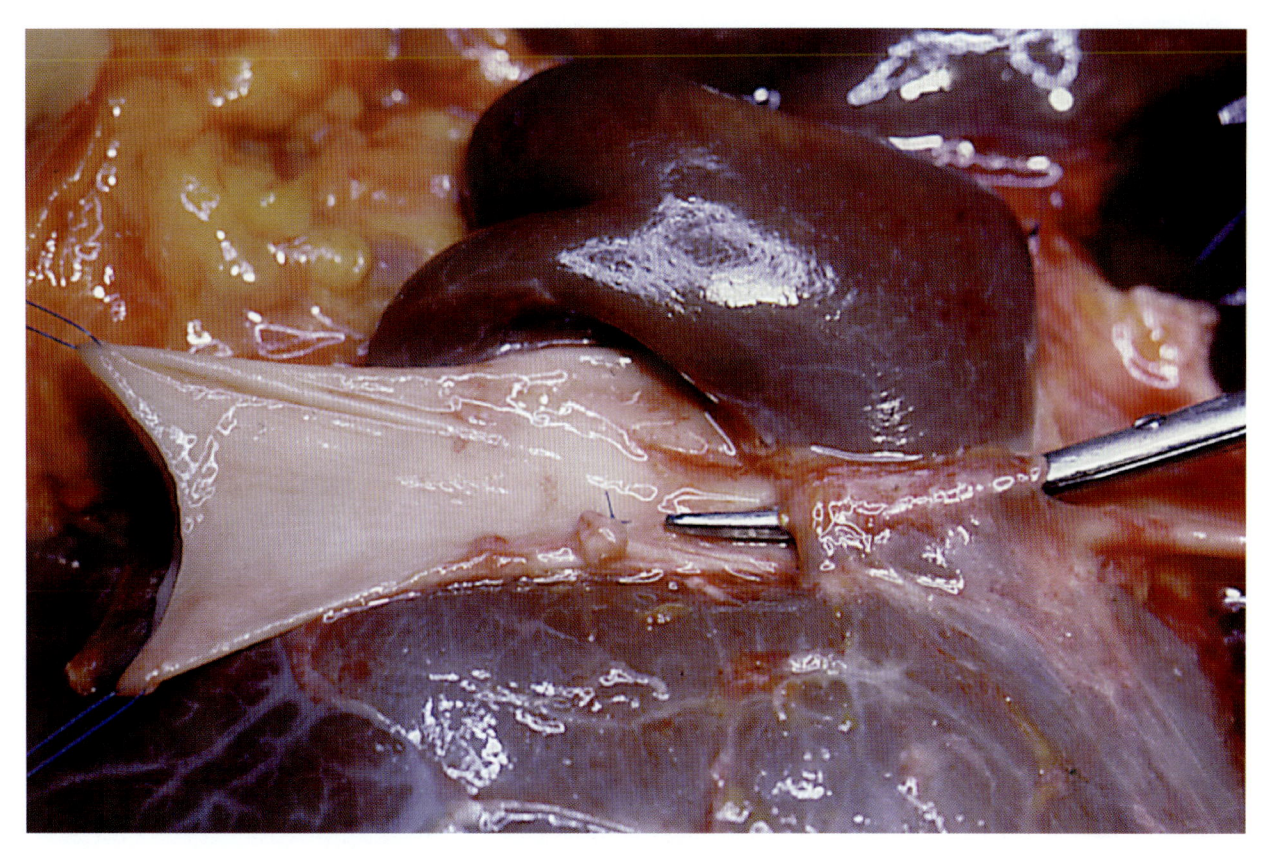

Figure 11.1 – *Posterior aspect of the left part of the caudate lobe (segment 1) in a liver graft. Scissors indicate the dorsal ligament which stretches between the caudate lobe and segment 7.*

Surgical anatomy

The caudate lobe corresponds to the portion of the parenchyma situated behind the Glissonian hilum and in front of the vena cava. It is an independent functional and anatomic unit, consisting of two parts, one situated to the left of the vena cava, which corresponds to the Spigel lobe in the strict sense, or Couinaud's segment 1 (***Figure 11.1***). The second part, or right caudate lobe, extends in front and to the right of the vena cava and terminates at the bottom, with an elevation situated between the right end of the hilum and the anterior aspect of the vena cava, known as the caudate process (this portion of parenchyma has also been defined as Couinaud's segment 9).[2] These two portions, right and left, are joined together by a narrow parenchymal bridge that forms the caudate isthmus.[3] The anterior margin of the right portion of the caudate lobe is delimitated by the course of the posterior right portal pedicle. The medial margin of the caudate lobe is the ligamentum venosum, a remainder of Arantius' duct, stretching between the umbilical portion of the left portal vein and the inferior border of the left hepatic vein, at the confluence with the vena cava. The upper part of the caudate lobe corresponds to the inferior border of the trunk of the three hepatic veins. The right margin of the caudate lobe is less clear and has no precise borders with the parenchyma of segments 8 and 7. A plane, passing between the right posterior branch of the portal vein and the lower border of the right hepatic vein at its outlet into the vena cava, is generally taken as defining the right border of the caudate lobe (***Figures 11.2 and 11.3***). These anatomical features are clearly visible, on ultrasound (***Figure 11.4***).

The two portions of the caudate lobe, right and left, have two independent Glissonian pedicles arising from the right and left

103

TECHNIQUES IN LIVER SURGERY

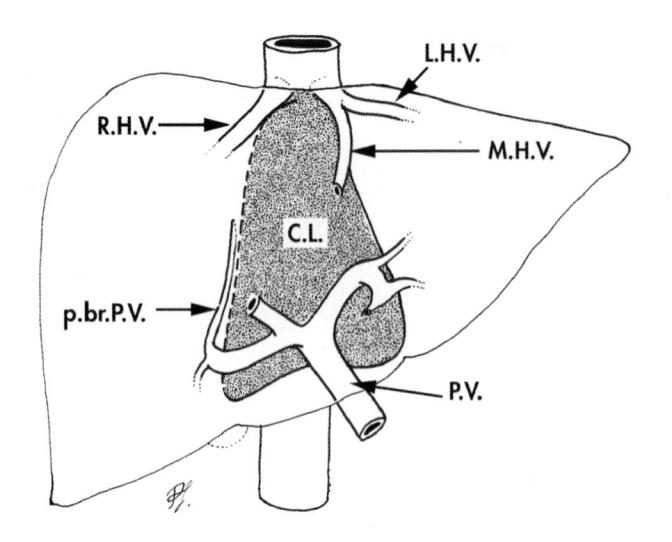

Figure 11.2 – *Landmarks of the caudate lobe (C.L.). P.V.=portal vein, p.br.P.V.=right posterior portal branch and lower margin of the right hepatic vein trunk marks the right border of the caudate lobe.*

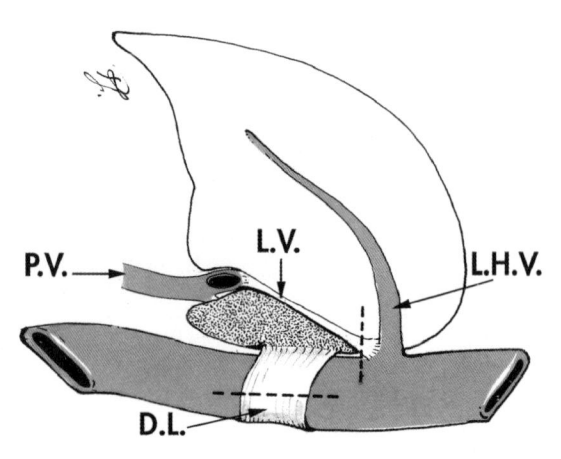

Figure 11.3 – *Diagramatic view of the caudate lobe from the left side. The ligamentum venosum (L.V.) and the dorsal ligament (D.L.) of the vena cava fix the caudate lobe and their division constitutes the key point for the complete detachment of segment 1. P.V.=portal vein trunk, L.H.V.=left hepatic vein.*

Figure 11.4 –
Echographic anatomy of the caudate lobe.
a) Transverse inferior scan. The two parts, right and left, of the caudate lobe (C.L.) can be identified, bordered on the right by the right posterior portal branch (p.br.P.V.) and on the left by the lesser omentum (l.o.). A right inferior hepatic vein flowing into the vena cava (V.C.) can also be seen.
b) Transverse scan on a higher plane, passing over the portal bifurcation. At this level there are no anatomical limits between the caudate lobe and the right hemiliver.
c) Sagittal scan showing the relationship of the caudate lobe with the left hepatic vein (L.H.V.). The ligamentum venosum (L.V.) which divides the caudate lobe from the left lobe of the liver can be seen.

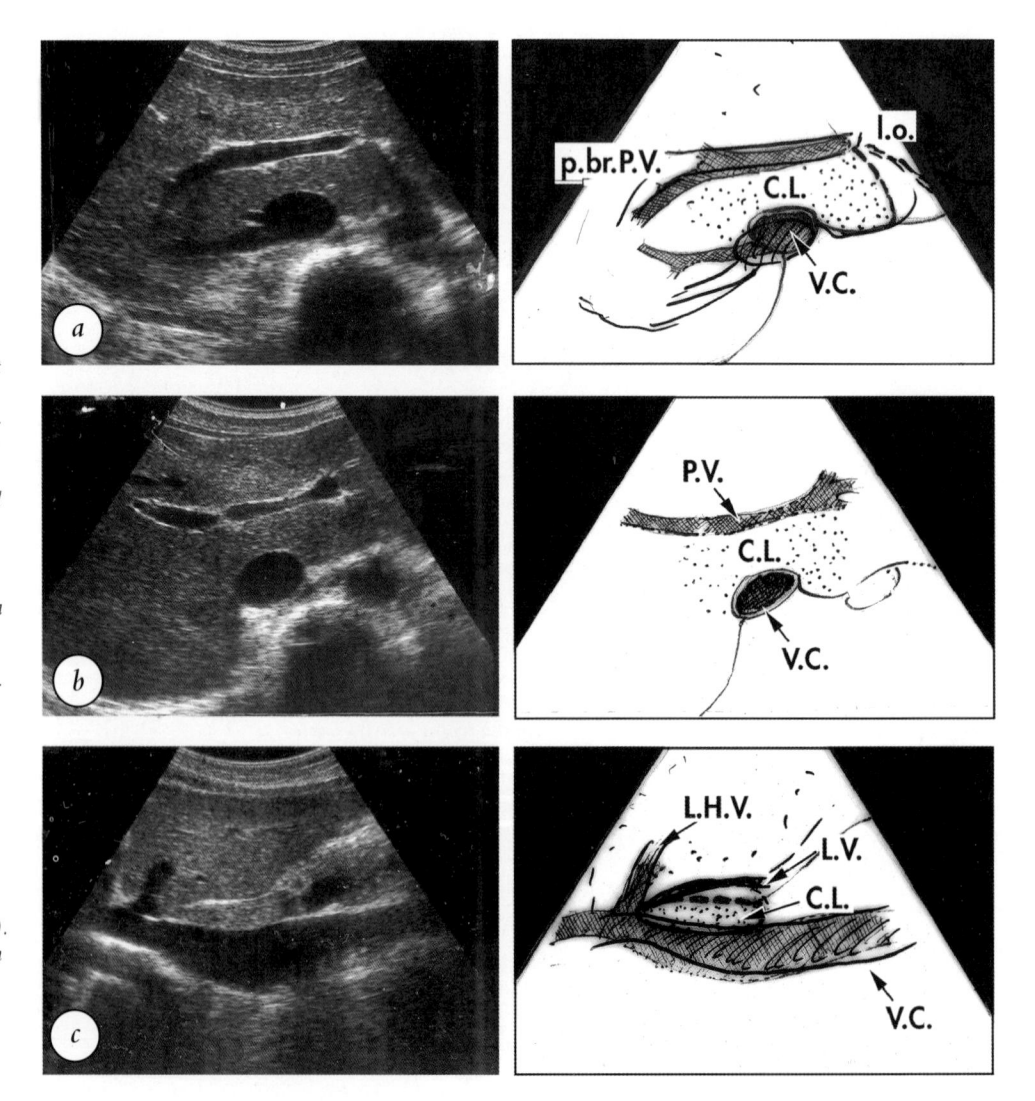

104

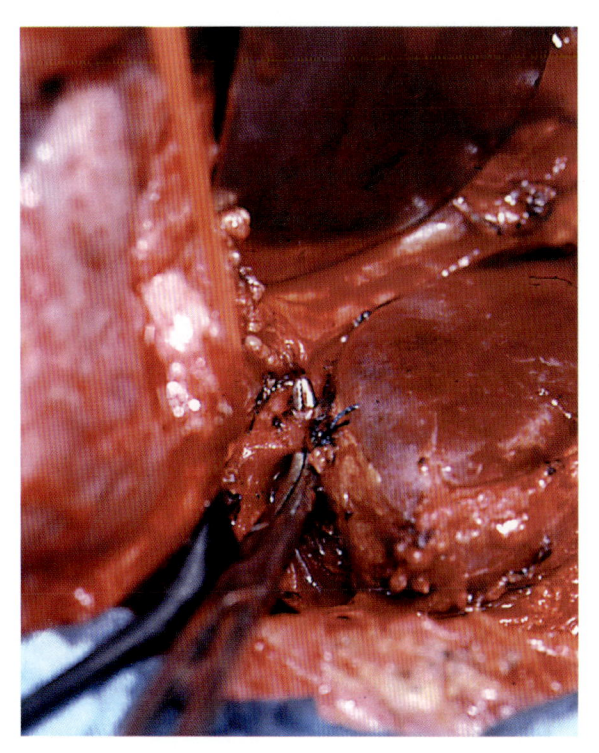

Figure 11.5 – *Ligation of the left portal branch of the caudate lobe. The lesser omentum is divided and the left lobe of the liver lifted upwards and towards the right. The dissector encircles the left portal Spigelian branch.*

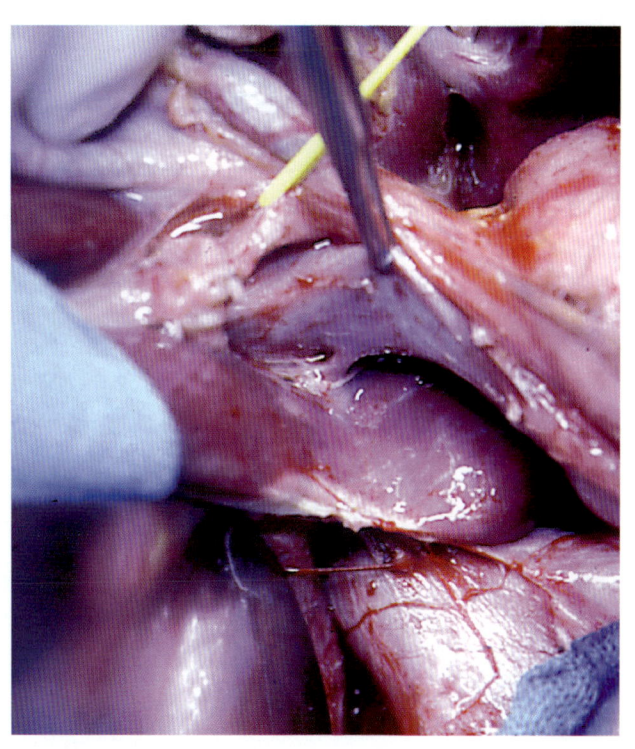

Figure 11.6 – *Right portal branch for the caudate lobe. The posterior peritoneal layer of the hepatoduodenal ligament is divided and the right branch of the portal vein is exposed and lifted. The short Spigelian branch is clearly visible, running between the posterior aspect of the right portal branch and the caudate process.*

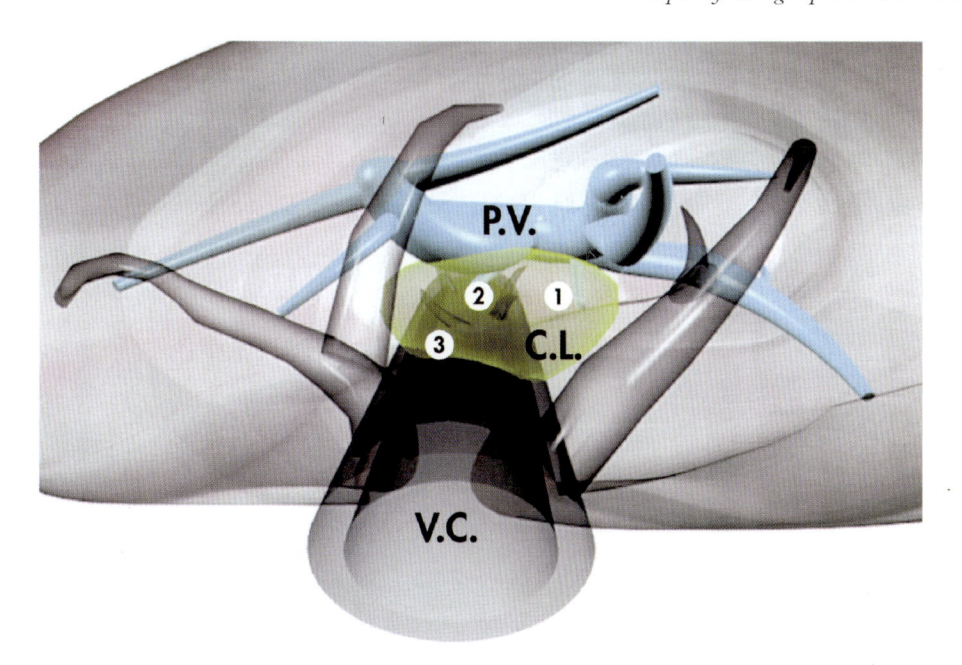

Figure 11.7 – *Diagram of the portal pedicles and the hepatic veins of the caudate lobe seen from above. The caudate lobe (C.L.) is colored yellow, the portal vein (P.V.) light blue and the vena cava (V.C.) dark blue. The two right (1) and left (2) portal branches of the caudate lobe and some Spigelian veins (3) are also shown.*

hemisystems. A constant branch arises from the left branch of the portal vein, and its extra-hepatic course (about 2 cm from the bifurcation) is clearly visible (**Figure 11.5**). The right pedicle may arise from either the right branch of the portal vein or the right posterior segmentary branch (**Figure 11.6**). Mizumoto[10] has described the anatomical variations of caudate lobe vascularization. From a practical point of view it is important to stress that the left branch is a constant feature which arises from the posterior aspect of the left branch of the portal vein and which must be preserved in a conventional left hepatectomy, and of a right, less evident branch, which can arise from the posterior aspect of the right branch of the portal vein and which may be damaged during a right hepatectomy on ligation of the right Glissonian pedicle (**Figure 11.7**).

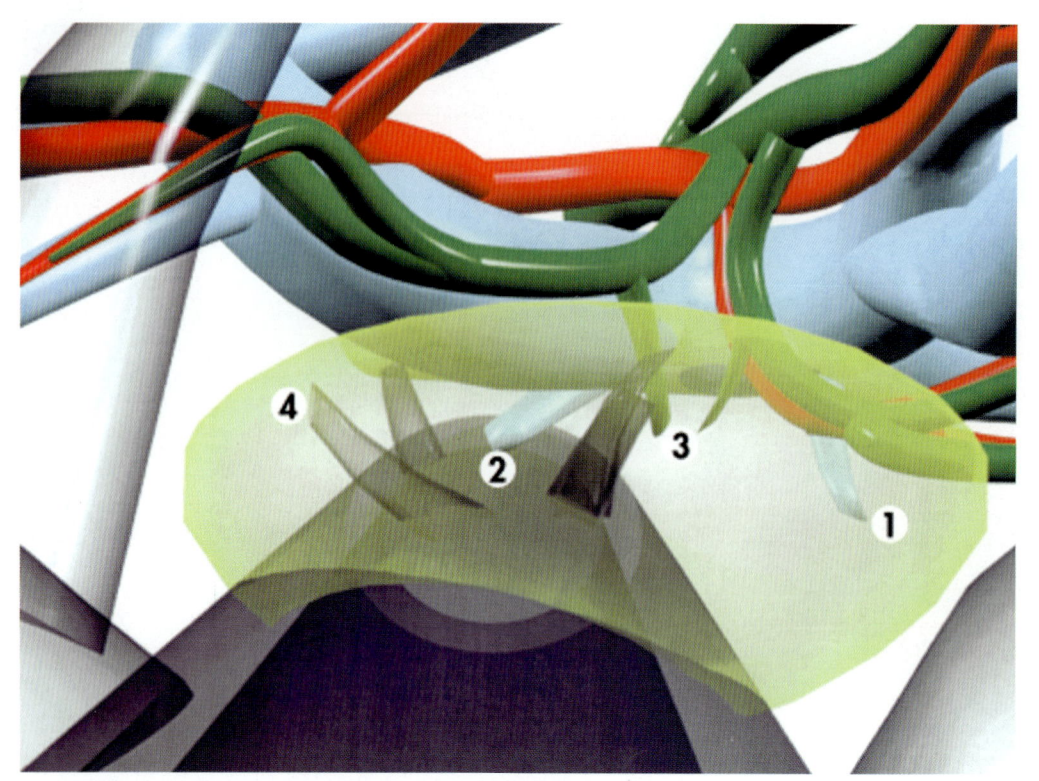

Figure 11.8 – *Diagram of the anatomy of the caudate lobe. The vena cava is colored dark blue, the portal branches light blue, the biliary ducts green and the artery red.*
1) right portal branch for the caudate lobe,
2) left portal branch, 3) right and left biliary ducts,
4) Spigelian hepatic veins.

Arterial circulation is less evident and may present anatomical variations. Generally speaking, however, there are two arterial pedicles, one arising from the left branch of the hepatic artery and one from the right branch.

Biliary drainage of the caudate lobe is through a constant branch which drains posteriorly into the left bile duct and a less evident branch draining into the right posterior segmentary duct close to the biliary confluence (**Figure 11.8**). The close relationship of the caudate lobe bile ducts with the biliary bifurcation are the basis of the constant involvement of the caudate lobe in hilar cholangiocarcinoma (Klatskin tumor). This relationship explains the need for resection of the caudate lobe, associated with resection of the biliary tract, in surgery for cholangiocarcinoma localized at the hepatic hilum, whenever the biliary bifurcation is removed.[8]

Venous drainage of the caudate lobe is directly into the vena cava through a variable number of veins, generally 2-6, which run from the posterior surface of the liver into the vena cava (**Figure 11.7**). This independent venous drainage explains the possibility of direct drainage of the Spigel lobe in the event of obstruction of the main hepatic veins, as for example in Budd-Chiari syndrome in which the caudate lobe develops compensatory hypertrophy which represents a typical diagnostic element.

The deep site of the caudate lobe and the absence of precise landmarks indicating its margins with the remainder of the right hemiliver make resection of the caudate lobe particularly demanding from a technical point of view. The anatomical relationship between the caudate lobe and the biliary bifurcation are of particular relevance. Resection of hilar cholangiocarcinoma cannot be considered oncologically complete unless resection of the caudate lobe is included. Invasion of the caudate lobe may also be a frequent occurrence in the presence of neoplasms of the posterior segments of the liver. The caudate lobe can also be the primary site of a hepatic tumor, hepatocarcinoma or benign tumor. Resection of the caudate lobe can be performed during a right or left hepatectomy, segmentary resection of segments 4 or 5. An isolated resection of the caudate lobe is a more technically complex procedure.

SURGERY OF THE CAUDATE LOBE

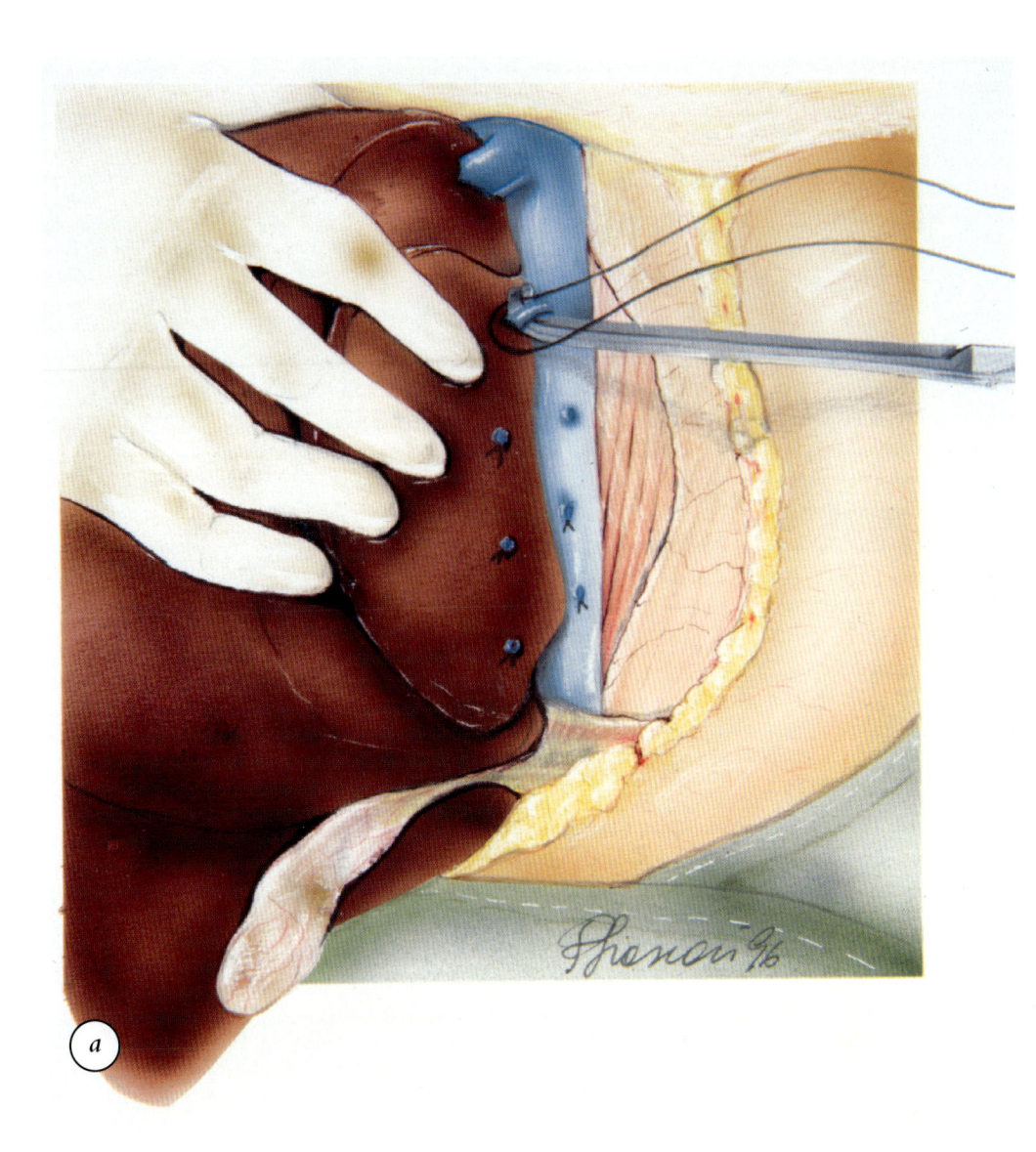

Figure 11.9 –
Left hepatectomy and caudate lobectomy.
a) *Ligature of the Spigelian veins. After dividing the lesser omentum and the posterior peritoneal layer, the caudate lobe is turned upwards and to the right, exposing the Spigelian veins which are divided from the bottom upwards.*
b) *Ligation of the Glissonian pedicles. The vascular structures are divided close to the bifurcation in order to include the pedicles for the left part of the caudate lobe, while the left hepatic duct is divided more distally. The liver is dissected along the Cantlie line.*

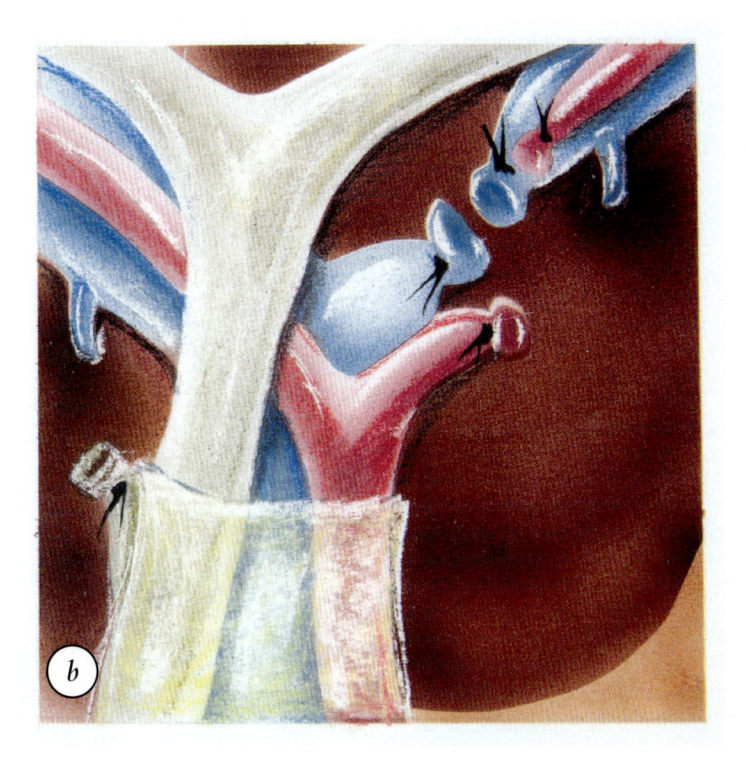

Left hepatectomy extended to the caudate lobe

This technique is indicated for primary tumors or metastases of the caudate lobe of such dimensions that isolated resection of segment 1 is not possible. Another typical indication is represented by cholangiocarcinoma of the biliary confluence, involving mainly the left hepatic duct: the tendency of these tumors to spread along the bile ducts of the caudate lobe makes resection of segment 1, associated with left hepatectomy, obligatory. The liver is completely mobilized and the right and left triangular ligaments, the falciform ligament and the lesser omentum are divided (***Figure 11.9a***). The dorsal ligament of the vena cava which holds the caudate lobe posteriorly is also divided. The peritoneal reflection layer which extends from the caudate lobe to the posterior peritoneum of the lesser sac is dissected, exposing the left aspect of the vena cava. The caudate lobe is elevated to expose the accessory hepatic veins which are ligated and divided. These veins vary in number, the largest being situated in the most cranial portion of the caudate lobe. The Spigelian veins are ligated with a Prolene® 4-0 transfixed stitch on the caval aspect and closed with metal clips on the hepatic aspect.

The left Glissonian pedicle is prepared extra-parenchymally, as for a conventional left hepatectomy: the portal and arterial branches are ligated at the level of the bifurcation in order to include the pedicles for the caudate lobe (*Figure 11.9b*). The parenchyma is divided along the ischemic demarcation line. Having reached the plane of the hilum, the left hepatic duct is encountered and divided immediately proximal to the bifurcation (in the event of hilar cholangiocarcinoma, the entire common bile duct is included in the resection and dissection is performed distal to the bifurcation, on the right hepatic duct or on the two anterior and posterior dividing branches). Only the caudate lobe now remains to be divided which at this level, posterior to the bifurcation of the hilum, is reduced to a thin parenchymal bridge which can be easily dissected if the vena cava has already been detached on both the right and the left (*Figure 11.10*). The last stage of the hepatectomy includes division of the middle hepatic vein and the *en bloc* removal of the left hemiliver (plus the biliary tract in the event of cholangiocarcinoma) and of the caudate lobe. Biliary leakage is checked by injecting air or methylene blue from the cystic duct.

The right part of the caudate lobe is more difficult to remove using a left-sided approach. In the presence of a tumor of the biliary confluence, resection of this portion is easier after the right hepatic duct has been divided distally to the bifurcation, within the parenchyma (at this point the hepatic duct has usually already split into the anterior-paramedian and postero-lateral ducts). Prior ligation of the right Spigelian branch arising from the right portal branch leads to ischemic demarcation of the right caudate lobe which identifies the parenchymal division line. The accessory hepatic veins must also be divided on the right margin of the retrohepatic vena cava. The parenchyma situated posterior to the portal bifurcation, corresponding to the right part of the caudate lobe, can thus be removed *en bloc* together with the remaining resection portion. Clamping of the hepatic pedicle is necessary for this last stage.

Right hepatectomy extended to the caudate lobe

This operation is indicated for infiltration of the caudate lobe by a posterior hepatic tumor. Another typical indication is hilar cholangiocarcinoma involving the right hepatic duct. The approach from the right side certainly makes it easier to remove the caudate lobe completely, including the left and right parts. The description of this technique refers to the case in *figures 11.11-13* of a cholangiocarcinoma of the biliary bifurcation. The access route consists of a subcostal J incision. The liver is completely mobilized, dividing the right and left triangular ligaments, the falciform ligament and the lesser omentum. To the right, division continues until the bare area is completely uncovered, fully exposing the right adrenal gland and the right margin of the vena cava. The most cranial portion of the vena cava must be mobilized by dividing the dorsal ligament of the vena cava which fixes the caudate lobe posteriorly. Once this ligament has been divided the confluence of the right hepatic vein can be exposed and encircled with tape (*Figure 11.12*). When the posterior aspect of the liver is lifted, the accessory hepatic veins are exposed. These veins vary in number and, as they are surrounded by loose connective tissue, dissection with a ligature carrier is straightforward. These veins are sutured and divided. Detachment of the caudate lobe from the vena cava is easier working from the bottom upwards. The left portion of the caudate lobe must also be detached from the vena cava; the liver is turned from the left towards the right, the peritoneal reflection layer is divided on the left margin of the caudate lobe and the short Spigelian veins are divided on the same side. When the posterior surface of the caudate lobe has been detached on both the right and the left, dissection continues as far as the Glissonian hilum.

The first stage is the division of the distal common bile duct above the pancreatic margin (fresh frozen section of the resection margin is systematically carried out when dealing with Klatskin tumors). The lymph nodes of the hepatic pedicle and the entire connective tissue of the pedicle are removed, completely skeletonizing the hepatic artery and the portal vein as far as the bifurcation. The left hepatic

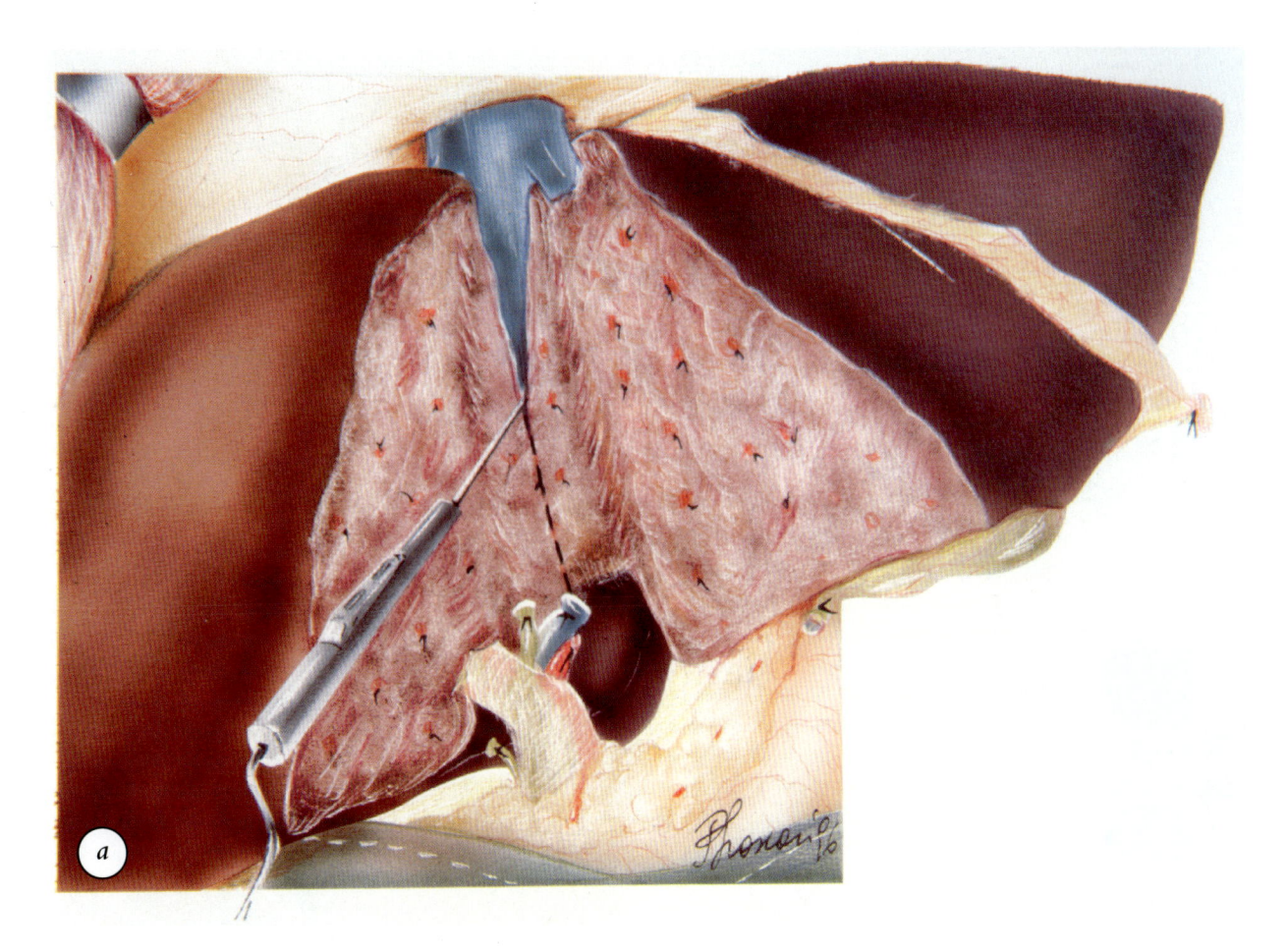

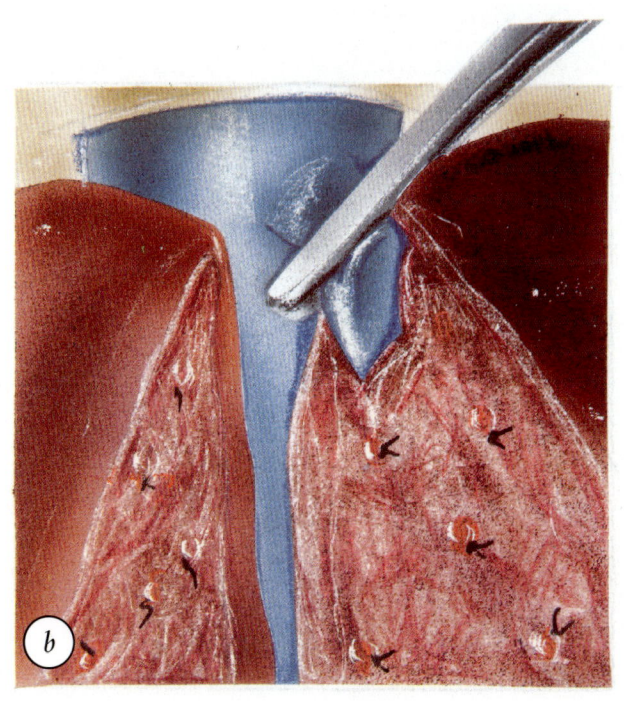

Figure 11.10 – *The caudate lobe is exposed posteriorly to the plane of the hilum. Resection of the left part of the caudate lobe is made easier by previously detaching it from the vena cava by division of the Spigelian veins. The thin bridge of parenchyma situated between the right and left parts of the caudate lobe is divided **a)**. Finally the common trunk of the left hepatic vein is clamped and divided **b)**.*

TECHNIQUES IN LIVER SURGERY

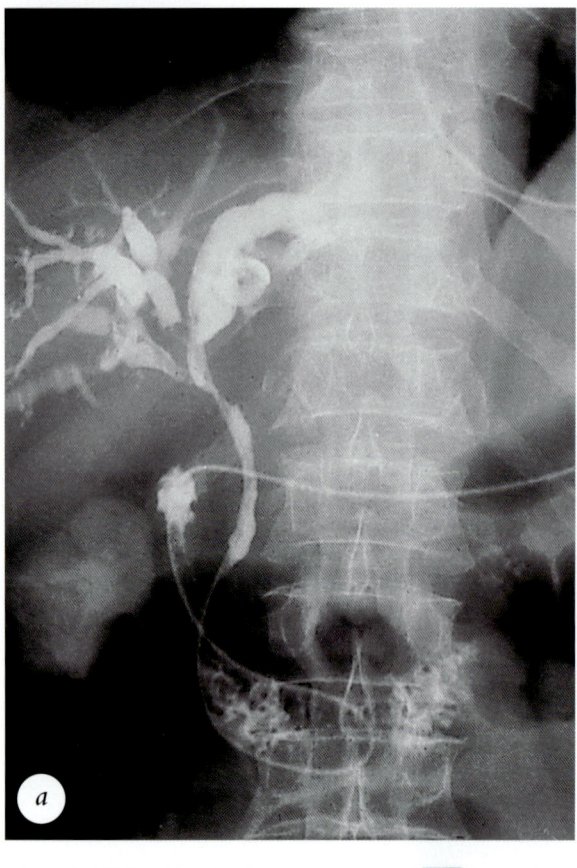

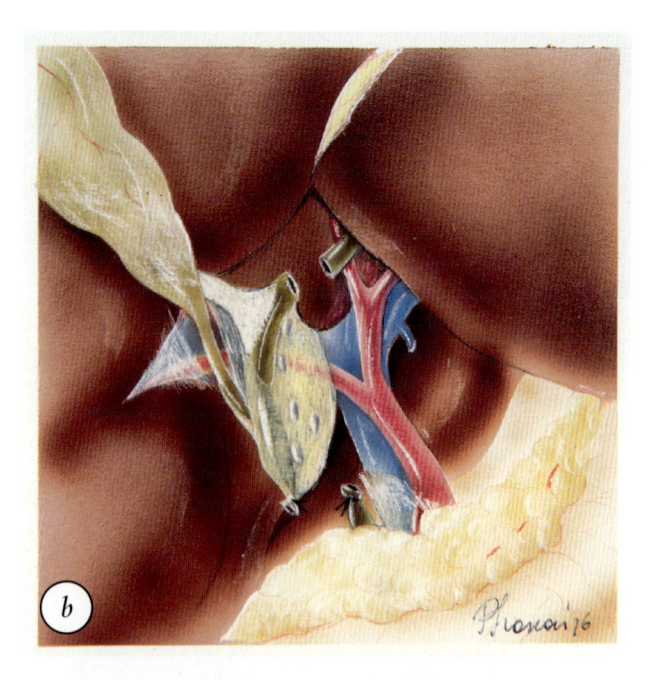

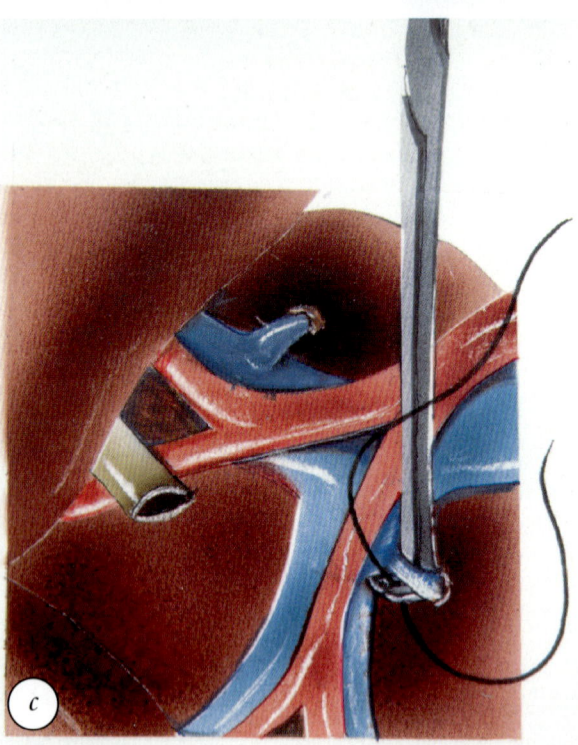

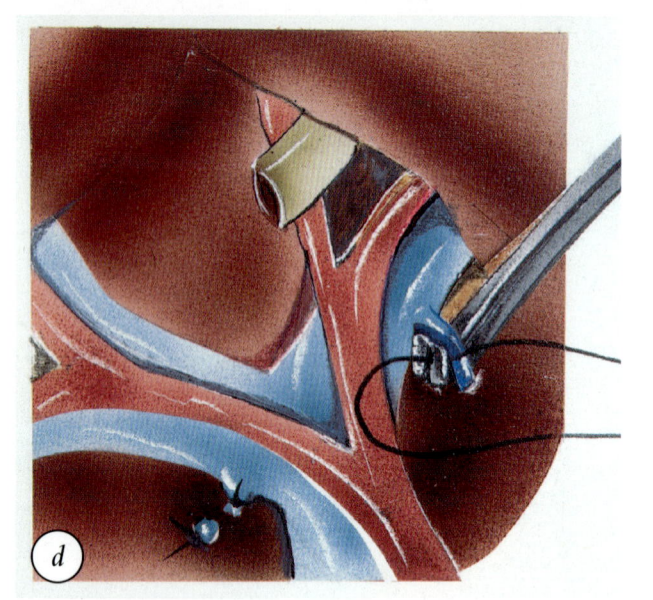

Figure 11.11 – **a)** *Right hepatectomy and total caudate lobectomy for Klatskin tumors.* **b)** *The distal common bile duct has been divided. The hepatic artery and portal vein have been skeletonized from the lymphatic tissue. The left hepatic duct has also been divided distally. The right and left portal Spigelian branches are now ligated and sutured* **c, d).**

SURGERY OF THE CAUDATE LOBE

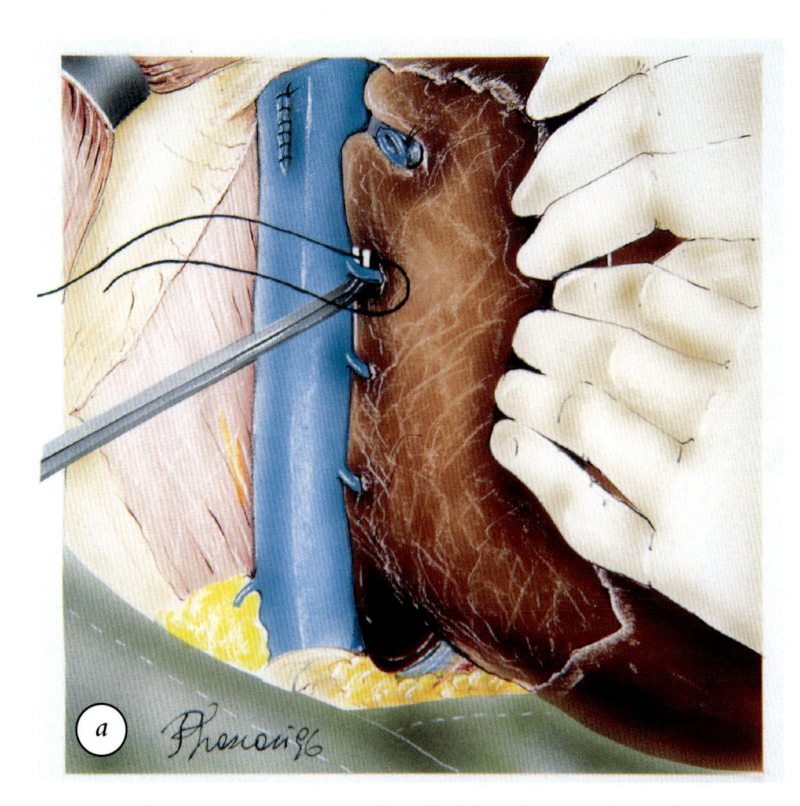

Figure 11.12 – *Right hepatectomy and total caudate lobectomy.* **a)** *After division of the right branches of the hepatic artery and the portal vein and of the right hepatic vein, the hepatic veins of the caudate lobe are divided, detaching the posterior aspect of the caudate lobe from the right aspect of the vena cava.* **b)** *Detachment of the left part of the caudate lobe.*

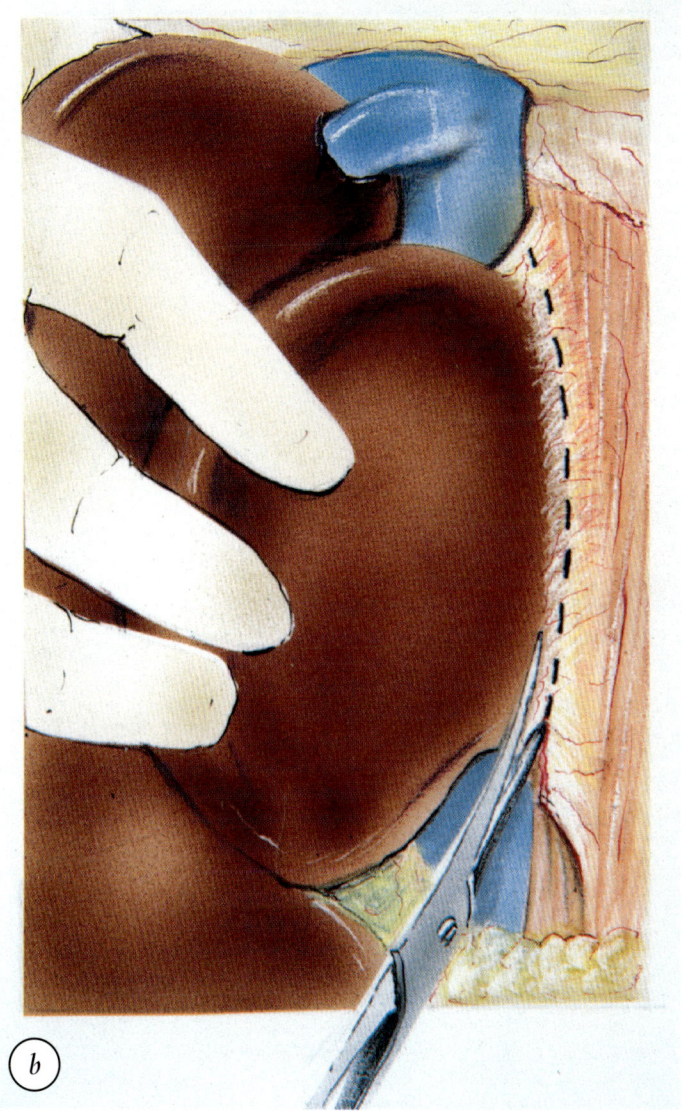

duct is divided distally to the tumor (a fresh frozen section of the resected margin is taken at this stage). Once the right branch of the portal vein has been detached, on its posterior aspect, the short branch for the right part of the caudate lobe is identified. This vein is ligated and divided. Isolation of the left Spigelian portal pedicle is easier. This branch is clearly visible on the lateral aspect of the left branch of the portal vein and is ligated and divided. The right arterial and portal branches are interrupted as for a conventional right hepatectomy. The right hepatic vein, previously isolated, is also clamped, divided and sutured.

Division of the parenchyma continues along the gallbladder–vena cava line as far as the hilar plane. Preliminary division of the left hepatic duct and left Spigelian portal branch exposes the left part of the caudate lobe which remains

TECHNIQUES IN LIVER SURGERY

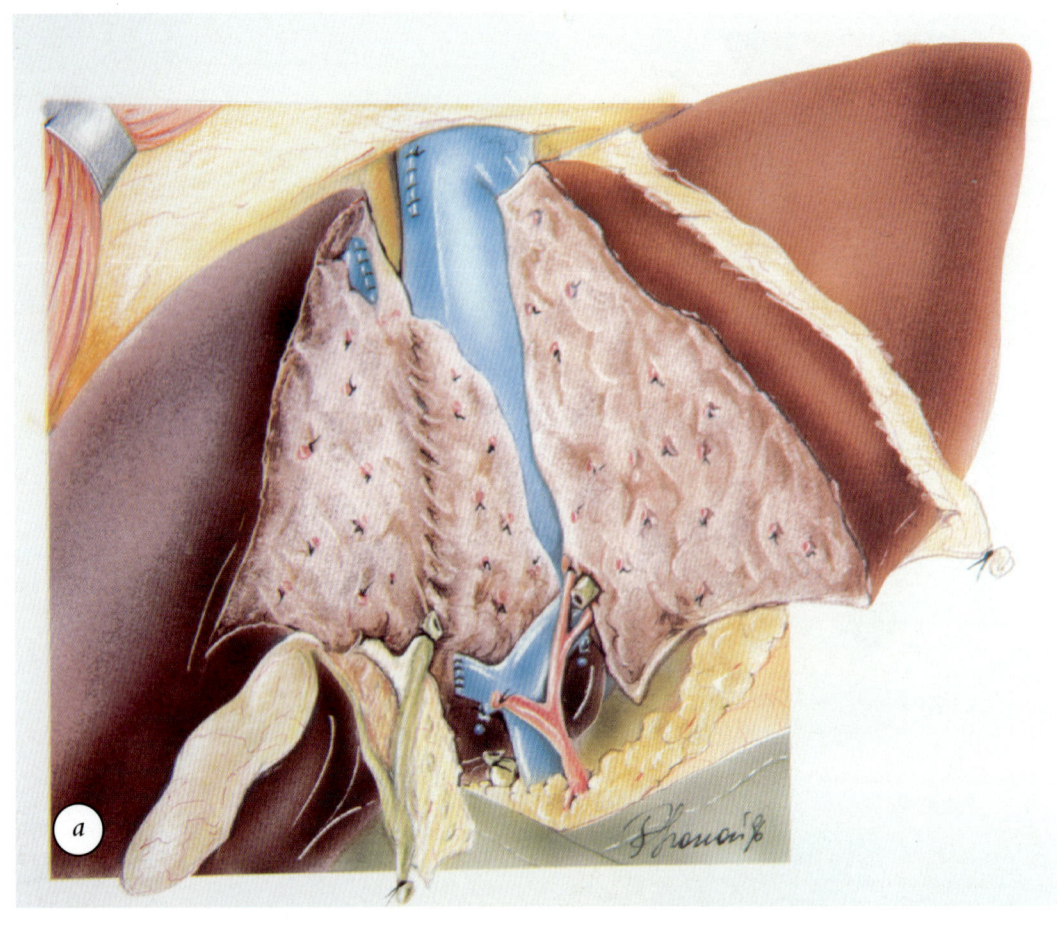

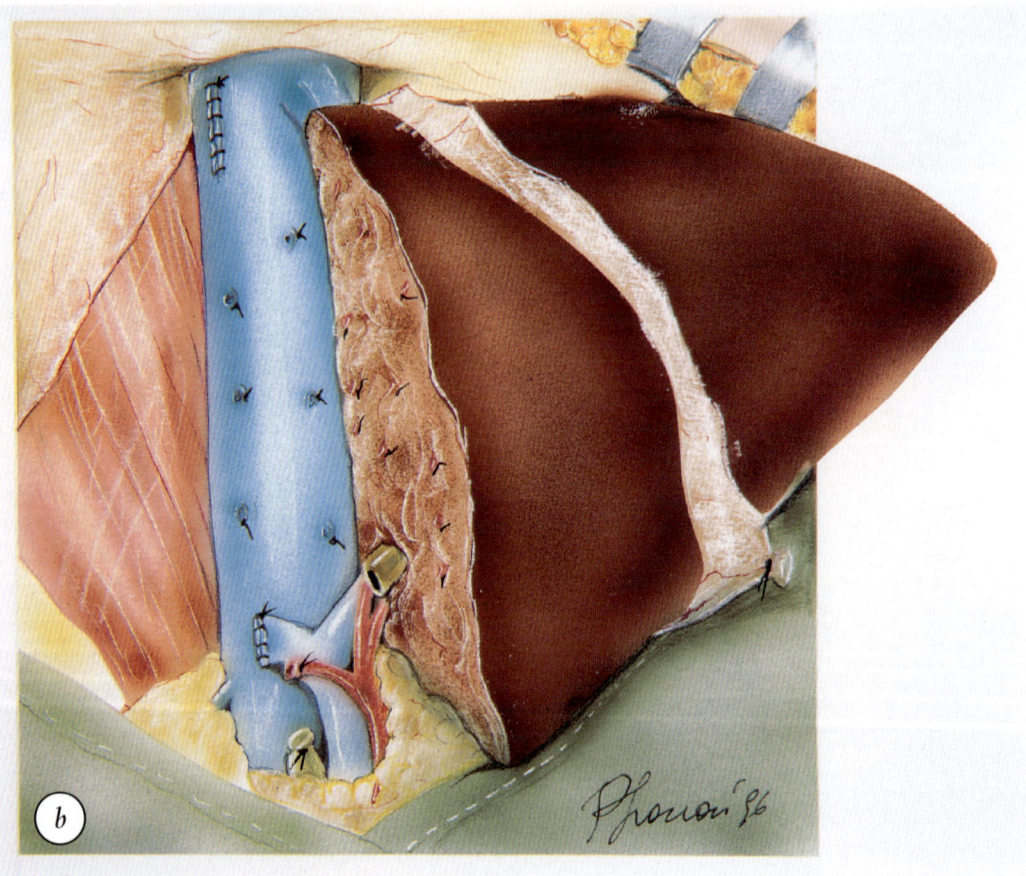

SURGERY OF THE CAUDATE LOBE

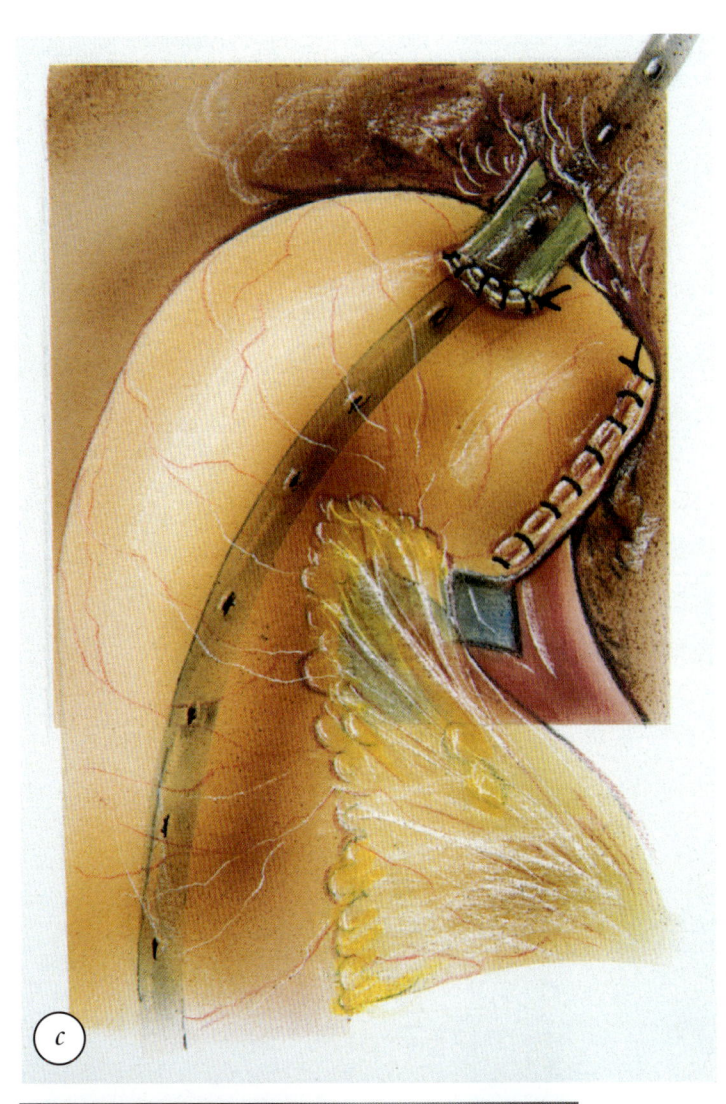

Figure 11.13 – *Right hepatectomy and total caudate lobectomy,* **a)** *Prior detachment of the anterior aspect of the vena cava makes the final stage of the hepatectomy easier* **b)**. **c)** *This is followed by cholangiojejunostomy with a Roux en Y loop on a Silastic stent.* **d)** *Cholangiographic control.*

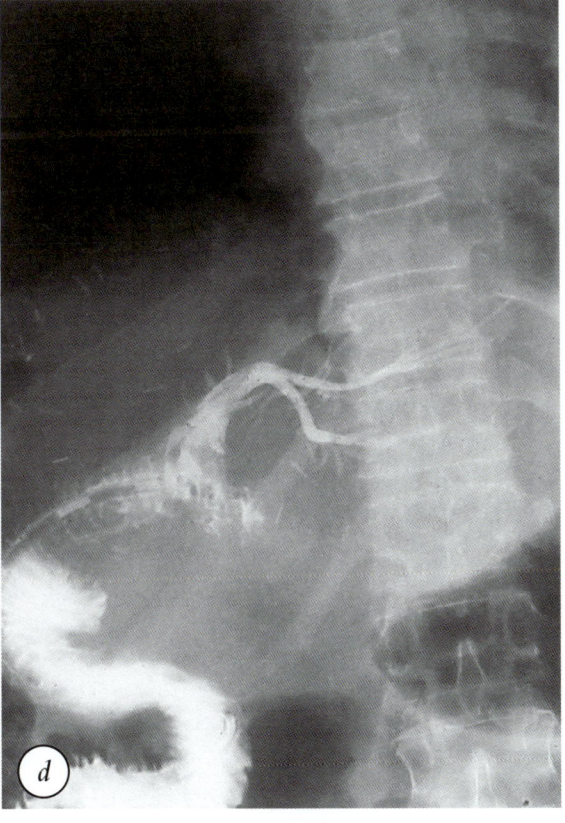

attached to the left hemiliver by the fibrous tissue which corresponds to Arantius's ligament which can be easily divided. At this stage the surgeon's left hand is placed in front of the vena cava, and pulling the left portion of the caudate lobe towards the resected portion. These last stages of the operation are performed with the hepatic pedicle clamped to minimize blood loss. The procedure is completed with anastomosis between the left hepatic duct and a Roux loop of jejunum on a Silastic stent, which is made to drain through the loop about 20 cm from the anastomosis (*Figure 11.13c-d*).

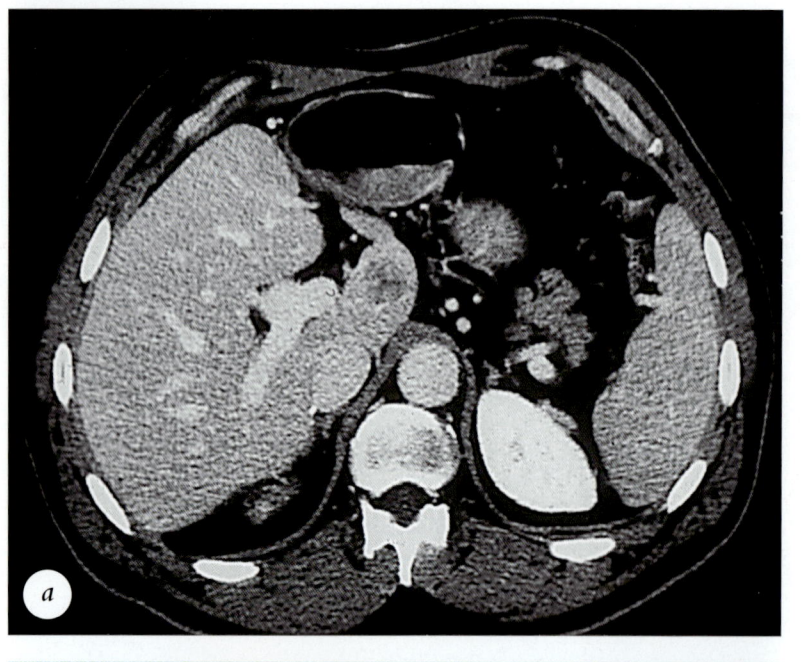

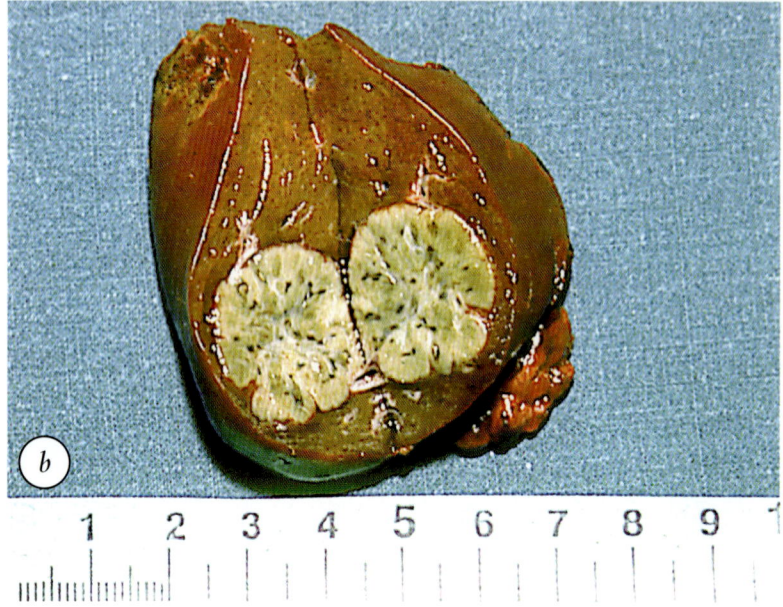

Figure 11.14 – *Isolated resection of segment 1 for metastasis of sarcoma of the eye, which arose nine years after resection of the primary tumor.*
a) Pre-operative CT scan.
b) Resected specimen.

Isolated resections of the caudate lobe

Resection of the left part of the caudate lobe may be indicated for benign tumors, such as adenomas, for malignant tumors localized in the caudate lobe, such as hepatocarcinoma, on cirrhosis, due to the need for limited resection in these cases, or for some metastatic lesions (*Figure 11.14*). The liver is completely mobilized on both the right and left. The right accessory hepatic veins are ligated and divided, the dorsal ligament of the vena cava is divided and the vena cava is prepared above and below the liver, for total vascular exclusion in the event of hemorrhage. The portal pedicle for the caudate lobe is ligated following the left branch of the portal vein along its left aspect. The left part of the liver is lifted upwards and to the right to expose the posterior aspect of the hilum where, inside the Glissonian sheath, the biliary and arterial structures for the caudate lobe are identified, ligated and divided. The caudate process is lifted and the Spigelian veins are ligated, freeing the anterior aspect of the vena cava as far as the outlet of the left hepatic vein, which represents the upper limit of the caudate lobe. The left part of the caudate lobe is now only attached by a thin bridge of parenchyma situated in front of the vena cava which can be easily dissected.

Isolated complete resection of the caudate lobe, including the paracaval portion and the caudate process, without removing other parts of the parenchyma, has occasionally been reported and are extremely complex procedures.[1,4-8,11] All these techniques require extensive exposure of the caudate lobe with complete mobilization of the liver and the retrohepatic vena cava. Finally, the liver is divided along the axis of the sagittal fissure.[5] The Glissonian branches leading to the caudate lobe are ligated on the posterior aspect of the Glissonian hilum. On the left, the caudate lobe is easier to detach after division of the fibrous cord which corresponds to Arantius's ligament. On the right, division of the parenchyma is more arbitrary, remaining between the posterior Glissonian pedicle and the vena cava in the parenchyma of segments 6 and 7. Clamping of the hepatic pedicle is indispensable during this stage of the dissection. Makuuchi[7] uses intraoperative ultrasound to identify the posterior Glissonian pedicle, injecting a dye to stain the parenchyma of segments 6 and 7 and find the correct limit for anatomical resection. Complete mobilization of the liver on the left and the right and exposure of the vena cava are the main preliminary stages for this complex and delicate hepatectomy.

REFERENCES

1. Bartlett D, Fong Y, Blumgart LH. Complete resection of the caudate lobe of the liver: technique and results. *Br J Surg* 1996; **83:** 1076-1081.
2. Couinaud C. The paracaval segments of the liver. *J Hep Bil Pancr Surg* 1994; **2:** 145-151.
3. Dodds WJ, Erickson SJ, Taylor AJ, Lawson TL, Stewart ET. Caudate lobe of the liver: anatomy, embryology and pathology. *Am J Radiol* 1990; **154:** 87-93.
4. Elias D, Lasser Ph, Desrennes E, Makarios N, Jang Y. Surgical approach to segment I for malignant tumors of the liver. *Surg Gynecol Obstetr* 1992; **175:** 17-24.
5. Kosuge T, Yamamoto J, Takayama T, Shimada K, Yamasaki S, Makuuchi M, Hasegawa H. An isolated complete resection of the caudate lobe, including paracaval portion for hepatocellular carcinoma. *Arch Surg* 1994; **129:** 280-284.
6. Leruth J, Grunwez JA, Blumgart LH. Resection of the caudate lobe of the liver. *Surg Gynecol Obstetr* 1990; **171:** 160-162.
7. Makuuchi M, Kawasaki S, Takayama T, Kumon M. Caudate lobectomy. In: Lygidakis NY and Makuuchi M. *Pitfalls and complications in the diagnosis and management of hepatobiliary and pancreatic disease.* Thieme, Stuttgart, 1993. pp. 124-132.
8. Miyagawa S, Makuuchi M, Chisuwa H, Lygidakis NS. Resection of a large liver cell adenoma originating in the caudate lobe. *Hepato Gastroenterol* 1992; **39:** 173-176.
9. Mizumoto R, Kawarada Y, Suzuki H. Surgical treatment of hilar cholangiocarcinoma of the bile duct. *Surg Gynecol Obstetr* 1986; **162:** 153-158.
10. Mizumoto R, Suzuki H. Surgical anatomy of the hepatic hilum with special reference to the caudate lobe. *World J Surg* 1988; **12:** 2-10.
11. Yamamoto J, Takayama T, Kosuge T, Yoshida J, Shimada K, Yamasaki S, Hasegawa H. An isolated caudate lobectomy by the transhepatic approach for hepatocellular carcinoma in cirrhotic liver. *Surgery* 1992; **111:** 699-702.

TECHNIQUES IN LIVER SURGERY

SECTION IV

Techniques with Vascular Involvement

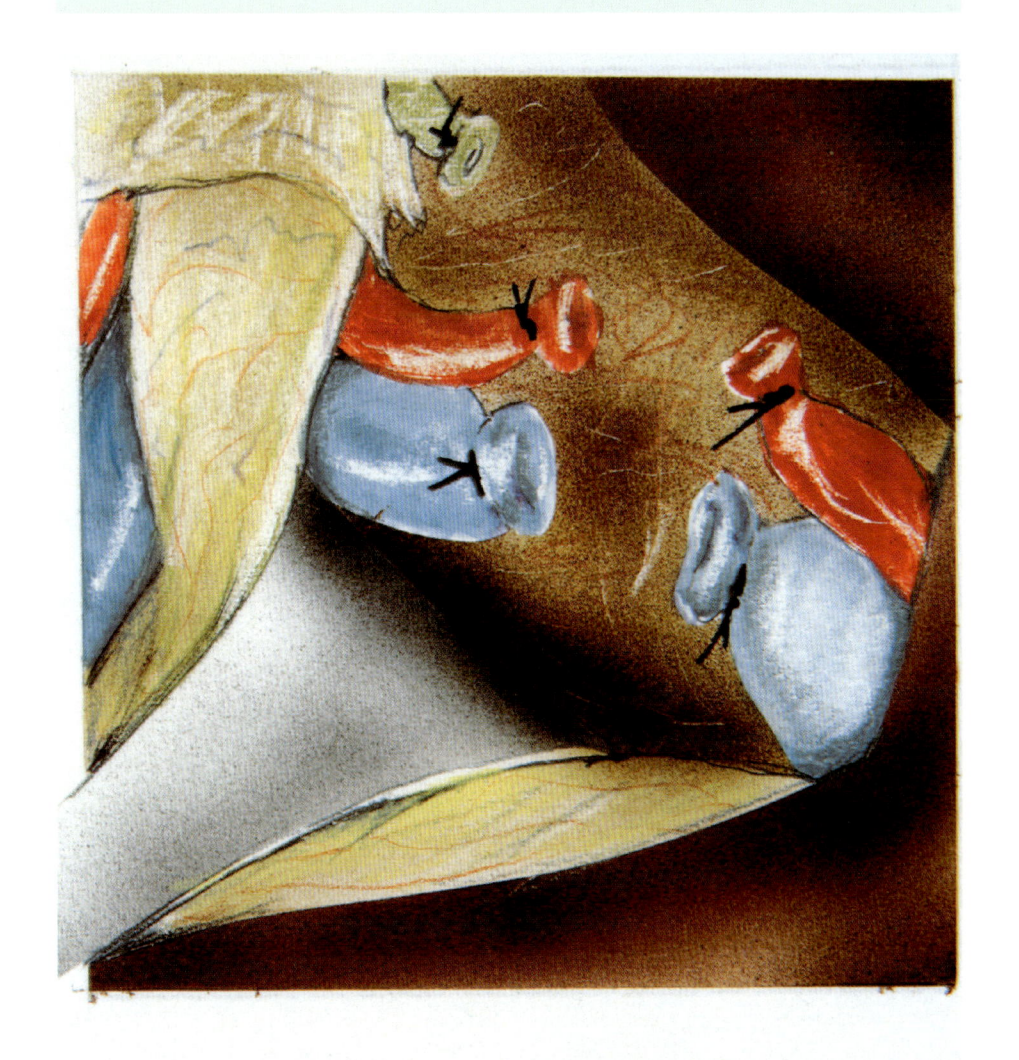

12

Total Vascular Exclusion of the Liver

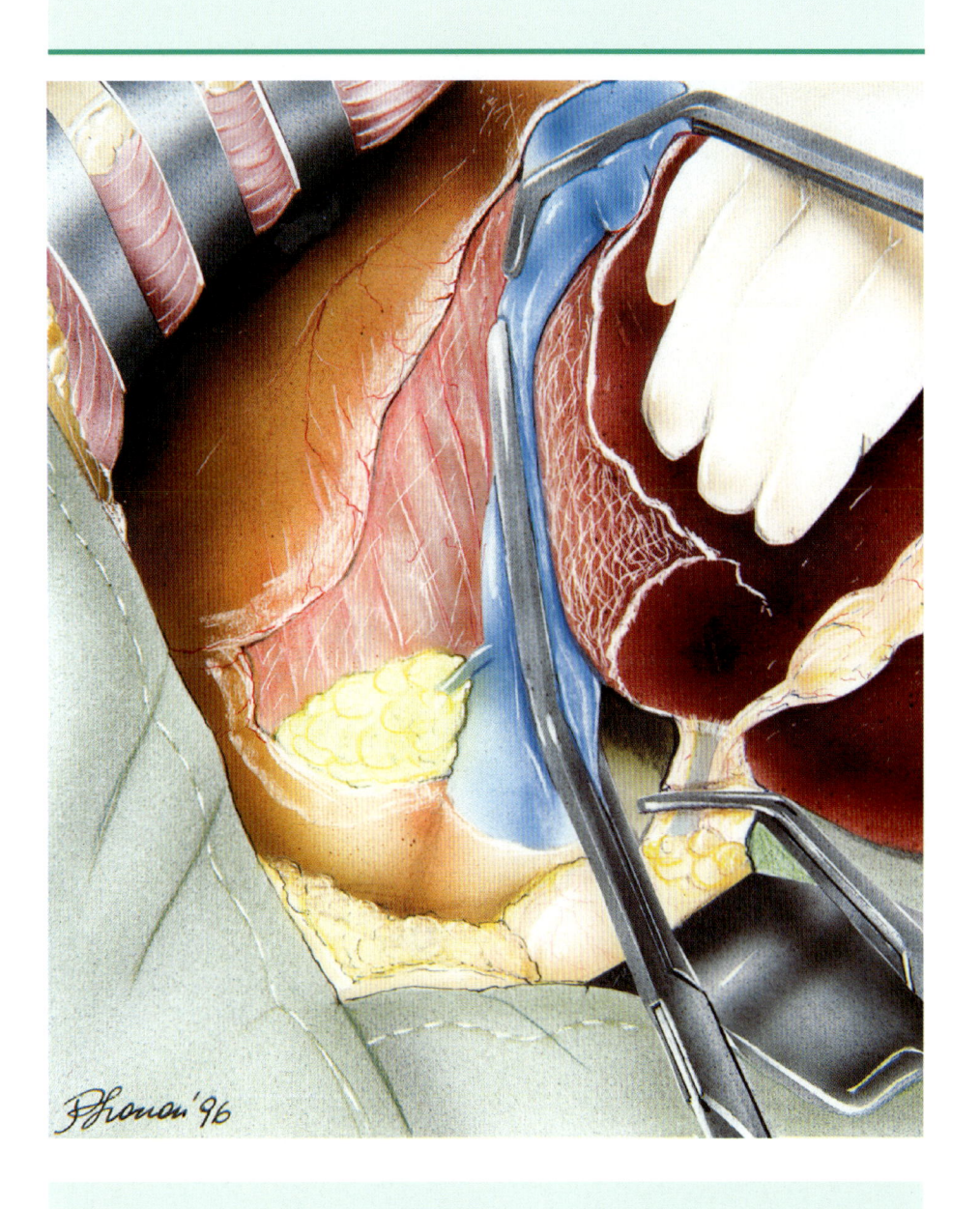

The technique of total vascular exclusion of the liver, introduced by Healey and popularized by Huguet, consists of clamping the hepatic pedicle at the hilum and the vena cava above and below the liver to exclude hepatic inflow from the Glissonian pedicle and outflow from the vena cava. Vascular exclusion makes it possible to operate on a completely bloodless parenchyma. This includes elective procedures, such as resection of neoplastic lesions, which infiltrate the vena cava or the caval-hepatic vein confluence, relative indications, which include all situations involving a particular risk of hemorrhage, such as large posterior tumors or lesions involving both hemilivers requiring extended hepatectomy, and resection of tumors of the caudate lobe which might damage the vena cava.

Vascular exclusion was used in our department in 21 cases out of 800 hepatectomies (2.5%), adopting highly selective indications which essentially included caval infiltrations, tumors involving the suprahepatic confluence or large suprarenal tumors infiltrating the liver.[4]

The hemodynamic consequences of total vascular exclusion of the liver are; a decrease in cardiac index from 30 to 60%, a decrease of pulmonary arterial pressure, and an increase in heart rate and peripheral vascular resistance which compensates for the effects on systemic arterial pressure.[3] Various elements are involved in modifying the individual response to vascular clamping, such as the volume of circulating blood and cardiac function in addition to the presence of porto-systemic and caval-caval collateral circulations and the intensity of the vasoconstrictor response. Individual variations in response to clamping necessitate a clamping test before starting transection of the liver.[7] Complete anesthesiological monitoring, including determination of cardiac index and pulmonary capillary pressure, is essential in planning operations with total vascular exclusion. Before beginning the clamping test, any hypovolemia or pre-existing anemia must be corrected. During the clamping test interference with anesthetic drugs must be excluded. The accepted limit is a reduction in arterial pressure of not more than 30% below the pre-clamping value. Hemodynamic tolerance to clamping is generally good, as long as specific measures are observed, and with close cooperation and understanding with the anesthetic team. In patients with correct vascular filling and without anemia, hemodynamic intolerance to clamping may depend on a pre-existing cardiopathy or on chronic treatment with beta blockers, which alter the vasoconstrictor response and reduce heart rate. Most of the time, however, the hemodynamic drownback is due to an incorrect clamping technique, as a result of which the liver continues to receive a quantity of blood that remains trapped in the parenchyma, creating a situation of hemodynamic sequestration. In these conditions, the blood generally originates from a collateral of the vena cava, the posterior diaphragmatic vein or the right suprarenal vein, not included in the caval clamping. In this case, the liver appears congested and a resection performed under these conditions can cause severe hemorrhage. Hemodynamic intolerance to clamping in the absence of a technical problem or incorrect anesthesiological support is rare and is only observed in patients with ischemic cardiopathy, or cardiopathy induced by prolonged chemotherapy, or by the use of beta blockers which reduce cardiac adaptability to reduced blood flow. True hemodynamic intolerance to clamping, with a drop in cardiac index of more than 50%, may indicate the need to clamp the aorta below the diaphragm. It should nevertheless be stressed that prolonged aortic clamping involves a significant risk of renal and intestinal ischemia. Another more logical solution in such cases is the application of a venous bypass fed by a Bio-Pump, as commonly used in liver transplants. Out of 21 cases of total vascular exclusion of the liver in our department, only once was hepatectomy abandoned, after a clamping test in a 65-year-old patient with ischemic cardiopathy.

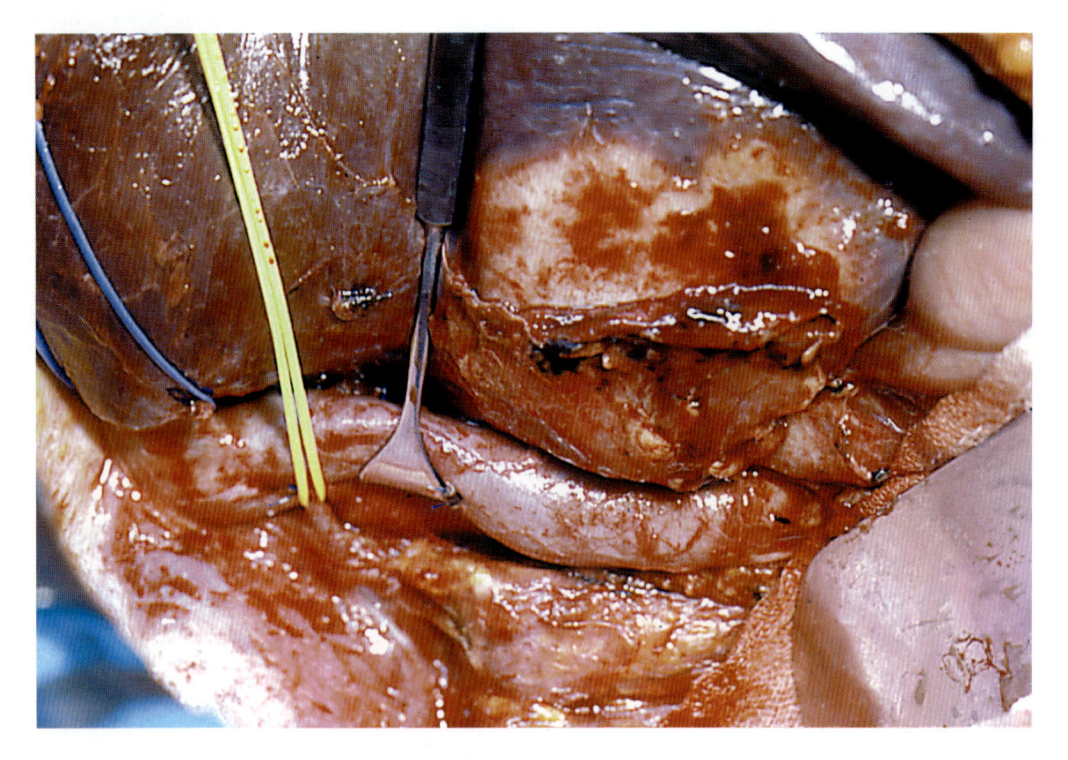

Figure 12.1 – *Posterior diaphragmatic vein (encircled with yellow tape) which drains into the posterior aspect of the vena cava, immediately below the trunk of the right hepatic vein (encircled with a blue tape) in a patient with a large tumor of segment 6 extended to the caudate lobe.*

Normal hepatic parenchyma will tolerate vascular exclusion for up to 45 minutes.[6,8,9] Huguet and Hannoun have recently shown that clamping can be prolonged, in particular situations, for even longer than an hour.[5,8] Initial hepatic function must be normal. Vascular exclusion in cirrhotic patients[2] and mainly in patients with biliary obstruction must be considered very carefully.[10] A randomized study was carried out by Belghiti to evaluate the effects of total vascular exclusion with respect to pedicular clamping in a series of non-cirrhotic patients submitted to major hepatectomy. It was not possible to perform total vascular exclusion in 5 out of 46 patients due to poor hemodynamic tolerance. No differences were observed between vascular exclusion and pedicular clamping in terms of intraoperative blood loss, of the need for transfusions and of the increase in transaminases and creatinine in the post-operative period. There was, however, a greater number of post-operative complications in the total vascular exclusion group.[1] Vascular exclusion is nevertheless a complex procedure which requires adequate anesthesiological support and should be reserved for special situations of more difficult hepatectomies, especially in the presence of caval involvement by hepatic tumors.

Technique

The technique of vascular exclusion involves extensive mobilization of the retrohepatic vena cava. The dorsal ligament of the vena cava must be divided completely to expose the vein and determine the presence of a posterior diaphragmatic collateral which may drain more distally into the vena cava (***Figure 12.1***). The peritoneum which covers the left margin of the vena cava is divided and left in contact with the vein which is then encircled with tape above and below the liver. The inferior clamp, positioned first, must be placed very obliquely so as to exclude the right suprarenal vein. A long De Bakey clamp is particularly suitable for this purpose. A clamp is then placed on the hepatic pedicle. The possible presence of a left hepatic artery on the superior aspect of the hepatogastric ligament must be ascertained and if present clamped separately. Clamping of the suprahepatic vena cava is then carried out, including a portion of the diaphragm, taking care to occlude the right and left hepatic veins and the posterior diaphragmatic vein with the clamp. It is important that the ends of the two caval clamps touch each other, thereby excluding all the venous collaterals (***Figure 12.2***). At times, as a result of particular

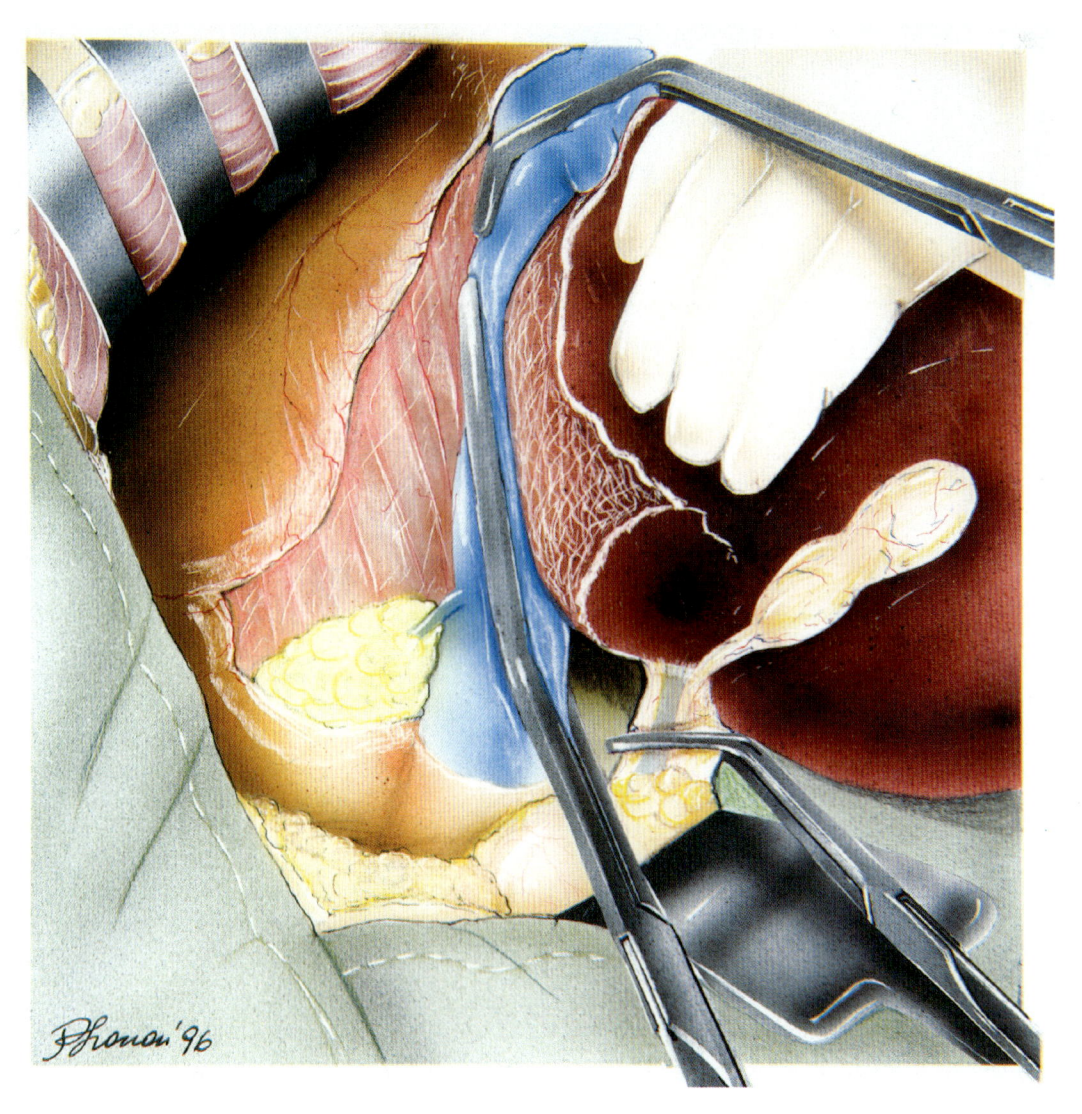

Figure 12.2 –
Position of the clamps for total vascular exclusion of the liver.

situations in the presence of large tumors which infiltrate the vena cava or the adrenal loggia, exposure of the retrohepatic vena cava is not easy and the distal clamp must be positioned without having identified the right adrenal vein. The clamping test with evaluation of the appearance of the liver is particularly useful in such cases.

REFERENCES

1. Belghiti J, Ballet T, Zante E, Ashehoug J, Noun R, Sauvanet A. Portal triad clamping versus total vascular exclusion for major liver resection. A randomized study. *Ann Surg* 1996; **224**: 155-161.
2. Bismuth H, Castaing D, Garden OJ. Major hepatic resection under total vascular exclusion. *Annals of Surgery* 1989; **210**: 13-19.
3. Delva E, Barrbeousse JP, Nordlinger B et al. Hemodynamic and biochemical monitoring during major liver resection with use of hepatic vascular exclusion. *Surgery* 1984; **95**: 309-318.
4. Grazi GL, Mazziotti A, Jovine E, Cavallari A. Total vascular exclusion of the liver: selective use, extensive use or abuse? *Arch. surg*. In press.
5. Hannoun L, Borie D. Delva E, Jones D, Nordlinger B, Parc R. Liver resections with normothermic ischemia exceeding one hour. A ten year experience. *Br J Surg* 1993; **80**: 1161-1165.
6. Huguet C, Nordlinger B, Galopin JJ, Bloch P, Gallot D. Normothermic hepatic vascular occlusion for extensive hepatectomy. *Surg Gynecol Obstetr* 1978; **147**: 689-693.
7. Huguet C, Addario-Chieco P, Gavelli A, Arrigo E, Harb J, Clement R. Technique of hepatic vascular exclusion for extensive liver resection. *Am J Surg* 1992; **163**: 602-605.
8. Huguet C, Gavelli A, Addario-Chieco P, et Al. Liver ischemia for hepatic resection: where is the limit? *Surgery* 1992; **11**: 251-259.
9. Nagasue N, Yukaya H, Ogawa Y, Hirose S, Okita M. Segmental and subsegmental resections of the cirrhotic liver under hepatic inflow and outflow occlusion. *Br J Surg* 1985; **72**: 565-568.
10. Thomas PG, Baer HU, Matthews JB, Gertsch P, Blumgart LH. Post-operative hepatic necrosis due to reduction in hepatic arterial blood flow during surgery for chronic biliary obstruction. *Dig Surg* 1990; **7**: 31-33.

13

Liver Resections with Involvement of the Retrohepatic Vena Cava

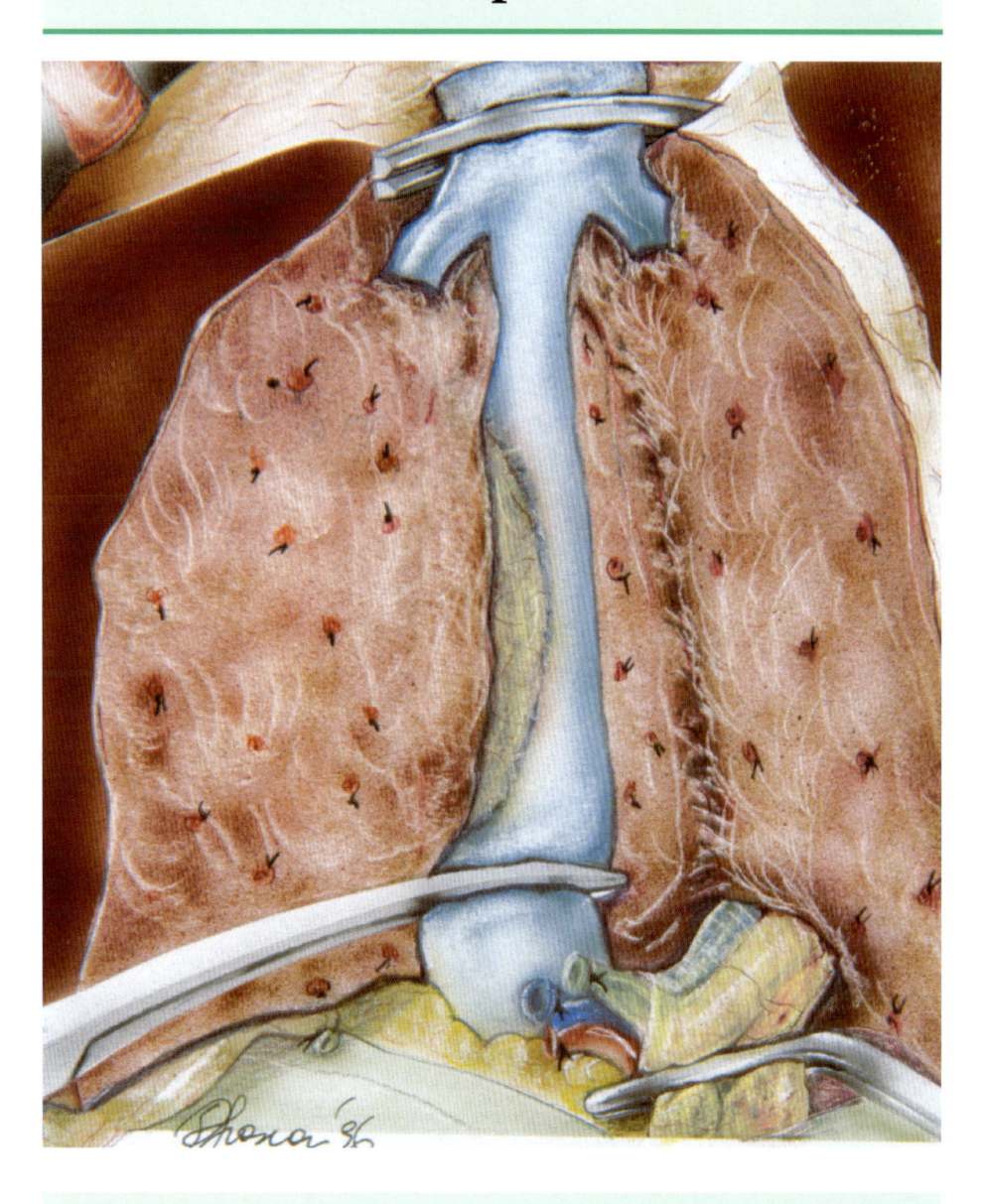

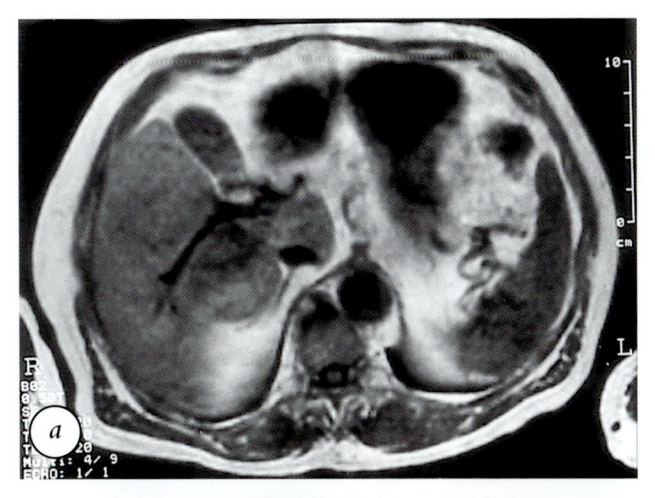

Figure 13.1 – *Hepatocellular carcinoma in a patient with chronic hepatitis. Right lateral bisegmentectomy with partial resection of the IVC.*
a) *Pre-operative MRI showing the tumor, located in segment 6 adjacent to the wall of the vena cava.*
b) *Clamping of the lateral arterial and portal pedicles with ischemia of segments 6 and 7.*
c) *Clamping of the vena cava in the zone infiltrated by the neoplasm and en bloc resection of segments 6 and 7, together with a part of the infiltrated caval wall. The vena cava was sutured directly with a Prolene 4-0 whipstitch.*
d) *The operative field at the end of the resection.*

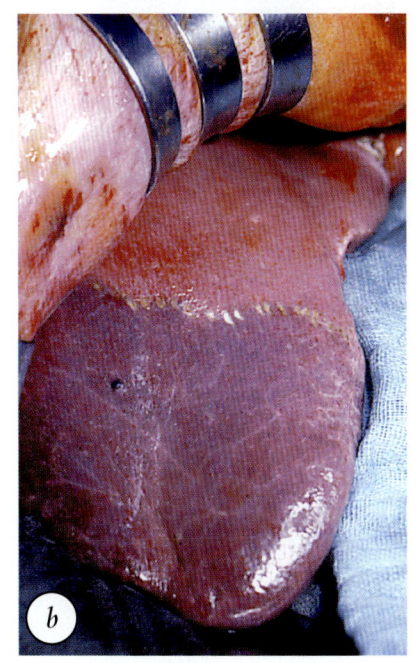

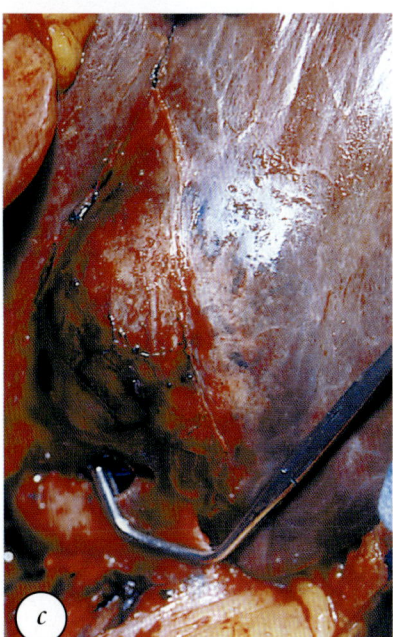

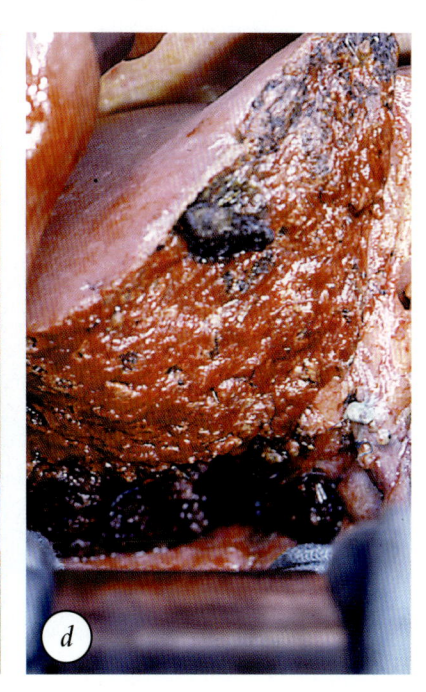

Invasion of the vena cava may occur in posterior tumors of the liver, localized in segments 6, 7 and 8 or in the caudate lobe. A complete thrombosis of the vena cava is rarely an indication for resection. The most appropriate indication is infiltration of the wall of the vena cava as the result of an adjacent tumor of the posterior aspect of the right lobe or the caudate lobe.[2-5] Pre-operative radiological assessment must clarify the extent of the invasion of the vena cava, the involvement of the main hepatic veins and the relationships with the hilar structures in addition to the intrahepatic extent of the tumor. Magnetic resonance imaging with sagittal and transverse scans provides the greatest amount of information. Cavography is advisable, as is arteriography to exclude arterial and portal involvement of the remaining segments of the liver. These examinations are very useful in establishing the presence of an intraluminal involvement but do not make it possible to assess the exact extent of the vessel wall infiltration. Operative strategy is often changed during the operation itself as a result of surgical exploration or intraoperative ultrasound, which is particularly useful in these situations to assess the extent of the tumor and the extent of the infiltration of the vena cava in relation to the convergence with the hepatic veins.

Involvement of the vena cava requires total vascular exclusion of the liver. Some limited infiltrations of the caval wall can, however, be resected with lateral clamping of the vein wall, without total interruption of the caval flow (***Figure 13.1***). In our experience, caval involvement during liver resection was observed in 1% of hepatectomies (8/800).[6] In 6 cases, partial resection of the caval wall was

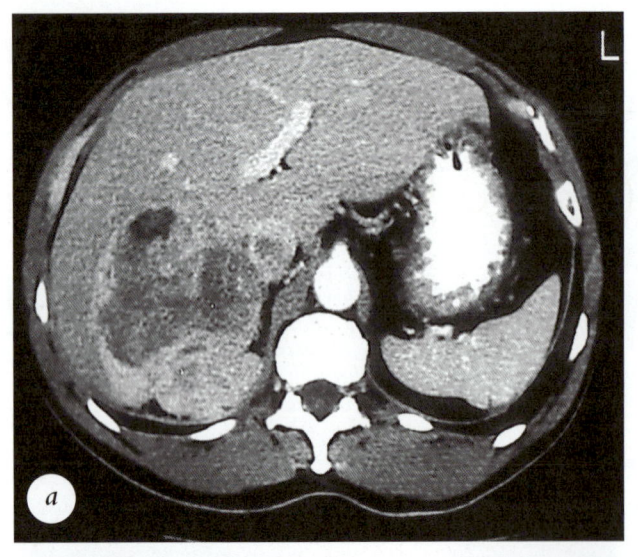

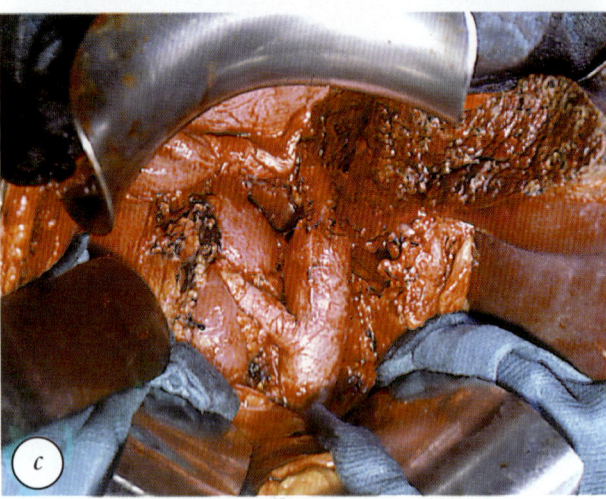

Figure 13.2 – *Adrenal paraganglioma with infiltration of the right lateral segments of the liver and of the retrohepatic vena cava. Right hepatectomy and caval resection under total vascular exclusion.* ***a)*** *Preoperative CT scan showing the tumor and a thrombus in the caval lumen.* ***b)*** *Cavography showing the extent of the caval infiltration and the intraluminal thrombus.* ***c)*** *The operative field after right hepatectomy and resection of a portion of the caval wall 3 cm long and 1.5 cm wide. The vena cava was sutured with a Prolene® 4-0 whipstitch. Total vascular exclusion was applied at the end of parenchymal dissection, just before resection of the caval wall infiltrated by the tumor, thus limiting vascular exclusion to 35 minutes.* ***d)*** *Surgical specimen comprising en bloc the adrenal tumor, the right hemiliver and the caval wall.*

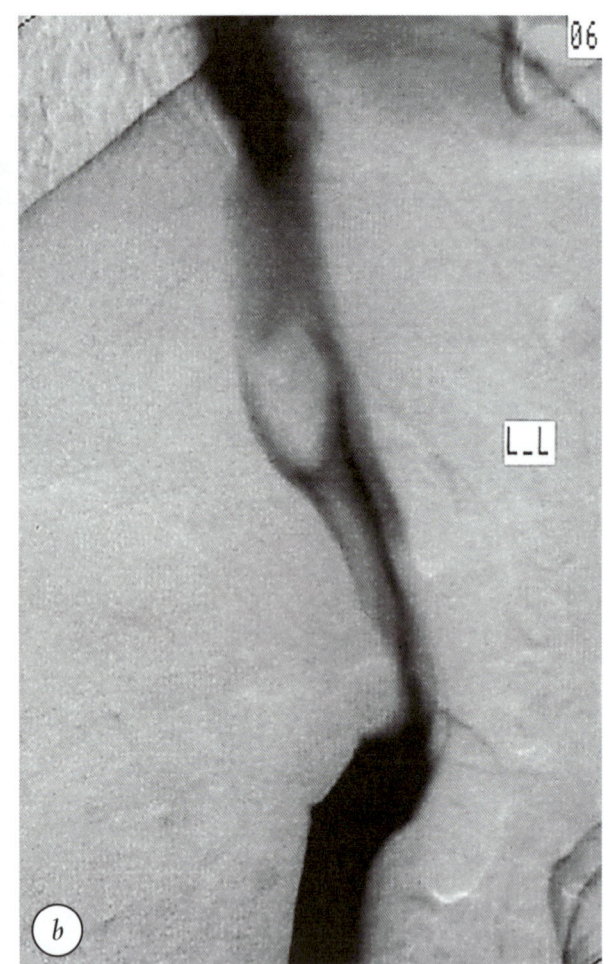

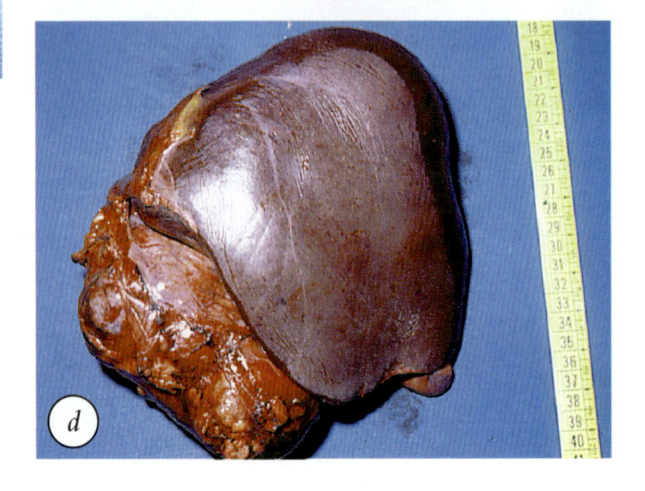

performed with direct suturing (4 cases with total vascular exclusion - ***Figure 13.2*** - and 2 with lateral clamping of the retrohepatic vena cava). In two cases, complete resection and prosthetic reconstruction of the vena cava was carried out as described below. For partial infiltration of the wall, in which direct suturing could result in stenosis of the caval lumen, a patch of saphenous vein can be used, as described by Broelsch.[1] Resection of the vena cava with prosthetic reconstruction is indicated for more extensive infiltration, when more than half the circumference of the vein is involved, or the wall is involved longitudinally or in cases of infiltration with endoluminal thrombus (***Figures 13.3-7***). The 2 cases treated with caval reconstruction were, respectively, metastases from colonic cancer and hepatocarcinoma in a non-cirrhotic liver. In both cases the post-operative period was uneventful. One presented with pulmonary metastases 1 year after surgery and the other is in good health without signs of recurrence, at the time of writing, 16 months after the operation.

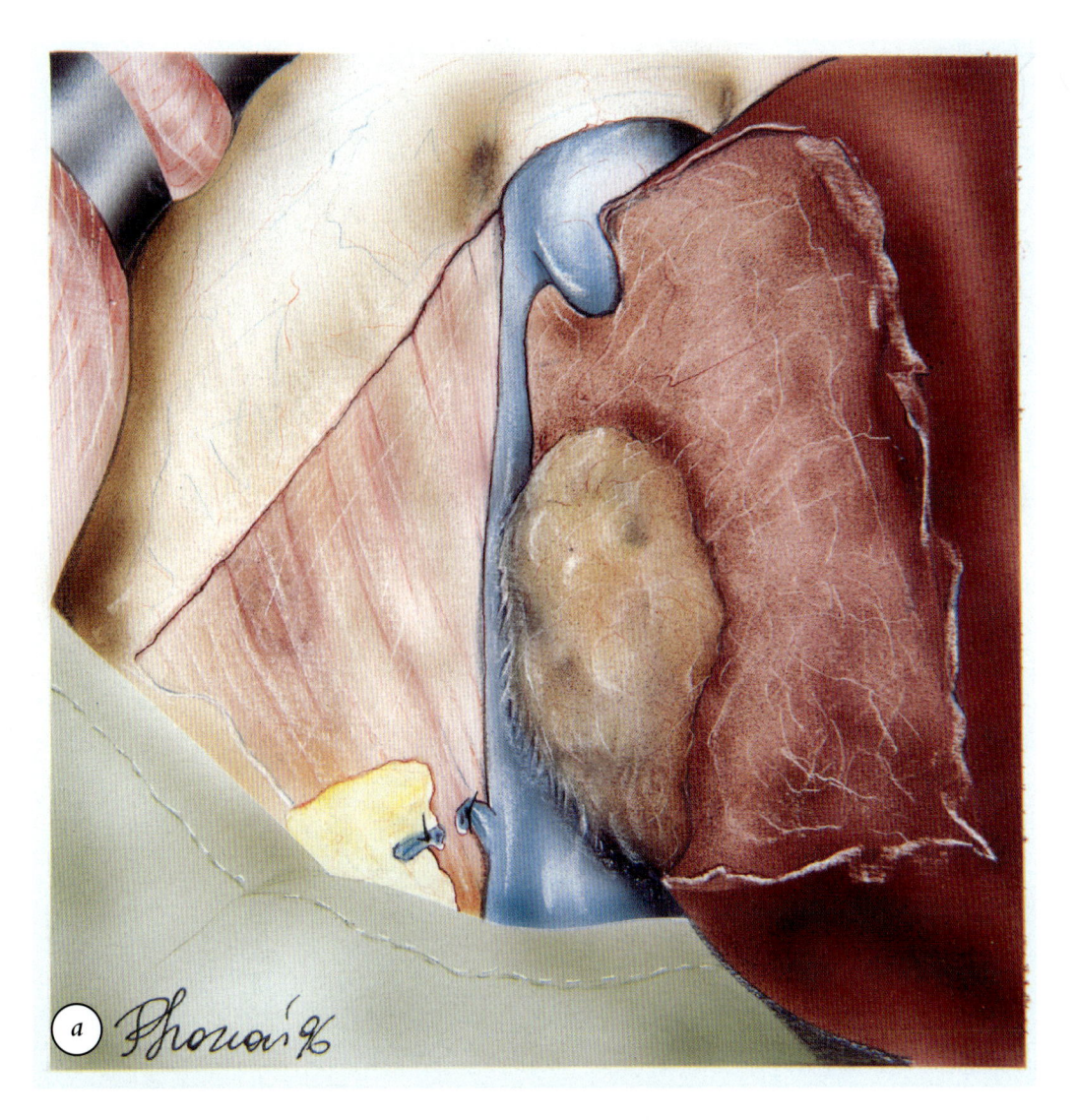

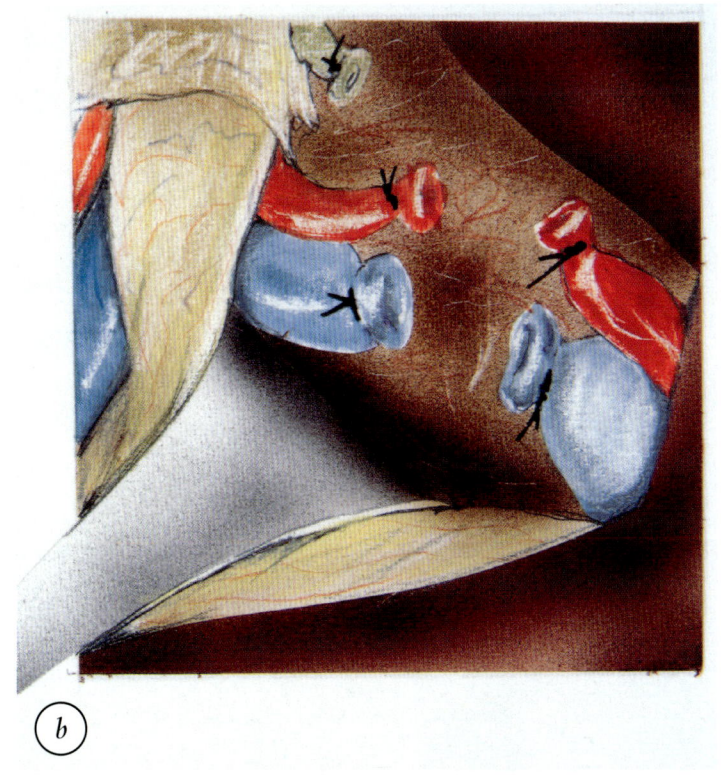

Figure 13.3 – ***a)*** *Mobilization of the right hemiliver and freeing of the lateral margin of the vena cava. The anterior wall of the vein is infiltrated by the neoplasm.*
b) *Ligation of the vascular pedicles for the right hemiliver.*

Technique

The liver must be completely mobilized with division of the falciform ligament and the right and left triangular ligaments (**Figure 13.3a**). The vena cava below and above the liver is isolated and encircled with tape in preparation for vascular exclusion. The hilar stage proceeds as for a conventional right hepatectomy (**Figure 13.3b**). Division of Glisson's capsule and of the parenchyma continues until the plane of the Glissonian hilum is reached. During this stage it is not necessary to clamp either the vena cava or the Glissonian pedicle, thus reducing the ischemic time as much as possible.

TECHNIQUES IN LIVER SURGERY

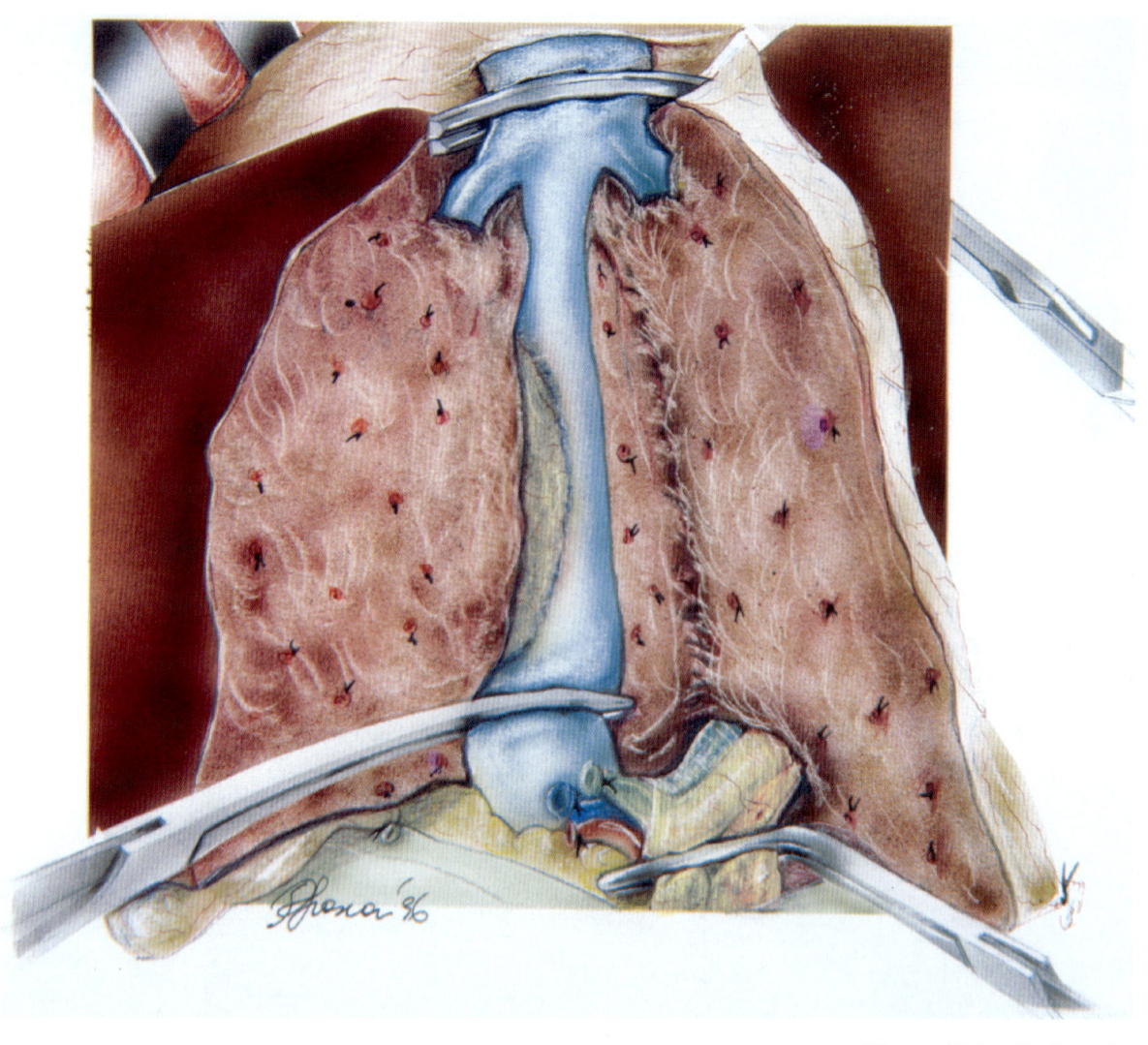

Figure 13.4 – *Total vascular exclusion of the liver.*

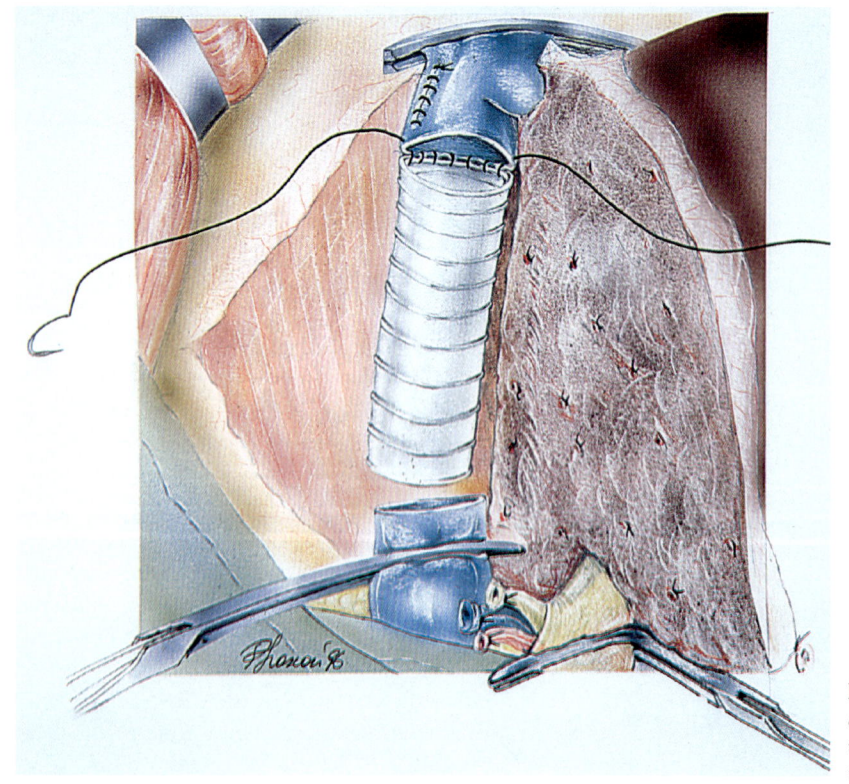

Figure 13.5 – *Proximal anastomosis of the vena cava with Gore-Tex® armed prosthesis under total vascular exclusion.*

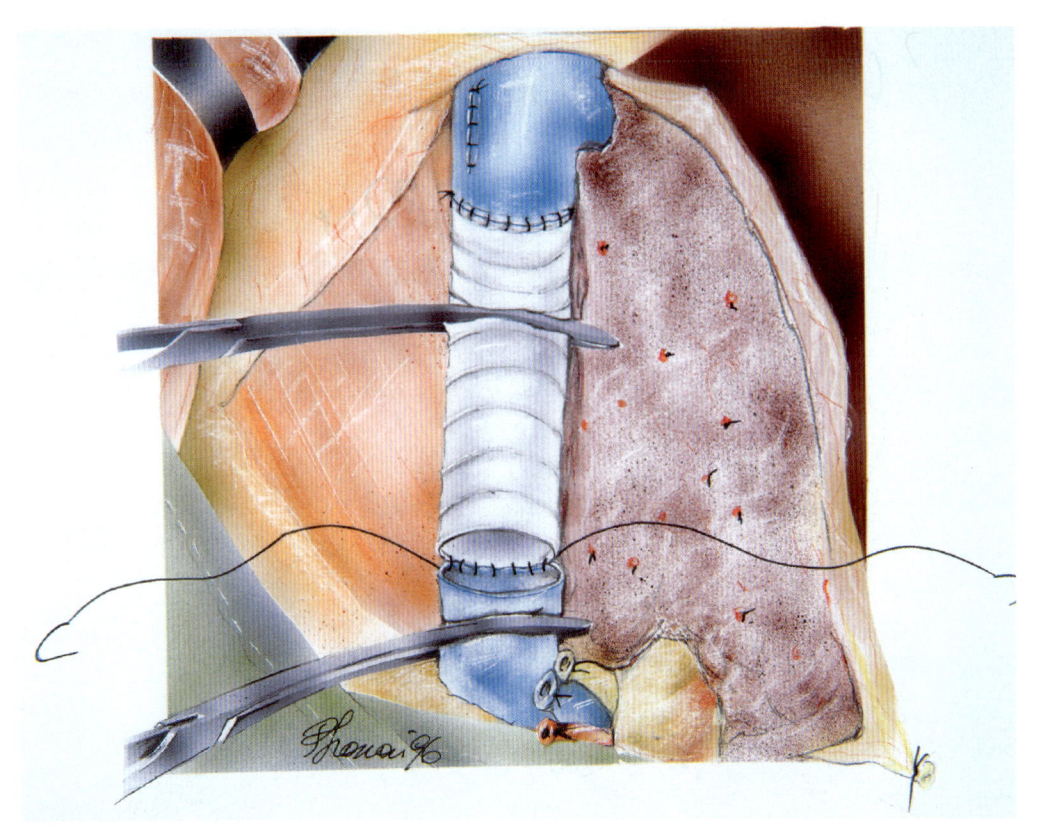

Figure 13.6 – *On completion of the proximal anastomosis the suprahepatic clamp is moved directly onto the prosthesis and the clamp on the hepatic pedicle at the hilum is removed.*

Vascular exclusion begins after resection has passed the hilar plane, according to the technique described below. A De Bakey clamp is first placed on the subhepatic vena cava, followed by a clamp on the hepatic pedicle and finally a clamp on the suprahepatic vena cava (**Figure 13.4**). As dissection continues upwards, the right hepatic vein is identified in segment 8, where it is clamped and divided. The anterior aspect of the vena cava is then gradually freed and can be divided below the confluence with the middle and left hepatic vein. Inferior resection of the vena cava is performed immediately below the liver and the right hemiliver can be removed *en bloc* with the tumor and with the entire segment of infiltrated vena cava. If there is enough space between the trunk of the hepatic veins and the upper limit of the caval infiltration, another vascular clamp can be placed on the vena cava immediately below the trunk of the hepatic veins so that the suprahepatic caval clamp and the Glissonian pedicle clamp can be opened, thus ending vascular exclusion of the liver. Only the vena cava is now still clamped and vascular exclusion of the liver is thus limited to 30-35 minutes. If, on the other hand, there is no adequate safety margin for a second caval clamp below the convergence of the hepatic veins, the first part of caval reconstruction can be continued with total vascular exclusion (**Figure 13.5**) and the caval clamp can be moved on to the prosthesis after proximal caval anastomosis has been completed (**Figure 13.6**).

For reconstruction of the vena cava, an armed Gore-Tex® prosthesis is used, slightly smaller in diameter than the vena cava, taking care to eliminate the first two rings of the prosthesis to make the anastomosis softer (**Figure 13.7**). Proximal anastomosis and subsequently distal anastomosis are fashioned with a Prolene® 3-0 whipstitch. Before completing distal anastomosis and removing the clamps, air must be removed from the prosthesis by temporarily opening the clamp to allow a backflow of blood through the vascular graft. By means of these measures vascular exclusion of the liver can be limited to a safety period not exceeding 50 minutes. We have never had to resort to hypothermic lavage of the liver or use a venous bypass. This possibility should, however, be borne in mind and the vascular access for

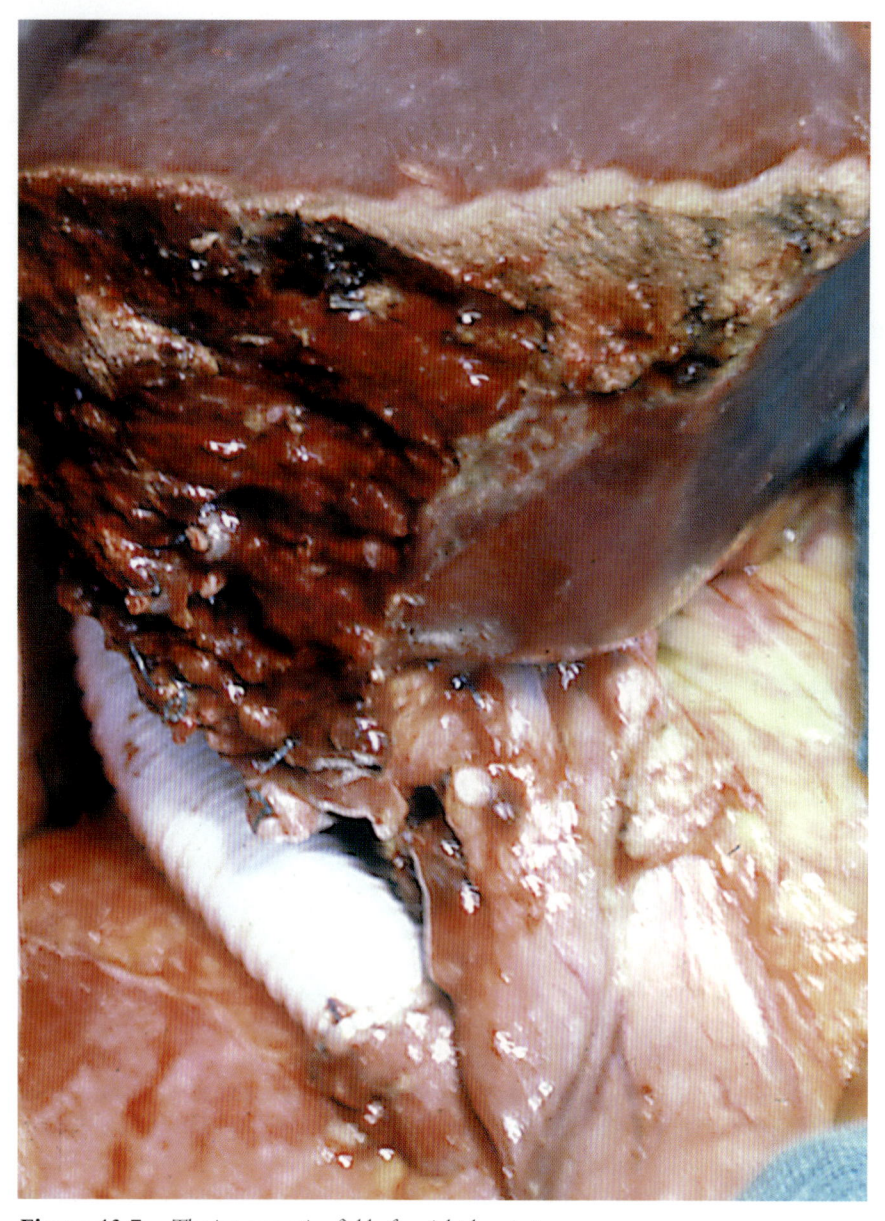

Figure 13.7 – *The intraoperative field after right hepatectomy and prosthesis replacement of the vena cava.*

bypass positioning (saphenous vein and left axillary vein) should be appropriately prepared before exclusion, in order to deal with the hemodynamic drownback during clamping. Biopumps with a heparinized wall circuit, commonly used in transplant surgery, should be prepared in the operating theater when planning this type of surgery which involves lengthy periods of vascular exclusion of the liver.

REFERENCES

1. Broelsch C. *Atlas of Liver Surgery*. Churchill Livingstone, New York, 1993.
2. Iwatsuki S, Todo S, Starzl TE. Right trisegmentectomy with a synthetic vena cava graft. *Arch Surg* 1988; **123:** 1021-1027.
3. Kumada K, Shimahara Y, Fukuki K, Itoh K, Morokawa S, Ozawa K. Extended right hepatic lobectomy: combined resection of inferior vena cava and its reconstruction by a PTFE graft (Gore-Tex). *Acta Chirurgica Scan* 1988; **154:** 481-483.
4. Miller CM, Schwarz ME, Nishizaki T. Combined hepatic and vena cava resection with autogenous caval graft replacement. *Arch Surg* 1991; **126:** 106-108.
5. O'Malley KJ, Stuart RC, McEntee BP. Combined resection of the inferior vena cava and extended right hepatectomy for leiomyosarcoma of the retrohepatic cava. *Br J Surg* 1994; **81:** 845-846.
6. Pierangeli F, Mazziotti A, Grazi GL *et al*. Hepatectomies with total resection of inferior vena cava. *HBP Surgery* 1996; **9 (suppl.2):** 107.

TECHNIQUES IN LIVER SURGERY

SECTION V

General Aspects of Liver Resection

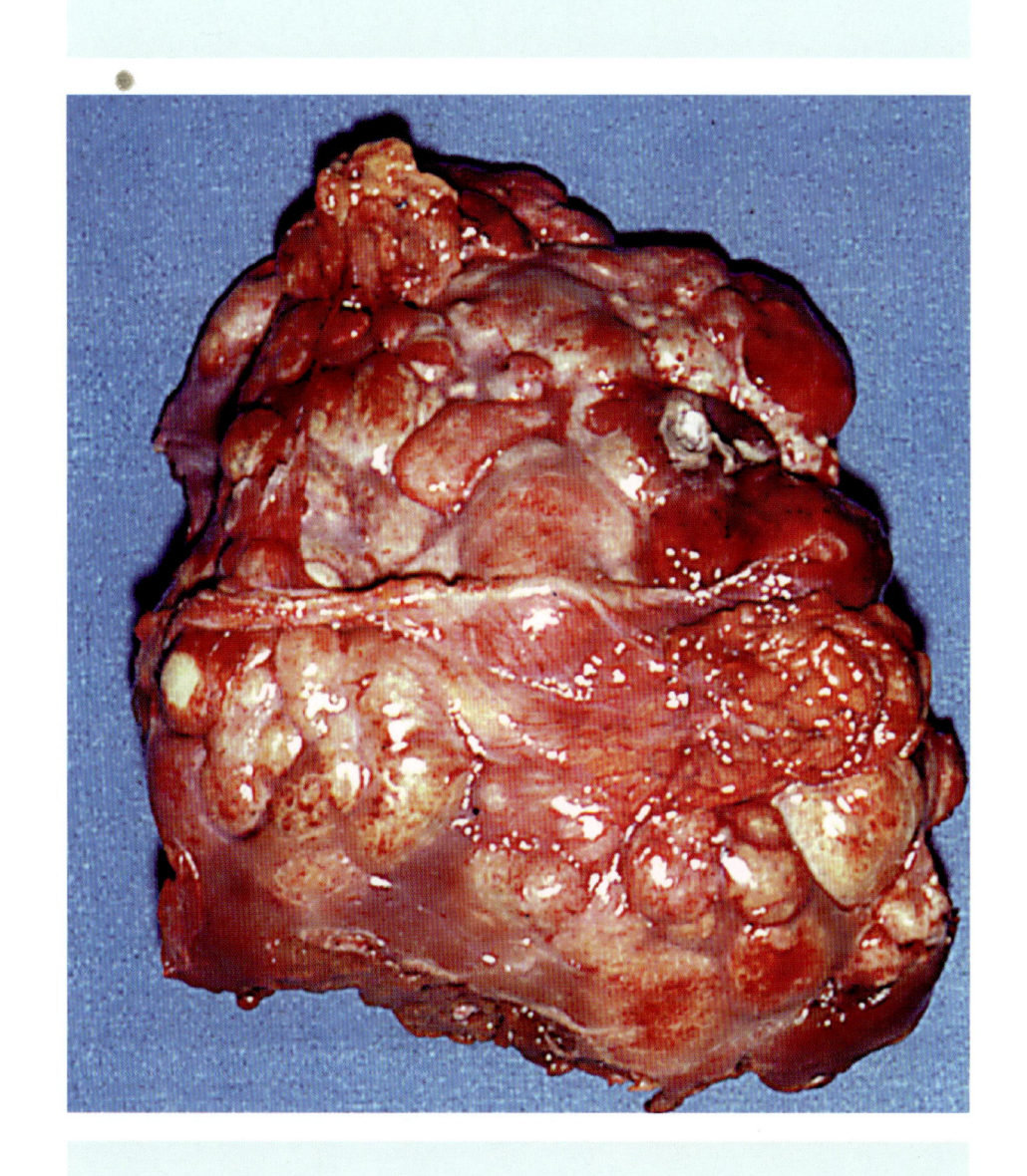

EUD a.te. 10
Systolisher Druck unter 80 mp Hp

14

Resection Technique

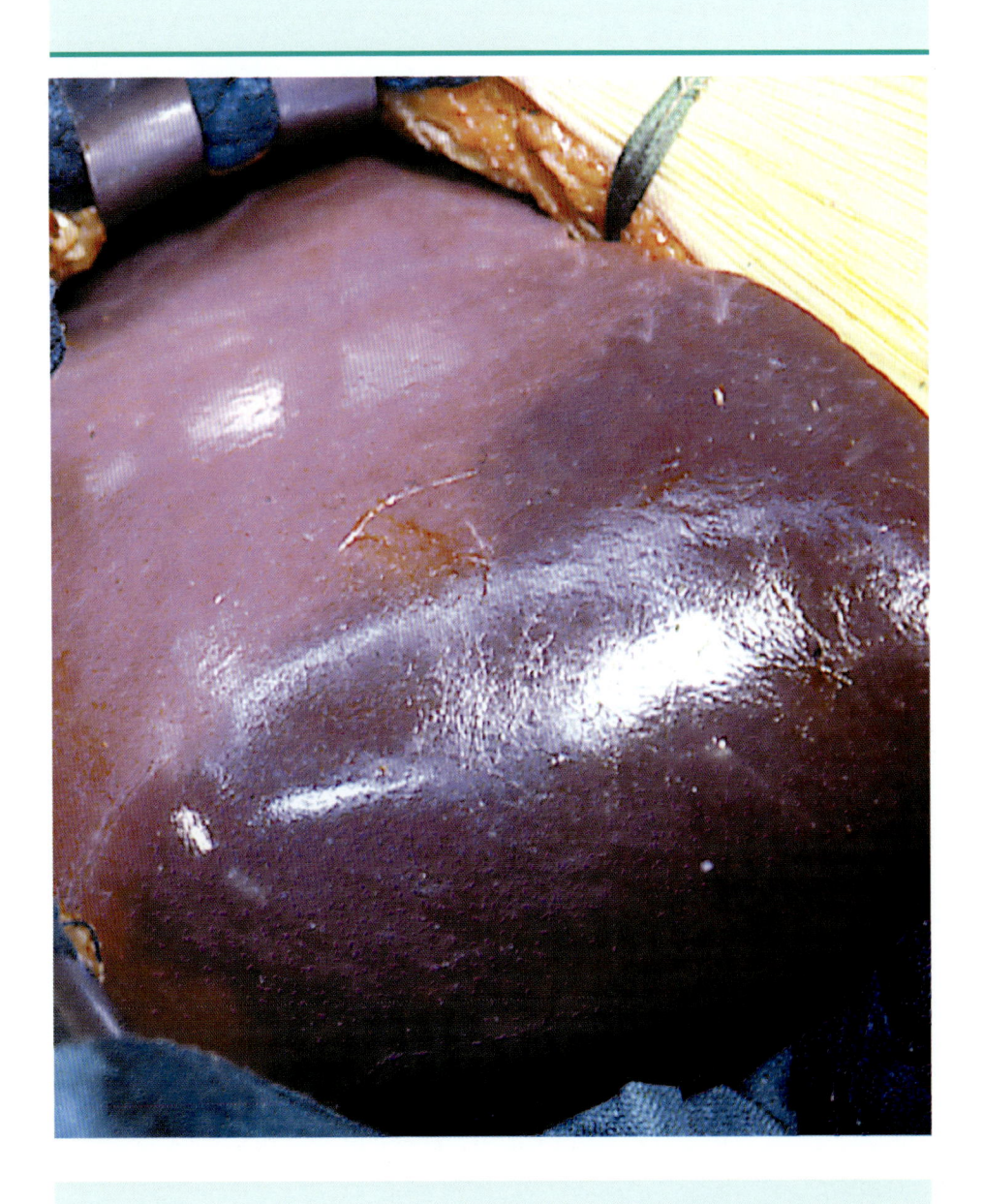

RESECTION TECHNIQUE

Once the Glissonian capsule has been cut by cautery, the parenchyma must be divided gradually to identify the vascular-biliary structures which must be electively ligated before being divided. The easiest way to carry out parenchymal division, with respect to the intrahepatic vessels, is to crush small portions of the parenchyma with the tip of a Kelly forceps. The more resistant vascular-biliary structures are divided as follows: the smaller vessels are coagulated by cautery, while the larger pedicles are ligated with fine threads (Vicryl® 3-0) and then divided. Clips can also be used to close the small pedicles. This procedure is undoubtedly easier and is preferable when division has to be performed quickly, for example during vascular clamping or emergency hepatectomy for trauma. Clips do, however, require a certain amount of care to make sure that the vessel is completely closed since the clip must be placed on a perfectly transverse plane. It is also necessary to make sure that the clips are not accidentally removed during subsequent maneuvers. The same result as division with forceps can be obtained with the 'finger crushing' method. This is, however, a less precise method and may not be so easy in the deeper parts of the resection. Identification and ligature of the intrahepatic Glissonian pedicles is easy since these structures are enclosed in connective tissue, even at their peripheral extremities. The hepatic veins, on the other hand, are much more delicate and are easily torn, retracting into the parenchyma causing secondary hemorrhage. The numerous small collaterals arising from the main branches of the hepatic veins are also easily torn, causing the formation of small defects which can lead to widespread bleeding when venous pressure increases. To prevent such hemorrhages from the main hepatic branches it is advisable to avoid dissection along the walls of the main hepatic veins and to always leave a small portion of parenchyma between the vein and the resection plane.

Use of the *ultrasound dissector* has not met with great success in hepatic surgery. Its function is based on the physical principle of fragmentation of the biological tissues with a probe vibrating at high frequencies (23 or 24 kHz). The probe is equipped with irrigation and aspiration systems. The effect of tissue fragmentation is more intense in collagen-poor tissues and should be carried out selectively on the parenchyma, avoiding the biliary and vascular structures. Adjustment of the amplitude of the oscillations provides different power levels of tissue dissection. Lower levels are appropriate for normal hepatic parenchyma and higher levels for fibrotic livers or for extra-Glissonian structures, such as the main bile ducts or the hepatic venous trunks. Parenchymal division performed with an ultrasound dissector is decidedly more accurate and safe, permitting meticulous exposure of the vascular and biliary pedicles, but it is unquestionably slower compared with conventional dissection using Kelly forceps. We have found no real advantage in using the ultrasound dissector, except in isolating segmentary pedicles in 'difficult' segmentectomies, particularly for isolation of the right paramedian pedicle in segmentectomies of segments 5 and 8, dissection of the intrahepatic bile ducts and dissection of the pericystium in hydatid liver cysts. Bearing in mind the high cost of the equipment, the purchase of an ultrasound dissector does not seem advisable except in centers where advanced hepato-biliary surgery is carried out.

The *waterjet dissector* consists of a handpiece that can emit a variable pressure jet of physiological solution, adjusted by the operator on a control panel. Dissection takes place by means of pressurized waterjet fragmenting the soft tissues (parenchyma, adipose tissue) while preserving the connective tissues. Like the ultrasound dissector, the pressure of the waterjet can be adjusted (from 0 to 50 kg/cm2) with a flow that can reach 43 ml/min. The device is equipped with an aspiration system and costs less than an ultrasound dissector. The small size of the handpiece and its light weight certainly make it easy to use and no particular training is necessary for the use of this equipment. This dissector makes it possible to achieve an extremely uniform resection, with minimal histological signs of hepatocyte degeneration, and to leave all intraparenchymal structures measuring more than 0.2 mm in diameter undamaged.[1] The use of this instrument can hinder hemostasis from minor sources due to the formation of air bubbles which prevent a perfectly clear view of the operating field. In addition, the formation of spurts of water mixed with blood necessitates the constant use of an aspirator and protective systems for the surgical team. Its role in cirrhotic or highly fibrotic livers remains undecided.

Hemostasis and biliostasis of resected areas

The identification and meticulous ligature of the vessels during resection is the best way of ensuring hemostasis of the resected portion and of preventing pre- and post-operative bleeding. Sutures including small portions of parenchyma, generally in Vicryl® 4-0, complete hemostasis. Electrocoagulation is sufficient for the smaller vessels. Hemostasis is thus usually easily achieved in the presence of a linear resection with a regular surface. Hemostasis may be problematic in cirrhotic livers or when the resected surface is uneven or in the presence of tears where the vascular pedicles retract into the parenchyma. In these cases, wider suture stitches can be used and tied to pieces of fibrin sponge to prevent further tearing of the parenchyma. The systematic use of through-and-through U stitches, including large portions of the parenchyma (the so-called 'mattress suture'), should be avoided as they may cause tissue necrosis with consequent hepatic sequestration, biliary fistulae or abscesses.

Biological glues have not, in our experience, been of any major practical use. Synthetic glues, such as cyanocrylate, despite having strong adhesive strength, are of little use as they are difficult to handle, requiring a completely dry resected surface and can lead to an intense inflammatory reaction.[8] Fibrin glue, the most commonly used, consists of human plasma concentrates which facilitate the final stage of the physiological process of coagulation. The protein concentrates are dissolved with aprotinin and then applied at the same time as a thrombin solution. The efficacy of fibrin glue has formed the subject of various clinical and experimental studies. One recent randomized study in 77 patients showed no significant differences in morbidity between patients treated with and without fibrin glue; the former did however present a minor loss of fluids from the abdominal drainages with a reduced concentration of bilirubin in the drainage liquid.[7]

The *Argon beam* coagulator represents a significant advantage compared with the standard electrocoagulator. It generates radiofrequencies at a coaxial flow of Argon, an inert and non-inflammable gas, to allow the electrical current to form an arc through the gas and achieve a focal coagulative necrosis of the tissues touched by the beam. It is the action of this current, rather than the gas itself, which causes the coagulation effect. This is represented visually by a blue-colour flame. Necrosis is possible of a thin and constant layer of parenchyma, of around 2.5 mm. As the Argon reduces the quantity of local oxygen, carbonization is less compared with a conventional electrocoagulator. The handpiece is perpendicular with respect to the surface to be coagulated and does not come into direct contact with it: this allows the instrument to be used like a paintbrush on the surface to be treated. As the depth of the effect is relatively constant, unlike a standard electrocoagulator, it makes it possible to achieve hemostasis even on irregular surfaces, frequently encountered in hepatic surgery. The flow of gas allows blood to be removed from the tissue, permitting a better view of the surgical field. The Argon beam coagulator is more efficient for small surface hemorrhage than the conventional electrocoagulator, causing less damage to the surrounding tissues and the vascular pedicles.[10] Another recently reported advantage of the use of the Argon coagulator is the treatment of the resected surface in cases of segmentectomies with an unsatisfactory resection margin from the limit of the tumor.[11] The study of the hemostatic effect obtained with various techniques in laboratory animals has shown that the Argon beam coagulator reduces blood loss, the time necessary to achieve satisfactory hemostasis and the depth of cellular damage compared with biological glues or suturing.[9] We have used this coagulator in numerous hepatic resections, mostly in cirrhotic patients and in liver transplants. We found it easy to use, requiring no particular handling technique either in the operating theater or in the surgical field. The Argon coagulator makes

COMPLICATIONS	NO. OF CASES	RE-OPERATIONS	DEATHS
Major			
Hemoperitineum	6	6	0
Subphrenic abscesses	23	7	0
Hepatic insufficiency	21	2★	13 (8)
Digestive hemorrhage	5	0	3 (3)
Biliary fistulae	23	2	0
Minor			
Ascites	64 (52)	0	0
Pulmonary complications	52	7	0

Numbers in parentheses indicate cirrhotic patients.
★Two patients with severe hepatic insufficiency after extensive resection underwent transplantation.

Table 14.1 - *Post-operative complications after hepatic resections (800 cases) with systematic use of abdominal drainage.*

it possible to achieve thorough hemostasis of the hepatic parenchyma and avoids the undesired effects observed with the extensive use of the conventional coagulator.

Biliostasis of the resected surface is equally important in preventing post-operative biliary fistulae and subphrenic abscesses. In the event of biliary leakage from the resected surface, it is particularly useful to inject air or a diluted solution of methylene blue from the cystic duct, closing the common bile duct distally with the fingers or with a smooth clamp. These procedures, together with cholangiography by the same route, are obligatory when there is a suspected lesion of a bile duct during resection or in surgery for hydatid cysts which involves a high risk of biliary lesions (see Chapter 21). Biliary leakage points on the resected surface must be sutured with Vicryl® 3-0 stitches. It remains doubtful whether external drainage of the bile tract can prevent post-operative biliary fistulas. In some retrospective studies, no decrease was observed in biliary fistulae or subphrenic abscesses in cases with biliary drainage.[4,6] In our department, external biliary drainage is recommended in patients with dilated bile tracts, in accidental lesions of the bile tracts and in surgery for complex hydatid cysts when it is necessary to leave a large part of pericystium in place.

To drain or not to drain after hepatic resection

In the last few years the necessity for systematic drainage after liver resection surgery has been the subject of some controversy. The arguments against its use are that it may be responsible for bacterial contamination causing intraperitoneal abscesses, that it is not effective in preventing the formation of intra-abdominal collections, and that it can cause ascitic fistulae in cirrhotic patients.[5] One recent randomized study in 81 patients who underwent elective hepatic resection with and without drainage showed that the percentage of post-operative intra-abdominal complications (subphrenic collections, hematomas, biliary collections) was identical in both groups; a higher percentage of infected intra-abdominal collections was observed in the patients with drainage.[2] The arguments against the systematic use of drainage were not confirmed by other clinical series which instead stress the usefulness of drainage in the prompt diagnosis of post-operative hemorrhage and in avoiding re-operation in the event of intra-abdominal hematoma or biliary fistulae from the resected surface, which can heal spontaneously if appropriately drained.[3]

Abdominal drainage continues to be systematically used in our department without any specific complications linked to its use. The rate of post-operative complications observed (**Table 14.1**) has proved to be identical to, if not lower than, cases of resection without drainage reported by the literature, particularly as far as septic complications are concerned. Ascitic fistulae in cirrhotic patients were always resolved with medical treatment. This complication can easily be prevented by early removal of the drainage tubes and by the systematic application of a purse-string suture around the drainage hole. Eighteen cases of biliary fistulae originating from the resected surface healed spontaneously, after leaving the drainage tubes in place for longer than 3 weeks. The systematic use of drainage after hepatic surgery seems to be a safe method of checking for post-operative hemorrhages or collections. Drainage is useful in preventing certain post-operative complications such as biliary fistulae and the formation of hematomas and does not appear to be directly responsible for post-operative septic complications.

REFERENCES

1. Baer HU, Maddern GJ, Blumgart LH. New water-jet dissector: initial experience in hepatic surgery. *Br J Surg* 1991; **78:** 502-503.
2. Belghiti J, Kabbei M, Sauvanet A, Vilgrain V, Panis Y, Fékété F. Drainage after elective hepatic resection. A randomized trial. *Ann Surg* 1993; **218:** 748-753.
3. Bona S, Gavelli A, Huguet C. The role of abdominal drainage after major hepatic resection. *Am J Surg* 1994; **167:** 593-595.
4. Fékété F, Guillet R. Traumatismes du foie. In: "Chirurgie 1980". Masson, Paris. 1980.
5. Franco D, Karaa A, Meakin JL *et al*. Hepatectomy without abdominal drainage: results of a prospective study in 61 patients. *Ann Surg* 1993; **218:** 748-753.
6. Lucas CE, Walt AJ. Analysis of randomized biliary drainage for liver trauma in 189 patients. *J Trauma* 1972; **12:** 925-929.
7. Noun R, Elias ., Balladur P, Bismuth H, Parc R, Lasser PH, Belghiti J. Fibrin glue effectiveness and tolerance after elective liver resections: a randomized trial. *Hepato Gastroenterol* 1996; **43:** 221-224.
8. Portoghese M, Acar C, Jebara V et Al. Alterations de la paroi vasculaire dues aux colles chirurgicales. *Etude expérimentale Presse Méd* 1991; **21:** 1154-1156.
9. Postema RR, Plaisier T, Kate FJW, Terpstra OT. Hemostasis after partial hepatectomy using argon beam coagulation. *Br J Surg* 1993; **80:** 1563-1565.
10. Rusch VW, Schmidt JR, Shoji Y, Fujimura Y. Use of the Argon beam electrocoagulator for performing pulmonary wedge resections. *Ann Thorac Surg* 1990; **49:** 287-291.
11. Yamagata M, Matsumoto T, Ikeda Y, Hayashi H, Sugimaki K. Recurrence on the resection line of hepatocellular carcinoma in the antero superior subsegment of the liver. The effect of Argon beam coagulator. *Hepato Gastroenterol* 1995; **42:** 9-12.

15

Evaluation of the Hepatic Functional Reserve

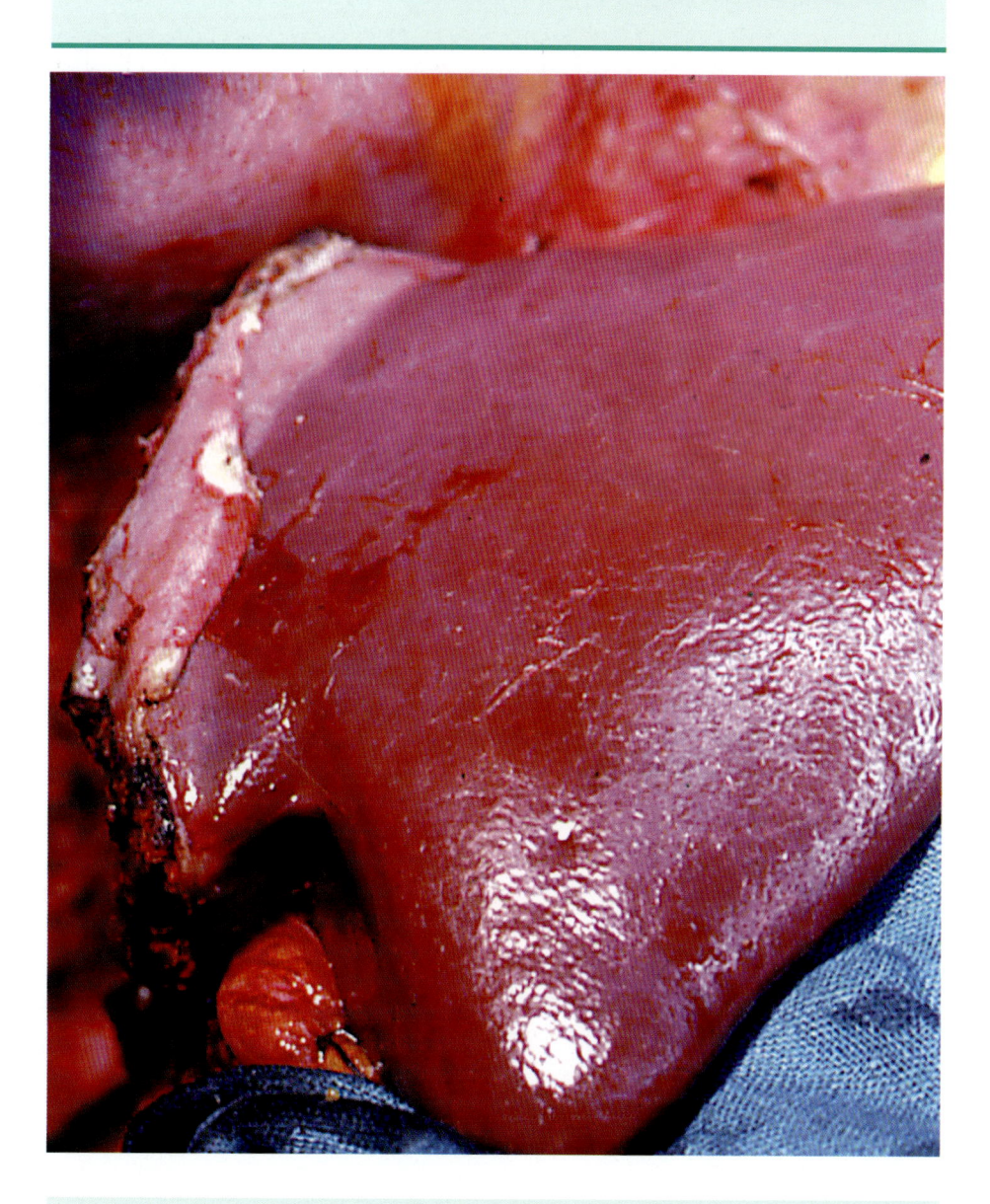

Restleber 0,5% des Körpergewichtes
≙ CT | 20-30% der Leber |
          der Rest

normale Leber 4-5% des Gewichtes (Körper)
  1 Liter Galle / die mit Druck 10-30 cm H2O
  1,5 Liter Blut / Minute

	MEGX (ng/ml)	NO. OF CASES	SURGERY	POST-OP. COMPLICATIONS
Child A (80 cases)				
	>50	8	8	0
	25-50	56	24	5 (21%)
	<25	16	15	11 (73%)
Child B and C (32 cases)				
	>50	0	0	0
	25-50	2	0	0
	<25	30	3	3 (100%)

Table 15.1 – *Evaluation of MEGX in cirrhotic patients (112 cases). Fifty of these patients underwent segmentary liver resection for hepatocarcinoma.*

Pre-operative evaluation of hepatic function is essential in the planning of liver resection, especially in cirrhotic patients. The Child-Pugh classification is the easiest and commonest method of quantifying the degree of liver insufficiency by considering the levels of bilirubin, albumin and prothrombin activity, and the presence of encephalopathy and evaluation of nutritional status. However, the evaluation made by the Child classification is not always complete and correct.[1] The levels of bilirubin and of serum albumin can be independent of hepatic function. The prothrombin activity can be affected by an altered intestinal absorption of vitamin K and can be corrected by parenteral administration of the vitamin. The assessment of encephalopathy and nutritional status can be observer-dependent.

In the last decade, many studies have tried to quantify the degree of derangement of liver function with more reliable functional tests. The aminopyrine breath test, the indocyanine green clearance test, the redox tolerance test[6] and the conventional galactose test have been the most commonly employed methods. However, all these techniques are more complex and have shown no real advantage when compared with the conventional Child classification.[7]

More recently, based on the experience of donor evaluation for liver transplantation,[5] the lidocaine-MEGX test was introduced to assess liver function in cirrhotic patients. The lidocaine is metabolized almost exclusively (97%) from the hepatocytes by the P-450 cytochromes to monoethylglycinexilidide. Fifteen minutes after an i.v. bolus injection of 1 mg/kg of lidocaine, a venous blood sample is taken and the MEGX rate is assessed by immunofluorescence assay (FPIA). MEGX values over 50 ng/ml are considered normal, between 25 and 50 ng/ml intermediately reduced and below 25 ng/ml greatly reduced. The injection of lidocaine at the doses required for the test is free of side effects.

In our department,[2,3] 200 patients with various liver pathologies were assessed by the lidocaine test in association with other conventional tests, including the Child classification. 112 of the patients were cirrhotic (95% of whom had an altered MEGX rate) while only 20% of the non-cirrhotics had a reduced MEGX rate. In contrast, using the Child classification in the group of cirrhotic patients (80 of whom were candidates for liver resection and thus had 'good' residual liver function) 73% of cases had elevated bilirubin, and less than 50% of cases had reduced albumin and prothrombin activity. The sensitivity, specificity and diagnostic accuracy of the lidocaine test in detecting the presence of cirrhosis were 95.5%, 79.5% and 84.4% respectively. Moreover, the MEGX values did not always correlate with the Child classification (*Table 15.1*). Eighty patients in the cirrhotic group were Child A. Only 8 of these had an MEGX value below 50 ng/ml, while 16 had greatly reduced (<25 ng/ml) MEGX values. The MEGX values were constantly reduced in the Child B and C patients. In this last group (32 cases) no patient had an MEGX rate over 50 ng/ml. 50of the cirrhotic patients underwent segmentary liver resection for hepatocarcinoma. In the patients with reduced MEGX levels, the incidence of post-operative complications linked to hepatic insufficiency (ascites, infections, jaundice) was greater than in patients with higher MEGX values and unrelated to the extent of liver resection.

The lidocaine test can also be of use in cases of acute hepatic insufficiency due to fulminant hepatitis or of hepatic insufficiency as a result of extensive resection. In these conditions the test allows rapid evaluation of the hepatic damage, unaffected by the infusion of liquids or fresh plasma which can alter conventional laboratory parameters. The data relative to evaluation of hepatic insufficiency after extensive liver resections have been published by our group[4]: after extended right hepatectomy due to severe trauma of the liver the MEGX rate was markedly reduced at an early stage, preceding the neurological alterations and the more common laboratory tests and giving important information for the appropriate timing of emergency liver transplantation with favorable outcome.

The lidocaine test appears to be a highly sensitive means of diagnosing the presence of a chronic liver disease and is more reliable than the Child classification in quantifying the extent of hepatic insufficiency. 'Functional' evaluation in cirrhotic patients must, however, always include the study of other organs, such as the heart, lungs and kidneys. Diabetes can also affect the incidence of post-operative complications. These complications also relate to other factors which depend on the operation *per se* in terms of surgical trauma, such as prolonged clamping of the hepatic pedicle, devascularization of areas of the parenchyma, the quantity of parenchyma removed with the tumor and the need for intra-operative transfusion.

REFERENCES

1. Conn. A peek for Child classification. *Hepatology* 1981; **1:** 673-676.
2. Ercolani G, Mazziotti A, Grazi GL *et al*. Evaluation of the liver function with the lidocaine (MEGX) test. Proceedings 2nd World IHPBA Congress, Bologna, 1996, Vol. 1, pp. 143-147.
3. Gozzetti G, Mazziotti A. Cosa c'è di nuovo in chirurgia epatica. Proceedings 97th Congress of Italian Society of Surgery, 1995, Rome, 1995, Vol. 1 pp. 175-230.
4. Gozzetti G, Mazziotti A, Jovine E, Grazi GL. Trapianto di fegato per trauma. *Chirurgia* 1994; **7:** 848-851.
5. Oellerich M, Ringe B, Gubernatis G *et al*. Lignocaine metabolite formation as a measure of pretransplant liver function. *Lancet* 1989; **1:** 640-642.
6. Ueda I. Mori K, Sakai Y *et al* Noninvasive evaluation of cytochrome-C-oxidase activity of the liver. Its prognostic value for hepatic resection. *Arch Surg* 1994; **129:** 303-308.
7. Zoedler T, Ebener C, Becker H, Roehr H. Evaluation of liver function tests to predict operative risk in liver surgery. *HPB Surgery* 1995; **9:** 13-18.

16

Tolerance of Liver Ischemia

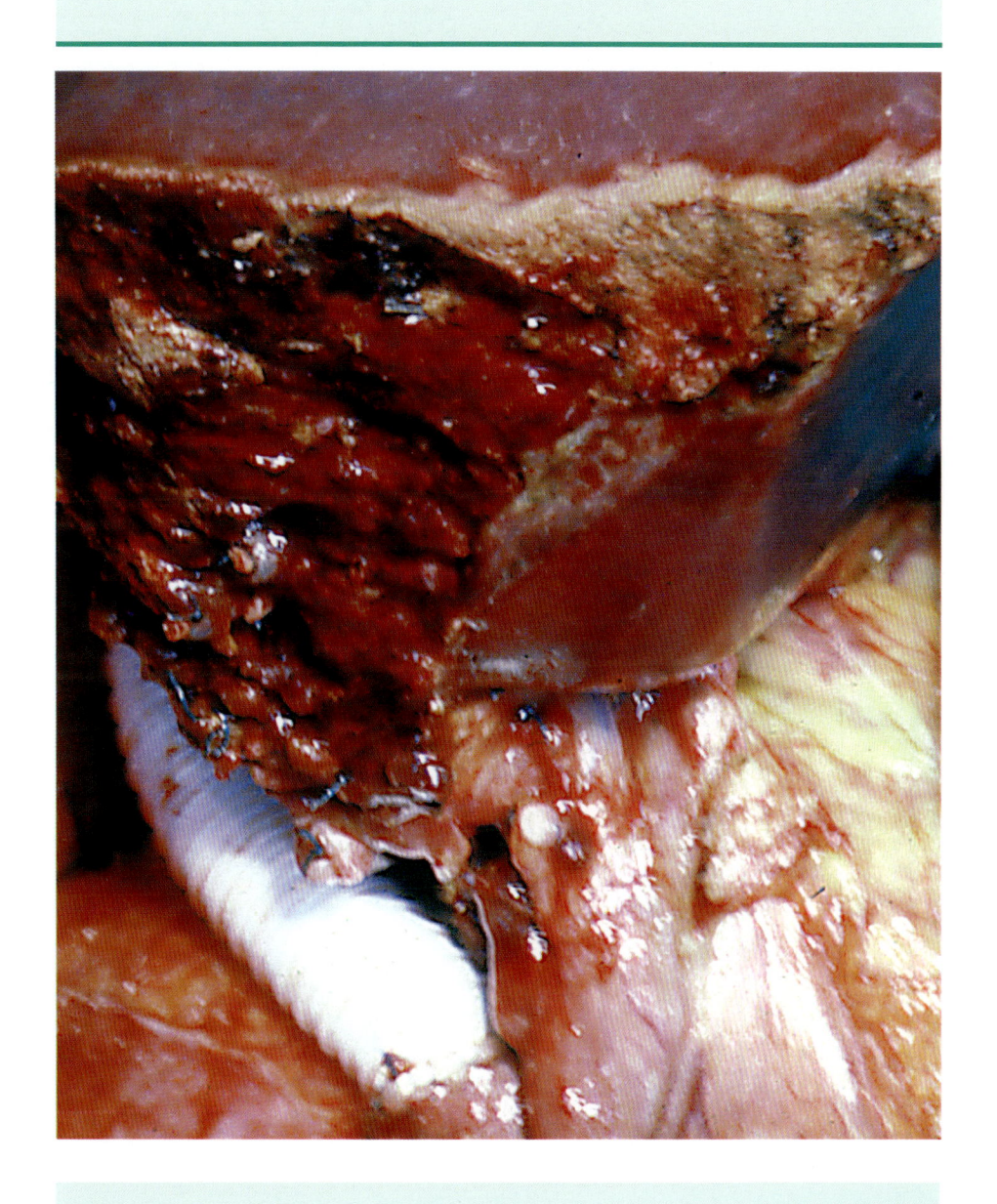

The liver has been widely shown to have good tolerance to normothermic ischemia, even for periods of more than an hour[4,6] In patients with a normal liver and normally perfused the temporary clamping of the hepatic pedicle at the hilum (Pringle's maneuver) does not cause major hemodynamic repercussions.[1] Effects caused by clamping lasting up to 60 minutes include an increase in cytonecrosis enzymes up to 10-13 times the normal levels, and also an increase in bilirubin and alkaline phosphatase. These values all return to normal within 1 week after operation and do not appear to be dependent on the length of clamping time if the ischemic periods is less than 60 minutes.[4,6]

Clamping of the pedicle is an extremely useful maneuver in hepatic surgery as it limits blood loss and reduces the need for transfusion which represent one of the main factors associated with post-operative morbidity.[3] However, the data regarding the tolerance of the liver to ischemia refer to clinical or experimental experiences in normal livers. In livers affected by chronic hepatitis, cirrhosis, chronic cholestasis or massive steatosis, prolonged ischemia can cause severe damage to the parenchyma and be responsible for post-operative hepatic insufficency. In order to limit ischemic damage Makuuchi[9] proposed intermittent clamping of the hepatic pedicle followed by brief periods of reperfusion. The protective effect of intermittent clamping has been demonstrated in clinical series[2] and in experimental studies in rats,[7] and is now widely used in clinical practice in the surgery of cirrhotic livers. This has not been confirmed in other recent clinical studies.[5,12] Knowledge of the hepatic damage caused by ischemia-reperfusion remains incomplete.

To test whether intermittent clamping represents a true advantage in terms of preventing hepatic damage and in order to define the physiopathological mechanisms responsible for ischemia-reperfusion damage, our group carried out a series of experimental studies. These include in vitro studies on isolated cells, ex vivo studies on isolated and perfused rat livers and in vivo experiments. The results confirmed that in experimental animals, periods of intermittent ischemia reduce cellular damage in terms of an increase in cytonecrosis enzymes and also reduce energy depletion and tissue antioxidant status, compared with periods of continuous ischemia of the same duration. The reperfusion is also characterized by a reduced formation of free radicals of oxygen and reduced liberation of cytonecrosis enzymes.[10]

One recent randomized clinical study demonstrated the improved tolerance of intermittent compared with continuous clamping in terms of a post-operative increase of cytonecrosis enzymes and, in cirrhotic patients, in terms of an increase in bilirubinemia and of the appearance of post-operative hepatic insufficiency.[11]

Hemihepatic vascular occlusion, i.e. the selective clamping of the right or left Glissonian pedicle, depending on the site of the parenchymal resection, has been proposed to limit the effects of hepatic ischemia.[8] The arterial and portal branches for the right or left left hemiliver are isolated extraparenchymally and are clamped with a bulldog clamp to prevent blood loss during parenchymal resection. This technique can be electively adopted in segmentectomies and is described in detail in Chapter 6. The method is commonly employed in resection of the lateral segments. One particular application is central hepatectomy which can be performed by clamping the right and left Glissonian pedicles alternately during the parenchymal resection of the right and left hemi-livers respectively. This method seems particularly advisable in patients with impaired liver function or with cirrhosis.

REFERENCES

1. Delva E, Camus Y, Nordlinger B et al. Vascular occlusion for liver resections. Operative management and tolerance to hepatic ischemia. *Ann Surg* 1989; **209**: 211-218.
2. Elias D, Desrennes E, Lasser P. Prolonged intermittent clamping of the portal triad during hepatectomy. *Br J Surg* 1991; **78**: 42-44.

3. Gozzetti G, Mazziotti A, Grazi GL et al. Liver resections without blood transfusions. Br J Surg 1995; **82:** 1105-1110.

4. Hannoun L, Borie D, Delva E et al. Liver resection with normothermic ischemia exceeding 1h. Br J Surg 1993; **80:** 1161-1165.

5. Hardy KJ, Tancheroen S, Shulkes A. Comparison of continuous versus intermittent ischemia-reperfusion during liver resection in an experimental model. Br J Surg 1995; **82:** 833-836.

6. Huguet C, Gavelli A, Chicco A et al. Liver ischemia for hepatic resections: where is the limit? Surgery 1992; **111:** 251-259.

7. Isozaki H, Adam R, Gigon M, Szekely AM, Shen M, Bismuth H. Experimental study of the protective effect of intermittent hepatic pedicle clamping in the rat. Br J Surg 1992; **79:** 310-313.

8. Makuuchi M, Mori T, Gunven P et al. Safety of hemihepatic vascular occlusion during resection of the liver. Surg Gynecol Obstet 1987; **164:** 155-158.

9. Makuuchi M, Mori T, Gunven P, Yamazaki S, Hasegawa H. Experimental study of protective effect of intermittent hepatic pedicle clamping in the rat. Br J Surg 1992; **79:** 310-313.

10. Nardo B, Gasbarrini A, Mazziotti A, Bernardi M, Cavallari A. Reduction of rat hepatic ischemia/reperfusion injury by intermittent anoxia. Proceedings 2nd World IHPBA Congress, Bologna 1996. Monduzzi, Bologna, 1996, pp. 139-142.

11. Pierangeli F, Jagot P, Farges O, Sauvanet A, Jany S, Belghiti J. Intermittent or continuous hepatic pedicle clamping. A randomized study. (Abstract). HPB Surg 1996; **9** (Suppl. 2): 25.

12. Quan D, Wall WJ. The safety of continuous hepatic inflow occlusion during major liver resections. Liver Transpl Surg 1996; **2:** 99-104.

17
Intra-operative Ultrasound

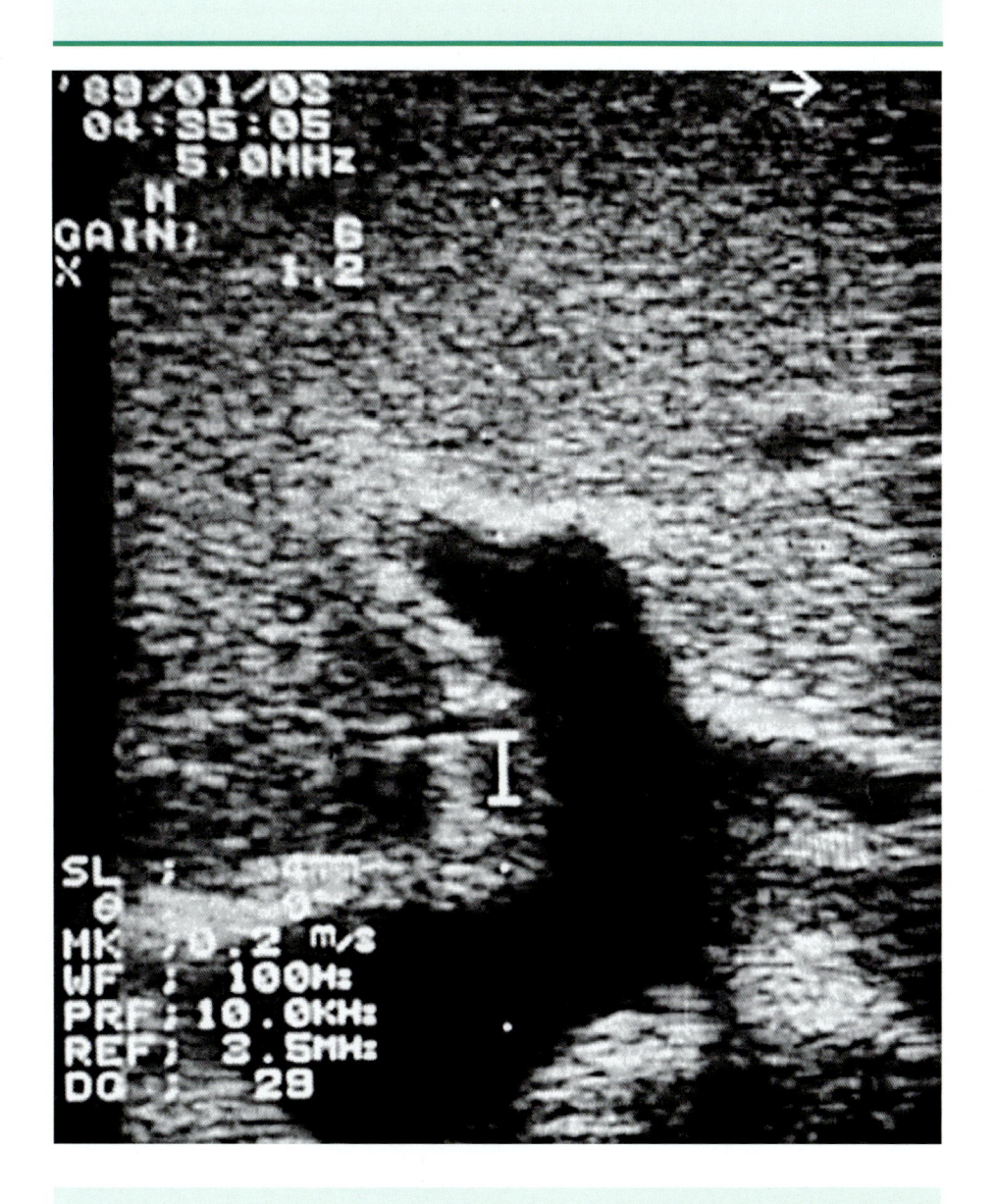

Liver surgery is an interesting and widely used application of intra-operative ultrasound (IOU). IOU can detect the presence of lesions, determine their anatomical location with regards to any adjacent vessels and provide an overall assessment of the lesion's extent. This information can be obtained at the start of the operation, minimizing unnecessary tissue dissection, traumatic surgical maneuvers and the use of contrast medium.

Instrumentation and exploration technique

IOU equipment is a conventional ultrasound device. It is advisable to limit its dimensions so that it can be used in small operating rooms and is easily moved and managed (adjustment of the 'gain' and 'gray scale', freezing of the images, etc., are performed by a nurse and not by a specialized technician). The apparatus should also have a screen large enough for the surgeon to be able to see the ultrasound image from one meter away. The probes must be small enough to be introduced into the abdominal cavity through a small incision, easily sterilized and with a sufficient cable length (about 2 m). Linear array probes are most commonly used for hepatic surgery (convex or sectorial probes are generally used in pancreatic and biliary surgery). These probes have a T aspect with the field of vision along the inferior horizontal bar of the T (the resulting images are rectangular with the superior part corresponding to the contact zone of the probe). They can easily be hand-held by the surgeon and are completely in contact with the hepatic surface in order to pass along the anterior and lateral aspects of the liver. The width of the probes varies from 3 to a maximum of 10 cm. The larger probes have a wider field of vision and are very useful for correct spatial topographic evaluation of the lesions with respect to the surrounding vascular structures but require adequate subcostal access. Smaller 3 cm probes have a narrower field of vision, with the disadvantage of providing a very confined picture of the parenchyma and a more difficult topographic evaluation of the lesions. Their use is mandatory in the case of mini laparotomy for an initial exploration, median laparotomy or lower umbilical laparotomy when exploration of the liver is advisable during surgery for colorectal tumors. Ultrasound frequency ranges from 5 up to 10 MHz. The 5 MHz probe is a good compromise between resolution power and maximum depth of exploration[9] and is most commonly used for liver surgery.

The probe is placed directly on the liver surface and manipulated by the surgeon. The surgeon performing the investigation interprets the IOU images. The examination may need to be repeated during the operation, e.g. in assessing the resection margins during liver tumor surgery. It would be time-consuming for a radiologist to spend several hours in the operating room and it is therefore necessary for the surgeon to learn how to perform and interpret ultrasound. Liver lesions situated superficially are more difficult to detect with ultrasound, because immediately below the probe there exists an artifact called the 'band effect' which conceals the area immediately below Glisson's capsule. To overcome this, a water barrier can be placed between the probe and the liver surface (e.g. a finger of a surgical glove filled with saline solution) in order to move away from the focal zone. Doppler probes can occasionally be moved to measure vessel flow. Verifying the patency of portosystemic anastomosis or arterial anastomosis during liver transplantation (*Figure 17.1*) of the graft is an uncommon application[9] and the usefulness of this application remains questionable. Other special probes for laparoscopic surgery have recently been adapted for the detection of bile duct stones or for the search for occult liver metastases in surgery for digestive tumors.[5,16,18,21,23,25,26] The probes are sterilized by liquid or gas.

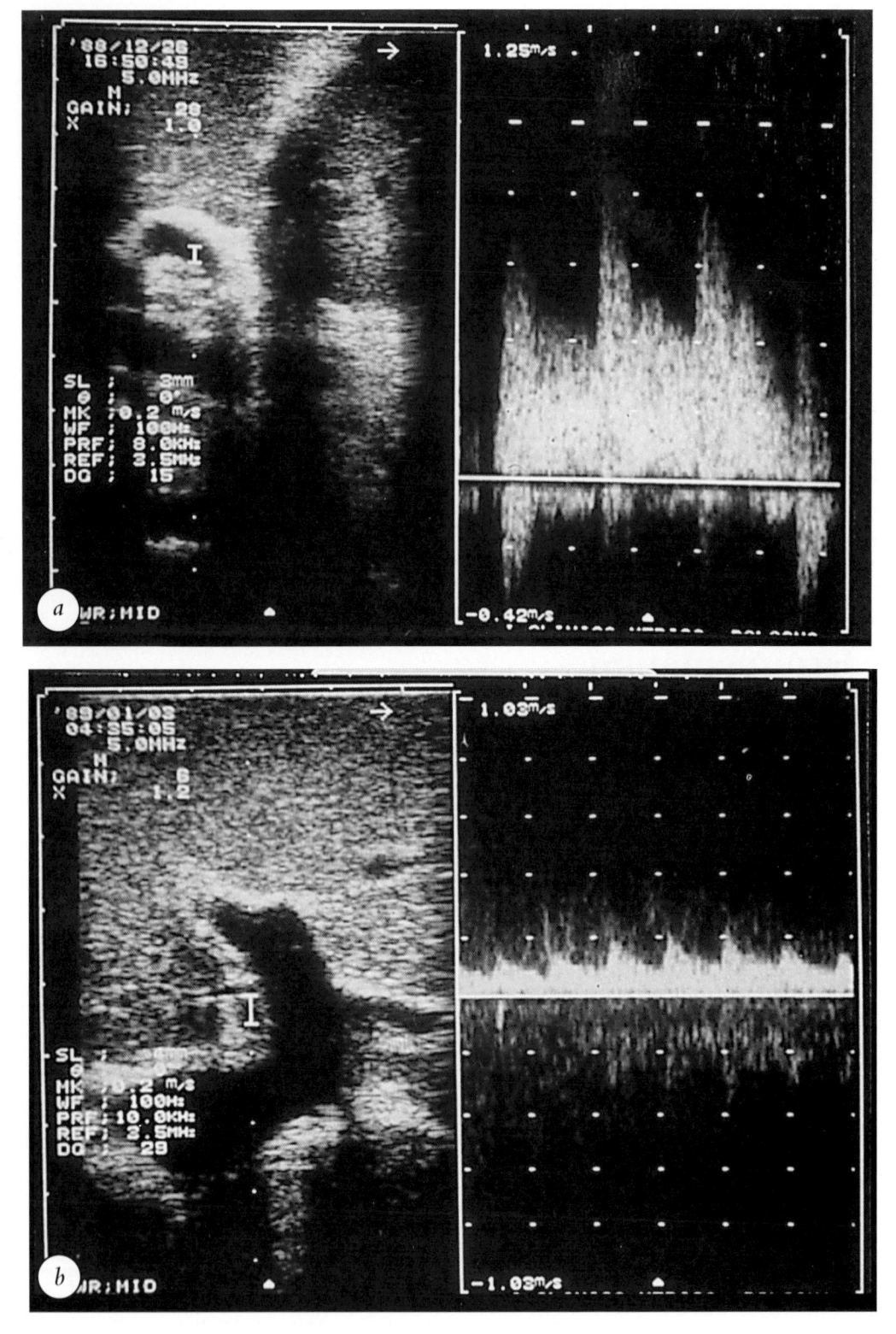

Figure 17.1 – *Intraoperative echo-Doppler control of hepatic artery anastomosis during liver transplantation.* ***a)*** *Probe positioned at the level of the trunk of the hepatic artery.* ***b)*** *Probe positioned at the level of the left branch of the hepatic artery.*

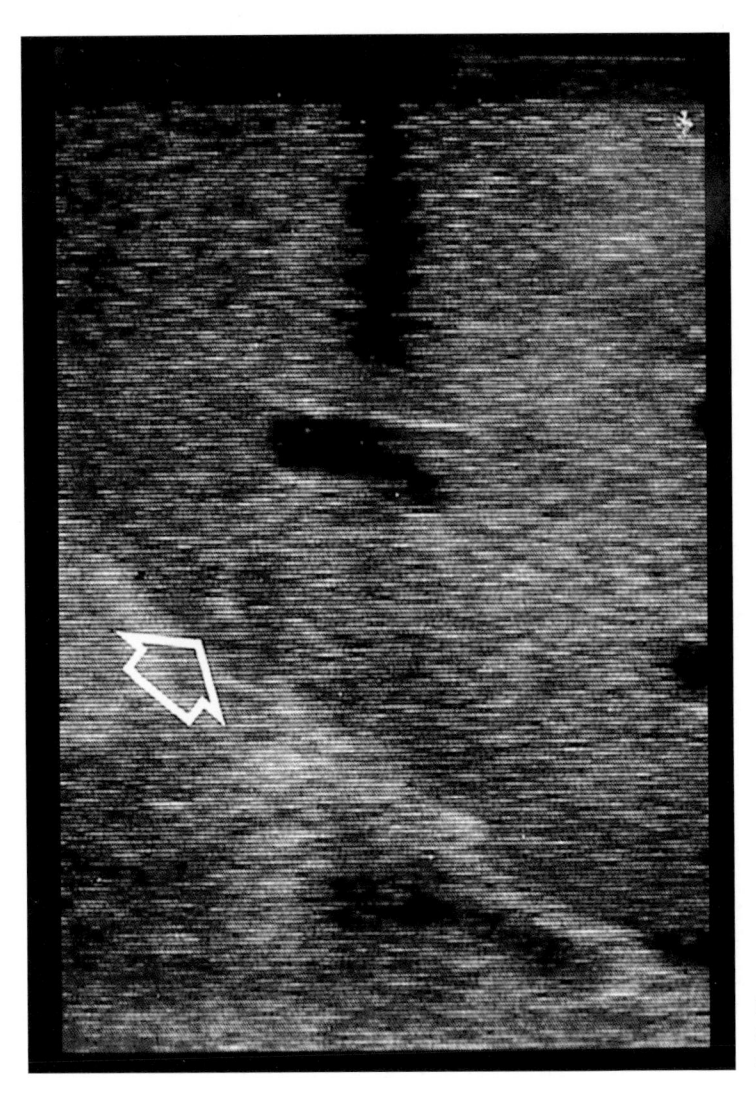

Figure 17.2 – *Small (0.5 cm) occult metastasis (white arrow) detected by intraoperative ultrasound.*

Hepatic ultrasound exploration

No preliminary division of the liver ligaments is needed to carry out a complete ultrasound exploration of the liver. The examination can be performed through a small laparotomy incision which is large enough for the surgeon's hand to pass through. As in the case of colorectal tumors, median laparotomy can also be performed. Systematic exploration of the liver should include both lobes, the portal branches to each segmentary branch and the courses of the main hepatic veins from their origins to the confluence in the vena cava. Care must be taken at this point to note any anatomic variations such as the presence of accessory hepatic veins. Exploration of the posterior segment can be performed without dividing the triangular ligament, if care is taken in moving the probe obliquely to include the furthest posterior portion of the parenchyma in the field of vision.

Contributions of IOU in liver surgery

DIAGNOSIS OF INTRAHEPATIC TUMORS

Lesions of about 1 cm or less are the limit of conventional radiological methods, including abdominal ultrasound, CT, MRI and angiography. Such lesions can also escape surgical exploration of the liver especially when they are deeply located within the parenchyma or in the presence of cirrhosis. The higher resolution capability of intra-operative probes allows lesions as small as 4 or 5 mm to be detected (***Figure 17.2***). Several reports and our own observations confirm the higher sensitivity of IOU compared with CT, pre-operative ultrasound and angiography for small lesions in normal or cirrhotic livers.[4,8,9,11,17]

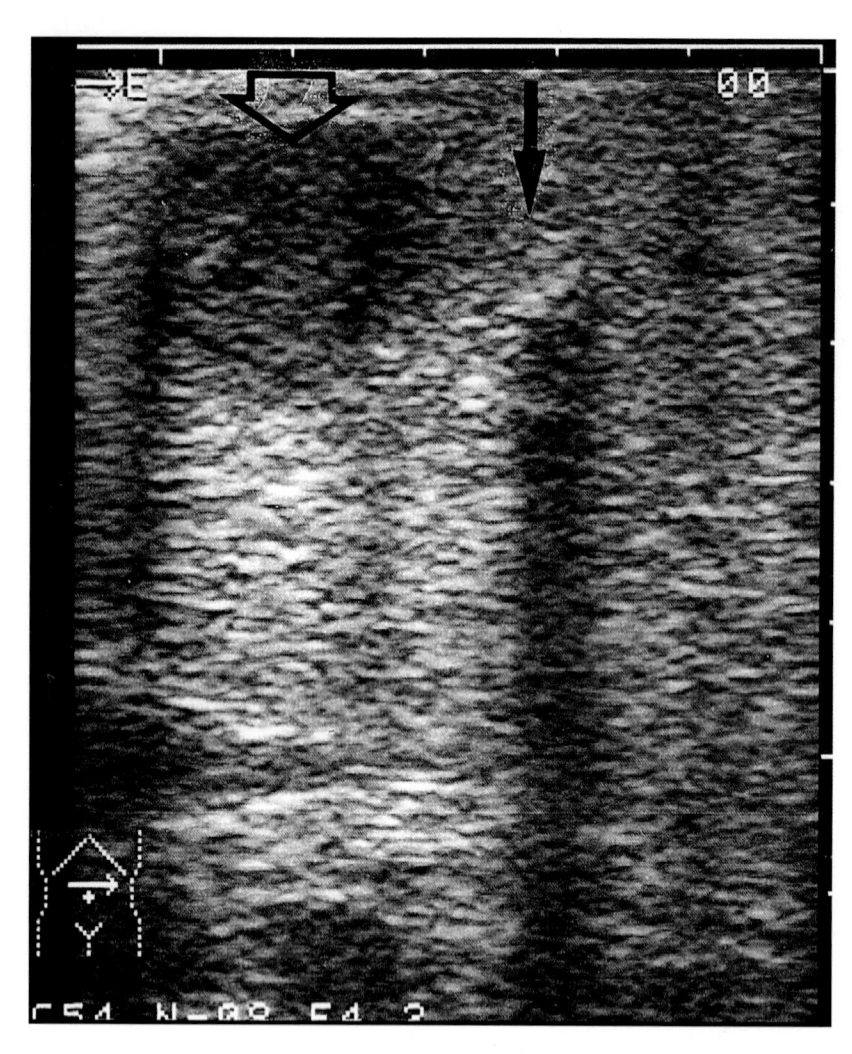

Figure 17.3 – *Control of resection margin by intraoperative ultrasound. Wedge resection of a small liver metastasis (line arrow). A sterile dressing has been placed on the resection plane, appearing as an echogenous image (black arrow) with a posterior shadow cone*

DETECTION OF OCCULT LIVER METASTASES

The importance of occult liver metastases detected by IOU during surgery for colorectal tumors becomes evident when considering that most of the patients operated on for these tumors do not routinely undergo extensive radiological studies if pre-operative ultrasound has not shown evidence of liver lesions; 5-10% of unsuspected liver lesions has been reported with IOU.[2,3,13,15,20,24] In our experience, IOU examination was particularly helpful in surgery for tumors of the pancreas, when pre-operative exploration and surgical exploration are hampered by the presence of cholestasis: the information provided radically affects surgical strategy, preventing unnecessary operations, such as pancreatectomy, in the presence of previously occult hepatic metastases.[9]

SURGERY FOR HEPATOCELLULAR CARCINOMA ON CIRRHOSIS

Surgery for hepatocellular carcinoma on cirrhosis has become extremely common in western countries due to the increasing frequency of this disease and to the detection of small subclinical tumors by the extensive use of screening methods such as ultrasound and tumor markers. The experience of surgeons from Eastern countries and recent data from European centers[7,10] show that the risk of resections in cirrhotic livers is acceptable if the residual liver function is carefully assessed and removal of non-tumor parenchyma is as conservative as possible. This suggests the need for precise localization of the tumor which is often not palpable within the cirrhotic parenchyma.[1,19,22] In these cases IOU is essential in order to visualize the tumor and its relationship with the intrahepatic vessels. Special techniques have been described for echo-guided resection in cirrhotics. For small tumors the surrounding parenchyma can be tattooed[9] or mapped.[12] Makuuchi introduced the injection of methylene blue in the portal branch to allow visualization of the correct anatomical limits of the segment to be removed.

RESECTION MARGIN CONTROL

During resection, ultrasound is usually repeated to verify the plane of the parenchymal division with respect to the limit of the tumor to ensure a sufficient resection margin. The importance of preserving a margin of at least 1 cm has been emphasized many times for the surgery of hepatic metastases[6,8,14] and hepatocarcinoma. In cases of tumor removal with margins less than 1 cm, recurrence has been found to be significantly higher (51%) compared with hepatectomy (33%) or after segmentectomy (30%).[8,10] The correct resection plane is often difficult to evaluate during liver resection, especially in cirrhotic livers. With IOU it is much easier to identify the distance from the tumor margin. To achieve this it is necessary to place an echogenic material, such as a surgical clamp or a piece of gauze, in the resection margin to verify whether the direction of the resection plane is correct to ensure an adequate distance from the lesion (**Figure 17.3**).

REFERENCES

1. Bismuth H, Castaing D, Garden OJ. The use of operative ultrasound in surgery of primary liver tumors. *World J Surg* 1987; **11**: 610-614.
2. Boldrini G, De Gaetano AM, Giovannini I *et al.* The systematic use of operative ultrasound for detection of liver metastases during colorectal surgery. *World J Surg* 1987; **11**: 622-627.
3. Charnely RM, Morris DL, Dennison AR, Amar SS, Hardcastle JD. Detection of colorectal liver metastases using intraoperative ultrasonography. *Br J Surg* 1994; **78**: 45-48.
4. Clarke MP, Kane RA, Steele G *et al.* Prospective comparison of preoperative imaging and intraoperative ultrasonography in the detection of liver tumors. *Surgery* 1989; **106**: 849-855.
5. Cuesta MA, Meijer S, Borgstein PJ, Sibinga Mulder L, Sikkenk AC. Laparoscopic ultra sonography for hepatobiliary and pancreatic malignancy. *Br J Surg* 1993; **80**: 1571-1574.
6. Ekberg H, Tranberg KG, Anderson K *et al.* Pattern of recurrence in liver resections of colorectal secondaries. *World J Surg* 1987; **11**: 541-547.
7. Franco D, Capussotti C, Smadja C *et al.* Resection of hepatocellular carcinoma. Results in 72 European patients with cirrhosis. *Gastroenterology* 1990; **98**: 733-738.
8. Gozzetti G, Mazziotti A. Expectations and possibilities of liver resections for metastases. In: Lygidakis N, Tytgat GNJ. (Eds), *Hepatobiliary and Pancreatic Malignancies*. Thieme, Stuttgart, pp. 183-190, 1989.
9. Gozzetti G, Mazziotti A, Bolondi L, Barbara L. *Intraoperative ultrasonography in hepatobiliary and pancreatic surgery.* Kluwer, Dordrecht, 1989.
10. Gozzetti G, Bell L, Capussotti L, Mazziotti A *et al.* Liver resections for hepatocellular carcinoma in cirrhotic patients. *Ital J Gastroenterol* 1992; **24**: 105-110.
11. Gunven P, Makuuchi M, Hasegawa H *et al.* Preoperative imaging of liver metastases. Comparison of angiography, CT scan and ultrasonography. *Ann Surg* 1985; **202**: 573-579.
12. Hasegawa H, Yamasaki S, Makuuchi M, Le Thai B. Nouvelle technique d'hépatectomie utilisant l'échographie péropératoire et des aiguilles de réperage intraparenchimateuses. Technique du géomètre. *J Chirurgie* 1988; **125**: 278-284.
13. Herman K. Intraoperative ultrasound in gastrointestinal cancer. An analysis of 272 operated patients. *Hepato-Gastroenterol* 1996; **43**:565-570.
14. Hughes KS, Simon R, Soughrabodis S *et al.* Resection of the liver for colorectal carcinoma metastases: a multi-institutional study of pat terns of recurrence. *Surgery* 1986; **100**: 278-284.
15. Machi J, Isamoto H, Yamashiti Y *et al.* Intraoperative ultrasonography in screening for liver metastases from colorectal cancer: comparative accuracy with traditional procedures. *Surgery* 1987; **101**: 678-684.
16. Machi J, Sigel B, Zaren HA *et al.* Technique of ultrasound examination during laparoscopic cholecystectomy. *Surg Endosc* 1993; **7**:544-549.
17. Makuuchi M. Abdominal intraoperative ultrasonography. Igaku Shoin, Tokyo, 1987.
18. Murugiah M, Paterson-Brown S, Windsor JA, Miles WFA, Garden OJ. Early experience of laparoscopic ultrasonography in the management of pancreatic carcinoma. *Surg Endosc* 1993; **7**: 177-181.
19. Nagasue N, Suchio S, Yakaya H. Intraoperative ultrasonography for the surgical treatment of hepatic tumors. *Acta Chir Scand* 1984; **150**: 311-316.
20. Rafelsen SR, Kronborg O, Larsen C, Fenger C. Intraoperative ultrasonography in detection

of hepatic metastases from colorectal cancer. *Dis Col Rectum* 1995; **38:** 355-360.
21. Santambrogio R, Bianchi P, Opocher E *et al*. Ecografia intraoperatoria laparoscopica. *Chirurgia* 1996; **9:** 203-209.
22. Shen JC, Lee S. Sung JC *et al*. Intraoperative hepatic ultrasonography. An indispensable procedure in resection of small hepatocellualr carcinoma. *Surgery* 1985; **97:** 97-103.
23. Stiegmann GV, McIntyre RC, Pearlman NW. Laparoscopic intracorporeal ultrasound. An alternative to cholangiography. *Surg Endosc* 1994; **8:** 167-172.
24. Stone MD, Kane R, Bothe A, Jessup JM, Cady B, Steele GD. Intraoperative ultrasound imaging of the liver at the time of colorectal resection. *Arch Surg* 1994; **129:** 431-435.
25. Yamamoto M, Stiegmann GV, Durham J *et al*. Laparoscopic guided intracorporeal ultrasound. An alterantive to cholangiography? *Surg Endosc* 1993; **7:** 325-330.
26. Yamashita Y, Kurokiji T, Hayashi J, Kimitsuki H, Hiraki M, Kakegawa T. Intraoperative ultrasonography during laparoscopic cholecystectomy. *Surg Laparosc Endosc* 1993; **3:** 167-171.

18

Indications for Liver Resection

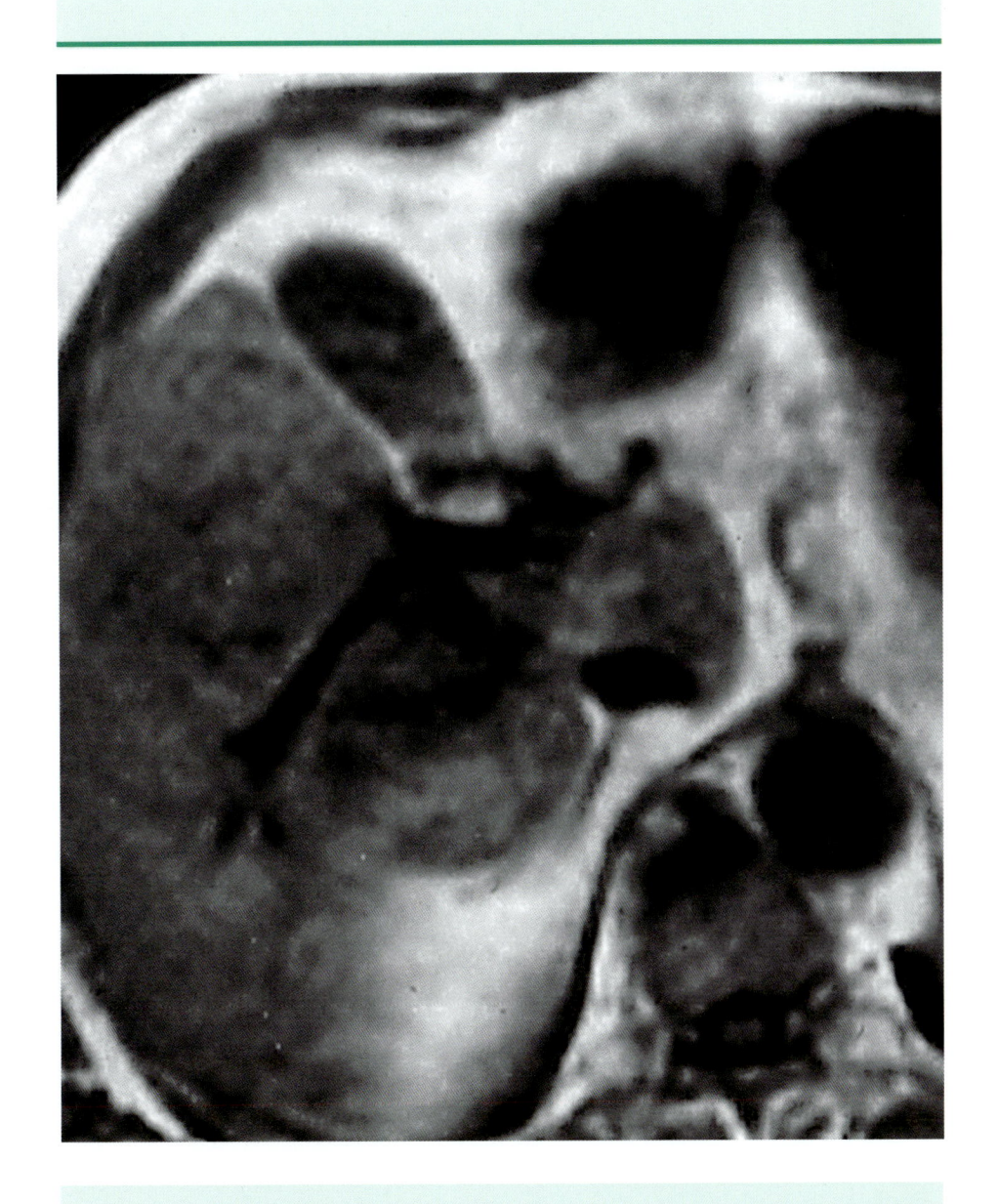

Primary malignant tumors

Hepatocarcinoma is one of the most common indications for hepatic resection. A rapid increase in the incidence of this type of tumor has been recorded in the last few years in European countries, probably related to the spread of hepatitis B and C virus infections.[6] The increasing use of screening methods for hepatic tumors (ultrasound and tumor markers) now makes it possible to detect subclinical cases of hepatic tumors more frequently and represents one of the main factors that has determined the rising request for hepatic resection surgery.[7]

An elective indication for resection is the uninodular type of hepatocarcinoma. The multifocal type, extension to both lobes, infiltration of the adjacent organs and the hepatic hilum, thrombosis of the portal vein or of the vena cava and the presence of lymph node or extrahepatic metastases are contraindications for this type of surgery and the pre-operative work-up is intended to exclude these. Partial infiltration of the wall of the vena cava can be taken into consideration for a resection with vascular reconstruction.

Hepatic cirrhosis is only a relative contraindication due to functional insufficiency and inability of the cirrhotic liver to regenerate. In the last few years case series of hepatic resection of cirrhotic livers have considerably increased, even in Western populations[10,11] Careful evaluation of the operative risk must be made in these cases and surgery should only be performed in patients with good functional reserve. Resection must preserve as much parenchyma as possible. This type of surgery can only be performed in cirrhotic patients with the help of intraoperative ultrasound, which makes it possible to identify the site of the tumor (which usually cannot be palpated inside a cirrhotic parenchyma) and its relationships with the intrahepatic vessels. The specific indications and the surgical technique problems for hepatocarcinoma associated with cirrhosis are described in Chapter 7.

The overall result of hepatic resection for primary liver tumors has shown improvement in the most recent case studies. Operative mortality in non-cirrhotic liver resections has fallen in most case series to acceptable levels of around 1%.[12] Evaluation of long-term results is more difficult, as the cases reported in the literature are often limited and are without a precise classification of the grading of the tumor. The best results have been recorded for asymptomatic tumors, with limited size, an expansive type of growth and without vascular infiltration of the areas surrounding the tumor; 5-year survival for these types of lesions can exceed 40%.[11] In cirrhotic patients the operative mortality is notably higher, even though it has fallen to less than 5% in the most recent case series.[19] Five-year survival is higher in patients without symptoms, with single tumors and in the absence of intravasal neoplastic thrombosis.[19] Long-term recurrence in cirrhotic livers is extremely frequent[1] and this greatly limits the expectations for this type of surgery in young patients. The most rational indications for resective surgery are older patients with non-progressive cirrhosis and good functional reserve, without the risk of hemorrhage from esophageal varices and with peripherally sited single tumors, in whom resection can be performed without removing large amounts of hepatic parenchyma. The indication for resection must however be considered in relation to the therapeutic alternatives: alcoholization, chemoembolization and transplantation.[2,8,17]

Metastatic tumors

Hepatic metastases are another common indication for liver resection. The most relevant indications are metastases from colorectal tumors or digestive endocrine tumors, with carcinologically complete resection of the primary tumor, and with no other local or systemic sites of tumor spread. Resection is indicated less frequently for extradigestive neoplasms such as tumors of the ovaries, breast, kidneys, testicles and leiomyosarcoma of the soft tissues. In certain selected cases, with curative type resection, results have been observed similar to those obtained in colorectal carcinoma.[14,25,30] A particular indication is metastases from digestive endocrine tumors, including pancreatic apudoma. The palliation of symptoms achieved in these cases and the good results in long-term survival encourage an aggressive approach, even for multiple metastases. Metastases from gastric tumors are a doubtful indication;[22] resection for metastases from pancreatic carcinoma should not be considered.

The extent of the resection for metastases is determined by the volume and by the number of the metastases; massive or multiple lesions in a hemiliver require major hepatectomy. In the more usual case of isolated metastasis, the current trend is to perform segmentectomies or wedge resections which include at least 1 cm of healthy liver tissue. As far as synchronous metastases are concerned, the current tendency is not to perform a major hepatectomy at the same time as resection of the primary tumor. One-stage combined resections certainly involve a higher rate of morbidity and do not seem to offer better long-term results.[29] The most common approach is to remove the primary tumor and postpone liver surgery for 2-3 months, after starting chemotherapy and completing the diagnostic work-up.

The limits of the resection based on the number of intrahepatic lesions vary according to the attitude of the surgical unit. Although the maximum operable number of metastases is usually accepted as being 4, patients with 5 or 6 lesions or even more do occasionally undergo surgery. This seems to depend on whether the operation can be correctly performed from a technical point of view and with a radical aim (good peritumoral margin, no extrahepatic diffusion).

Five-year survival for hepatic resections for metastases from colorectal carcinoma ranges from 20 to 40%. The factors which most affect prognosis are grading of the primary tumor, number of metastases and time interval between exeresis of the primary tumor and appearance of the metastases; the most favorable situation is represented by unilobar metachronous metastases.[23]

Benign tumors

Some clinical studies have contributed to our knowledge of the natural history of benign tumors of the liver and thus define the surgical indications, particularly for angiomas, the most frequent benign tumors found in the liver.[4] The risk of complications from angiomas (rupture, growth in volume) is much less than was once thought: spontaneous rupture of hepatic angiomas is truly exceptional (less than 1% for large angiomas). The tendency to increase in size, which can now be monitored with ultrasound, is very rare. The prevailing tendency in most liver surgery centers is now to limit the surgical indication to symptomatic angiomas or those with a documented tendency to enlarge, in addition to the (very rare) cases of spontaneous angioma rupture,[12] or following biopsy or surgical maneuvers.

Focal nodular hyperplasia is also generally considered a benign condition and surgical indication for this disease is currently limited either to the (rare) certainly symptomatic cases or when radiological examinations and percutaneous biopsy do not permit diagnosis to be made with certainty. Adenomas, on the other hand, involve a high risk of rupture with hemoperitoneum or intrahepatic hematomas[15,16] and a possible risk of neoplastic degeneration.[9,26,27] The risk of an adenoma rupturing does not depend on the size of the lesion.[13] nor on the fact that the patient stops taking oral contraceptives.[5] Surgery should be undertaken for hepatic adenomas, even in asymptomatic cases.

In benign tumors, the type of resection depends on the site and the size of the lesion. For lesions of limited dimensions and sited peripherally, hemi-nucleations are indicated, staying close to the capsule which is present particularly in angiomas. For large lesions or those involving an entire hemiliver, we prefer to perform typical hepatectomies which leave a linear resection plane, more limited than in a wedge resection which follows the margin of the tumor, and make hemostasis easier to carry out. Ligation of the Glissonian pedicles also reduces the size of the tumor and makes mobilization of the liver and resection easier.

Klatskin tumors

These tumors pose complex treatment problems which are the subject of controversy.

Radical surgery is accompanied by more favorable results than palliative treatment, (e.g. biliary-intestinal shunts or biliary drainage[3,21,24,28]). Resection can be proposed for tumors localized at the biliary bifurcation, without lymph node or hepatic metastases. The surgical techniques, described in Chapter 24, include perihilar wedge resection, resection of the caudate lobe and resection of the bile tract with bilioenteric reconstruction on a Roux loop, and right or left hepatectomies, again accompanied by resection of the caudate lobe, if the right or left bile ducts are involved. In the commoner cases of tumors of the biliary bifurcation, resection includes segment 4 and the caudate lobe. The latter must always be removed due to the close relationship between the biliary bifurcation and the caudate lobe. The Spigel lobe is the elective site of neoplasm relapse, if left in place, after resection of a tumor of the hilum. Recent data suggest better long-term results with aggressive resection for tumors of the biliary bifurcation.[20]

Other less frequent indications for hepatic resection include rare benign tumors,[4] congenital cystic dilations of the bile tract, some hydatid cysts (see Chapter 21), intrahepatic lythiasis with segmentary involvement and sarcomas of the liver, the latter having an extremely poor prognosis.

REFERENCES

1. Belghiti J, Panis Y, Farges O, Benhamou JP, Fékété F. Intrahepatic recurrence after resection of hepatocellular carcinoma complicating cirrhosis. *Ann Surg* 1991; **214**: 114-118.
2. Bismuth H, Cliche L, Adam R, Castaing D. Surgical treatment of hepatocellular carcinoma in cirrhosis: liver resection or transplantation? *Transpl Proc* 1993; **25**: 1066-1067.
3. Cameron JL, Pilt HA, Zinner NJ, Kanfman SL. Management of proximal cholangiocarcinoma by surgical resection and radiotherapy. *Am J Surg* 1990; **152**: 91-98.
4. Cavallari A, Mazziotti A, Grazi GL, Jovine E et al. Benign and borderline liver lesions. Proceedings 2nd World IHPBA Congress, Bologna 1996. Monduzzi, Bologna, 1996, Vol. 1, pp. 175-181.
5. Cheng PN, Shiann JS, Lin XZ. Hepatic adenoma: an observation from asymptomatic stage to rupture. *Hepato-Gastroenterol* 1996; **43**: 245-248.
6. Colombo M, Kuo G, Choo QL et al. Prevalence of antibodies to hepatitis C virus in Italian patients with hepatocellular carcinoma. *Lancet* 1989; **2**: 1006-1008.
7. Consensus Report. Early diagnosis of hepatocellular carcinoma in Italy. *J Hepatol* 1992; **14**: 401-403.
8. Farmer DG, Rosove MH, Shaked A, Busuttill RW. Current treatment modalities for hepatocellular carcinoma. *Ann Surg* 1994; **219**: 236-247.
9. Gordon SC, Reddy RL, Livingstone AS, Jeffers LJ, Schill ER. Resolution of a contraceptive steroid-induced hepatic adenoma with subsequent evolution into hepatocellular carcinoma. *Ann Int Med*. 1986; **105**: 547-549.
10. Gozzetti G, Mazziotti A, Cavallari A et al. Clinical experience with hepatic resections for hepatocellular carcinoma in patients with cirrhosis. *Surg Gynecol. Obstetr* 1988; **166**: 503-510.
11. Gozzetti G, Mazziotti A, Grazi GL, Jovine E. Surgical experience with 168 primary liver cell carcinomas treated with hepatic resections. *J Surg Oncol* 1993; **3**: 59-61.
12. Gozzetti G, Mazziotti A, Grazi GL, Jovine E, Pierangeli F, Gallucci A, Morganti M. Liver resections without blood transfusions. *Br J Surg* 1995; **82**: 1105-1110.
13. Flowers BF, McBurney RP, Vera SR. Ruptured hepatic adenoma: a spectrum of presentation and treatment. *Am Surg* 1990; **56**: 381-383.
15. Kelly D, Lehrer D, Emre S, Guy S, Sheiner P, Miller C, Schwartz M. Liver resections for metastases of non-colorectal origin. Proceedings 2nd World IHPBA Congress, Bologna 1996. Monduzzi, Bologna, 1996, Vol. 1, pp. 381-384.
16. Kerlin P, Davis L, McGill DB, Weiland LH, Adson MA, Sheedy PF. Hepatic adenoma and focal nodular hyperplasia: clinical, pathological and radiological features. *Gastroenterology* 1983; **84**: 994-1002.
17. Langer J, Langer B, Taylor B et al. Carcinoma of the extrahepatic bile ducts: results of an aggressive approach. *Surgery* 1985; **98**:752-759.
18. Livraghi T, Bolondi L, Buscarini L et al. No treatment, resection and ethanol injection in hepatocellular carcinoma: a retrospective analysis of survival in 391 patients with cirrhosis. *J Hepatol* 1995; **15**: 77-80.
19. Mazziotti A, Jovine E, Grazi GL et al. Spontaneus subcapsular rupture of hepatic hemangioma. *Eur J Surg* 1995; **161**: 687-689.
20. Mazziotti A, Grazi GL, Jovine E et al. Expectations, possibilities and limits of liver resections for hepatocellular carcinoma in cirrhotic patients. Proceedings 2nd World IHPBA Congress, Bologna 1996. Monduzzi, Bologna, 1996, Vol. 1, pp. 239-246.
21. Principe A, Lugaresi ML, Mazziotti A, Lords R, Masetti M, Cavallari A. Klatskin tumors: assessment of resectability and therapeutic alternatives. Proceedings 2nd World IHPBA Congress, Bologna 1996. Monduzzi, Bologna, 1996, Vol. 1, pp. 901-907.
21. Rossi R, Heiss F, Beckmann C, Braasch J. Management of cancer in the bile duct. *Surg Clin North Amer* 1985; **65**: 59-78.
22. Saito A, Korenaga D, Sakagauchi Y, Ohno S, Ichiyashi Y, Sugimaki K. Surgical treatment for gastric carcinomas with concomitant hepatic metastasis. *Hepato-Gastroenterol* 1996; **43**: 560-564.

23. Scheele J, Stang R, Altendorf-Hoffmann A, Paul M. Resection of colorectal liver metastases. *World J Surg;* 1995; **19:** 59-71.
24. Schoenthaler R, Philips T, Castro J, Efird JT, Better A, Way LW. Carcinoma of the extrahepatic bile ducts. The University of California at San Francisco experience. *Ann Surg* 1994; **219:** 267-274.
25. Schwartz SJ. Hepatic resection for non-colorectal, non-neuroendocrine metastases. *World J. Surg* 1995; **19:** 72-75.
26. Tao LC. Oral contraceptive-associated liver cell adenoma and hepatocellular carcinoma. *Cancer* 1991; **68:** 341-347.
27. Tesluck H, Lawrie J. Hepatocellular adenoma: its transformation to carcinoma in users of oral contraceptives. *Arch Pathol Lab Med* 1981; **105:** 296-299.
28. Van der Hul RL, Johans PW, Lamers JS, Veeze-Kuijpers B, Blankenstein MV, Terpstra OT. Proximal cholangiocarcinoma: a multidisciplinary approach. *Eur J Surg* 1994; **160:** 213-218.
29. Vogt P, Raab R, Ringe B, Pichlmayr R. Resection of synchronous liver metastases from colorectal cancer. *World J Surg* 1991; **15:** 62-67.
30. Wolf RF, Goodnight JE, Frag DE, Schneider PD. Results of resection and proposed guidelines for patient selection in instances of non-colorectal hepatic metastases. *Surg Gynecol Obstetr* 1991; **173:** 454-460.

19

Pre-operative Portal Embolization

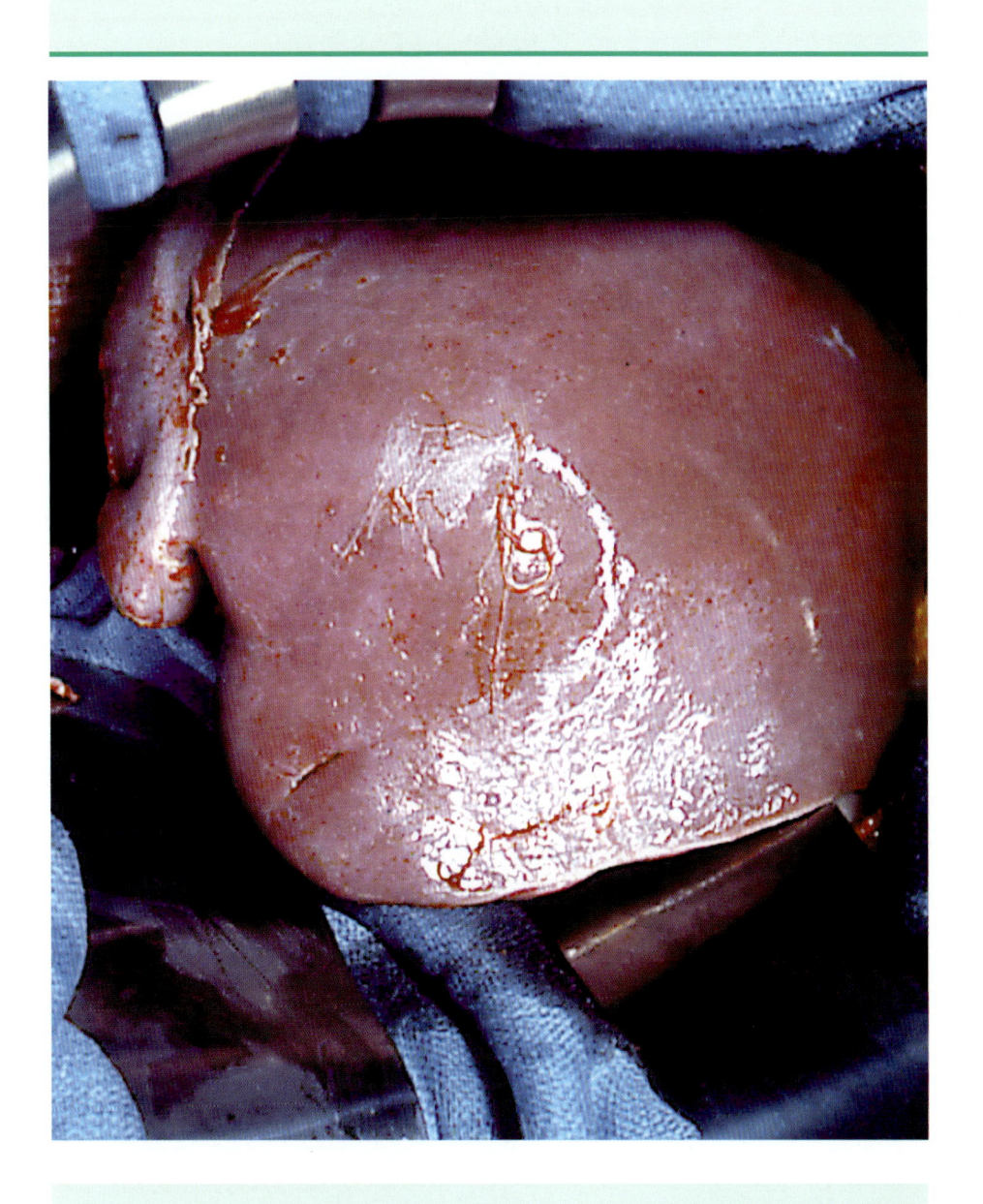

Conventional right hepatectomy is perfectly tolerated by a normal liver. Even hepatectomies for trauma, when all the excised parenchyma is healthy, are not complicated by signs of hepatic insufficiency unless prolonged ischemia of the parenchyma, hypotension or portal thrombosis has occurred. The risk of hepatic insufficiency after hepatectomy exists, however, in cholestatic livers or in the presence of chronic liver disease and cirrhosis. The risk must be considered in cases of extended hepatectomy, involving one or more segments of both hemi-livers, particularly in the presence of a centrally located tumor, when the part to be excised includes a significant amount of healthy parenchyma, or if the contralateral hepatic lobe is not hypertrophic.

Embolization of a portal branch in order to determine compensatory hypertrophy of the contralateral hepatic lobe in planning an extended hepatic resection has been proposed by Kinoshita[5] and Makuuchi.[7] The physiological grounds for this procedure are based on the effects of the portal flow on hepatic regeneration. Ligation of a portal branch in experimental animals leads to atrophy of the corresponding hemiliver and hypertrophy of the contralateral one.[10] The same phenomenon is known in man in cases of neoplastic thrombosis of a portal branch in tumors of the hepatic hilum[11] The effects of experimental portal embolization have been studied by Tanaka: one week after embolization the contralateral liver doubles its weight on average, with a parallel increase in the mitotic index and in the DNA synthesis of hepatocytes and an almost double increase in the number of Kupffer cells.[12]

The preferred technique for embolization is the trans-hepatic percutaneous route with insertion of a catheter pushed from Rex's recess as far as the right branch or the anterior and posterior dividing branches of the portal vein. The most commonly used embolization substances are gelfoam, cyanocrylate and metal coils with gelfoam. We prefer to use metal coils which have the advantage of easy radiological control.

Tolerance to embolization is good. From a clinical point of view, no deaths or complications linked with the method have been reported. A slight fever reaction is reported in most cases, disappearing spontaneously within 3-7 days.[1,6] A slight increase is always observed in cytonecrosis enzymes in the first few days after embolization.[6] The maximum increase in size of the remaining liver is achieved about 40-50 days after embolization with gelfoam and within the first month using cyanocrylate. The size of the remaining liver increases greatest after cyanocrylate (a mean of 69%) compared with gelfoam (between 20 and 50%), probably due to the greater embolizing effect of cyanocrylate. A period of 3-4 weeks, therefore, seems to be the ideal time that should be allowed to elapse between embolization and hepatectomy. Hypertrophy is observed in both non-cirrhotic livers and in cirrhotic patients. The increase in volume is more limited in diabetic patients.[9] Several clinical series come from the Far East[3,4,8,9,12] and from some European centres.[1,2] More than 100 cases had been reported in the literature by the end of 1994. All the clinical studies report good tolerance to embolization; the compensatory hypertrophy of the contralateral liver is particularly evident when embolization proves to be complete. The post-operative morbidity and mortality reported after hepatectomy preceded by embolization are perfectly acceptable considering that these are cases of extended resection. The rare cases of post-operative mortality reported refer only to cirrhotic patients after right hepatectomy.[6]

The indications for pre-operative portal embolization are extended hepatectomies in the presence of a remaining liver reduced in size. In the presence of a non-cirrhotic liver, such hepatectomies preserve only segments 2 and 3. An ideal indication consists of large tumors localized in the central segments of the liver involving removal of a significant mass of healthy tissue (*Figure 19.1*). One indication is

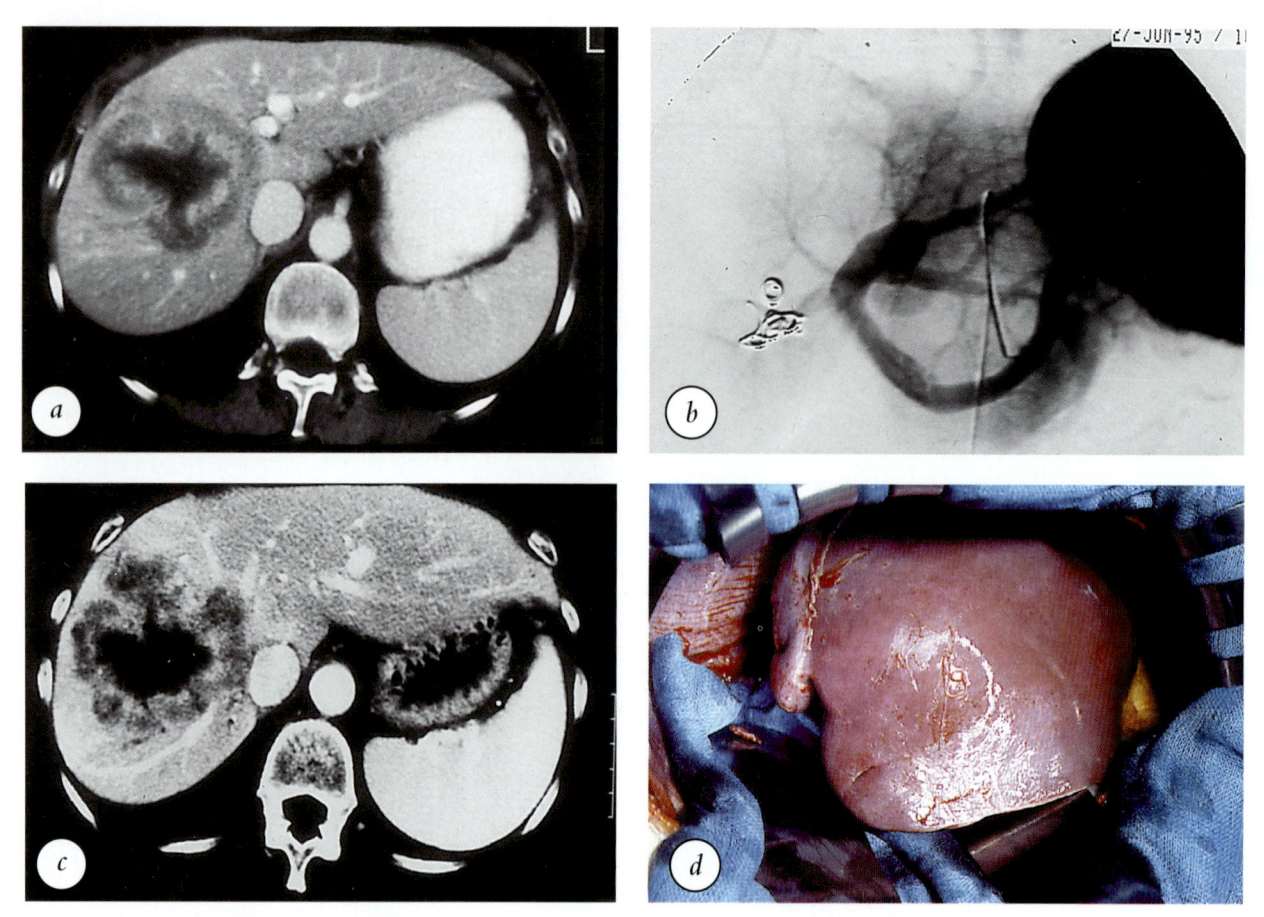

Figure 19.1 – *Pre-operative portal embolization for large metastases in the central segments of the liver. **a)** Pre-operative CT: the lesion occupies segments 4, 5 and 8. **b)** Angiographic control after embolization of the right branch of the portal vein with injection of metal coils and gelfoam. **c)** CT control 20 days after treatment. The hypertrophy of the left lobe is evident. **d)** One month after embolization the patient underwent right hepatectomy extended to include segment 4. The post-operative period was totally uneventful.*

cholangiocarcinoma of the hepatic hilum requiring hepatectomy extended to the caudate lobe and bilio-enteric anastomosis.[4,9] In such cases, the risk of hepatic insufficiency linked to the parenchymal resection is exacerbated by the cholestasis. The method is advisable when planning a major hepatectomy in a cirrhotic liver [6] or in the presence of multiple lobar hepatic metastases requiring an extended right hepatectomy associated with wedge resections on the left lobe.[3]

REFERENCES

1. De Baere Th, Roche A, Vavasseur D *et al.* Portal vein embolization: utility for inducing left hepatic lobe hypertrophy before surgery. *Radiology* 1993; **188**: 73-77.

2. Elias D, Roche A, Vavasseur D, Lasser Ph. Induction d'une hypertrophie d'un petit lobe gauche hépatique avant hépatectomie droite elargie, par embolization portal droite préopératoire. *Ann Chir* 1992; **46**: 404-410.

3. Kawasaki S, Makuuchi M, Kakazu T *et al.* Resection of multiple metastatic liver tumors after portal embolization. *Surgery* 1994; **6**: 674-677.

4. Kawasaki S, Makuuchi M, Miyagawa S, Kakazu T. Radical operation after portal embolization for tumor of hilar bile duct. *J Am Coll Surg* 1994; **178**: 480-486.

5. Kinoshita H, Sakai K, Hirohashi K, Igawa S, Yamasaki O, Kubo S. Preoperative portal vein embolization for hepatocellular carcinoma. *World J Surg* 1986; **10**: 803-807.

6. Lee KC, Kinoshita H, Hirohashi K, Kubo S, Iwasa R. Extension of surgical indications for hepatocellular carcinoma by portal vein embolization. *World J Surg* 1993; **17**: 109-115.

7. Makuuchi M, Thai BL, Takayasu K *et al.* Preoperative portal embolization to increase the safety of major hepatectomy for hilar bile duct carcinoma: a preliminary report. *Surgery* 1990; **107**: 521-529.

8. Makuuchi M, Kosuge T, Lygidakis N. New possibilities for major liver surgery in patients with Klatskin tumors or primary hepatocellular carcinoma: an old problem revisited. *Hepato-Gastroenterol* 1991; **81**: 329-336.

9. Nagino M, Niunura Y, Kamiya J *et al.* Changes in hepatic lobe volume in biliary tract cancer patients after right portal vein embolization.

Hepatology 1995; **21:** 434-439.
10. Rous P, Larimore L. Relation of the portal blood to liver maintenance. *J Exp Med* 1920; **31:** 609-632.
11. Takayasu K, Muramatsu Y, Shima Y, Moriyama N, Yamada T, Makuuchi M. Hepatic lobar atrophy following obstruction of the ipsilateral portal vein from hilar cholangiocarcinoma. *Radiology* 1986; **160:** 389-393.
12. Tanaka H, Kinoshita H, Hirohashi K, Kubo S, Lee KC. Increased safety by two stage hepatectomy with preoperative portal vein embolization in rats. *J Surg Res* 1984; **57:** 687-692.

TECHNIQUES IN LIVER SURGERY

SECTION VI

Surgery for Liver Cysts and Trauma

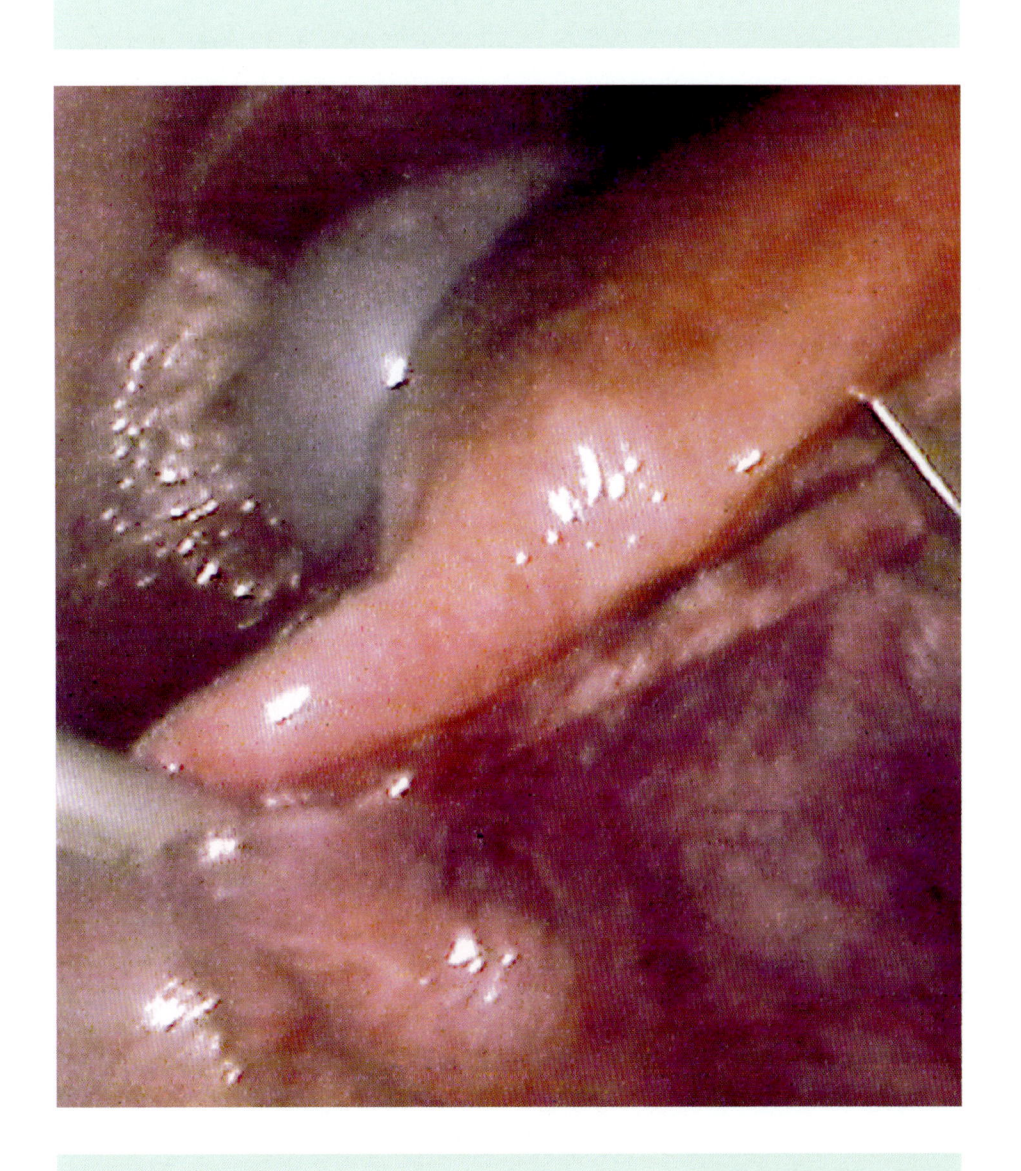

20

Surgery for Non-parasitic Liver Cysts

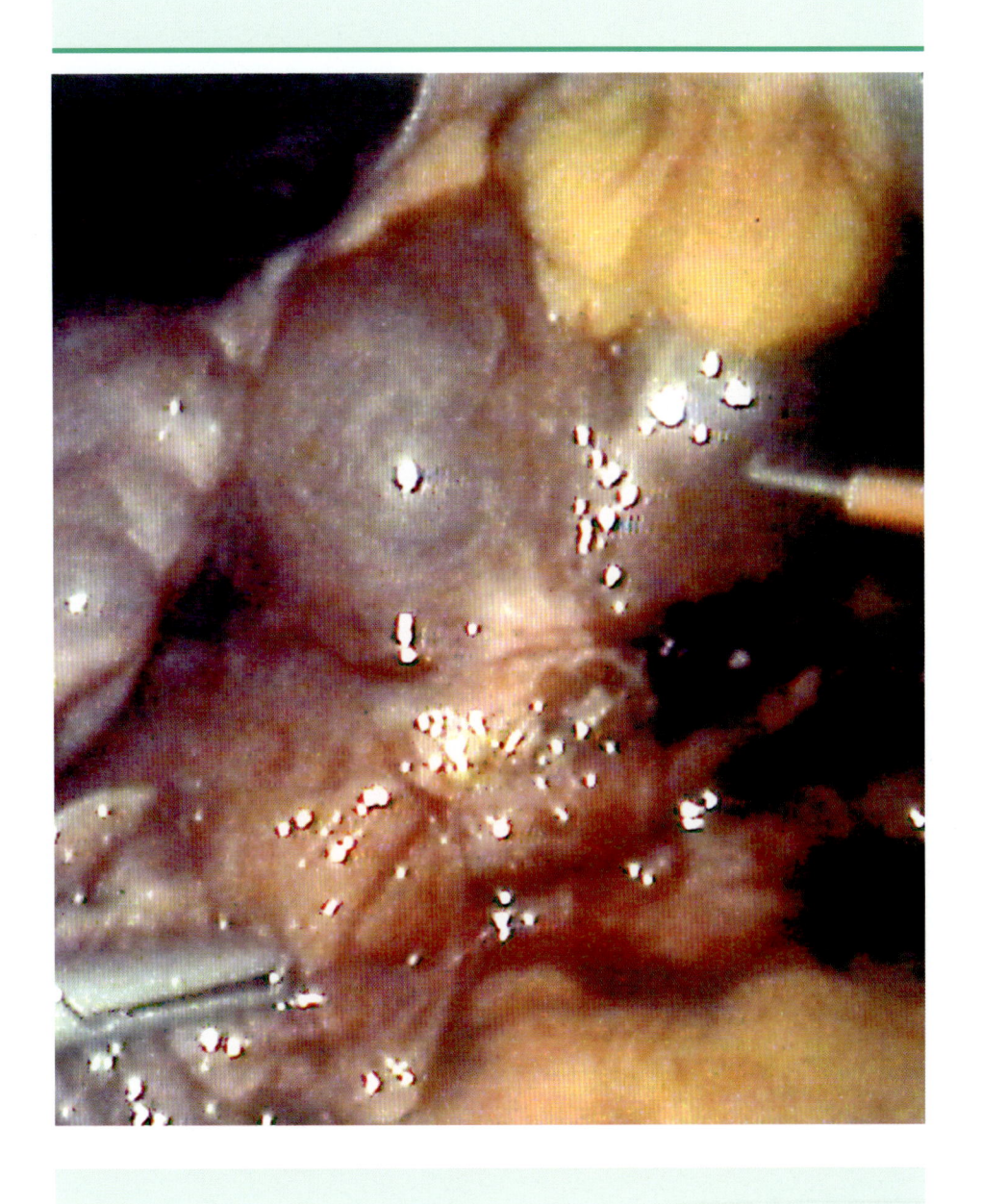

SURGERY FOR NON-PARASITIC LIVER CYSTS

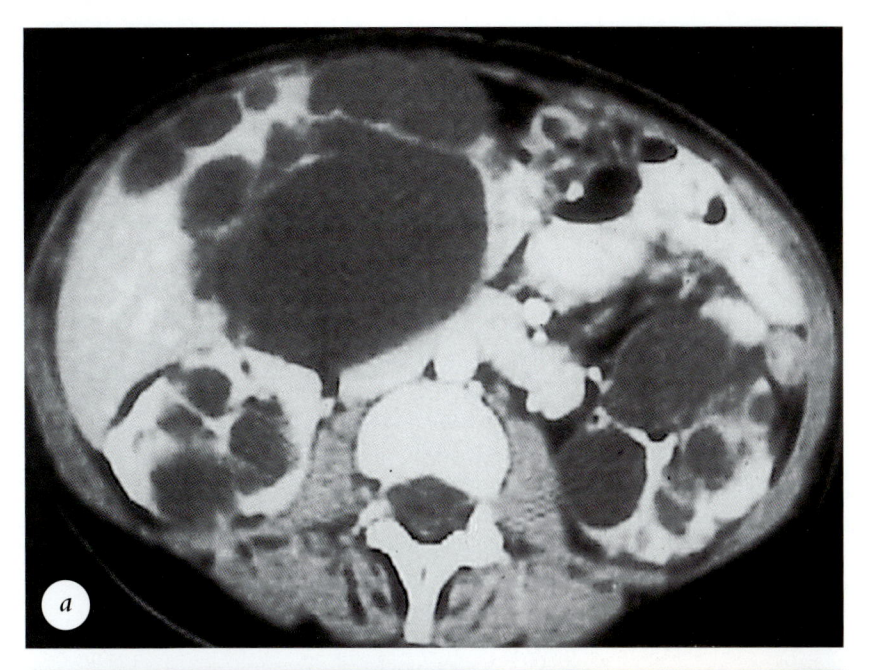

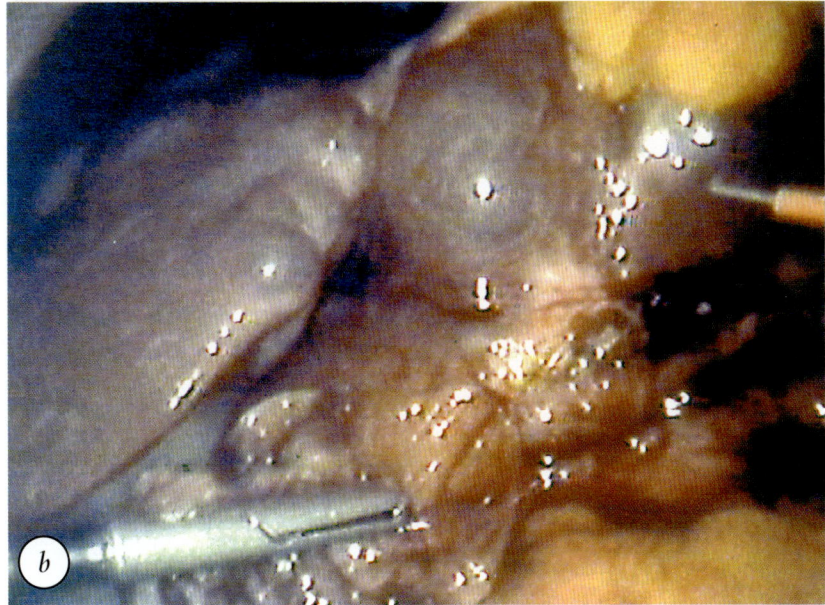

Figure 20.1 – *Polycystic liver and kidney disease. The liver cysts were more than 10 cm in diameter and reached the lower abdominal quadrants, causing abdominal tension.* **a)** *CT scan.* **b)** *Laparoscopic view. Puncture aspiration of the cysts.*

Serous cysts of the liver are a congenital condition and originate from anomalous bile ducts, not in communication with the bile tract. These cysts have an epithelial coating similar to that of the bile ducts, giving rise to the term 'biliary cysts' sometimes used in literature. They contain serous liquid not bile and are almost always asymptomatic. Treatment is only required for the (rare) symptomatic forms. The treatment of choice is echo-guided percutaneous aspiration with alcohol injection of the cavity. An alternative possibility is opening of the cyst and extensive removal of the most peripheral portion of the cyst wall to prevent recurrence. This type of operation can easily be performed by laparoscopy.[2]

Polycystic liver disease is a rare congenital ailment transmitted as an autosomal dominant character, more frequent in females. It is part of a syndrome of multi-organ cystic malformation affecting kidneys, liver, pancreas, spleen, lungs, ovaries, parathyroid, pituitary and peritoneum. It is associated in 50% of cases with polycystic kidneys in adults. The cysts may be present in only one lobe or extend throughout the liver, in the form of multiple small lesions, large 'dominant' cysts (which can be over 10 cm in diameter) (***Figure 20.1***), or as mixed forms with minute cysts in conjunction with dominant ones. The disease may become symptomatic in up to 15% of cases when the cysts reach significant dimensions which alter the shape of the liver. Compression causes symptoms such as abdominal tension, a sense of heaviness, or pain when the cysts are complicated by hemorrhage, infection, jaundice due to biliary obstruction or liver failure due to complete replacement of the liver parenchyma.

Treatment is indicated only for the symptomatic or complicated forms of polycystic liver disease and varies according to the anatomo-clinical forms of the disease. Treatment ranges from fenestration of cysts which grow to particularly large dimensions and become 'dominant', developing in clusters and leaving large areas of the parenchyma unaffected, to hepatic resections for cysts with a prevalently segmentary or lobar development, and even to liver transplantation when the disease involves the entire liver and leads to progressive hepatic insufficiency[7] (2 cases in our transplant series).

Fenestration as proposed by Lin,[4] which involves wide opening of the superficial cysts and treatment of the deeper cysts, is the procedure which has had the widest acceptance[1,6,8] and appears indicated in the case of 'dominant' symptomatic or complicated cysts. This procedure can be easily performed laparoscopically by surgeons expert both in hepatic surgery and in laparoscopic techniques, with the same characteristics described for the open methodology. The value of laparoscopy and the treatment of simple serous cysts or polycystic liver disease has been confirmed.[2]

Laparoscopic fenestration

The procedure is performed under general anesthesia. Induction of the pneumoperitoneum can be performed from the left side, under ultrasound control, to avoid accidental puncture of the cysts, or with the open laparoscopy technique by a Hasson trocar. We use four trocars,[3,5] one 10 mm infraumbilical trocar for the laparoscope, one 5 mm trocar on the right side, one 5 mm trocar in the epigastrium and one 10 mm trocar in the left hypochondrium, at a site lower than the ones for standard laparoscopic cholecystectomy. The puncture/aspiration system is positioned in the epigastric trocar, the grasper is inserted in the right trocar to expose the cyst, while the scissors are used through the trocar in the left upper quadrant of the abdomen and connected to the uni- or bi-polar cautery which is the instrument mainly used to perform this procedure. After aspiration of the serous content of the cyst (*Figure 20.1*), the wall is excised at approximately 1 cm from the hepatic margin, coagulating progressively during the resection or selectively with uni- or bi-polar coagulation (*Figure 20.2*). Inside the cavity of the most superficial cyst the deeper cysts are tackled with the same aspiration/emptying procedure and resection of the most external portion of the cyst wall. The smaller superficial cysts are opened with a coagulating hook. In some cases a fifth trocar can be inserted in the right flank to allow mobilization of the right lobe of the liver, adherent to the diaphragm as a result of the inflammatory reaction caused by the infected cyst and the previous percutaneous drainage. A grasper is inserted through this fifth port, allowing the liver to be pushed medially and downwards to divide adhesions with the diaphragm. After dissection of the liver, the cyst is identified and its content suctioned to prevent contamination of the peritoneal cavity. The cyst is then opened and a large portion of the exposed wall is excised to completely unroof the cavity. Other superficial cysts, both in the right and left lobes, with a clear serous content, are emptied, opened and a portion of the wall is excised with coagulating scissors. A drain is recommended after this procedure, through the hole of the right subcostal trocar. The drain should be left in place for about 24 hours and then removed to prevent ascitic losses which are common after fenestration of liver cysts either laparoscopically or with open surgery.

The immediate results of such operations for polycystic liver disease are generally good, eliminating the symptoms which indicated the operation. Laparoscopic fenestration has the advantage of being less invasive than conventional surgery and allows easier dialysis for patients with concomitant renal failure. An additional advantage is the formation of fewer intra-abdominal adhesions, allowing easier re-operation in the event of recurrence. The real problem remains the high percentage of long-term cyst recurrence in other segments of the liver, a common occurrence even after major open surgery. The patient must be informed of this risk of recurrence before the operation which must in any case be proposed as a symptomatic and palliative measure.

Complications and pitfalls

The formation of ascites is possible after fenestration of liver cysts. The ascites is proportional to the number of cysts opened and to the quantity of cystic wall left in place. Ascites depends on the production of serous fluid by

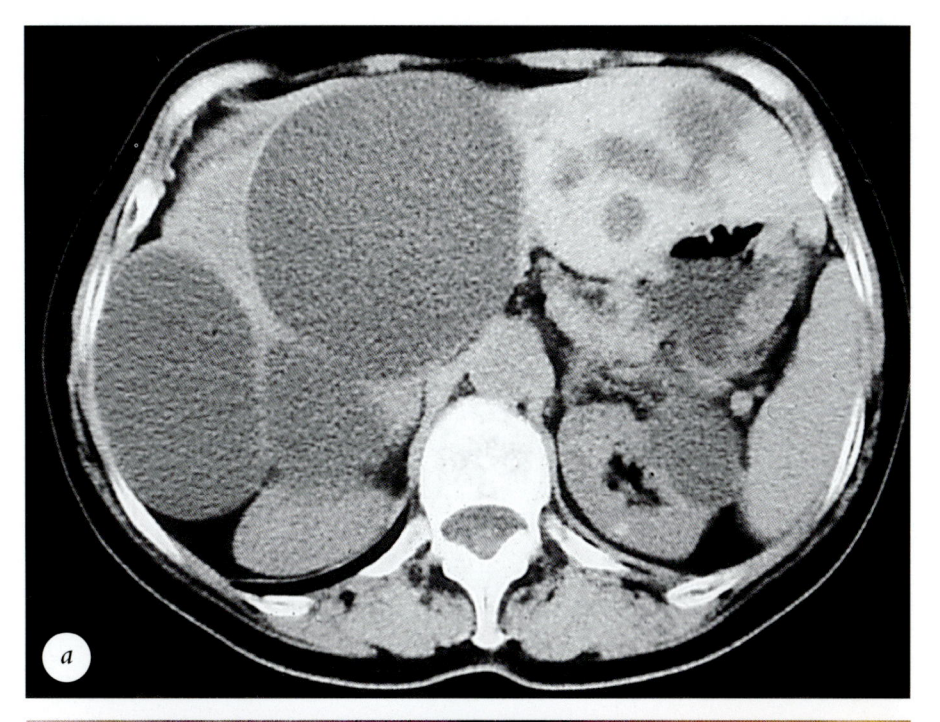

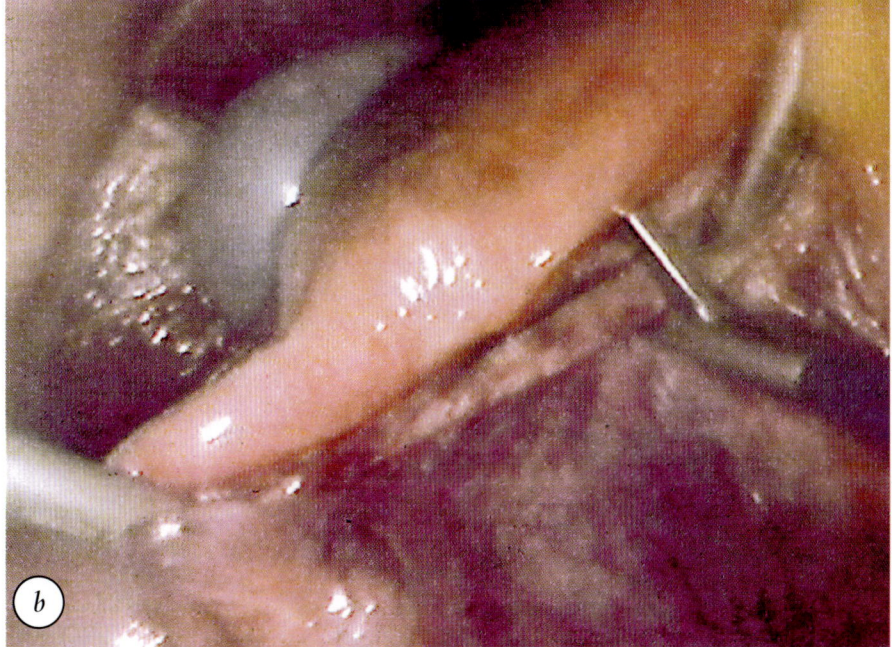

Figure 20.2 – *Large 'dominant' cysts that have developed mainly in the right hemiliver. **a)** CT scan. **b)** Laparoscopic view. After aspiration of the contents the external wall of the cyst is resected with a coagulator. Access to the deeper cysts is obtained through the opening made in the more superficial cysts.*

the epithelial cells that line the cystic cavity. The production of this fluid is not affected by the administration of diuretics. Since the epithelium which lines the cells is the biliary type, its secretion is affected by the hormonal stimuli that normally regulate the secretion of biliary mucosa. Gastric secretion inhibitors, such as octreotide, are effective in reducing the production of fluid by cysts opened with fenestration. A wide excision of the cystic wall and cauterization of the cavity are nevertheless highly advisable in preventing the onset of post-operative ascites.

The long-term results show a high tendency towards reformation of the liver cysts in the months following surgery. Recurrence is proportional to the extent of the resection of the cystic wall, but depends above all on the type of polycystosis. More satisfactory results can only be expected in the presence of large 'dominant' cysts which develop towards the surface of the liver, leaving extensive portions of the parenchyma unaffected, or in the presence of cysts which extend in a cluster from a liver segment. The results will certainly be disappointing in the case of cysts that involve all segments of the liver and in massive hepatic polycystosis.

REFERENCES

1. Armitage NC, Blumgart LH. Partial resection and fenestration in the treatment of polycystic liver disease. *Br J Surg* 1984; **71(3):** 242.
2. Fabiani P, Katkhouda N, Jovine E, Monjel J. Laparoscopic fenestration of biliary cysts. *Surg. Laparosc. Endosc* 1991; **1(3):** 162.
3. Gozzetti G, Mazziotti A. Laparoscopic fenestration for polycystic liver. In: Meinero M, Melotti G, Mouret Ph "Laparoscopic surgery. The Nineties". Masson, Milan, 1993, pp. 348-353.
4. Lin TY, Chen CC, Wang SM *et al*. Treatment of non-parasitic cystic disease of the liver: a new approach to therapy with polycstic liver. *Ann Surg* 1968; **168(5):** 921.
5. Mazziotti A, Gigot GF, Jovine E, Morganti M, Ajuero V, Gozzetti G. Chirurgia laparoscopica per fegato policistico. *Chirurgia* 1992; **5:** 175-179.
6. Newman KD, Torres VE, Rakela J, Nagorney DM. Treatment of highly symptomatic polycystic liver disease. *Ann Surg* 1990; **212(1):** 30.
7. Turnage RH. Eckhauser E, Knol JA, Thompson NW. Therapeutic dilemmas in patients with symptomatic polycystic liver disease. *Am Surg* 1988; **54:** 365.
8. Starzl TE, Reyes J, Tzakis A, Mieles L, Todo S, Gordon R. Liver transplantation for liver polycystic disease. *Arch Surg* 1990; **125:** 575-577.

21

Surgery for Liver Hydatidosis

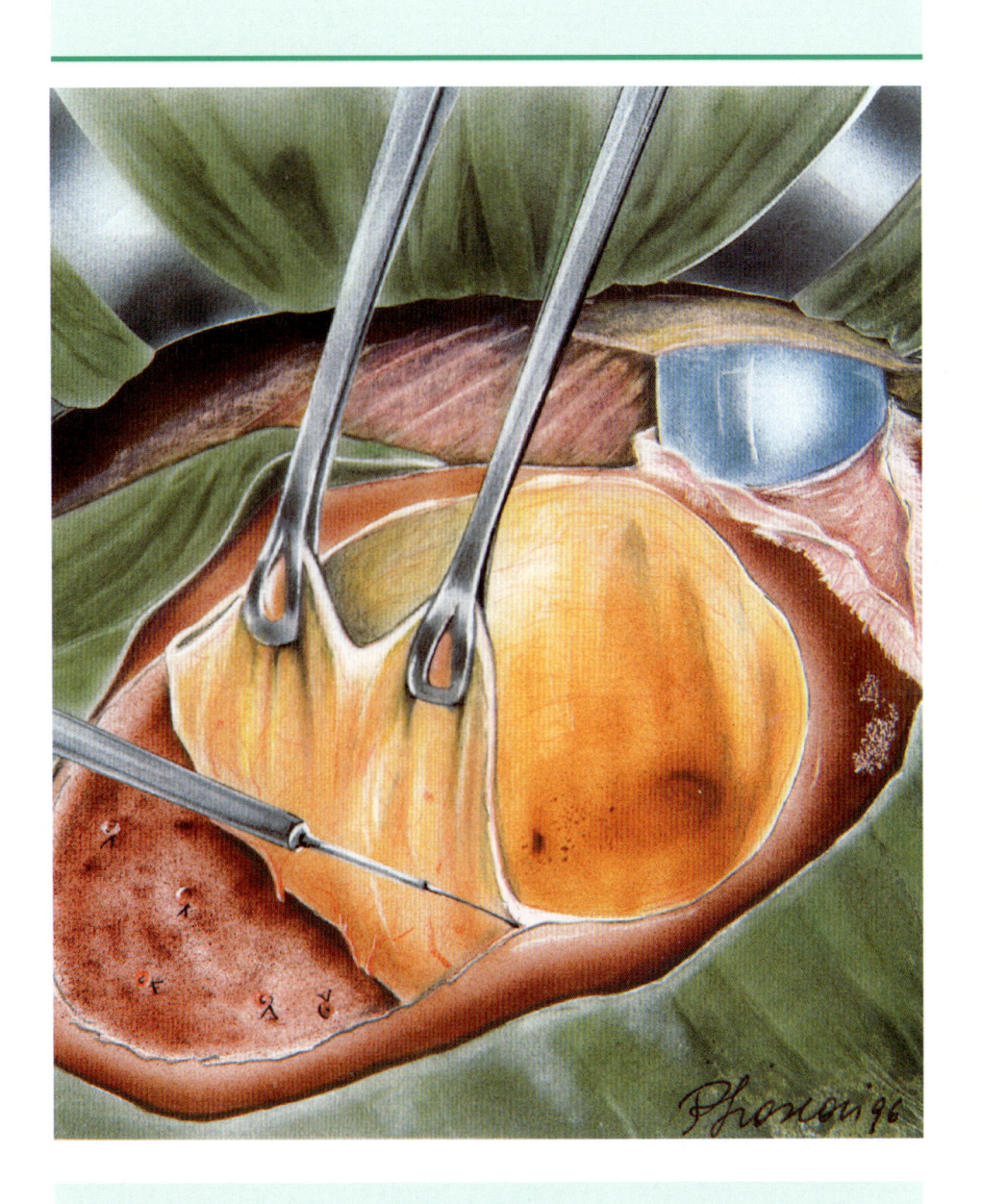

Hepatic hydatidosis is still an endemic disease in Mediterranean countries and may occasionally be found in the UK, North America and continental European countries. The eggs of *Echinococcus granulosus* reach the liver through the portal circulation and develop into cysts; the daughter cysts germinate from an internal 'proligerous' membrane and determine the progressive growth of the cysts. A fibrous capsule, the pericystium, forms around the cysts and becomes progressively thicker, coming into close contact with the vascular-biliary structures of the surrounding parenchyma. As the cysts grow the hepatic vessels are compressed and displaced, greatly altering the intrahepatic anatomy. In particular, the compression affects the bile ducts whose walls can become eroded within the pericystium or inside the cyst; the erosion of the bile duct wall is the basis for the formation of biliocystic fistulae which are very frequent in the larger hydatid cysts. Passage of bile into the cysts is generally observed, while a reverse flow of the cystic material into the bile ducts is much rarer. The presence of bile causes an alteration of the parasite biology, leading ultimately to its death, and an increase in the inflammation around the pericystium which is responsible for its sclerosis and calcification.

The erosion of the wall of the bile ducts adhering to the pericystium explains how the bile ducts frequently[7,19,23,25] (in over 50% of the cases of larger cysts in our experience) open up when the cysts are emptied and the pressure inside the cavity disappears. This phenomenon is responsible for the formation of biliary fistulae inside the cyst wall and must always be borne in mind during surgery to prevent the onset of post-operative biliary fistulae. The development of daughter cysts outside the proligerous membrane, through the pericystium, towards the surrounding parenchyma (exogenous vesiculation) is much rarer.

While no treatment is required for dead calcified cysts, and percutaneous drainage can be successfuly employed in the (rare) forms of uncomplicated unilocular young cysts,[13,17] surgery remains the treatment of choice in most cases. Medical treatment with mebendazole, flubendazole and albendazole has shown a very limited efficacy in hydatid cysts in adults, and it is extremely common for cysts to remain alive even after 12 months of medical treatment.[2,10-12,26] Excision of the cyst and the pericystium can theoretically be defined as 'radical' surgery, to eliminate the cyst and overcome the problems of the remaining cavity, the site of post-operative complications[5,20,22,23] Total cystopericystectomy is however often difficult for technical reasons, especially for the larger cysts which penetrate the parenchyma or for central liver cysts. Sub-total pericystectomies leave the deepest part of the pericystium in place and are a compromise to be adopted in the most complex, large cysts situated in the parenchyma and in close contact with the intrahepatic structures. Liver resection may exceptionally be required in particular situations - multiple cysts of a hemiliver or localized in the left lobe, or cysts which take up an entire peripheral hepatic segment. Surgical technique must be based, case by case, on careful consideration of the site of the cyst, its relationship with the intrahepatic vascular-biliary structures and the condition of the pericystium, bearing in mind that hydatidosis is a benign disease and that the patient must not therefore be exposed to a high operative risk.

Total pericystectomy

Total pericystectomy is, theoretically, the ideal treatment for hepatic hydatidosis: complete excision of the pericystium favors the healing process of the remaining cavity, reduces post-operative morbidity and recurrence due to exogenous vesiculation. However, the larger the cyst and its intrahepatic development, the more difficult the operation is to perform, requiring particular experience in liver surgery. The operative risk of pericystectomy is particularly high in deeply-rooted cysts at the level of the hilum.

The operative technique for total pericystectomy is illustrated in *Figure 21.1*. A J or subcostal

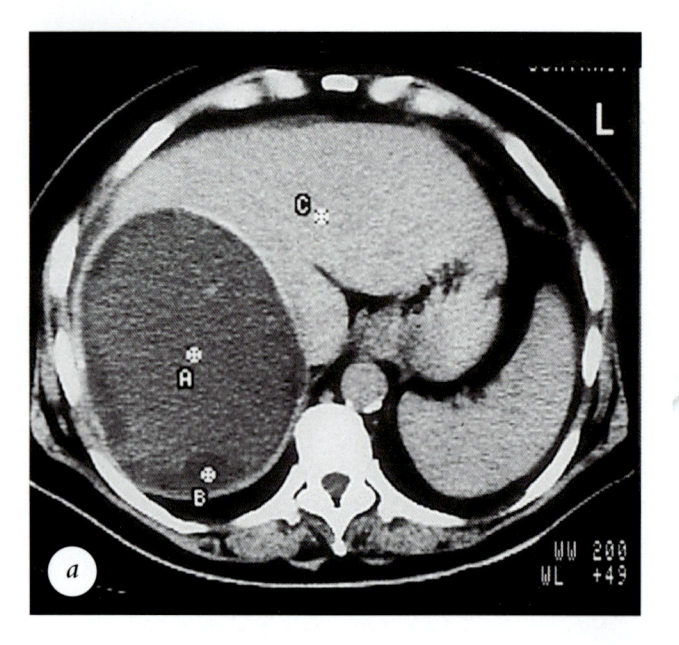

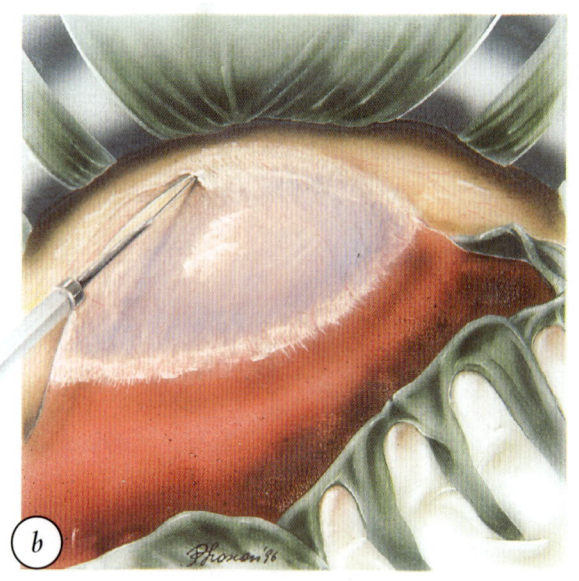

Figure 21.1 – *Total pericystectomy for hydatid liver cyst.* **a)** *Pre-operative CT: the cyst occupies the posterio-superior part of the right lobe of the liver.* **b)** *Dissection by cautery of the fibrous adherences with the diaphragm. The abdominal cavity is protected by dressings soaked in hypertonic saline solution.* **c)** *Dissection of Glisson's capsule along the edge of the cyst.*

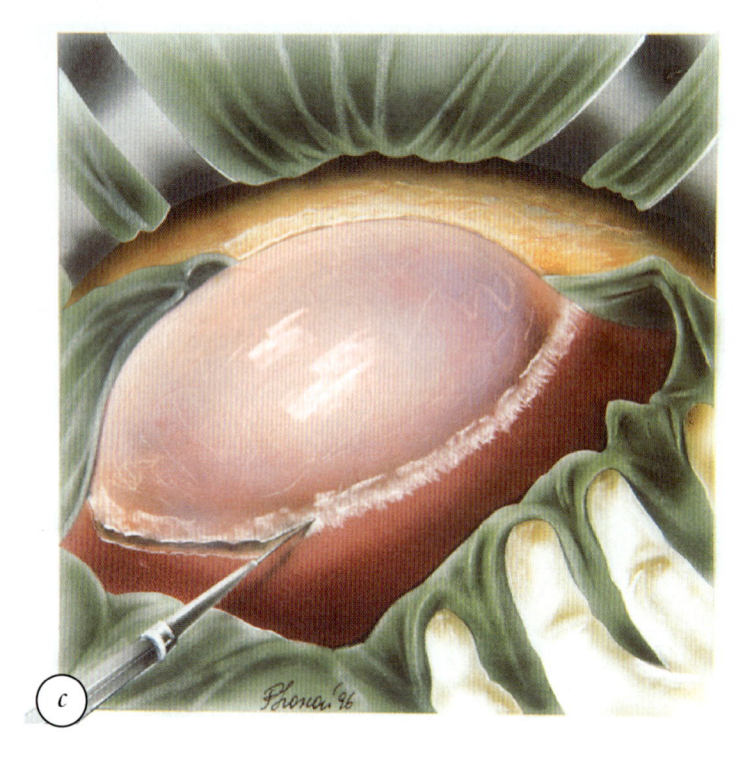

bilateral incision is made, depending on the site of the cyst. The first stage consists of dissecting the adhesions which are always present between the cyst and the diaphragm (**Figure 21.1b**). Before starting mobilization (which may risk rupturing the cyst) the liver must be isolated and the peritoneal cavity protected to prevent spilling of the hydatid liquid and peritoneal dissemination of the parasite. Hypertonic saline is the safest scolicidal solution; formol solutions which are extremely irritant and damaging for the bile ducts are nowadays not used. Dressings soaked in saline solution must not be placed in direct contact with large areas of the peritoneum so that massive absorption of sodium is avoided, or osmolarity alterations which may result in hyperosmolar coma. Dissection of the pericystium from the parenchyma, after incision of Glisson's capsule by cautery (**Figure 21.1d**), must be carried out gradually to detach the vascular-biliary pedicles which adhere to the pericystium and must be dissected carefully and progressively (**Figure 21.1e**). This dissection can be carried out with a Kelly clamp or with an ultrasound knife which makes it easy to

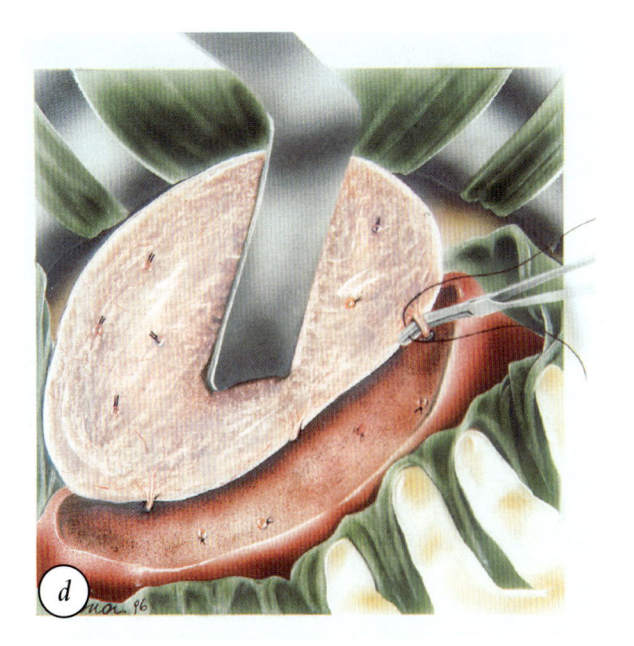

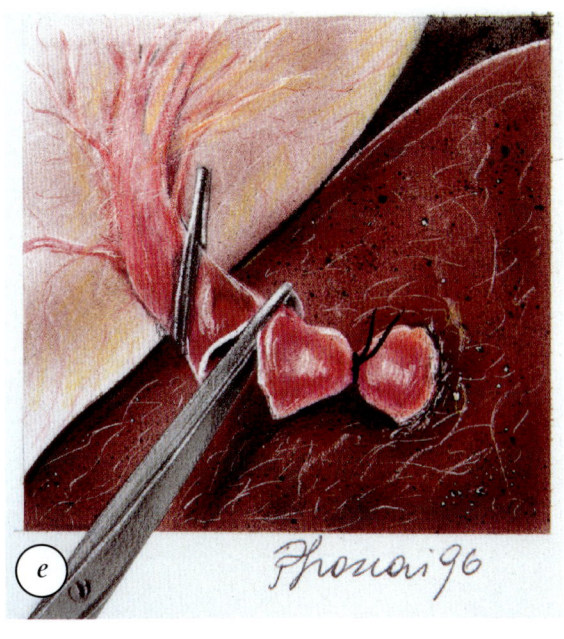

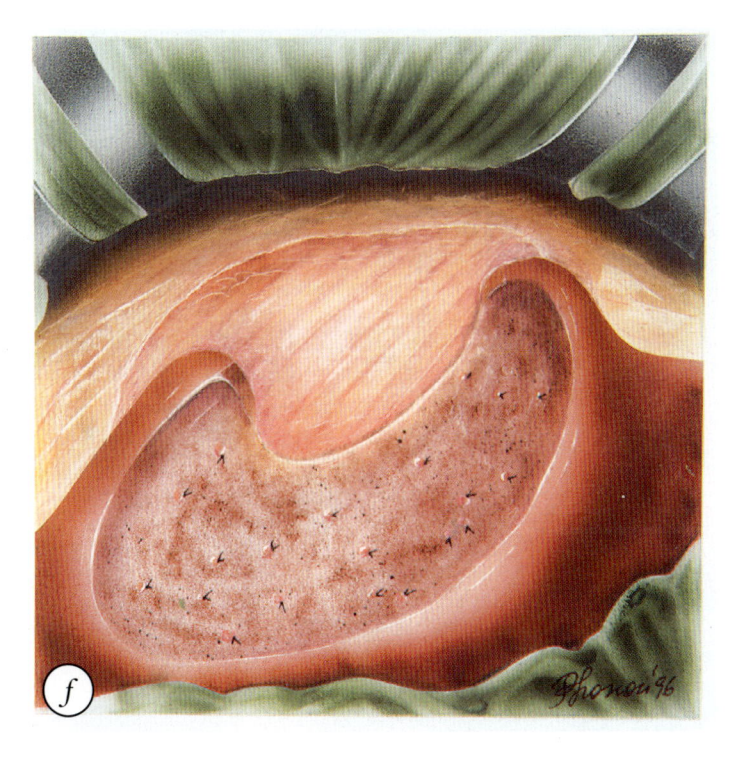

Figure 21.1 continued –
d) *Progressive dissection of the cyst from the hepatic parenchyma with ligature of the vessels adhering to the pericystium **e)**.*
f) *The raw surface of the liver after total pericystectomy*

identify the cleavage plane. Vessels that have to be divided should be ligated or sutured with Vicryl® 3-0 stitches. Particular care should be taken with the dissection of the suprahepatic pedicles with thinner and more fragile walls. Some more superficial parts of the parenchyma may be devitalized and must be removed with partial *'à la demande'* resections. At the end of a total pericystectomy the raw surfaces of the liver are similar to those of a resection wedge after conventional hepatectomy (***Figure 21.1f***) and should be treated as already described in Chapter 14, paying particular attention to biliary leaks: the use of methylene blue as a control, injected into the gallbladder by puncture or in the cystic duct if the gallbladder has to be removed, is a very useful procedure in hydatid surgery.

The opening of the cysts can facilitate pericystectomy in the case of larger cysts. The cysts are emptied by puncture and, after ensuring that the surgical field is fully protected, completely opened. Traction is exerted on the pericystium to detach it from the parenchyma progressively, working inwards until it is completely removed (*open cyst total pericystectomy*).

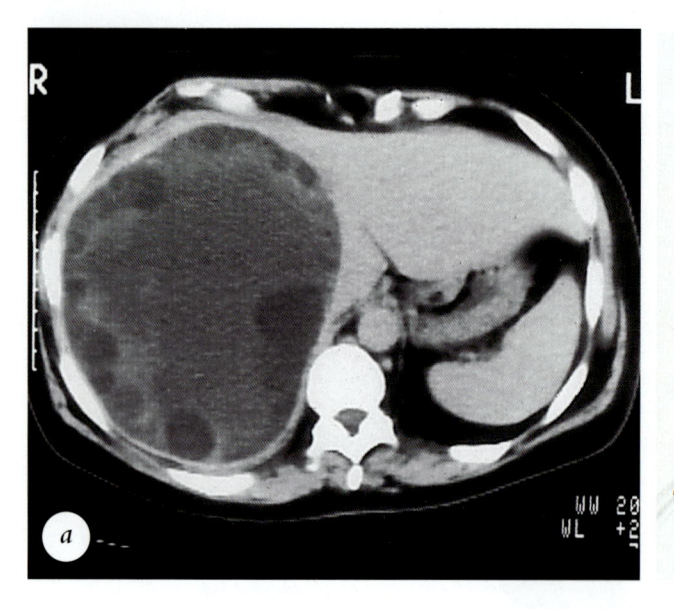

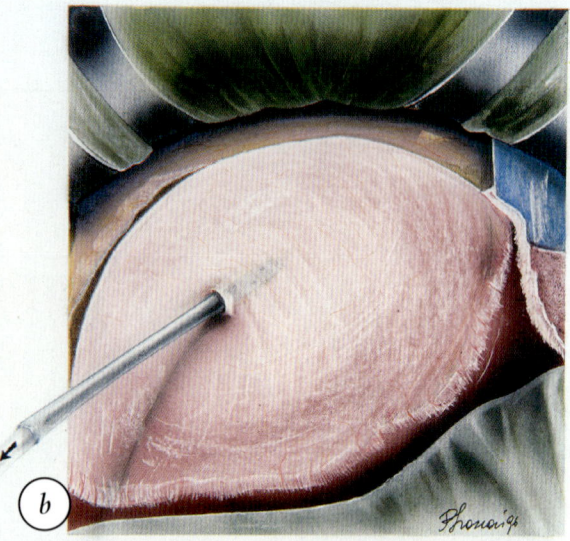

Figure 21.2 – *Sub-total pericystectomy for hydatid liver cyst. **a)** Pre-operative CT: the cyst occupies practically the entire right lobe of the liver. **b)** Aspiration by puncture of the liquid contents of the cyst. **c)** The cyst wall is opened and the daughter cysts are aspirated.*

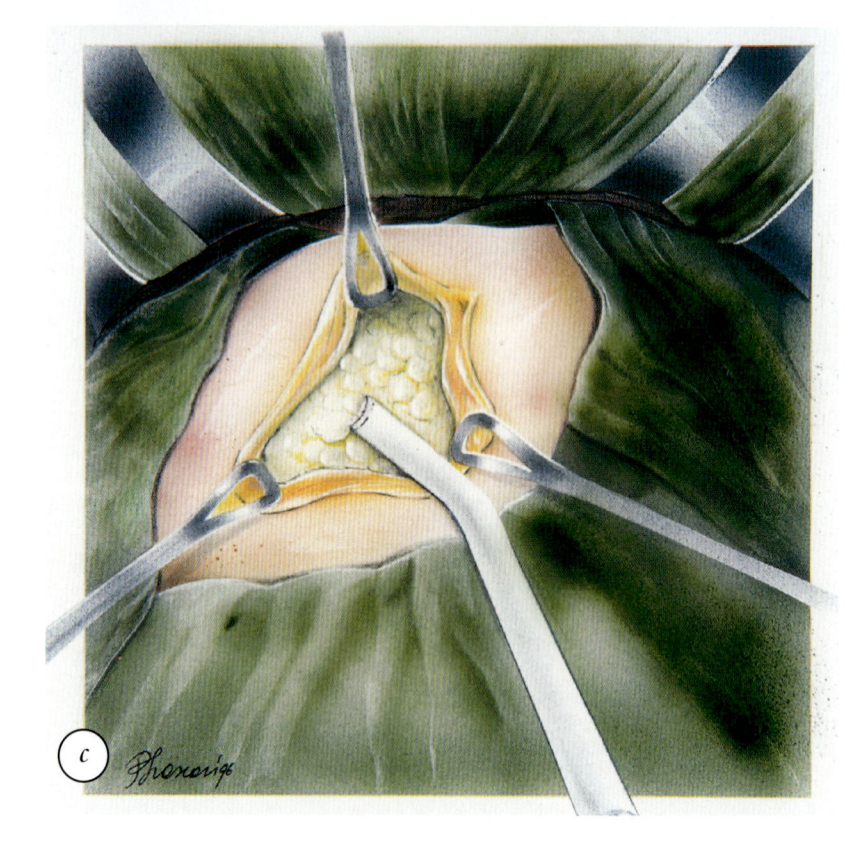

Sub-total pericystectomy

The technique is illustrated in **Figure 21.2** and represents the most rational choice for larger cysts with extended intrahepatic development. After sectioning the diaphragmatic adherences, exposing the outermost part of the pericystium and protecting the peritoneal cavity, the contents of the cyst are aspirated (**Figure 21.2b**) and then fully opened (**Figure 21.2c**). The cyst cavity is cleansed with saline solution without injecting the solution under pressure into the cavity. Dissection of the pericystium from the parenchyma continues posteriorly: the diaphragm is stretched as a result of development of the cyst and has a very thin wall which may easily open, generating a pneumothorax which can be detected during surgery or immediately afterwards. The pericystium is dissected from the parenchyma, proceeding inwards towards the deeper planes as far as a point which is considered safe to prevent lesions of the intrahepatic vascular lesions (**Figure 21.2d**). The vena cava can generally be

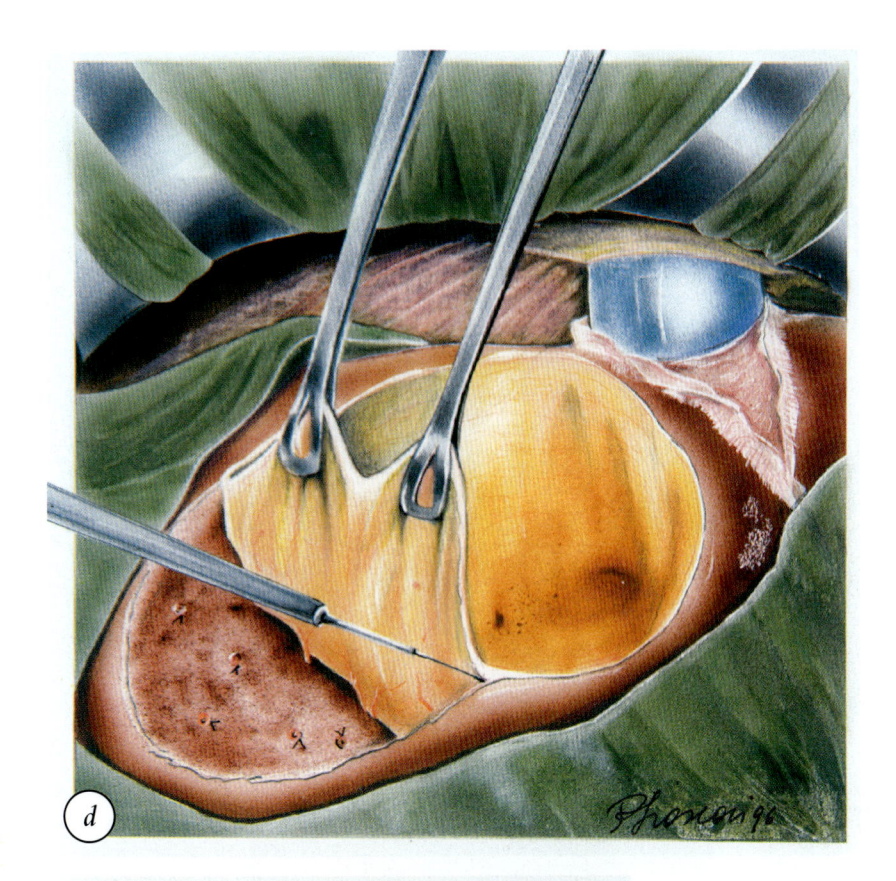

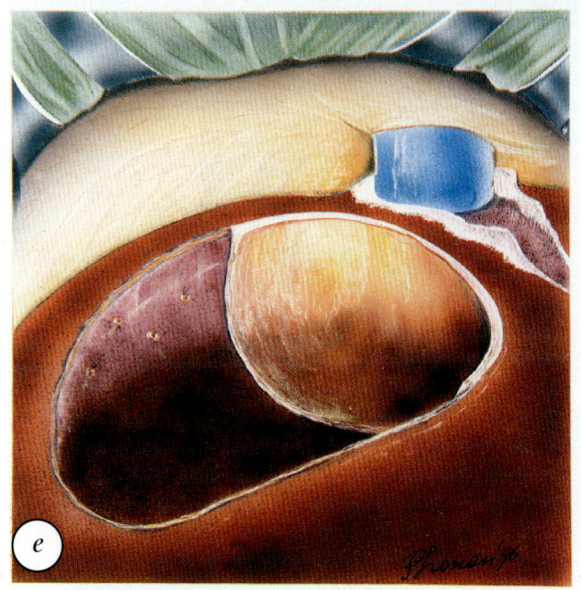

Figure 21.2 continued –
d) Dissection of the cyst wall from the hepatic parenchyma, leaving the portion of pericystium that adheres to the confluence of the right hepatic vein e).

easily detached from the pericystium, while the tougher adherences are encountered in correspondence with the Glissonian pedicles and it is here that the highest risks of hemorrhagic lesions or lesions of the bile ducts exist. The deepest part of the pericystium in the parenchyma is left in place after cleansing the cavity with saline solution (*Figure 21.2e*). Intraoperative ultrasound is extremely useful in these conditions, when intrahepatic anatomy is distorted by the cystic growth, to establish the safety margin for resection of the pericystium as it shows the exact point of adherence to the vascular pedicles (*Figure 21.3*). It is also useful to exclude the presence of exogenous vesiculation. Particular care must be taken to control biliary leakage: cholangiography by puncture of the gallbladder and methylene blue control must be systematic and the leakage points must be sutured with Vicryl® 3-0. The border areas of devitalized parenchyma must be removed to allow the remaining cavity to flatten where the omentum is placed to fill the cavity and prevent adherence with the intestine. One or two drainage tubes should be placed.

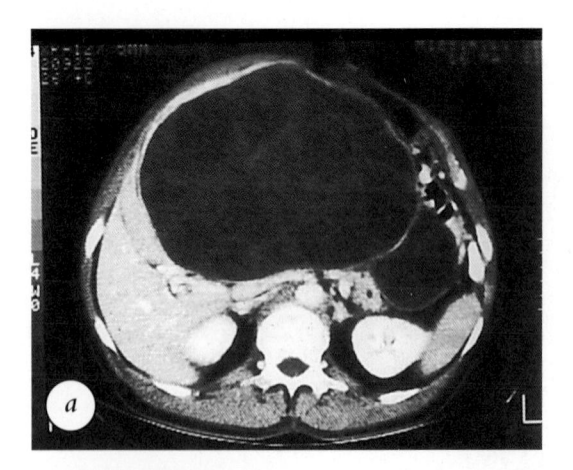

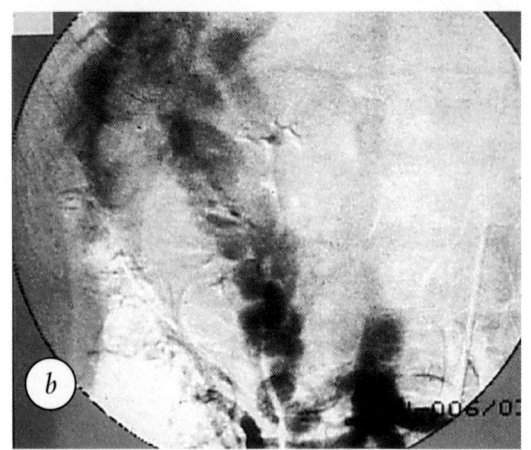

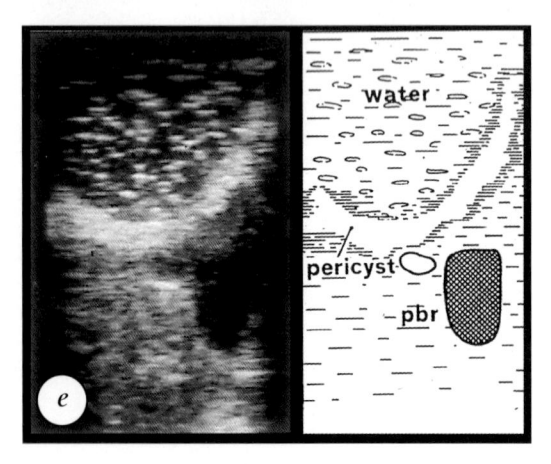

Figure 21.3 – *Massive hydatid liver cyst, sub-total pericystectomy with the aid of intra-operative ultrasound. The cyst has developed in the left hemiliver a); cavography reveals compression of the vena cava b) while mesenteric angiography shows a pseudo thrombosis of the portal vein c). After emptying of the cyst, the vena cava (vc.) and the intra-hepatic portal branches (p.br.) appear patent at intra-operative ultrasound d,e). These scans were obtained by inserting the US probes directly into the water-filled cystic cavity. Dissection of the pericystium proceeds, under IOU guidance, up to a safe distance from the main intra-hepatic vessels, such as the hepatic trunks visible in f), mhv=middle hepatic vein, rhv=right hepatic vein.*

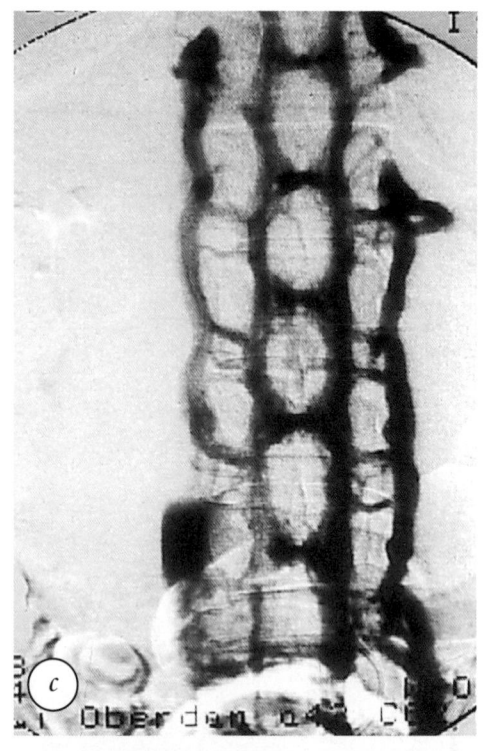

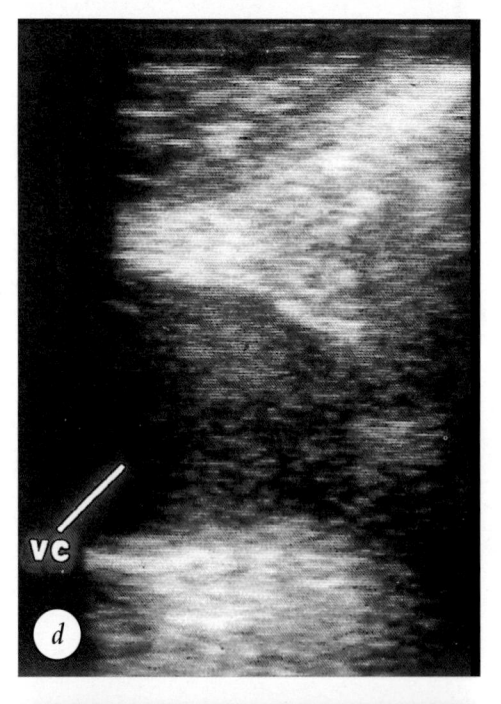

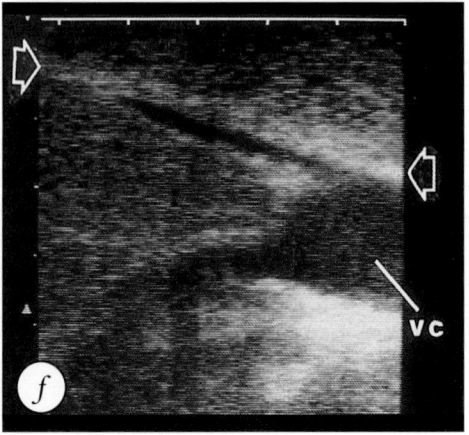

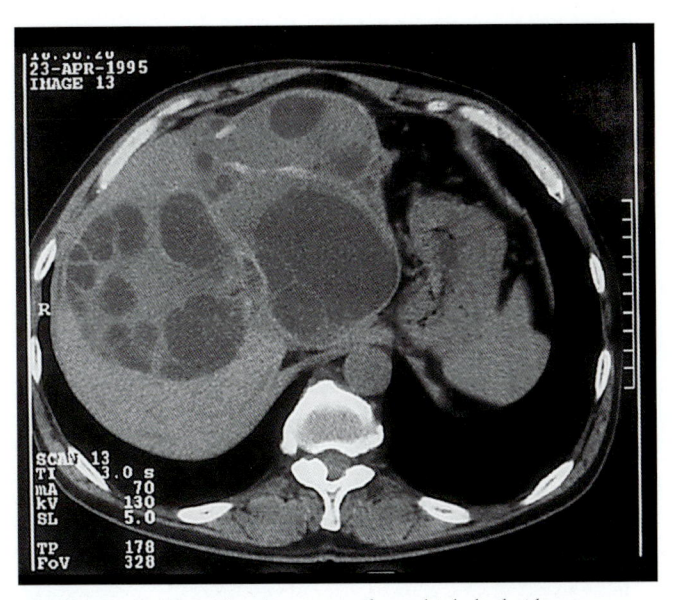

Figure 21.4 – *Partial pericystectomy for multiple hydatid cysts localized in various segments of the right lobe.*

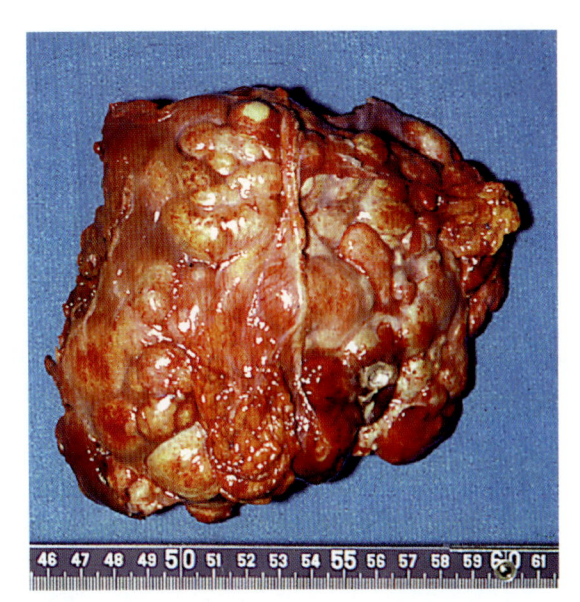

Figure 21.6 – *Hydatid cyst in the left lobe of the liver. Left lobectomy, resection specimen.*

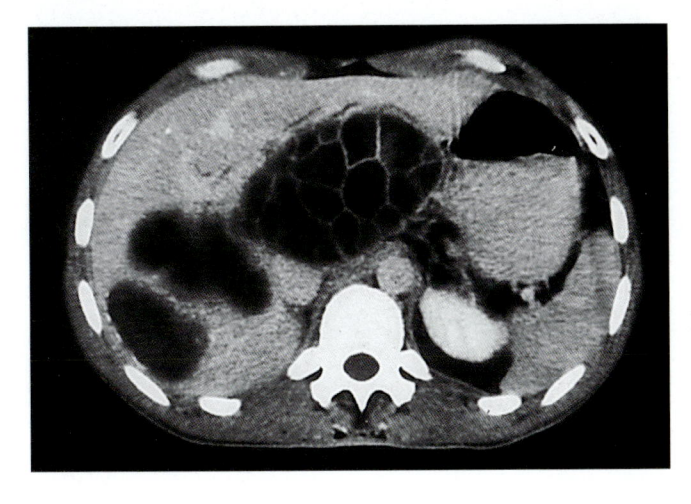

Figure 21.5 – *Multiple hydatid cysts localized in the right lateral segments and in the caudate lobe. Partial pericystectomy.*

Partial pericystectomy

This technique is used infrequently since a greater number of post-operative complications arise such as abscesses, biliary fistulae or recurrence of hydatidosis. This type of surgery is now limited to particular cases of cysts completely enclosed within the hepatic parenchyma or developed between the suprahepatic hilus and the Glissionian hilum, to cysts localized in the caudate lobe or to multiple intrahepatic localizations (***Figures 21.4 - 21.5***). The technique is quick and easy and consists of draining the cysts, cleansing the cavity and removing the most prominent wall of the pericystium. A large part of the cavity is thus left in place and must be filled with the omentum after controlling biliostasis. External drainage of the remaining cavity must be systematically carried out.

Liver resections

Standard hepatectomies should no longer be performed in liver hydatidosis surgery. The presence of a hydatid cyst greatly alters the intrahepatic anatomy and sometimes even the anatomy of the Glissonian and extra-suprahepatic pedicles due to the compression exerted by the cysts and the inflammatory adherences which form around the pericystium. Hepatectomy with elective extra-parenchymal ligation of the vascular pedicles is extremely dangerous in these cases because of the risk of vascular lesions and above all of biliary lesions. Hepatic resections are justified only in the case of cysts in the left lobe, when the entire second and third segments are involved and the parenchyma is replaced by the development of the cyst (***Figure 21.6***), and of cysts localized in the lower segments of the

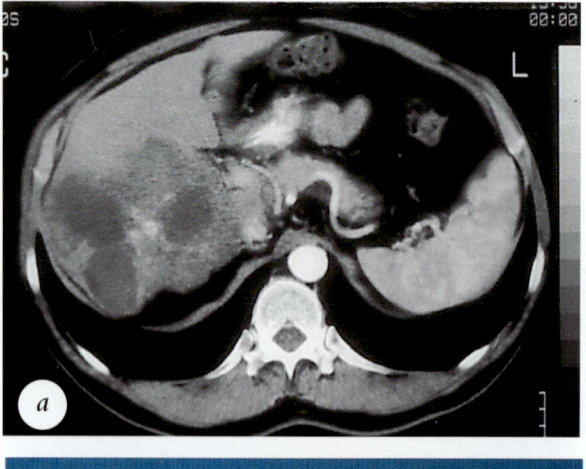

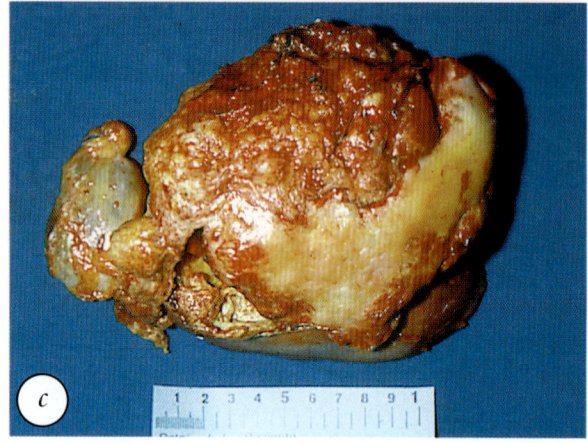

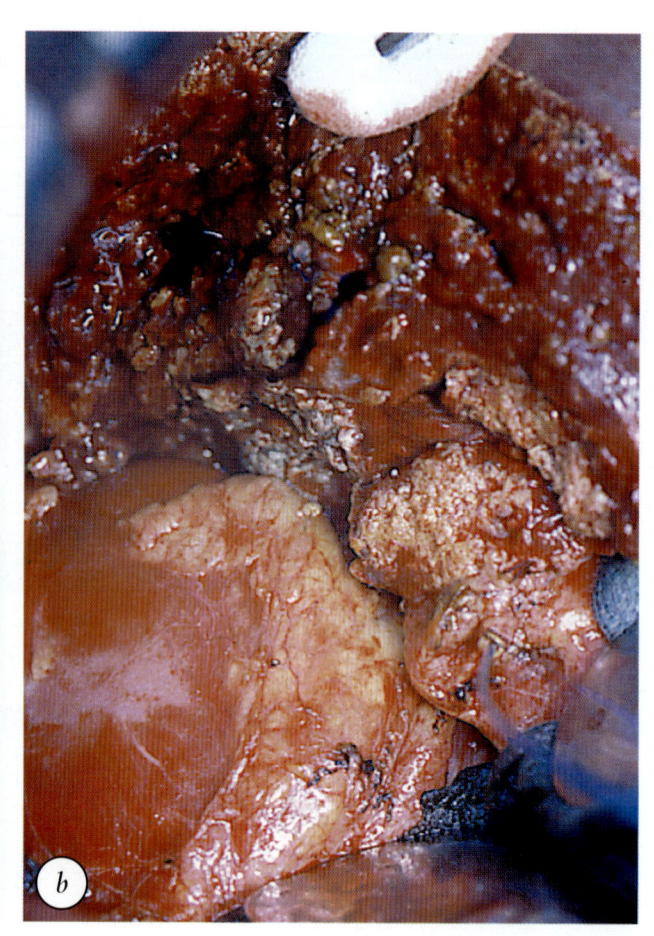

Figure 21.7 – *Hydatid cysts of segment 6. Segmentectomy 6. a) Pre-operative CT scan. b) Operating field after the atypical resection of segment 6. c) Resection specimen including the gallbladder.*

liver (**Figure 21.7**). In these cases, resection should be performed 'à la demande', with the aim of compensating a pericystectomy which would leave a deep residual cavity or portions of suspended or ischemic parenchyma.

There are basically two therapeutic approaches in dealing with hydatid liver disease: 'radical' techniques, with removal of the cysts and the pericystium, and a conservative approach such as partial pericystectomy. Important facts such as the reduction of post-operative morbidity and long-term recurrence constitute a strong argument for more 'complete' intervention (this term seems more appropriate than 'radical') involving removal of the cysts and the pericystium without leaving a residual cavity with fibrotic walls, the site of the main post-operative complications. This approach is supported by most surgeons working in endemic areas.[5,8,15,16,20,22,24] This type of surgery must, however, be employed prudently and selectively, and not performed indiscriminately for all locations of hydatid cysts of the liver. Our policy is to carry out total pericystectomy when technically feasible without risk, reserving conservative techniques for the more complex forms in which total pericystectomy is contraindicated, as we are convinced that the best results are obtained with careful selection of patients and attentive use of the various techniques available.

Complications

HEMORRHAGE

Unless a correct resection plan is followed, and especially if the pericystium is calcified, it is easy to damage the vascular pedicles adhering

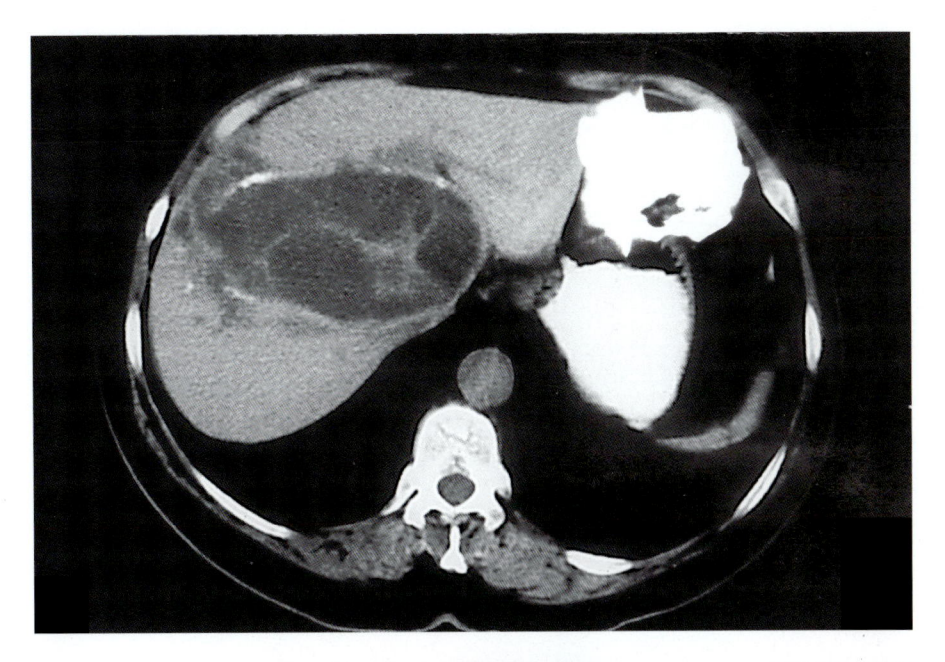

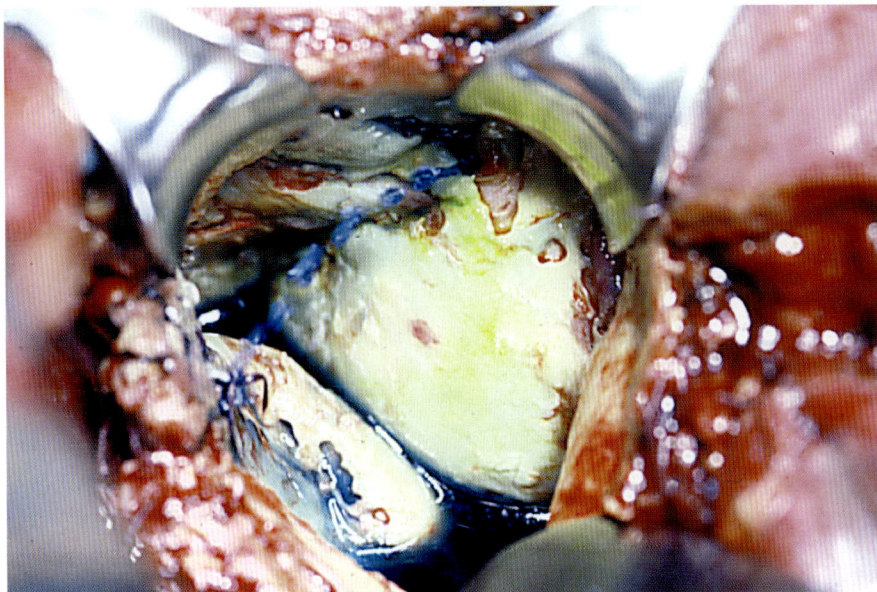

Figure 21.8 – *Biliary fistula seen by injection of methylene blue through the cystic duct.*
a) *Pre-operative CT scan: hydatid cyst of the middle segments of the liver.*
b) *After opening the cyst, injection of methylene blue through the cystic duct reveals a large biliary fistula which is sutured with Vicryl® stitches. Surgery consisted of a partial pericystectomy and filling of the residual cavity with omentum.*

to the pericystium and in particular the hepatic veins which have thinner walls and numerous collaterals. Dissection adhering to the plane of the pericystium is the best way of preventing these hemorrhages. More serious lesions may occur due to tears of the vena cava as a result of excessive traction of the pericystium or tearing of the accessory hepatic veins. These lesions are more complex because the presence of the pericystium makes direct hemostasis more difficult since it can only be performed after adequate exposure, plugging the hemorrhage and maintaining the patient under positive expiration end pressure to prevent the risk of air embolism.

LESIONS OF THE DIAPHRAGM

During dissection of the external wall of the pericystium the diaphragm may easily be opened, causing pneumothorax which may sometimes only be evident 1-2 days after surgery. In the event of a diaphragmatic lesion the air should be aspirated from the pleural cavity with a probe and the diaphragm closed with Vicryl® 0 sutures. Lesions with persisting pneumothorax require pleural drainage.

BILIARY FISTULAE

The development of cysts within the parenchyma leads to erosion of the biliary ducts adhering to the pericystium with formation of biliary fistulae opening inside the cavity after drainage of the cyst. These fistulae can be detected by injecting methylene blue in the gallbladder[6] or the cystic duct (**Figure 21.8**). We recommend the systematic use of this

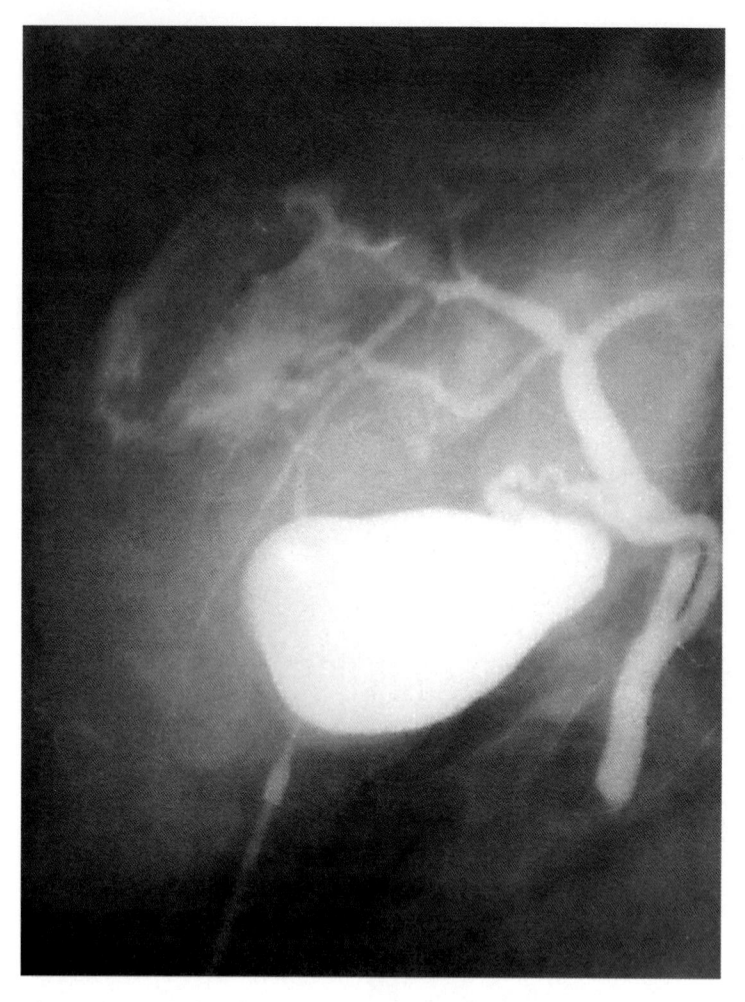

Figure 21.9 – *Biliary fistula shown with transcholecystic cholangiography after emptying a hydatid cyst of the right lobe of the liver.*

control and of cholangiography (***Figure 21.9***) to document the fistulae or to check for the presence - much rarer - of hydatid material which has migrated into the bile duct. Biliary fistulae recognized during surgery should be sutured with Vicryl® 3-0. In the event of multiple fistulae we prefer to remove the gallbladder and position a transcystic drainage to drain the bile duct and for post-operative checks; one or two drainage tubes should be systematically left in place in the remaining cavity in view of the possibility of biliary fistulae. Small fistulae drained through the abdominal tubes heal spontaneously in a few weeks (but may sometimes take several months!). Larger fistulae may require endoscopic intubation of the biliary system or re-operation. If a transcystic drainage has not been left in place, ERCP is indispensable in these cases to plan the most appropriate treatment.

SUBPHRENIC ABSCESSES

These may occur in the presence of biliary fistulae and a wide cavity with rigid walls due to the persistence of extensive portions of pericystium. These abscesses can be successfully treated with echo- and CT-guided percutaneous drainage.

LESIONS OF THE MAIN BILE DUCT

Lesions of the common bile duct and of the convergence of the hepatic bile ducts are a feared complication in pericystectomies or hepatic resections for cysts adhering to the hilum or to the hepatic pedicle. The bile duct can be very close to the pericystium as a result of the inflammatory process and anatomy can be significantly altered, making division or ligation of the bile duct difficult during surgery. Intra-operative cholangiography must be systematically performed in the presence of cysts which develop as far as the level of the hilum. A lesion recognized during the operation must be repaired with a Kehr tube. Lesions detected post-operatively must be treated with a perendoscopic stent when possible or with a Roux en Y loop bilioenteric anastomosis, a particularly difficult operation in these circumstances.

INTRAPERITONEAL DISSEMINATION OF HYDATID LIQUID

The peritoneal cavity must be carefully cleansed and washed with Betadine solution. Antiparasite treatment with Albendazol must be administered post-operatively for at least 3 months.

HYPEROSMOLAR COMA

This serious complication has rarely been reported.[15,27] It occurred in one case in our experience in hydatid hepatic and intraperitoneal cysts due to the massive absorption of sodium through the numerous dressings soaked in hypertonic saline solution placed in direct contact with the peritoneum. The patient died in spite of dialysis treatment. It is necessary to avoid direct contact of the dressings soaked in saline solution with the intestinal loops and extensive areas of the peritoneum. Sodium levels require careful review.

CAUSTIC SCLEROSING CHOLANGITIS

This is a rare and extremely serious complication of the surgical treatment of hepatic hydatidosis due to the irritant action on the biliary epithelium of scolicidal agents used to sterilize the cysts. In addition to formalin, hypertonic saline solutions, ethanol, silver nitrate and iodine solutions can generate secondary sclerosing cholangitis.[3,4,9] These substances pass from the cavity of the cysts through the biliary fistulae which are present in over 50% of larger cysts. The biliary lesions are very similar to those observed in primitive sclerosing cholangitis with progressive segmentary stenosis of the intra- and extra-hepatic bile ducts. Prevention of this serious complication is based on abolishing the practice of injection under pressure of scolicidal agents into the cyst. Sterilization of the cystic cavity can be safely carried out after drainage of the cyst and cleansing of the cystic wall with dressings soaked in hypertonic saline solution or in hydrogen peroxide.

INTRABILIARY RUPTURE

The passage of hydatid material into the biliary tract is a rare and serious complication, resulting in obstructive jaundice and cholangitis. It is advisable to relieve the obstruction before surgery by endoscopic papillotomy.[1] After drainage of the cysts and systematic removal of the gallbladder, the cystic biliary fistula must be identified by injecting methylene blue in the cystic duct and sutured with Vicryl® from inside the cavity. The hydatid material in the biliary tract must be removed by means of a choledochotomy and the common bile duct drained with a Kehr tube.[19] Hepatic resection is occasionally necessary to treat more complex forms with calcification of the cystic wall in which conservative treatment is not sufficient.

REFERENCES

1. Aeberhard P, Fuhrimann R, Strahm P, Thommen A. Surgical treatment of hydatid disease of the liver: an experience from outside the endemic area. *Hepato-Gastroenterol* 1996; **43**: 627-636.
2. Bahr R, Amman R, Bircher J. Die Chemotherapie der menschlichen Echinokokkose. *Chirurg* 1984; **55**:114-116.
3. Belghiti J, Benhamou JP, Houry S, Huguier M, Fèkètè F. Caustic sclerosing cholangitis: a complication of the surgical treatment of hydatid disease of the liver. *Arch Surg* 1986; **121**: 1162-65.
4. Belghiti J, Perniceni T, Kabbej J, Fèkètè F. Complications of perioperative sterilization of hydatid cysts of the liver. *Chirurgie* 1992; **117**: 343-6.
5. Belli L, Aseni O, Rondinara GF, Bertini M. Improved results with pericystectomy in normothermic ischemia for hepatic hydatidosis. *Surg Gynecol Obstetr* 1986; **163**: 127-32.
6. Bouzidi A. Kyste hydatique du foie. Editions techniques. Encycl Méd Chir (Paris, France), Hepatologie 1993; 7-023-A-10.
7. Bilge A, Sozuer EM. Diagnosis and surgical treatment of hepatic hydatid disease. *HPB Surgery* 1992; **6**: 57-64.
8. Cangiotti L, Giulini SM, Muiesan P, Nodari F, Begni A, Tiberio G. Hydatid disease of the liver: long-term results of surgical treatment. *G Chir* 1991; **12**: 501-504.
9. Castellano G, Moreno Sanchez D, Gutierrez T, Moreno Gonzalez F, Colina F, Solis Herruzo JA. Caustic sclerosing cholangitis. Report of four cases and a cumulative review of the literature. *Hepato-Gastroenterol* 1994; **41**: 458-470.
10. Davis A, Pawlowski ZS, Dixon H. Multicentric clinical trial of benzimizadolecarbamates in human echinococcosis. Bull. WHO 1986; **64**: 383-388.
11. El Mufti M. *Surgical management of hydatid disease*. Butterworth-Heineman, Oxford, 1989.
12. Gil Grande LA, Rodriguez Cabeiro F, Prieto JG *et al*. Randomized controlled trial of efficacy of albendazole in intra-abdominal hydatid disease. *Lancet* 1993; **342**: 1262-1272.
13. Giorgio A, Tarantino L, Francica G, Mariniello N, Aloisso T, Soscia F, Pierri G. Unilocular hydatid liver cysts: treatment with US-guided,

doubled percutaneous aspiration and alcohol injection. *Radiology* 1992; **184:** 705-710.

14. Gozzetti G, Mazziotti A, Bolondi L, Barbara L. *Intraoperative ultrasonography in surgery for liver tumors*. Kluwer, Dordrecht, 1989.

15. Grundmann R, Eitenmüller J, Pichlmaier H. Zur Indikation der verschiedenen Operationsverfahren bei Leberechinococcus. *Chirurg* 1981; **52:** 332-337.

16. Gruttadauria S, Marino G, Gruttadauria G. Development of echinococcosis; diagnosis and treatment over a 20 year period. Proceedings 2nd World IHPBA Congress, Bologna 1996. Monduz., Bologna, 1996, Vol. 1, pp. 207-210.

17. Kilicturgay S, Sadikoglu Y, Sauci G, Irgil C, Ozen Y, Bilgel H. Percutaneous aspiration and drainage of hydatid cysts. Is it helpful for diagnosis and treatment? Proceedings 1st European IHPBA Congress, Athens 1995. Monduzzi, Bologna, 1995, pp. 847-852.

18. Luder PJ, Witassek F, Weigand K, Ecker J, Bircher J. Treatment of cystic echinococcosis (Echinococcus Granulosus) with Mebendazole: assessment of bound and free drug levels in cyst fluid and of parasite vitality in operative specimens. *Eur J Clin Pharmacol* 1989; **28:** 279-289.

19. Lygidakis NJ. Diagnosis and treatment of intra-biliary rupture of hydatid cysts of the liver. *Arch Surg* 1983; **118:** 1186-89.

20. Magistrelli P, Masetti P, Coppola R, Messia A, Picciocchi A. Surgical treatment of the hydatid disease of the liver. *Arch Surg* 1991; **126:** 518-523.

21. Morel PH, Robert J, Rohner A. Surgical treatment of hydatid disease of the liver: a survey of 69 patients. *Surgery* 1988; **104:** 859-862.

22. Moreno Gonzalez E, Rico Selas P, Martinet B, Garcia Garcia I, Carato Palma F, Hidalgo Pascual M. Results of surgical treatment of hepatic hydatidosis: current therapeutic modifications. *World J Surg* 1991; **15:** 254-263.

23. Safioleas M, Mistakos E, Manti C, Katsikas D, Skalkeas G. Diagnostic evaluation and surgical management of hydatid disease of the liver. *World J Surg* 1994; **18:** 859-65.

24. Secchi MA, Pettinari R, Ledesma C *et al*. Hepatic hydatidosis. A multicentric study of surgical procedures in 971 cases. Proceedings 2nd World IHPBA Congress, Bologna 1996. Monduzzi, Bologna, 1996, Vol. 1, pp. 201-206.

25. Settaf A, Mansori F, Sefriani A, Slaoni A. Kystes hydatiques du foie. Classification à visée therapeutique et prognostique. 387 observations. Presse Méd 1994; 23: 362-366.

26. Valle M, Serafini D, Bernardini P Complications of hepatic hydatidosis. *Minerva Chir* 1992; **47:** 15-16.

27. Wanninayake HM, Brough W, Bullock N, Calne RY, Farman JV. Hypernatremia after treatment of hydatic cysts. *Br Med J* 1992; **284:** 1302-1303.

28. Woodtli W. Effects of plasma mebendazole concentrations in the treatment of human echinococcosis. *Am J Trop Med Hyg* 1985; **34:** 745-760.

22

Liver Trauma

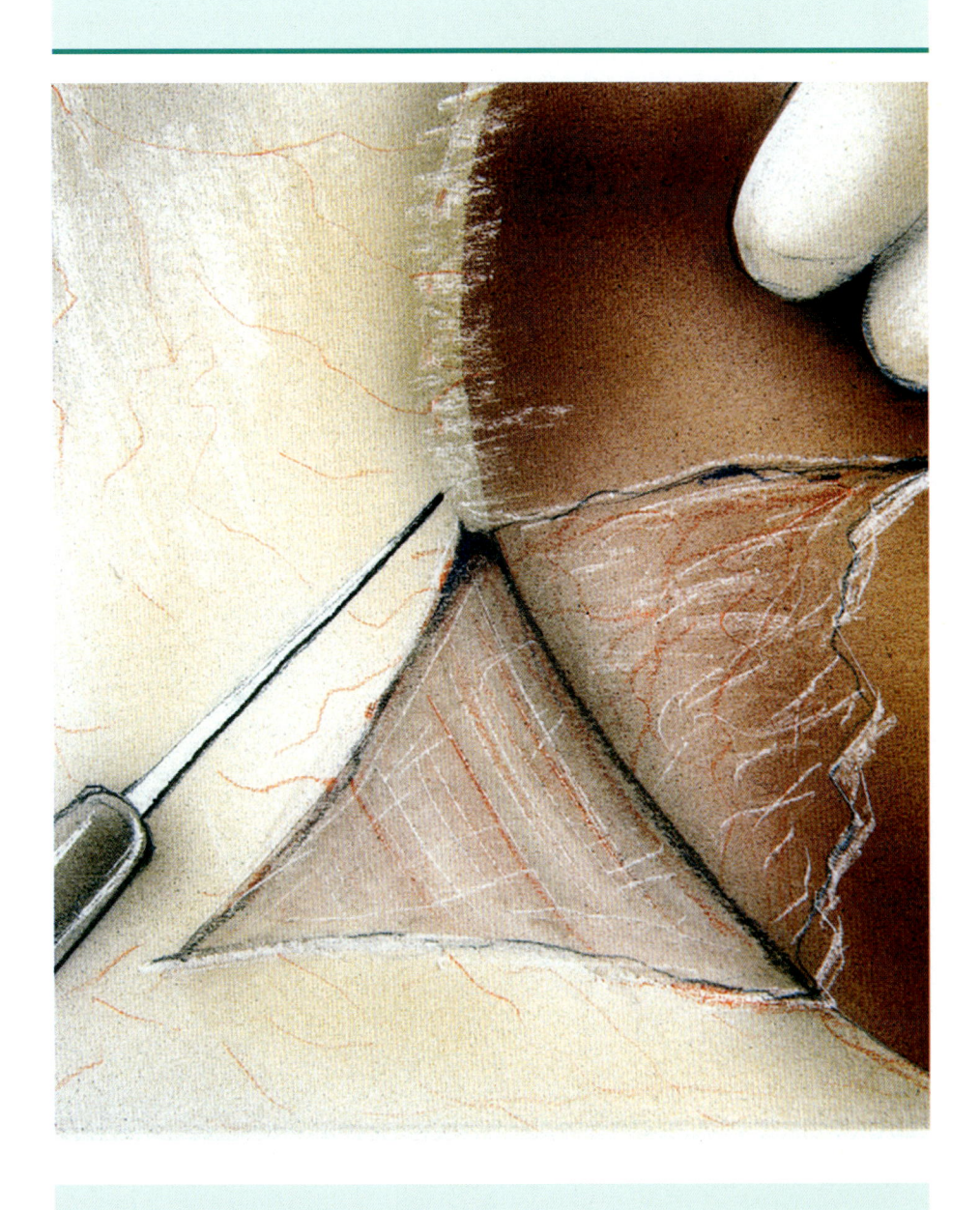

191

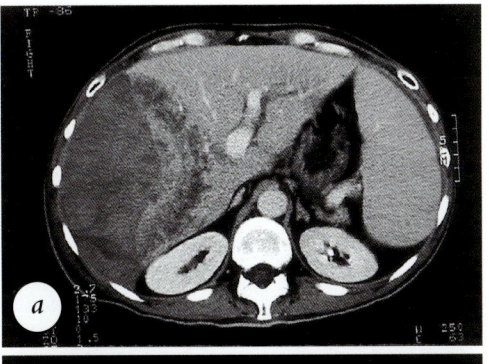

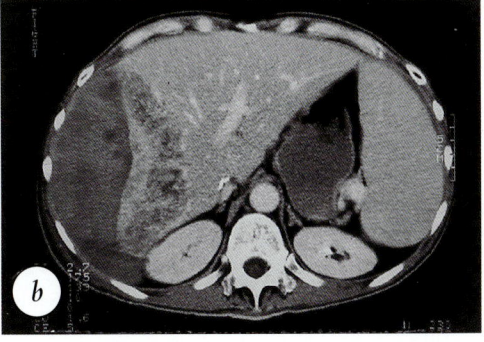

Figure 22.1 –
*Huge hepatic hematoma after blunt injury of the liver **a**). Spontaneous regression at CT control 2 months after the trauma **b**)*

Traumatic lesions of the liver are the result of either blunt or penetrating (less frequent) trauma of the abdomen. The trauma mechanism lies at the basis of the types of lesions that can be observed. In contrecoup lesions (falls from heights, abrupt braking – as in some motorcycle or car accidents) the liver can tear due to the tension on its attaching structures, the triangular ligaments, the round ligament and the caval-hepatic vein confluence, causing linear wounds close to the insertion of the ligaments and even detachment of the most posterior portions of a hemiliver and severe caval-hepatic vein lacerations. Compression trauma (falls on the right side, car accidents involving collision with the steering wheel, lesions caused by blows) lead to contusion of a hepatic lobe (usually the right), with lesions that can range from more or less deep lacerations of the capsule, to crushing of the parenchyma or to the formation of an intrahepatic hematoma. Penetrating wounds are rarer in current practice and vary according to the cause of the trauma (knife or gunshot wounds); their severity also depends on associated lesions of the intestine, diaphragm, intrathoracic organs or main abdominal vessels.

The diagnosis and approach to the patient depend on the presentation. Lesions to the liver are usually discovered intraoperatively in patients undergoing emergency surgery with clinical signs of shock and hemoperitoeum and in these cases the only diagnostic examination that can be carried out is ultrasound to confirm the presence of hematoperitoneum. Ultrasound is only exceptionally used to diagnose traumatic lesions of the liver apart from detection of intrahepatic hematomas. In patients who are stable hemodynamically and in whom hepatic lesions are clinically suspected, a CT scan and possibly angiography should be considered in addition to ultrasound.

The approach in emergency cases is median laparotomy which permits exploration of the entire abdominal cavity. After aspirating the blood, the liver and spleen are explored, and any hemorrhagic lesions are packed. The intestine, mesentery, bladder and retroperitoneum are then explored. In the event of lesions of the right lobe of the liver, the median incision is extended transversely towards the right. In exceptional cases, for more complex lesions involving the suprahepatic hilum, the incision can be extended to the thorax. Before completing exploration of the hepatic lesions it is necessary to ensure the hemodynamic stability of the patient, packing any sources of hemorrhage with sterile dressings until blood pressure is restored and the hemodynamic situation is adequately compensated. Only then can the dressings be removed and the extent of the hepatic lesions adequately evaluated.

Intrahepatic hematomas without intraperitoneal hemorrhage or signs of hemobilia do not require any treatment. The natural history of these lesions is decidedly favourable, with eventual absorption of the hematoma (***Figure 22.1***). If the hematoma is not responsible for active bleeding and is discovered during laparotomy exploration, it should not be opened. Packing with sterile dressings which could lead to ischemic necrosis or any other type of treatment is unnecessary.

Superficial capsular lacerations do not require any particular treatment. These lesions are often no longer actively bleeding at intervention. If bleeding persists in the decapsulated zone, hemostasis can be achieved with an Argon coagulator or simply by applying a fibrin sponge or spraying the area with Tissucol. Suturing is not recommended as this could enlarge the decapsulation. A gravity abdominal drainage tube can be left in place for 48 hours for safety's sake.

Deeper linear lesions with active bleeding or *stellate lesions* of the parenchyma must be explored and elective hemostasis attempted. If the lesion involves the right lateral segments or the hepatic dome, the liver should be mobilized after compression of the hemorrhage site with sterile dressings. Division of the ligaments makes it possible to move the liver forward and facilitates the application of hemostasis stitches without tension. The ideal treatment consists of elective hemostasis of the bleeding vessels with Vicryl® 3.0 stitches, including small portions of parenchyma around the bleeding vessels, or of elective ligation of the pedicles if these are visible inside the wound. If there is conspicuous hemorrhage during these maneuvers the hepatic pedicle should be clamped at the hilum (***Figure 22.2***). Clamping is indicated as long as the patient is hemodynamically stable and there are no signs of shock. Through-and-through U stitches are not advisable for treating hepatic lacerations. If the hemorrhagic lesion is deep, suturing does not ensure hemostasis. Through-and-through stitches can cause the formation of intrahepatic biliary collections, the basis for secondary hemobilia. Such stitches are also often a source of parenchymal necrosis and sequestration with the formation of post-operative infected areas or biliary fistulas.

In more complex *stellate lesions*, when hemostasis cannot be ensured by suturing and in the presence of diffuse parenchymal hemorrhage, the most rational approach is to apply perihepatic packing.[2,5,7,9] Temporary packing can also be applied to allow complete radiological evaluation and, if necessary, arrange for the patient to be transferred to a specialized liver surgery center. The liver must be appropriately mobilized so that packing can be uniformly placed around the entire lobe, avoiding excessive compression of the parenchyma which can lead to ischemic necrosis and compression on the vena cava which can impair venous drainage and renal insufficiency.[3] The packing should be kept in place for at least 3 days. An alternative to packing is the application of a Vicryl mesh® (Vicryl Knitted Mesh, Polyglactin 910, Ethicon) which is fixed under tension to Glisson's capsule, corresponding to the insertion of the hepatic ligaments, which is thicker and stitches can be applied.[14] The hemiliver involved must be mobilized, compressing the site of the hemorrhage. If the right hemiliver is affected, the mesh should be fixed on one side corresponding to the insertion of the right triangular ligament and on the other side at the insertion of the falciform ligament, with sufficient traction to control the hemorrhage. This procedure is indicated for venous hemorrhage that is not particularly deep or for extensive sub-capsular lesions. In one case it was successfully used for an extensive ruptured sub-capsular hematoma of the graft during liver transplant surgery (***Figure 22.3***).

Parenchymal lesions can lead to the destruction of extensive parts of the parenchyma and resection of the devitalized area is necessary. *Emergency resections* must be limited to cases in which hemostasis cannot otherwise be achieved, one example being atypical hepatectomies, following the spontaneous division lines on the parenchyma. Care must be taken not to leave devitalized zones of parenchyma whose vascular pedicles have been interrupted during extra-anatomical resections. Lesions of the left lobe are a particular indication for hepatic resection, especially if the insertion area of the round ligament is involved, where the adjacency of the Glissonian pedicle of segment 3 can cause major hemorrhage or biliary fistulas. Major hepatectomies are rarely required as a result of trauma. The most rational approach is to avoid major operations which remove a large mass of healthy tissue in patients already in a critical condition as a result of the trauma or from shock. In our center, conventional hepatectomies for trauma were carried out in 6 cases out of 48 surgically treated traumatic lesions. Three cases were right hepatectomies, 1 was a left hepatectomy and the other 2 were left lobectomies. The first case was a compression trauma caused by a car accident, with profound linear rupture of the right hemiliver and hemorrhage from a lesion of the right branch of the portal vein. The hemorrhage recurred dramatically every time the hepatic pedicle was unclamped and

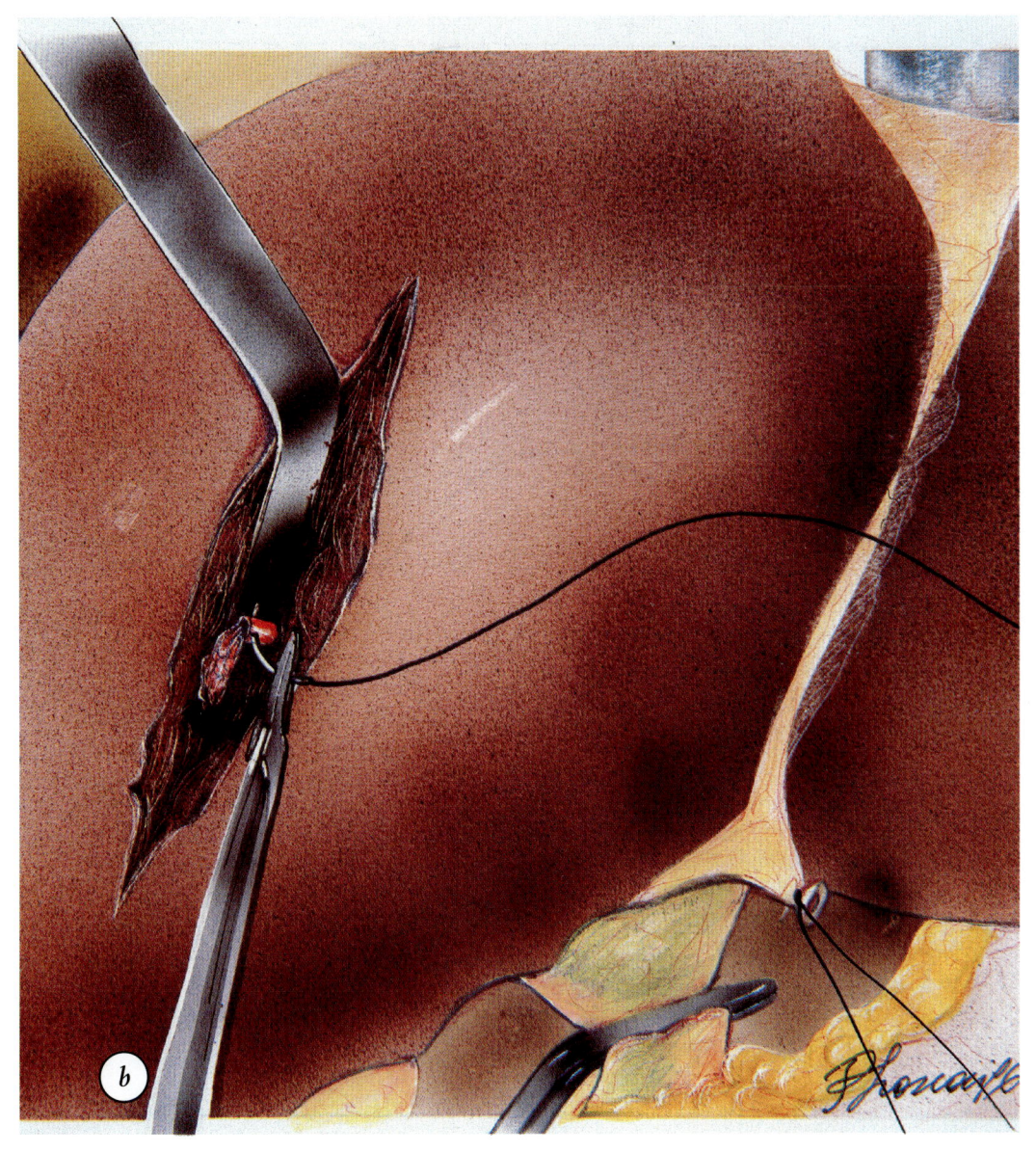

LIVER TRAUMA

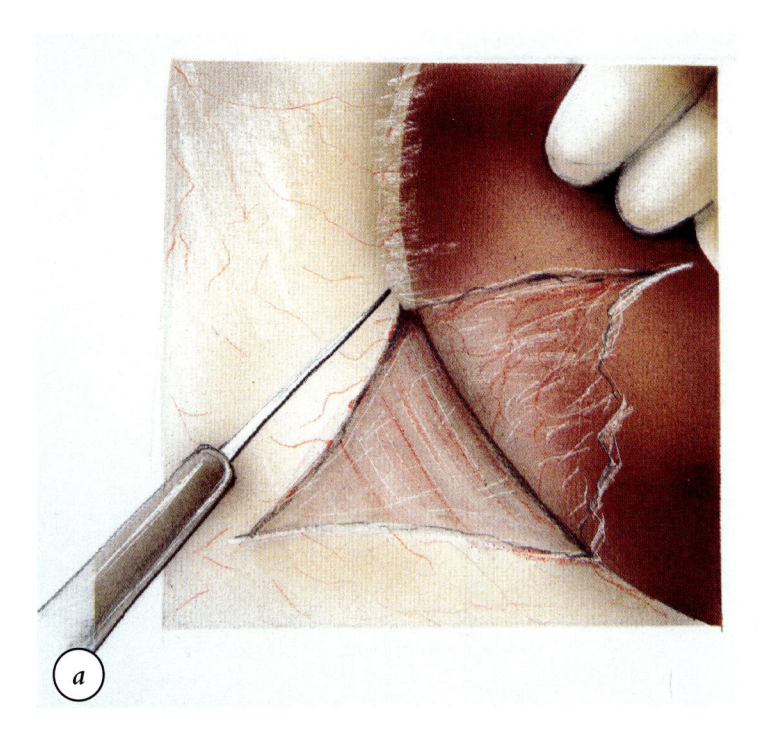

Figure 22.2– *Deep laceration of the liver due to blunt trauma. The right lobe is mobilized, compressing the hemorrhagic site **a)**. Elective hemostasis of the bleeding vessels is achieved by clamping of the hepatic pedicle **b)**. The hepatic laceration is left open and simply covered with omentum. Subhepatic drainage is systematically left in place.*

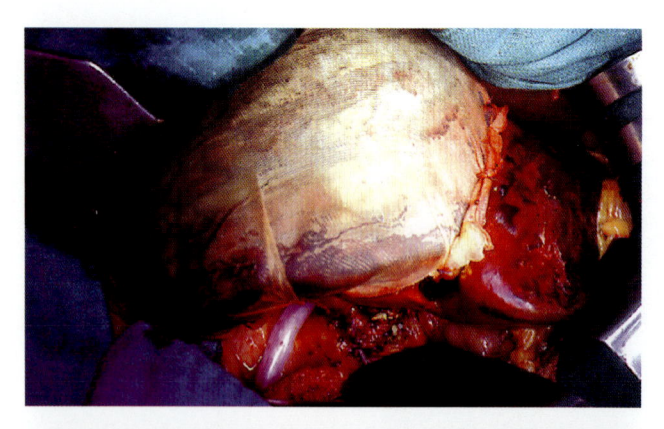

Figure 22.3 – *Application of Vicryl mesh for widespread subcapsular lesions due to blunt trauma. The right lobe is mobilized and the mesh is fixed between the insertion of the right triangular ligament, the gallbladder fissure and the insertion of the falciform ligament.*

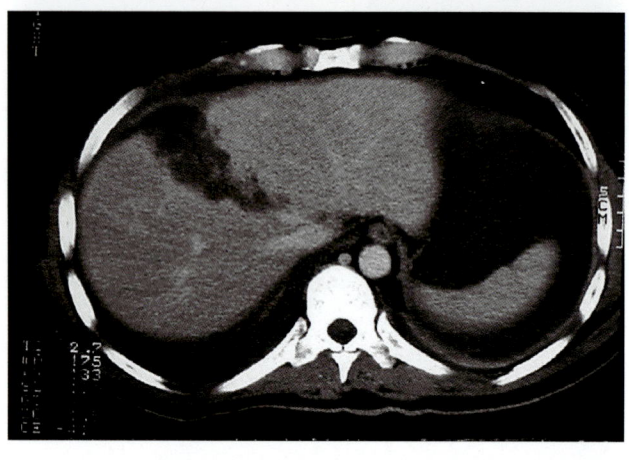

Figure 22.4 – *Blunt hepatic trauma with complete laceration of the parenchyma along the sagittal scissure plane. The left hepatic duct had been detached from the biliary confluence. After an initial inadequate attempt at hemostasis, the patient underwent left hepatectomy with suturing of the hepatic duct after positioning of a Kehr tube.*

hepatectomy was the only possibility given the site of the hemorrhagic lesion. In another two cases the hemorrhage could not be controlled by packing and hepatectomy was performed a few days after the first conservative treatment. One patient was treated seven days after blunt trauma which had caused deep parenchymal laceration along the Cantlie line, completely detaching the right and left hemiliver (**Figure 22.4**). After an initial attempt at hemostasis in another hospital, the patient was re-admitted with a choleperitoneum due to the laceration of the left hepatic duct at the level of the biliary bifurcation. During the re-operation it was not possible to perform a direct anastomosis on the damaged hepatic duct and a left hepatectomy was therefore carried out with suturing of the biliary tract on a Kehr tube. The remaining 2 cases in which a left lobectomy was performed were a penetrating wound and trauma caused by crushing. Although no deaths occurred, it must be stressed that major hepatectomy for trauma should only be performed when absolutely necessary, preferably at a specialized center and with the patient hemodynamically stable.

The most complex lesions that can occur in emergency situations are those involving the suprahepatic hilum. These demanding lesions are difficult to control with packing. In these circumstances, when the trunk of a hepatic vein is interrupted at the convergence, it is essential first of all to ensure manual compression of the hemorrhagic area before starting to mobilize the liver. Hypovolemia must be compensated and the patient placed under positive end expiratory pressure (PEEP) to prevent air embolism. At the same time the anesthetist must position a central venous route to allow rapid infusion of liquids and hemodynamic monitoring. The incision is extended to permit complete exposure. In the presence of posterior lesions and when it is not possible to apply a vascular clamp directly, it is advisable to free the vena cava above and below the liver, always exerting manual pressure at the site of the hemorrhage, and perform total vascular exclusion which can only be tolerated if circulating volume is restored. With the liver under vascular exclusion, the two lacerated stumps of the hepatic vein can be sutured. Ligation of the hepatic vein at its origin is well tolerated, due to the rapid formation of collateral drainage circulations.[1,8] In the last 15 years we have never resorted to other more complex procedures such as the application of caval shunts, the practical application of

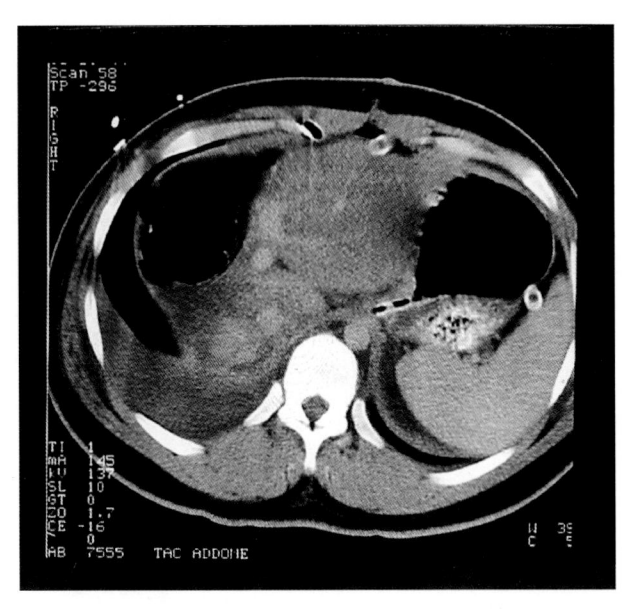

Figure 22.5– *Emergency extended right hepatectomy performed at another hospital due to blunt trauma with multiple lacerations of the right lobe. The patient had undergone prolonged clamping of the hepatic pedicle. Two days after the trauma the patient presented signs of progressive encephalopathy and became comatose on the third day. The patient was successfully transplanted 5 days after the trauma.*

which has, moreover, been rarely reported. The current tendency is to discourage the use of the these highly complex procedures which are associated with a very high degree of mortality.

Liver transplantation is also employed as a 'life-saving' procedure in patients with particularly complex liver trauma. Up to 1994 approximately 20 transplants for trauma had been described in the literature, including 1 case in our series (**Figure 22.5**).[4] The majority of these were emergency transplants for severe hepatic insufficiency after extensive resections or for biliary damage which could not otherwise be corrected. Only in a small number were performed to achieve otherwise impossible hemostasis: the entire parenchyma was removed in these cases, preserving the vena cava and constructing a portacaval shunt to ensure splanchnic venous return. Transplantation was performed a few days after total hepatectomy.[11]

The prognosis after hepatic trauma depends not only on the complexity of the lesions and the involvement of other organs (cranial trauma, thoracic trauma, bone fractures) but also on the promptness of the diagnosis, and often on the type of emergency treatment administered. It is important to stress that the treatment of certain post-traumatic complex lesions is one of the most difficult technical problems in hepatic surgery, requiring multidisciplinary cooperation between surgeons, anesthetists familiar with liver surgery, radiologists and operative angioradiologists. If the first emergency operation is performed in a district hospital, where all these skills are not available, the most correct approach is to apply effective packing for temporary hemostasis and to promptly contact the nearest center with major experience in liver surgery for the definitive treatment.

Complications

Post-traumatic hemobilia

Hemorrhage in the biliary tract can be caused by a direct vascular-biliary communication, as a result of penetrating wounds (the same mechanism is responsible for hemobilia from hepatic biopsy or percutaneous transhepatic drainage) and, more often, is a complication of liver trauma or the result of a traumatic lesion in an inadequately treated liver. In the latter case, the hemobilia may be a consequence of a

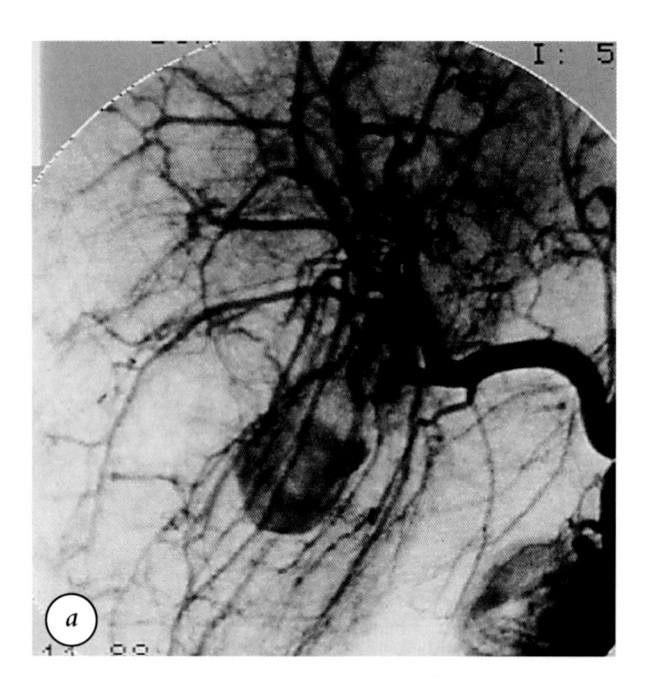

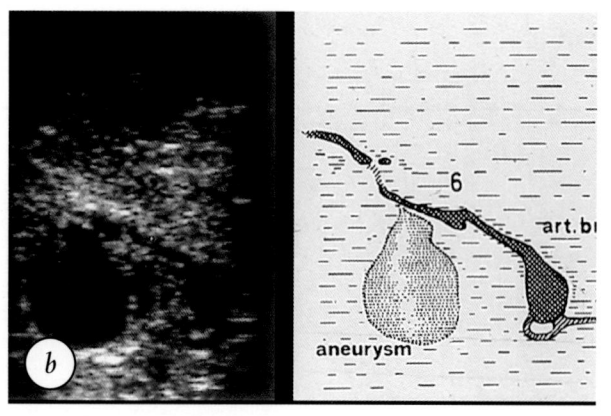

Figure 22.6 – *Blunt liver trauma due to a fall (attempted suicide). 14 days after the accident the patient presented a digestive hemorrhage. The patient was febrile. Abdominal ultrasound showed a distended gallbladder with echogenous material. Arteriography revealed the presence of a pseudoaneurysm in the arterial branch of segment 6* **a)**. *Blood culture was positive due to the presence of mycetes as a result of an infected intra-hepatic hematoma. During laparotomy, intraoperative ultrasound identified the pseudoaneurysm which originated from the arterial branch of segment 6 (art.br.6)* **b)**. *Surgery consisted of a segmentary echo-guided resection of segment 6.*

post-traumatic aneurysm of an intrahepatic arterial branch which ruptures in the biliary tract or of a parenchymal laceration which also involves the intrahepatic bile ducts. In our center, out of 21 cases of embolization which we observed 13 were patients who had received prior inadequate treatment of a liver trauma with application of superficial suturing for the treatment of a lesion which actually involved the parenchyma to a deeper level. The presence of a cavity below the suture, in which the hemorrhage and the loss of bile continue, forms an accumulation of blood which discharges into the biliary tract once a certain tension has been reached. The presence of bile is the basic reason for the failure of this type of lesion to heal spontaneously: the bile dissolves the local clot and prevents healing of the liver wounds.[12] This pathogenetic mechanism explains why gastrointestinal (GI) hemorrhages in hemobilia often occur in proportion to the progressive filling of blood and bile in the intraparenchymal lacerations which then empty into the bile ducts and their usually late onset - from a few days up to several weeks after the trauma. Hemobilia should be suspected in the event of GI hemorrhage in any patient who has suffered blunt trauma of the abdomen or in a patient with surgically treated liver trauma. Clinical diagnosis is easy in the presence of the classic symptoms: GI hemorrhage, pain in the right hypochondrium and jaundice. Ultrasound shows the presence of clots inside a distended gallbladder, possible distension of the biliary tract and the presence of an intrahepatic hematoma. CT is useful in identifying the site of the hematoma. Angiography should be systematically requested to evaluate the presence of aneurysms of the intrahepatic arterial branches or interruptions of the intraparenchymal vessels, or more rarely the site of an arterial fistula in the form of contrast medium leakage.

The treatment of hemobilia depends on the type of complex hepatic lesion with respect to former inadequate treatment. Hemobilia without hematoperitoneum can be successfully treated with arterial embolization. This treatment is indicated in particular for hemobilia caused by percutaneous transhepatic maneuvers or in the presence of a post-traumatic aneurysm. Embolization must be carried out distally, beyond the arterial bifurcation, and followed by antibiotic treatment to prevent the risk of septic complications linked to the ischemia. Lesions associated with a hepatic laceration and with hematoperitoneum require laparotomy with extensive opening of the cavity, debridement and elective hemostais. Removal of the gallbladder must be systematic and biliary leakage is controlled by the injection of methylene blue from the cystic duct.

The more complex lesions observed after initial emergency treatment for hemostasis should be treated at centres which specialise in liver surgery. Treatment can vary from opening of the cavity with débridement to segmentary liver resections (*Figure 22.6*) or to major hepatectomies in the presence of more extensive intraparenchymal cavities due to the interruption of main intrahepatic vessels.

Hepatic sequestration and infectious complications

The formation of hepatic sequestra is the result of 'mattress' sutures which devitalize portions of the parenchyma with secondary infection, to the interruption of segmentary vascular pedicles caused by the hemostasis of a deep lesion or to the formation of an intraparenchymal cavity after suturing of only the superficial layers. A full radiological work-up (CT, scintigraphy with marked leukocytes and often angiography) is required for complete evaluation of the lesion. Treatment consists of resection 'à la demande' of the devitalized areas, or of debridement with extensive opening and drainage of the cavity.

REFERENCES

1. Beppu M, Fukuzaki T, Mitani K, Fujimoti K, Taniguchi J. Hepatic segmentectomy with segmental hepatic vein sacrifice. *Arch Surg* 1990; **125:** 1170-1176.
2. Feliciano DV, Mattox KL, Burch JM, Bitondog CG, Jordan GL. Packing for control of hepatic hemorrhage. *J Trauma* 1986; **26:** 738-743.
3. Gadzijev EM, Stanisavljevic D, Wahl M, Butinar J, Grkaman Wahl J. Evaluation of the pressure of perihepatic packing in liver trauma. Proceedings of the 2nd World IHPBA Congress, Bologna 1996. Monduzzi, Bologna, 1996, pp.211-214.
4. Gozzetti G, Mazziotti A, Jovine E, Grazi GL. Liver transplantation for trauma. *Chirurgia* 1994; **7:** 848-851.
5. Hollands MJ, Little JM. Perihepatic packing: its role in the management of liver trauma. *Aust N Zel J Surg* 1989; **59:** 21-24.
6. Ivatury RR, Nallathambi M, Gundut Y, Constable R, Rohman M, Stahl WM. Liver packing for controllable hemorrhage: a reappraisal. *J Trauma* 1986; **26:** 746-753.
7. Krige JEF, Borhman PC, Terblanche J. Therapeutic perihepatic packing in complex liver trauma. *Br J.Surg* 1992; **79:** 43-46.
8. Ou QJ, Hermann RE. Hepatic vein ligation and preservation of liver segments in major resections. *Arch Surg* 1982; **122:** 1198-1200.
9. Pachter HL et al. Significant trends in the treatment of hepatic trauma. Experience with 411 injuries. *Ann Surg* 1992; **215:** 492-502.
10. Reed RE et al. Continuing evolution in the approach to severe liver trauma. *Ann Surg* 1992; **216:** 524-538.
11. Ringe B, Pichlmair R, Ziegler H et al. Management of severe hepatic trauma by two-stage total hepatectomy and subsequent liver transplantation. *Surgery* 1991; **109:** 792-795.
12. Sandblom P. Hemobilia. In: Blumgart LH *Surgery of the liver and biliary tract*. Churchill Livingstone, Edinburgh, 1994, pp. 1159-1274.
13. Sharp KW, Locicero RJ. Abdominal packing for surgically uncontrollable hemorrhage. *Ann Surg* 1992; **215:** 467-475.
14. Stevens SL, Maull KI, Enderson BL. Total hepatic mesh wrap for hemostasis. *Surg Gynecol Obstet* 1992; **175:** 181-182.

TECHNIQUES IN LIVER SURGERY

SECTION VII

Intra-arterial Chemotherapy

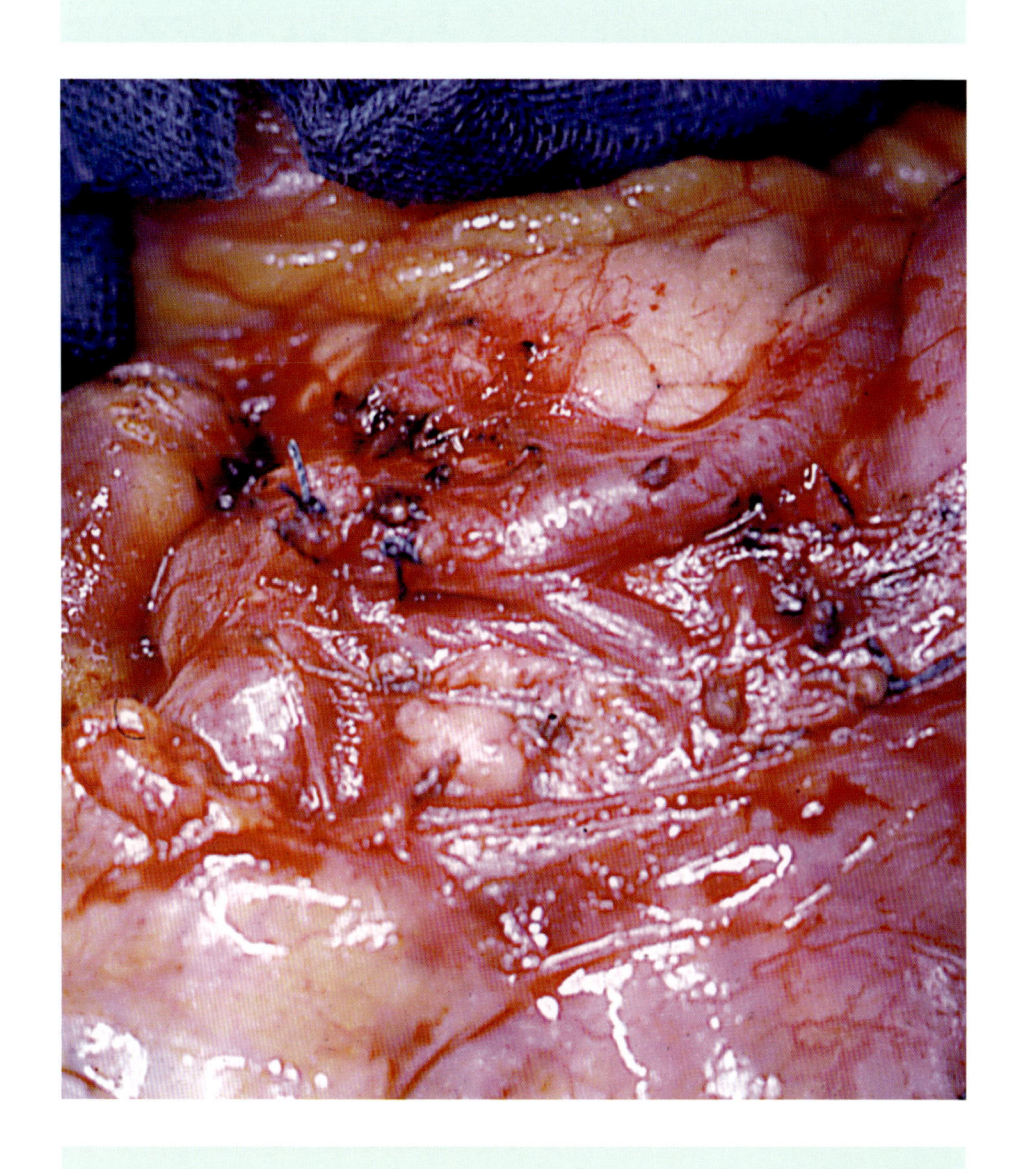

23

Intra-arterial Infusion for Locoregional Chemotherapy

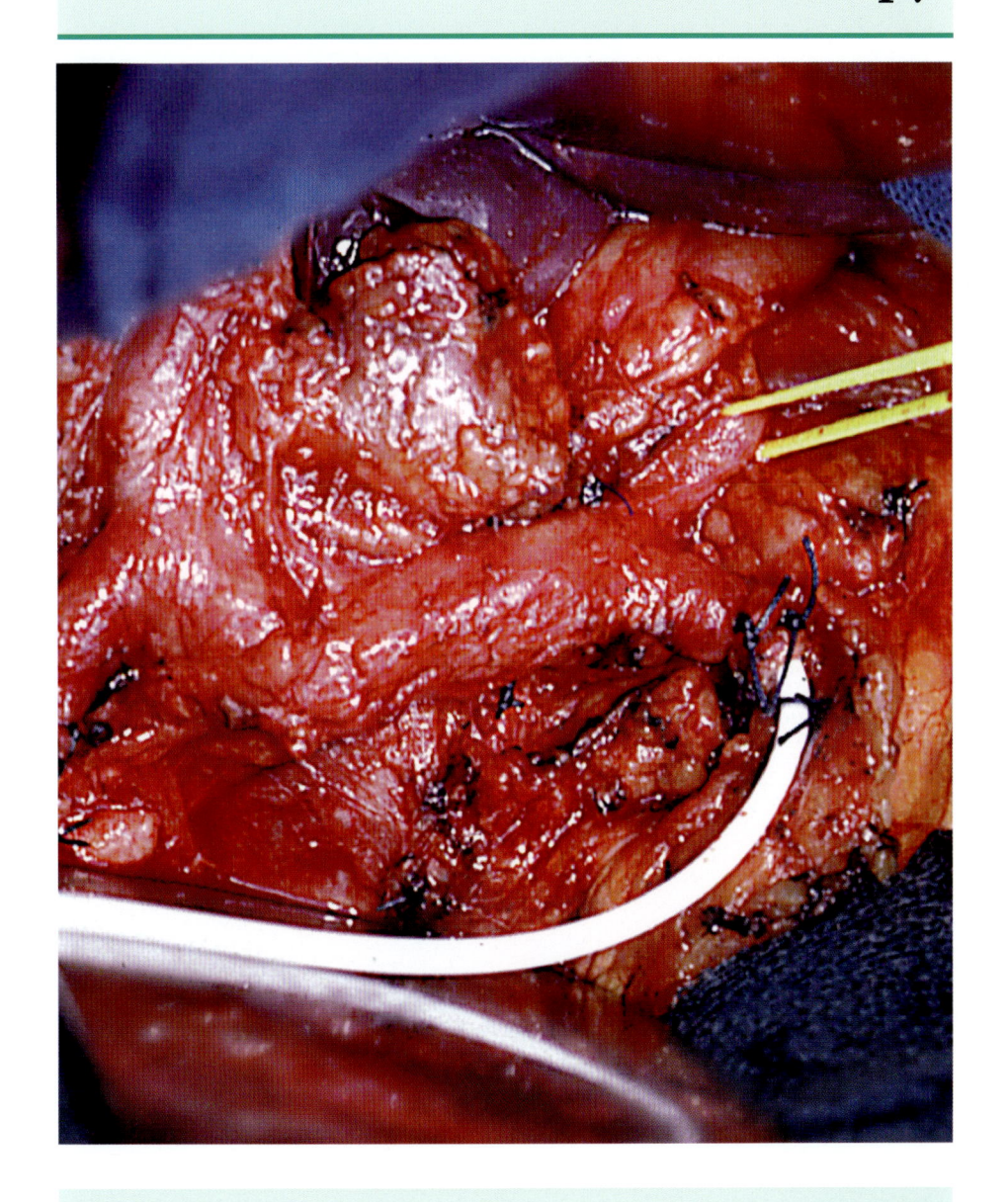

Hepatic intra-arterial chemotherapy is used to treat those patients with metastatic or primary liver cancer not eligible for liver resection. The rationale for this treatment is based on the high arterial vascularization of hepatic tumors and on the high concentration of drugs which can thus be dispatched directly to the tumor, greatly increasing the antitumoral effect and reducing the toxic side effects of chemotherapy.[6,20] The development of implantable devices has made infusion therapy feasible and practical in the outpatient setting. Two types of devices are used: pumps which make it possible to accumulate a certain quantity of drug which is then released on a continuous basis, or simple, smaller and more economical ports for periodic infusions.

The drugs most commonly used for intra-arterial infusion are 5-Fluorouracil (5-FU), 5-fluorouracil 2 deoxyuridine (FUDR), Bischlorethylnitrosurea, Mitomycin, Cisplatin and Adriamycin. All these drugs are metabolized by the liver on first passage giving an estimated increase of 2-fold for Adriamycin, 10-fold for 5-FU andmore than 100-fold for FUDR which is therefore one of the most commonly used drugs in hepatic intra-arterial chemotherapy. Randomized clinical studies demonstrate the superiority of intra-arterial chemotherapy with respect to systemic chemotherapy in metastases from colorectal carcinoma in terms of a greater response to treatment with a reduction in volume of the metastases and of the Carcino Embryogenic Antigen (CEA) values.[2,5,8,9,13,15,17,21] The objective data on prolongation of survival remain controversial and to date do not allow any definitive conclusions to be drawn. Furthermore, while intra-arterial chemotherapy may avoid some of the side effects of systemic chemotherapy, such as myelosuppression or gastroenteric disorders such as nausea and diarrhoea, it is not however without morbidity or pitfalls (see below). The main problem which can occur during continuous intra-arterial treatment is hepatobiliary toxicity, reflected by an increase in transaminase and cholestatic enzymes and which may lead to a clinical-pathological pattern similar to sclerosing cholangitis.[7]

The enthusiasm with which this method was first accepted has now become more restrained. Intra-arterial chemotherapy seems to be a rational proposal only in carefully selected cases of hepatic metastases, primitive non-resectable tumors without extrahepatic spread or lymph nodes metastases, involving less than 50% of the hepatic parenchyma. Patients with portal thrombosis are excluded, due to the risk of hepatic infarction, as are patients with cholestasis caused by infiltration of the bile ducts, due to the risk of infection and hepatic insufficiency.

Intra-arterial chemotherapy can be used in patients who have undergone hepatic resection for metastases in order to reduce the risk of intrahepatic recurrence and to improve survival. Two randomized shunts have been reported, demonstrating the effects of associated resection and intra-arterial chemotherapy treatment.[8,16] Both studies, carried out in patients with single or multiple metastases and subjected to hepatic resection, show that intra-arterial chemotherapy significantly increases 5-year survival and reduces tumor recurrence with a longer disease-free interval. Successful results of adjuvant locoregional chemotherapy combined with interleukin 2 immunotherapy have recently been reported in patients undergoing liver resections for metastatic cancers[12,16] Another more recent non-randomized study concerns hepatic intra-arterial chemotherapy associated with liver resection in patients operated on for hepatocarcinoma. More than half the patients treated were cirrhotics. The infusion consisted of a combination of 5-FU, adriamycin and mitomycin and the treatment was carried out at intervals for 10 months after the operation. The results of this study show an increase in survival and disease-free survival in patients treated with adjuvant chemotherapy.[14]

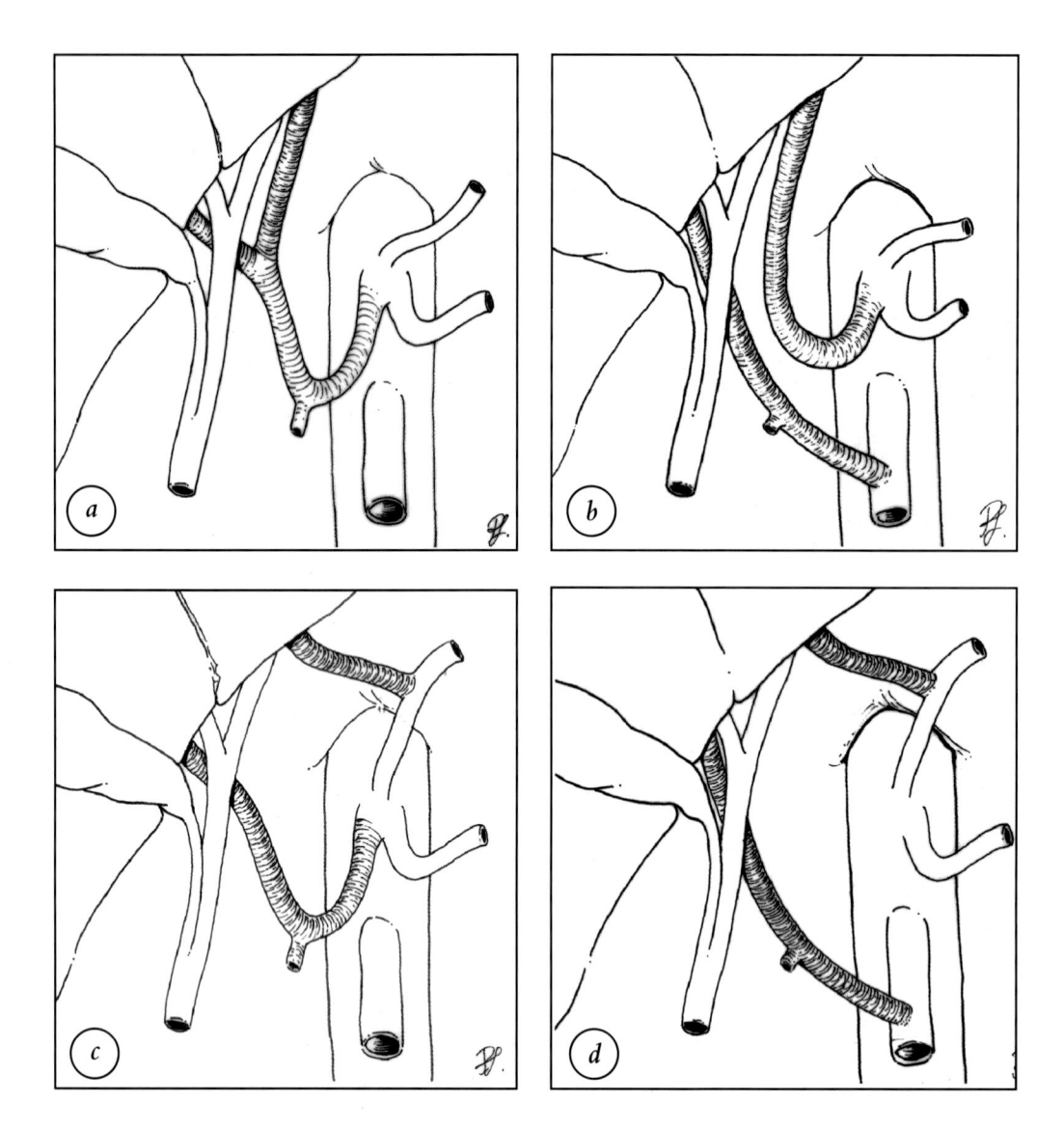

Figure 20.1 – *Anatomical variations of the hepatic artery. The modal arrangement **a)** with an arterial trunk that arises from the celiac trunk and bifurcates at the level of the hepatic pedicle into a right branch and a left branch is seen in about 75% of cases. The most frequent anomaly is the presence of a right hepatic artery **b)**, either accessory (if a right branch arising from the hepatic artery is also present) or aberrant (arising from the superior mesenteric artery. This anomaly is encountered in around 10% of cases. The anomalous artery runs posterior to the common bile duct, along the right margin of the portal trunk. A left hepatic artery arising from the left gastric artery **c)**, accessory or aberrant, is present in 10% of cases. This branch is clearly visible in the upper part of the hepatogastric ligament. In the remaining cases a common hepatic artery arising from the celiac trunk is absent. This is replaced by one or two branches, arising respectively from the superior mesenteric artery and from the left gastric artery **d)**. Much more rarely, the common hepatic artery may arise directly from the aorta.*

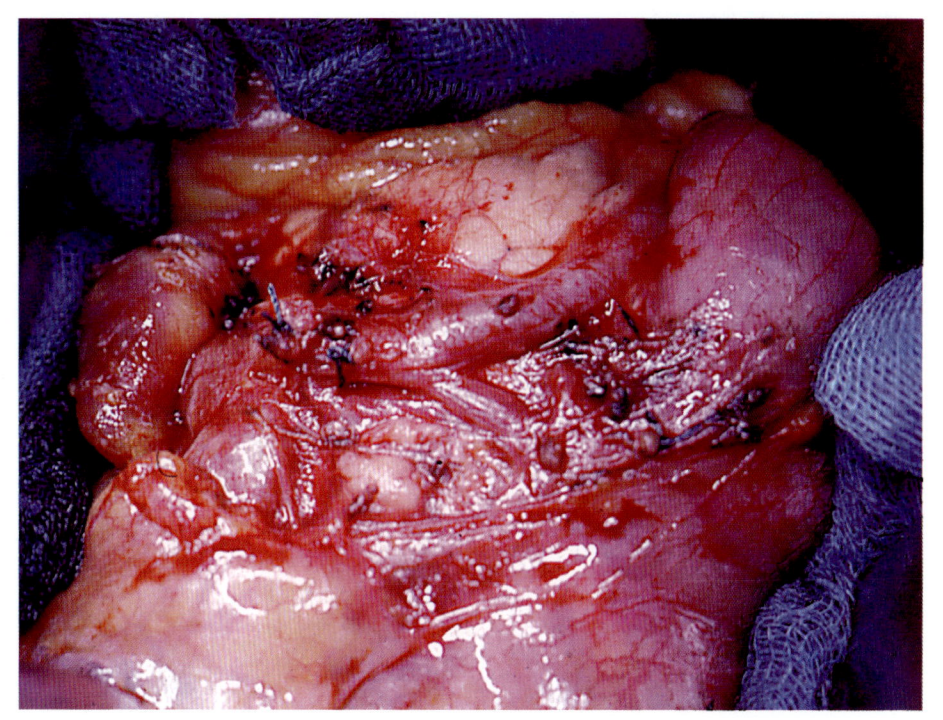

Figure 23.2 – *Preparation of the gastroduodenal artery for positioning of the catheter for intra-arterial hepatic chemotherapy. The pyloric vessels have been divided. The antro-pyloric region has been liberated and moved downwards. The gastroduodenal artery is followed from its outlet from the hepatic artery for about 3 cm. The superior pancreatic-duodenal branch which enters the pancreas is clearly visible on the posterior aspect of the gastroduodenal artery. This branch must be isolated to prevent misperfusion of the drug in the pancreas.*

We favor the use of adjuvant intra-arterial chemotherapy, especially after the resection of multiple hepatic metastases when the risk of recurrence is higher. The treatment has been carried out at the same times as hepatic resection in 25 patients in our department, without adverse effects. The analysis of long-term survival does not allow conclusive statements to be made although the incidence of intrahepatic recurrence at two years is below 20%, dedidedly lower than our historic series of liver resections for metastases.

Hepatic arteriography is advisable when planning surgery for intra-arterial device placement, in view of the frequency of anatomical variations of the hepatic artery. There are two types of arterial anatomic variations: accessory arteries and aberrant arteries. An *accessory artery* is an additional vessel when the normal right and left branches arising from the common hepatic artery are present. An *aberrant artery* is the arterial supply for the right or left hemiliver from another branch of the coeliac artery or the superior mesenteric artery and not the common hepatic artery. The most common anatomical variations of the hepatic artery which must be taken into consideration in the placement of intra-arterial devices are shown in *Figure 23.1*. The percentages of the anatomical variations reported in the figure are those described by Hiatt based on observations in 1000 liver donors for transplant.[3]

Technique

Surgical exploration must exclude the presence of extrahepatic metastases (lymph nodes of the hepatic pedicle, peritoneal metastases) which in our view contraindicate the placement of intra-arterial devices. Any anomalous arteries must be accurately identified: the left hepatic artery originating from the left gastric artery is found on the superior aspect of the gastrohepatic ligament and is easily visible. A right hepatic artery arising from the superior mesenteric artery follows a retroduodenal course and can be identified in the hepatic pedicle posterior to the common bile duct to the right of the portal vein in the lymphatic tissue which lies between these two vessels. Removal of the gallbladder is advisable to prevent clinical cholecystitis, especially when a pump for continuous chemotherapy is being inserted. The catheter is positioned in the hepatic artery through the gastroduodenal artery. This is isolated behind the duodenum after ligating the pyloric artery and all vessels leading to the upper margin of the duodenal bulb and gastric antrum to prevent delivery of the drug to the stomach. This antro-pyloric devascularization is essential.[1,4,19] Ligation of the pyloric vessels allows the duodenum to be moved downwards and to expose the gastroduodenal artery which is followed for about 2 cm from the junction with the hepatic artery and ligated distally. From the posterior aspect of the proximal portion of the gastroduodenal artery 1 or 2 small branches are commonly encountered, leading to the pancreas (*Figure 23.2*). These branches must be identified and ligated to prevent delivery of the drug to the pancreas. The common and the proper hepatic arteries must be mobilized for about 3 cm in order to identify and ligate the small branches leading to the gastric antrum.

The port and pump are placed in a subcutaneous pocket at a distance from the laparotomy incision, with a 3 cm contraincision at the level of the transumbilical line. Hemostasis of the subcutaneous pocket must be meticulous to prevent the formation of hematomas or collections. Care must be taken that the diaphragm of the pump is not in contact with the cutaneous incision. The pump is fixed with reabsorbable stitches to the fascia of the external oblique muscle. A quantity of subcutaneous tissue must be left above the pump to prevent skin ulceration during treatment. In obese patients the layer of subcutaneous fat makes access through the abdominal wall difficult and in such cases we prefer to fashion the pocket on the thoracic wall, above a rib, where palpation of the pump is easier. The catheter is brought through the abdominal aponeurosis in the abdominal cavity, ensuring that it lies straight and that the system is filled with heparin solution. The hepatic artery is clamped at the level of the junction with the gastroduodenal artery and the catheter is inserted in the latter through a small arteriotomy without going beyond the lumen of the hepatic artery to prevent the risk of arterial thrombosis. The catheter is fixed with a non-absorbable ligature. The correct position of the pump is checked by injecting a solution of methylene blue which should color the surface of the liver uniformly without impregnating other organs - the stomach in particular.

Access via the gastroduodenal artery is used for insertion of the catheter even in the presence of the most common anatomical variations of the hepatic artery. Anomalous arteries are ligated after carrying out a clamping test. When an anomalous vessel is clamped a portion of the liver may assume a cyanotic appearance; the liver usually returns to its normal color in a few minutes due to the rapid formation of collateral circulation. In rare cases signs of ischemia may persist after clamping an anomalous artery and a second port should then be inserted in the left gastric artery or in the splenic artery.[11,17]

Another fairly frequent condition, observed in about 10% of cases, is the early bifurcation of the right and left branches of the artery with a very short common hepatic artery, or the origin of the gastroduodenal artery from the right branch of the hepatic artery. In these cases, positioning of the catheter in the gastroduodenal artery does not ensure perfusion throughout the liver. The most rational access in such cases is to perfuse the entire hepatic arterial tree through the splenic artery. The splenic artery is isolated for about 2 cm to the left of the celiac trunk and ligated distally. The gastroduodenal and pyloric arteies are also ligated. The catheter is inserted through the splenic artery and advanced into the hepatic artery for about 2 cm to prevent displacement and to allow good perfusion of the drug (*Figure 23.3*). Ligation of the gastroduodenal, pyloric and splenic arteries does not have adverse effects. This access route from the splenic artery is also used in cases of thrombosis of the gastroduodenal artery after a previous failed application of the intra-arterial device.

An exceptional situation is represented by stenosis of the celiac triad and of the hepatic artery at its origin. In such cases the arterial blood flow to the liver is supplied by the gastroduodenal artery which is extremely hypertrophic and must be preserved. Cannulization must be carried out through the common hepatic artery and the end of the catheter must be positioned at the confluence with the gastroduodenal artery.

Complications

EXTRAHEPATIC PERFUSION

Correct positioning of the catheter and the quality of hepatic perfusion must be checked before beginning chemotherapy. This check is carried out a week after the operation with a technetium macroaggregated albumin scan, infusing 3-5 cl of Technetium 99 through the pump. It should be preceded by scintigraphy with conventional technetium, with i.v. injec-

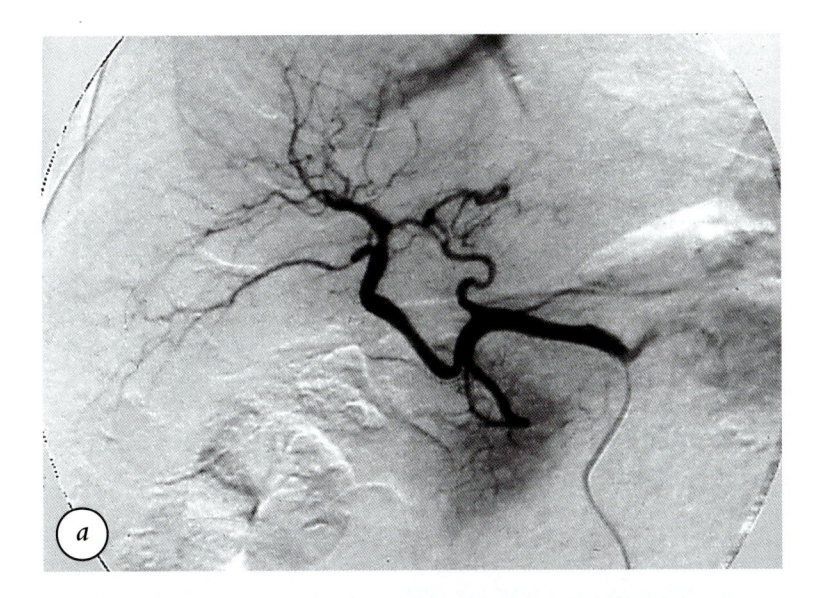

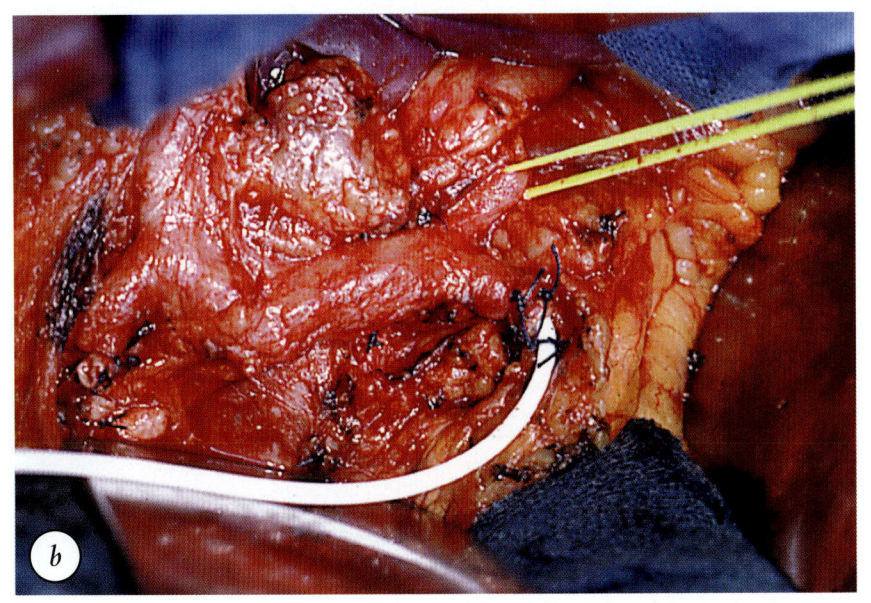

Figure 23.3 – *Positioning of the catheter for intra-arterial hepatic chemotherapy from the splenic artery. a) Early bifurcation of the hepatic artery with the gastroduodenal artery arising from the right branch. Selective hepatic angiography. b) The catheter is inserted in the splenic artery about 2 cm from its outlet. The distal part of the splenic artery is ligated. The catheter is then advanced into the lumen of the common hepatic artery. The gastroduodenal artery and the pyloric artery are ligated. The yellow tape elevates the left gastric artery.*

tion of the isotope, to evaluate the extent of the metastatic invasion of the liver. If extrahepatic accumulation of isotope is observed (most commonly in the stomach, head of the pancreas, spleen) chemotherapy should not be administered. The precise positioning of the catheter after adequate exposure of the hepatic artery and ligation of all the collaterals leading to the stomach and the duodenal-pancreatic collaterals of the gastroduodenal artery is the best way of preventing these complications. If extrahepatic perfusion of the isotope is observed, it is advisable to carry out angiography directly from the pump in order to try and identify exactly which collateral is responsible for the perfusion. Re-laparotomy with ligation of the collateral is the only way that chemotherapy treatment can be started.

INCOMPLETE PERFUSION

Incomplete perfusion of the liver during assessment with technetium microaggregated albumin scan may occur due to the presence of an anomalous artery not ligated during the operation or if the end of the catheter has been pushed too distally into the hepatic artery as far as one of the dividing branches, usually the left one. This problem can be avoided by performing pre-operative angiography to determine the presence of anomalous arteries. Intra-operative control of the positioning of the probe also safeguards against this complication. Arteriography through the pump makes it possible to define the cause of incomplete hepatic perfusion. In the presence of an anomalous vessel an attempt can be made with angiographic embolization. Malposition of the catheter must be corrected surgically.

GASTRO-DUODENAL ULCERS

Perfusion of a portion of the gastric antrum or the duodenum by the chemotherapy drugs can cause severe mucus ulcers which present clinically with intense epigastric pain at the commencement of antiblastic infusion and necessitates suspension of the treatment.[1] This is due to incomplete ligation of the collaterals for the duodenum, branches of the gastroduodenal or pyloric arteries or small collaterals leading to the gastric antrum.

THROMBOSIS OF THE HEPATIC ARTERY

This is a relatively rare complication which may be observed some time after the operation and which does not involve clinical consequences, apart from the need to stop treatment. Malposition of the catheter, pushed too far into the lumen of the artery, can contribute to arterial thrombosis. Incorrect management of the pump, by failing to flush with heparin solution, can also cause this complication.

THROMBOSIS OF THE CATHETER

Like the previous complication, thrombosis of the catheter makes injection of the drugs impossible. It is caused by a technical error such as the failure to flush the pump with heparin solution after each treatment or backbleeding into the catheter during the injection. In cases of recent thrombosis or incomplete thrombosis of the catheter, it may be possible to unblock the catheter by flushing the port with heparin solution. If the obstruction also involves the gastroduodenal artery, the catheter must be removed and repositioned in the hepatic artery through the splenic artery.

SUBCUTANEOUS POCKET INFECTION OR INFLAMMATION

Fashioning the subcataneous pocket must be performed under aseptic conditions and with careful hemostasis to prevent hematomas which can lead to a secondary infection. Prophylactic antibiotic treatment is always required for this procedure. Inflammation of the pocket is due to leakage of chemotherapy drugs which have an irritant or necrotic (Adriamycin) effect on the tissues. Infusions must be suspended until the inflammatory or infectious process has been completely resolved. In the event of suppuration or necrosis of the subcutaneous pocket, the only solution is removal of the pump.

HEPATO-BILIARY TOXICITY

The bile ducts are vascularized exclusively by the hepatic artery and are therefore extremely sensitive to the action of antiblastic drugs, some of which, such as FUDR, have a toxic effect on the biliary epithelium, especially if the infusion is continuous.[6,7] In laboratory terms, this toxicity is represented by increases in transaminase and cholestatic enzymes. The clinical pattern may lead to severe cholestasis with hepatomegaly and alterations of the bile ducts similar to those observed in sclerosing cholangitis. Initial alterations can be reversed by suspending the treatment with FUDR and the use of cortisone.

REFERENCES

1. Bible KC, Hatfield AK, Lansford CL, Kammer BA. Gastric ulceration as a complication of hepatic artery infusion chemotherapy. *South Med J* 1986; **79**: 755-757.
2. Chang AE, Schneider PD, Sugerbaker PH. A prospective randomized trial of regional versus systemic continuous 5-fluorodeoxyuridine chemotherapy in the treatment of colorectal liver metastases. *Ann Surg* 1987; **206**: 685-693.
3. Hiatt JR, Gabbay J, Busuttil RW. Surgical anatomy of the hepatic arteries: 1000 cases. *Ann Surg* 1994; **220**: 50-52.
4. Hohn DC, Stagg RJ, Price DC *et al*. Avoidance of gastroduodenal toxicity in patients receiving hepatic arterial 5-fluoro-2 deoxyuridine. *J Clin Orthol* 1985; **3**: 1257-1260.
5. Hohn DC, Stagg RJ, Friedman M *et al*. A randomized trial of continuous intravenous versus hepatic intra-arterial floxuridine in patients with colorectal cancer metastatic to the liver: the Northern California Oncology Group trial. *J Clin Oncol* 1989; **7**: 1646-1654.
6. Kemeny N, Daly J, Oderman P *et al*. Hepatic artery pump infusion: toxicity and results in patients with metastatic colorectal carcinoma. *J Clin Oncol* 1984; **2**: 595-600.
7. Kemeny MM, Battifora H, Blayney D *et al*. Sclerosing cholangitis after continuous hepatic artery infusion of FUDR. *Ann Surg* 1985; **202**: 176-180.
8. Kemeny MM, Goldberg D, Beatty D *et al*. Results of a prospective randomized trial of continuous regional chemotherapy and hepatic resection as a treatment of hepatic metastases from colorectal primaries. *Cancer* 1986; **57**: 492-498.
9. Kemeny N, Daly J, Reichman B *et al*. Intrahepatic or systemic infusion of fluorodeoxyuridine in patients with liver metastases from colorectal carcinoma: a randomized trial. *Ann Intern Med* 1987; **107**: 459-465.
10. Kemeny N, Cohen A, Bertino JR, Sigurdson ER, Botet J, Oderman P. Continuous intrahepatic infusion of floxuridine and leucovorin through an implantable pump for the treatment of hepatic metastases from colorectal carcinoma. *Cancer* 1990; **65**: 2446-2450.
11. Kemeny N, Sigurdson ER. Intra-arterial chemotherapy for liver tumors. In: Blumgart

LH *Surgery of the liver and biliary tract*. Churchill Livingstone, Edinburgh, 1994, pp. 1473-1491.

12. Lygidakis NJ, Ziras N, Parissis J. Resection versus resection combined with adjuvant chemo-immunotherapy for metastatic colorectal liver cancer. A new look at an old problem. *Hepato-Gastroenterol* 1995; **42:** 155-161.

13. Martin JK Jr, O'Conncell MJ, Wieand HS *et al*. Intra-arterial floxuridine *vs* systemic fluorouracil for hepatic metastases from colorectal cancer. A randomized trial. *Arch Surg* 1990; **125:** 1022.

14. Nakashima K, Kitano S, Kim YI, Aramaki M, Kawano K. Postoperative adjuvant arterial infusion chemotherapy for patients with hepatocellular carcinoma. *Hepato-Gastroenterol* 1996; **43:** 1410-1414.

15. Niederhunber JE, Ensminger W, Gyves J *et al*. Regional chemotherapy of colorectal cancer metastatic to the liver. *Cancer* 1994; **53:** 1336-1340.

16. Okuno K, Shigeoka H, Lee YS *et al*. Adjuvant hepatic arterial IL-2 and MMC, 5-FU after curative resection of colorectal liver metastases. *Hepato-Gastroenterol* 1996; **43:** 688-691.

17. Rayner AA, Kerlan RK, Stagg RJ *et al*. Total hepatic arterial perfusion after occlusion of variant lobal vessels: implications for hepatic arterial chemotherapy. *Surgery* 1986; **90:** 708-714.

18. Rougier L, Laplanche A, Huguier M *et al*. Hepatic arterial infusion of floxuridine in patients with liver metastases from colorectal carcinoma: long-term results of a prospective randomized trial. *J Clin Oncol* 1992; **10:** 1112-1118.

19. Shike M, Gillin JS, Kemeny N *et al*. Severe gastroduodenal ulcerations complicating hepatic artery infusion chemotherapy for metastatic colon cancer. *Am J Gastroenterol* 1986; **81:** 176-179.

20. Stagg R, Venook A, Chase J *et al*. Alternating hepatic intra-arterial floxuridine and fluorouracil: a less toxic regimen for treatment of liver metastases from colorectal cancer. *J Nat Canc Inst* 1991; **83:** 423-428.

21. Wagman LD, Kemeny MM, Leong L, Galvan M. A prospective randomized evaluation of the treatment of colorectal cancer metastatic to the liver. *J Clin Oncol* 1990; **8:** 1885-1893.

TECHNIQUES IN LIVER SURGERY

SECTION VIII

Biliary Tumors

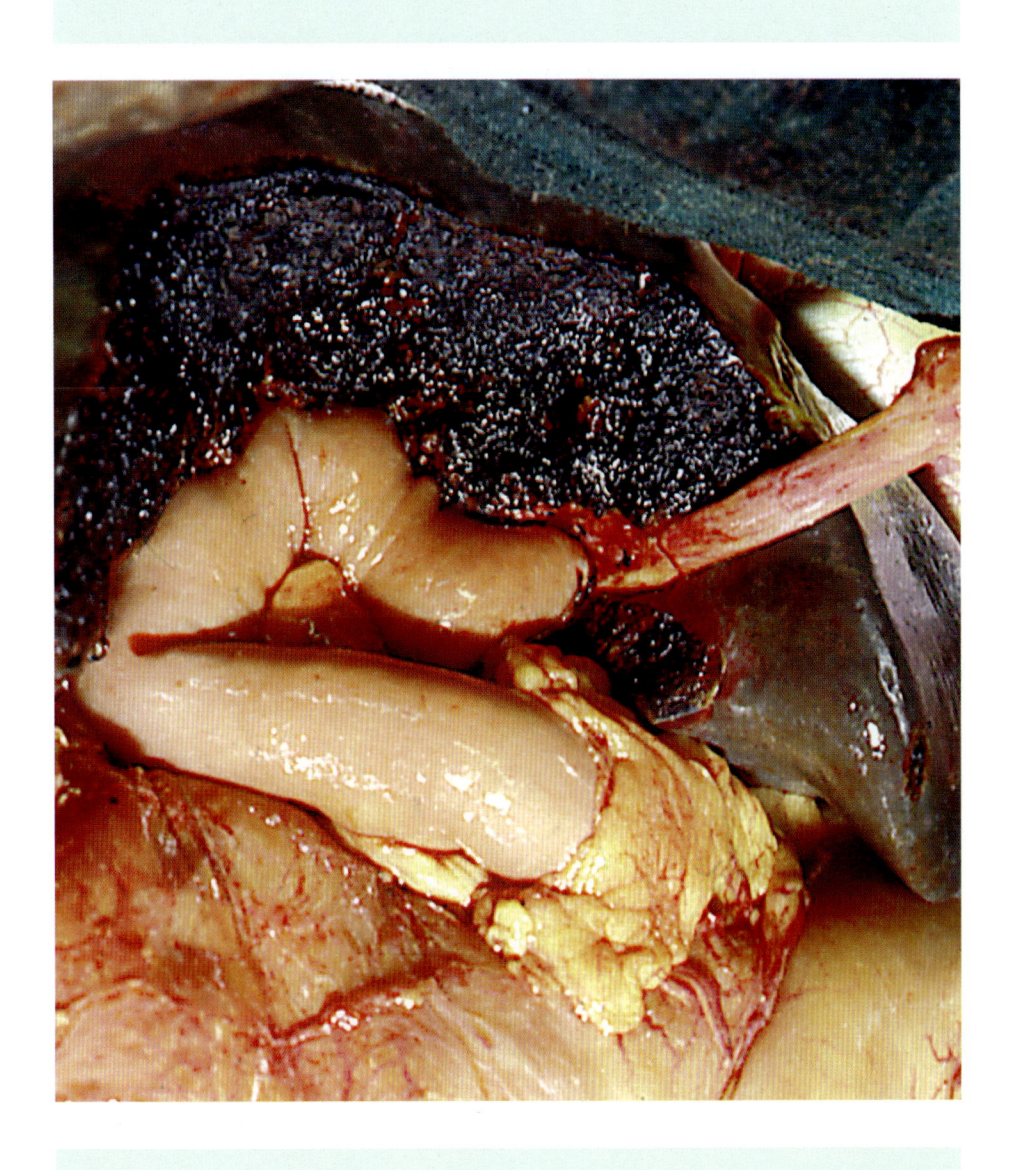

24

Resection of Hilar Cholangiocarcinoma

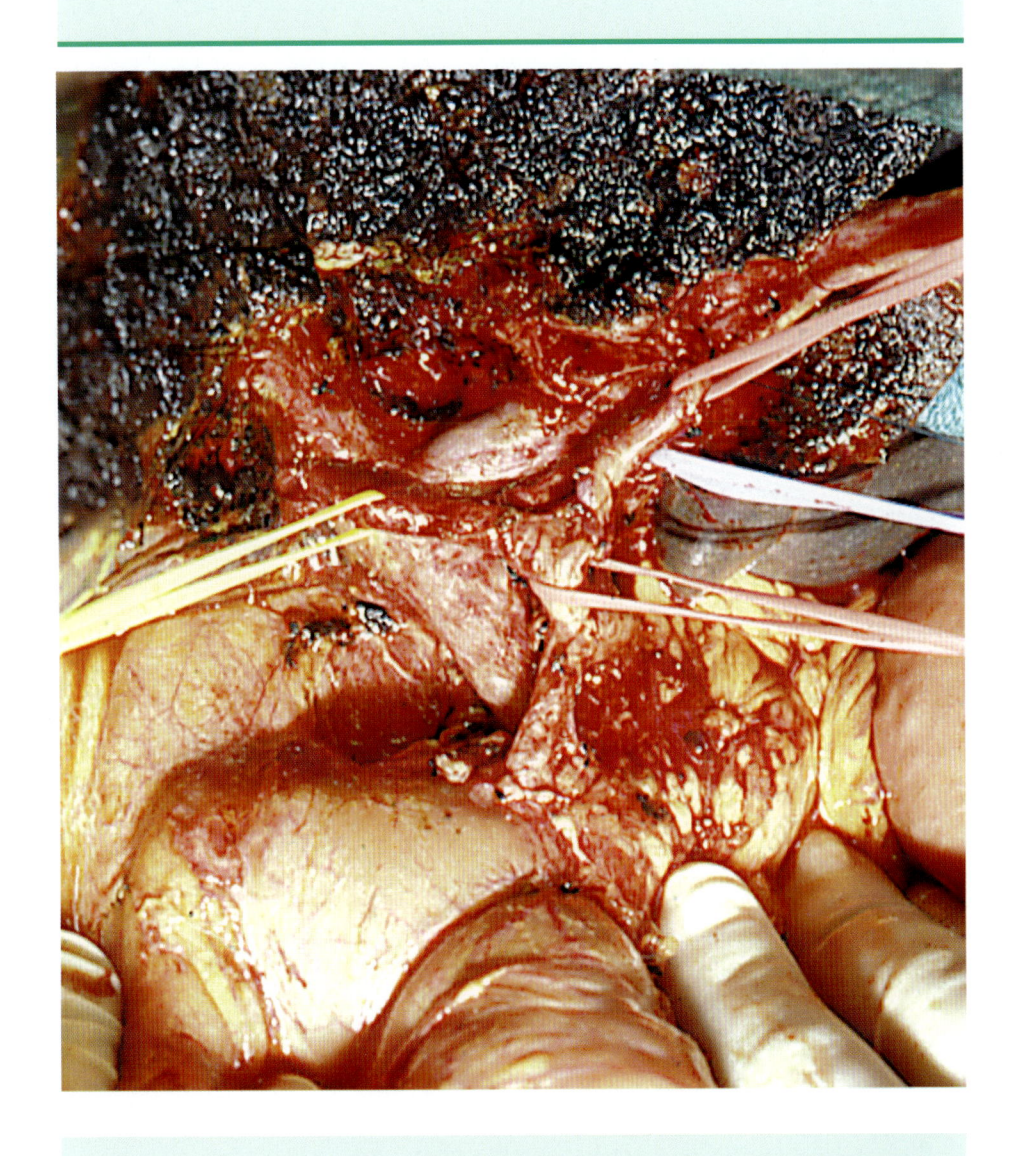

E. Moreno González, M. Hidalgo Pasqual, I. García García,
J.C. Meneu Diaz, A. González Chamozzo

The basic treatment of malignant tumors of the bile duct involves the resection *en bloc* of the biliary duct, the adjacent lymphatic tissue and the regional lymph nodes. If the surgery envisaged is theoretically to be curative, the excision should be sufficiently wide since any remaining malignant tissue will reduce both the possibilities of achieving a cure and the palliative nature of the surgery.

The importance of wide excision of the biliary tract

The tendency of carcinoma of the biliary tract to infiltrate in over 90% of patients requires total removal of the main biliary tract, even when dealing with tumors located in the confluence of the bile ducts. While it is possible to treat some patients with a more limited resection, if a segment of suprapancreatic common bile duct is left, it will neither benefit the patient nor reduce the technical difficulties at surgery, but will be a potential source of recurrence. If this biliary remnant is left, the portobiliary glands, which are often affected (28%) in tumors the confluence of the bile ducts, will not have been removed either.

Any sign of neoplastic infiltration of the intrapancreatic common bile duct at suprapapillary level will require extending the excision to include part of the head of the pancreas and duodenum. While this is not controversial in carcinoma of the common bile duct, in its lower or mid-third, there may be some disagreement in the presence of tumors of the confluence of the bile ducts. It is highly probable that resection of the confluence of the bile ducts will make it necessary either to extend the excision to cover the proximal hepatic tissue and extend surgery to include the resection of the paramedian segments together with Segment 1, or to perform a right or left hemihepatectomy - a far more serious matter if this is performed in association with a resection of the head of the pancreas and duodenum. Additionally, the increased surgical risk to the patient concerned as regards the prognosis of the disease localized in the confluence of the bile ducts has to be established, as well as the benefits of performing an associated pancreaticoduodenectomy.

Even if excision of the confluence of the bile ducts leads to the surgical removal (albeit theoretical) of the disease, irrespective of whether it is performed in association with hepatic resection or not, if there is infiltration of malignant cells in the common bile duct and adjacent pancreas, they cannot be left untreated.

Removal of the lymphatic system

Clearly, it is essential to remove all the lymphatic tissue enveloping the vascular structures in the hepato-duodenal ligament *en bloc* with the main biliary tract. These should not be separated but preserved with the lymphatic tissue, to facilitate anatomical identification by pathologists and avoid cellular dispersion in the event of lymphatic metastasis.

There may be grounds for greater controversy regarding lymphatic extension to the portobiliary groups of nodes, the nodes behind the head of the pancreas (which make it necessary to mobilize the duodenum and the pancreatic head), the right suprapancreatic or common hepatic artery groups, and the celiac groups, which envelop the celiac trunk and its distribution branches.

There is insufficient documentation of the incidence of lymphatic invasion in the right suprapancreatic and celiac groups, but it is estimated at between 15 to 25% in the former, and not more than 10% in the latter. This could rule out the benefit of dissecting the celiac trunk. None the less, since this technique involves no difficulty, if there is a risk of it being diseased, it should be removed.

It can be claimed that if distant nodes are affected, this casts a shadow on the surgical prognosis and reduces long-term survival. This might call for extemporaneous systematic histopathological study of the more distant nodes (behind the head of the pancreas and the celiac groups) which, moreover, are also connected to the retroperitoneal lymphatic tissue, thus favouring further dissemination of the disease if they are found to have been affected. There is currently a paucity of documentation available and the only valid conclusion would be for prospective studies to be set up to enable the data to be evaluated, and to attempt to render it as useful as possible. In any event, metastatic lymph adenopathies at the level of the celiac trunk should be a contraindication to procedures involving extensive hepatobiliary resection, sometimes including resection and reconstruction of vascular elements. Palliative techniques which do not involve surgical removal should be sought instead, although at the present time there have been no apparent advances made in combined chemotherapy.

Resection of vascular elements

Resection of the vascular elements infiltrated by the growth of the tumor should not be queried if the situation is observed during excision of the tumor. Once this procedure is underway, and there is no possibility of return or of abandoning, it if the infiltrated vascular segment is critical for the remaining liver, vascular reconstruction should always be carried out.

Infiltration of vascular elements undoubtedly worsens the prognosis, particularly if the portal vein is involved. However, excision of segments of the hepatic artery, or of the trunk or extrahepatic branches of the portal vein, should not increase the risk of the surgery, and from the technical viewpoint, reconstruction of the arterial or venous continuity is a straightforward procedure.

An issue which does, however, call for greater discussion is the preoperative study of the extent of the tumor, and the likelihood of vascular involvement, in terms of the value that can be placed on these results to contraindicate surgical treatment. Vascular involvement (infiltration, compression or thrombosis) is suspected when tumors are very large (they need only exceed 3 cm in diameter at hepatic hilum level to be so termed), when there is thickening of the vascular wall beside the tumor, or in conglomerates of adenopathies, and, finally, when vascular thrombosis is suspected, or atrophy of a lobe of the liver demonstrated (generally due to thrombosis of the ipsilateral portal branch).

While there is no overall agreement on the contraindications of resection of the tumor in the event of suspected vascular infiltration, it is generally agreed that, in this instance, hepatic arteriography or splenoportal arteriography should be performed, although the diagnostic imaging procedures (CT or MRI) combined with intravenous contrast or echo-Doppler duplex (US-Doppler-duplex) do not give sufficient topographic diagnosis to contraindicate surgical treatment.

If the angiographic study of a patient, who was otherwise healthy and well nourished, revealed thrombosis of one of the branches of the hepatic artery or portal vein, or if there was a reduction in calibre as a result of probable infiltration by the tumor of the hepatic artery or the portal vein, it is debatable whether or not surgery is recommended.

In a hypothetical case such as this, surgical exploration should be performed to confirm that excision is impossible. After this has been established, the most correct palliative treatment should then be performed, and would involve peripherical biliary diversion by cholangiojejuostomy. However, should it be contraindicated, then transtumoral external or external-internal drainage, or an expanding metal Wall-stent type, or soft transtumoral stent made of Teflon or silicone, should be installed during the same operation.

The main contraindications for performing surgery on malignant tumors of the confluence of the biliary tree are: major physical deterioration (which could be improved via parenteral nutrition and antibiotherapy, if necessary), multiple hepatic metastasis in both hepatic lobes, or very serious cardiopulmonary disease in an aged patient. In these groups of patients, percutaneous installation of catheters or transtumoral stents is indicated, under radiological control (CT or US).

Extending the excision to the hepatic parenchyma

The anatomical position of the confluence of the bile ducts is generally extrahepatic. Both hepatic ducts lead out of the hepatic parenchyma and immediately converge, coinciding with the bifurcation of the portal vein and resting on its front surface. Infiltration of one or more primary hepatic ducts will also involve extension to the adjacent hepatic parenchyma, although it is not always possible to detect this at macroscopic level. For this reason, resection of the hepatic parenchyma in contact with the infiltrated biliary surface should be the rule to follow in surgery of this kind. However, the particular layout of the portal ducts or spaces, in which an artery (a branch of the hepatic artery), a vein (a branch of the portal vein) and a bile duct run together along the whole length of the intrahepatic course, is a reminder that before infiltrating the hepatic parenchyma they infiltrate the connecting space surrounding these vascular biliary elements. This calls for investigation of the branches affected and their removal, if necessary, along with the tributary hepatic segments. This exacerbates the technical difficulties of the biliary resection and, more importantly, the extent of the hepatic parenchyma to be removed.

At the lower face of the liver, the hepatic tissue which makes contact with the confluence of the bile duct corresponds to Segment 1, which covers the back surface and upper portion of segment 4 (4B) and its mid-third or the limiting area between Subsegments 4A and 4B. Consequently, it is highly likely that tumor growth has led to the infiltration of these segments, calling for the resection of both, as well as the confluence of the bile duct, if neoplastic infiltration is suspected. However, at this level, the malignant growth could also invade the vascular structures linked to a hepatic lobe, and this would require extending hepatic resection to Segments 2 and 3, or 5 and 8, or, less frequently, to Segments 5, 6, 7 and 8, when it would be impossible to reconstruct the right portal vein.

If we observe how all the segments listed are connected to the confluence of the bile duct, it is clear that Segment 1 should always be removed, in a single block with the confluence of the bile duct, and that excision of the remaining segments will depend on the extent of the growth of the tumor, either to right or to left.

Removal of segment 1

With the patient in supine decubitus position, displacement of the left hepatic lobe in a cranioventral direction provides wide visualization of the surface of the gastrohepatic ligament and, consequently, the profile of segment 1 covering the whole of the ventromedial surface of the retrohepatic vena cava. The gastrohepatic ligament has to be sectioned to gain access for the dissection of segment 1. However, it should be remembered that an accessory hepatic artery, a branch of the coronary artery (left gastric) and the hepatic branch of the anterior vagus nerve, is often present in its proximal portion. Both structures can be sectioned. However, if the left gastric artery is wider in diameter, it should be established if it is the left hepatic artery, as in this case, its origin and course should be left intact until a decision is taken on whether any liver segment irrigated by this artery has to be maintained.

Mobilization of segment 1 starts with the section of the retroperitoneal surface in the limiting line between the medial edge of the segment and the surface of the retrohepatic vena cava, which is dissected in craniocaudal direction. The medial edge of segment 1 is displaced in a ventral direction, dissecting the anterior face of the vena cava and identifying in it the confluence of the hepatic veins (2 to 3), which form the direct venous drainage of this segment in the vena cava. These veins should not be occluded before the hepatopetal blood flow to this segment is occluded. Dissection of the branch of the hepatic artery and the corresponding portal vein is thus preferred, followed by its ligature and section, prior to mobilization.

In the case of tumors of the confluence of the bile ducts, the liberation of the posterior face of segment 1 can provide a route to explore the characteristics, limitations and extent of neoplastic infiltration, while dissection of the vascular biliary elements at hepatic portal level should not be performed before mobilizing the elements of the hepato-duodenal ligament.

Pre-operative biliary drainage

The main problem in the treatment malignant tumors affecting the biliary tract is its obstruction and the consequences of the icteric syndrome, in terms of the alteration of the hepato-cellular function, progressive hemorrhagic diathesis, alterations in the absorption and metabolization of nutrients, immunological deficiency (existing, but hard to quantify) and the risk of infection leading to sepsis which is often catastrophic.

If biliary decompression is recommended in

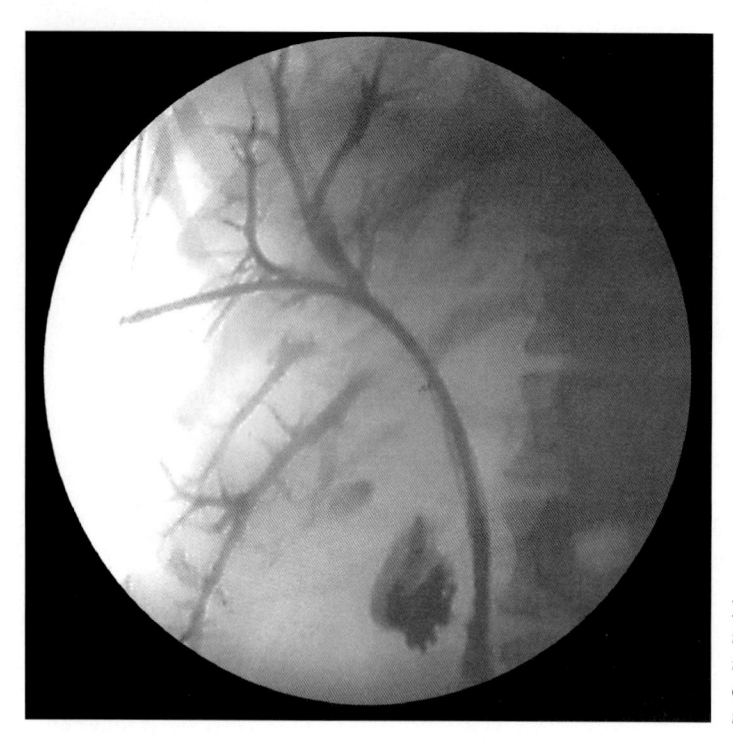

Figure 24.1 – *External-internal transparietohepatic percutaneous catheter in the obstruction of the biliary confluence due to malignant disease.*

the location of tumors which do not require hepatic resection, it is even so in the case of tumors of the confluence of the bile duct. Percutaneous biliary drainage is also helpful when performing a cholangiography, to determine the morphology of the intrahepatic biliary tree, to demonstrate where the tumor is located, the extent of infiltration of the primary hepatic ducts and segmentary branches, the possible dissociation of both intrahepatic trees and, in some cases, obstructions or irregularities in the intrahepatic biliary tree, which confirm the presence of implants in the biliary lumen or hepatic metastasis (*Figure 24.1*).

In any case, extrahepatic biliary drainage can cause dissemination of malignant tumor cells and metastasis at the parietal outflow orifice, a possibility which has been mentioned, in the literature but is not well documented. Furthermore, single external drainage via percutaneous puncture of the right hepatic lobe does not constitute a decompression route for the whole intrahepatic biliary tract, and segmentary branches may be obstructed at the level of the confluence on the corresponding primary hepatic duct. Consequently, several percutaneous drainages should be installed. As the diameter of a pigtail is not usually sufficient, except during the first few hours when there is high biliary tree pressure, drainage should be changed gradually until the maximum diameter is achieved some days later.

This more complicated manipulation can lead to cellular implants, infection of the biliary tract and the gall bladder. Although there is little documentation available, most accounts come from Japanese groups, who have substantial experience in segmentary percutaneous biliary drainage. An added advantage of multiple drainage is its use during surgery to assist in the identification of the segmentary branches affected, and in postoperative maintenance as transanastomotic drainages, if several anastomoses are performed between the intrahepatic branches and the Roux-en-Y loop, and generally used for the reconstruction of biliodigestive continuity. Finally, the different external drainages may help to confirm whether the biliointestinal anastomoses are hermetic, and assist cicatrization, avoiding transanastomotic biliary leakage when used during the initial post-operative period for multiple external drainage.

Technical difficulties aside, despite the possibility of cellular implants, hemobilia or other types of hemorrhage, if external drainage is used, this has to be maintained for at least 2 to 4 weeks. This increases the time spent in hospital, the risk of biliary infection, and the risk that during this period tumor growth will infiltrate vascular elements not previously affected, making some tumors irresectable or allowing more time for malignant cells to disperse through the lymphatic tree.

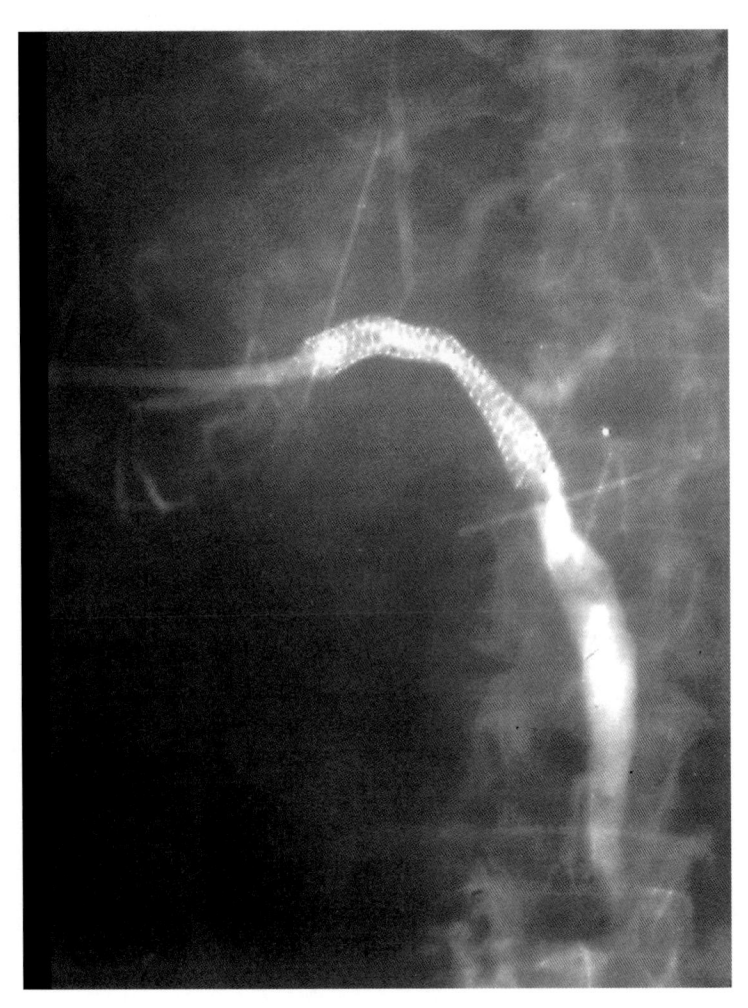

Figure 24.2 – *Wall-stent prosthesis installed by means of right transparietohepatic percutaneous puncture.*

For these reasons, the question of whether or not single or multiple external drainage of the biliary tree is recommended should be considered cautiously, on an individual basis, for patients needing percutaneous cholangiography for topographic diagnosis of the lesion, for those suffering from severe malnutrition, who should be maintained with parenteral nutrition for at least two weeks prior to surgery, or for high-risk patients suffering from severe hepatocellular involvement, due to progressive jaundice for long periods of time without specific diagnosis.

Temporary or permanent transtumoral prostheses

Over the past 5 years there has been a significant increase in the use of expanding prostheses (Wall-stent), well-installed either percutaneously or using endoscopic retrograde methods. A large number of patients suffering from obstructive jaundice caused by malignant lesions of the main or accessory biliary tract located at any level, have been referred directly from medical areas - where there has been incorrect or insufficient study of the extent of the tumor — to have permanent prostheses installed as their only treatment, without offering them the possibility of a more definitive treatment (**Figure 24.2**).

When installing a transparietohepatic percutaneous prosthesis, the different stages of the technique should be borne in mind. Initially, external drainage only is installed. 2 to 3 days later, when possible, this is converted to external-internal drainage, passing the lower end through the narrow lumen maintained in the area of infiltration of the tumor. 1 to 3 days later, the parieto-abdominal orifice and the segmentary conduit lumen are dilated, and the expanding prosthesis is inserted ensuring that its near and far ends are kept sufficiently clear of the limits of tumor infiltration. 3 to 7 days later, after confirming that contrast passes to the duodenum without any obstruction, biliary drainage is removed. Some interventional

Table 24.1 – *Results of wallstent prosthesis as only treatment*

COMPLICATIONS	PERCUTANEOUS TRANHEPATIC	ENDOSCOPIC TRANSPAPILLAR
Patients	132	26
Cholangitis	102 (77.3 %)	22 (84.6 %)
Malposition	19 (14.4 %)	1 (3.8 %)
Obstructionead	89 (67.4 %)	8 (30.8 %)
Replacement	26 (19.7 %)	–
Hospital Stay (Total follow-up)	2.8 m	1.6 m
Survival	4.8 m	3.1 m

radiologists prefer to maintain external drainage for 2 to 4 weeks, until reduction of the calibre of the dilated biliary tract is confirmed, thus avoiding the risk of a biliary fistula.

Installation of the expanding prosthesis through the retrograde route calls for an endoscopic cholangiography (ERCP) to be performed and, subsequently, a papillary sphincterotomy, if installation of the prosthesis is recommended, to provide sufficient calibre to allow the guide and then the prosthesis to pass through. This installation route is used less frequently because of the incidence of pancreatitis, infection, and hemorrhage, which, though infrequent, occurs in a greater percentage of cases than when the percutaneous method is used.

In both procedures, the far end of the prosthesis is left inside the duodenal lumen, extending past the papilla of Vater to assist the passage of bile juice. However, the wires in the prosthesis can separate, and this may lead to erosion of the surface of the duodenal wall.

All expanding prostheses meet with obstruction because of the growth of the tumor past the rods of the prosthesis and through the space between them, although in order for this to happen, the patient has to survive for 3 and 6 months after its installation. However, remains of desquamation from the surface of the tumor, the precipitation of biliary salts and acids, and residues of food which flow back from the duodenum through the open papilla, may lead to maintained (less frequent) or intermittent progressive obstruction (*Table 24.1*).

Obstruction and duodenum-biliary flow-back are the cause of ascending cholangitis, which occurs in almost all cases, with a greater or lesser degree of virulence, and calls for frequent stays in hospital, percutaneous cannulization of the prosthesis, cleansing of its lumen, sample-taking for cultures and antibiotic assay and, not infrequently, the installation of a new prosthesis through the lumen, which will have decreased in diameter (*Figure 24.3*). It is not unusual for the expanding prosthesis to displace the main biliary tract, compressing and obstructing the cystic-common bile duct confluence and causing cholecystitis.

While surgery for resection of the tumor from the confluence of the bile ducts is feasible after installation of an expanding prosthesis, the procedure is more complicated because of the extent of surrounding inflammatory reaction, which causes greater lymphatic flow and drainage, with node infarcts which can occasionally be mistaken for lymphatic metastasis. Moreover, the inflammatory reaction, itself may lead to pyephlebitis with laminar or complete portal thrombosis. This is always attributed to the growth of the tumor, rather than to the action of the displacement force of the wall of the biliary tract and reaction to a foreign body encrusted on the internal surface of the hepatic bile duct.

In some cases, hepatocellular function is affected and fails to recover completely, and for hemorrhagic diathesis to occur, which sometimes starts with biliary sepsis.

As a result, the installation of expanding prostheses should be performed by expert surgical teams, when surgical resection is considered impossible or involves high-risk, while an average survival rate of less than 6 months is

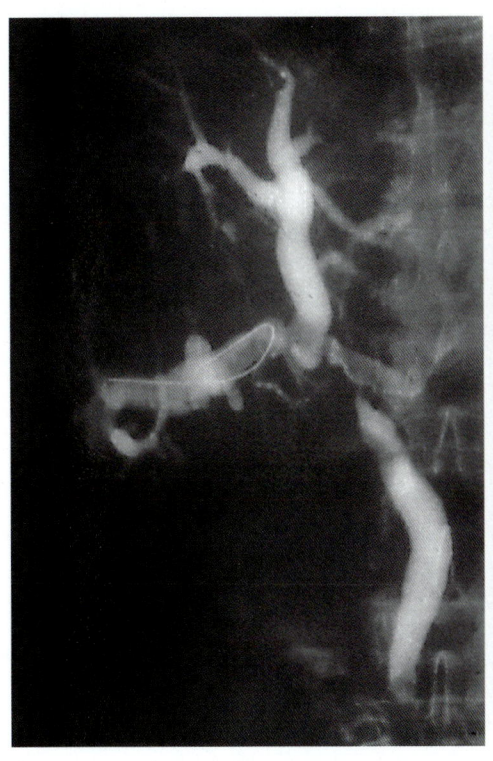

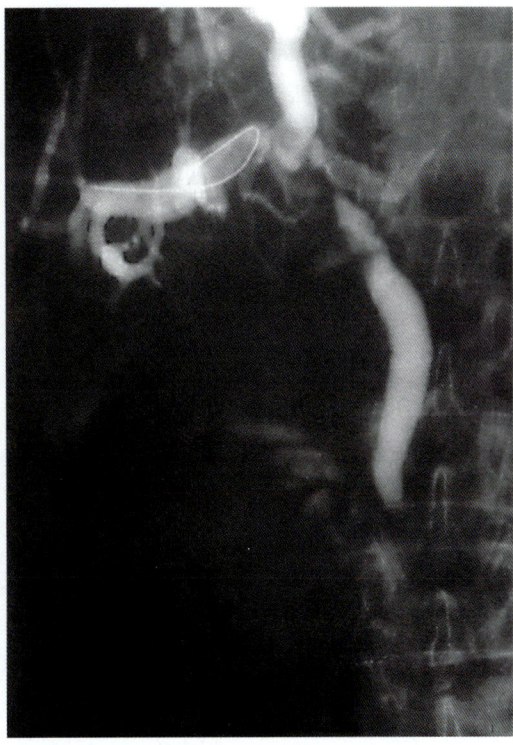

Figure 24.3 – *Wrongly-installed prosthesis at the biliary confluence level.*

Table 24.2 – *Peripheral cholangio-jejunostomy*

TECHNIQUE	PATIENTS	JAUNDICE RELIF	JAUNDICE RECURRENCE	CHOLANGITIS	AVERAGE SURVIVAL
Longmire	4	4	–	–	6.1 m
HEPP Soupault	16	16	4 (66.6%)	5 (71.4%)	7.3 m
Double	3	3	–	–	4.8 m
Cholecysto Cholangio	4	4	2 (33.3%)	2 (28.6%)	3.8 m
Total	27	27	6 (100%)	7 (100%)	5.5 m

accepted. However, consideration should be given to the fact that morbidity is equal or lower when peripheral cholangiojejunostomy is performed as a palliative measure, and that the survival rate is higher after this has been performed than it is after the installation of a prosthesis (***Table 24.2***).

Dissection of the hepatoduodenal ligament

Surgery should start with the inspection and palpation of the hepatoduodenal ligament, to identify the limits of the tumor, its mobility or infiltration of adjacent planes and elements, confirming the existence or absence of infiltration of vascular elements and, in particular, of the portal vein or its branches. The presence of inflammation on the surface of the common bile duct, or inflammation of the ligament itself, as well as atrophy of a hepatic lobe, are all elements indicating portal thrombosis.

Although some surgeons recommend wedge biopsy or puncture of the tumor, we do not recommend this practice. The search for malignant cells may prove to be negative, but would not exclude the presence of a carcinoma, while manipulation of the tumor could increase the risk of tumoral dispersion.

If distant metastases is ruled out, lymphatic or blood (hepatic metastasis) freeing of the duodenopancreatic block can start, exploring the posterior face of the cephalic portion of the pancreas, as well as the retroperitoneal juxta-aortic and juxta-caval lymphatic tissue, and checking the origin of the celiac trunk and the superior mesenteric artery. A biopsy is recommended if lymph node metastasis in the retroperitoneal space is suspected, since the prognosis will not change with the surgical excision.

After considering whether or not to proceed with the excision, dissection of the celiac trunk and the common hepatic artery can start, mobilizing the lymphatic tissue covering them, and displacing it. Thereafter, the gastroduodenal artery and its anterior and posterior branches are dissected, freeing the lymphatic tissue covering them, and keeping it all in a single block. The hepatic artery itself is dissected, occluding the branches that irrigate the main biliary tract.

The lymphatic tissue behind the head of the pancreas and the precaval lymphatic tissue is freed. The suprapancreatic common bile duct is dissected in a circular direction and sectioned longitudinally. The bile duct is occluded by vascular clamp and a cylinder of distal segment is taken out for fresh protein examination which will confirm the absence of neoplastic infiltration. The distal stump of bile duct is closed by continuous stitching, using long-lasting reabsorbable material.

On exercising traction in a cranial direction from the lower end of the biliary tract, circular dissection of the portal vein, of the hepatic artery itself and of its distribution branches, can be continued. If there is no neoplastic infiltration of these elements, the bifurcation of the portal vein is dissected, sectioning the 2 or 3 small veins which converge at this level and which come from the confluence of the bile duct. Thereafter, dissection of the left hepatic artery and its two branches, the left hepatic artery and middle hepatic artery, and the right hepatic artery with its anterior and posterior terminal branches which embrace the right primary hepatic duct, is performed. The cystic artery is occluded between ligatures and sectioned, and the gall bladder is separated from its hepatic bed.

Resection excluding the hepatic parenchyma

In malignant tumors of the confluence of the bile duct which do not extend through the primary hepatic ducts (*Figure 24.4*) it is sufficient to dissect the latter, ensuring a safety margin of 15 to 20 mm, and then to proceed with an independent section of both ducts and occasionally also the bile duct corresponding to segment 1 (*Figure 24.5*).

The adjacent hepatic parenchyma should be resectioned to ensure that areas in contact with the tumor are not overlooked. This excision only involves surgical removal of Glisson's capsule, which is reinforced at this level, and approximately 1 cm in depth of hepatic parenchyma.

Reconstruction by biliary anastomosis on the proximal end of a Roux-en-Y loop can be performed separately on the left hepatic duct and more distally, some 2 to 3 cm to the right. However, in some cases, the pronounced dilation and elongation of both ducts, and the thickening of their wall, permits the anastomosis of one hepatic duct with the other, forming a wide biliary stoma which could be increased in diameter by lengthwise section of the left hepatic duct. In this way a single biliojejunal anastomosis on the end of the jejunal loop ascending through a hole in the transverse mesocolon is sufficient. (*Figures 24.6-7*).

Extension of the resection to the left hepatic lobe

The tumor infiltrates the left hepatic duct more frequently than it will extend to the intrahepatic segmentary branches; the hepatic artery and left vein are occluded by tumor growth while the branch corresponding to segment 1 is also frequently affected.

The discovery of this neoplastic progression makes it necessary to ligate and section the left hepatic artery at its origin on the hepatic artery, itself and the left portal vein at portal bifurcation level. Then, displacing the main biliary tract and the lymphatic tissue to the left, the right hepatic artery is dissected as well as its anterior and posterior branches. The right portal vein is released from the lymphatic tissue covering it, which is maintained in a single block in contact with the confluence of the bile duct and the rest of the freed hepatoduodenal lymphatic tissue. Dissection of the right hepatic duct then proceeds to the confluence of the branches of the posterior segments, and is sectioned at this level to secure a 15 to 20 mm safety margin.

Thereafter, the retroperitoneal surface cover-

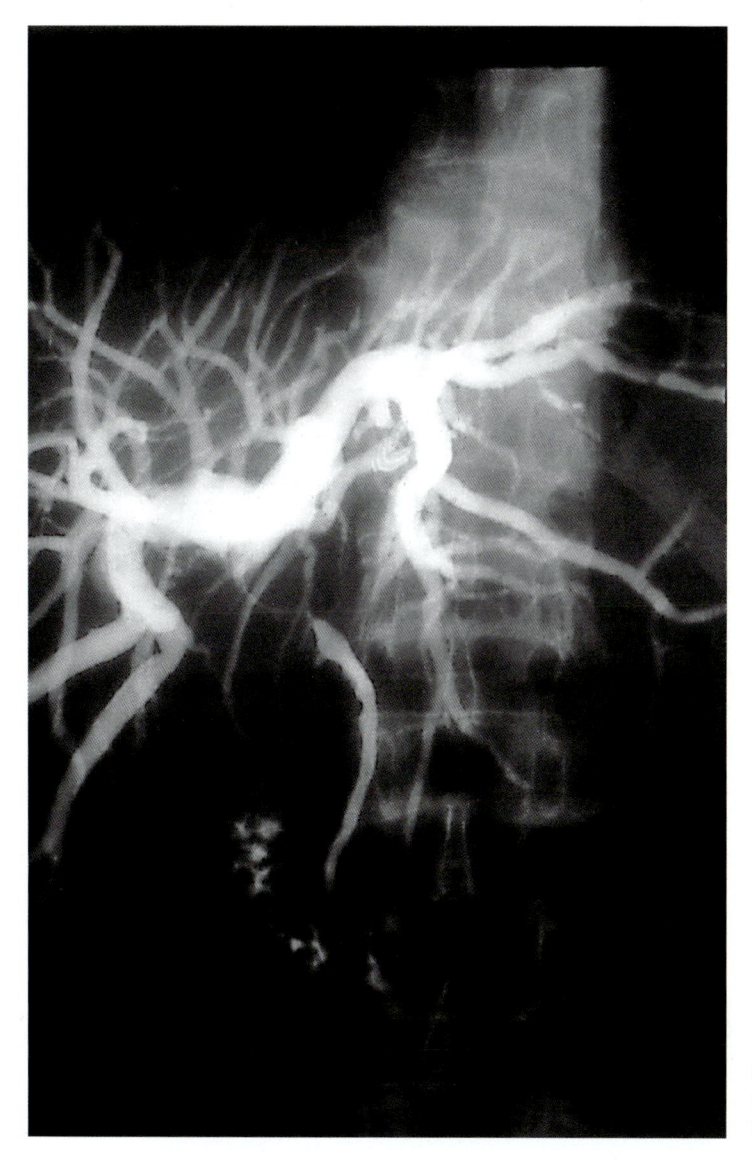

Figure 24.4 – *Transparietohepatic cholangiography showing malignant tumor of the biliary confluence.*

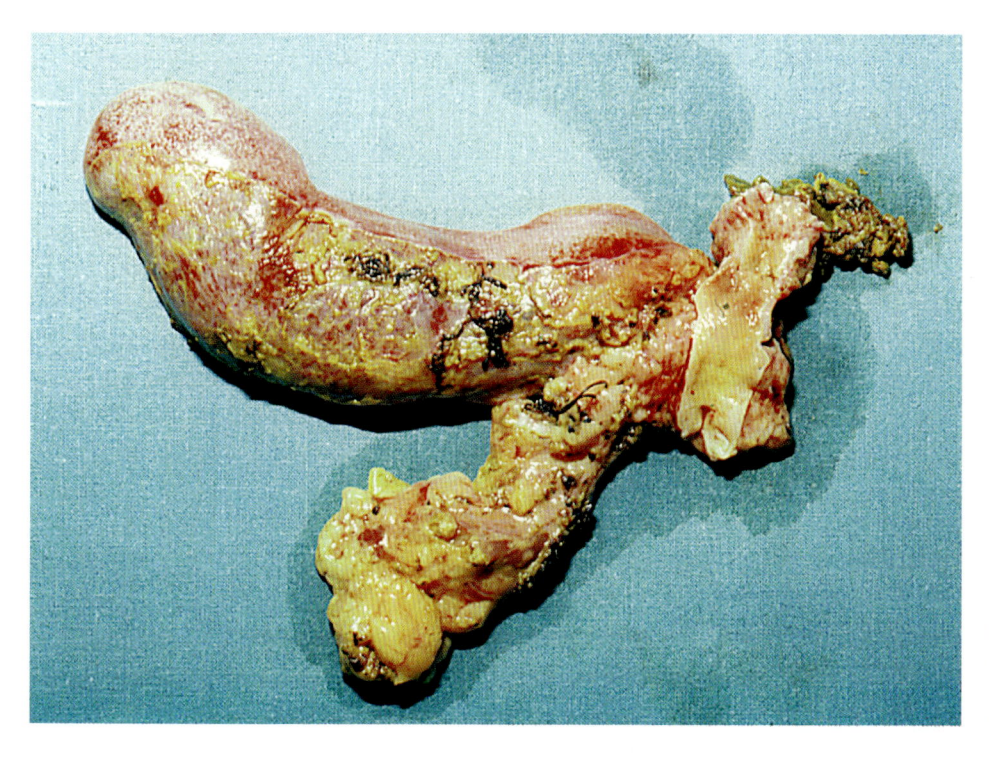

Figure 24.5 – *Carcinoma of the common hepatic duct. Resected specimen including the biliary confluence.*

TECHNIQUES IN LIVER SURGERY

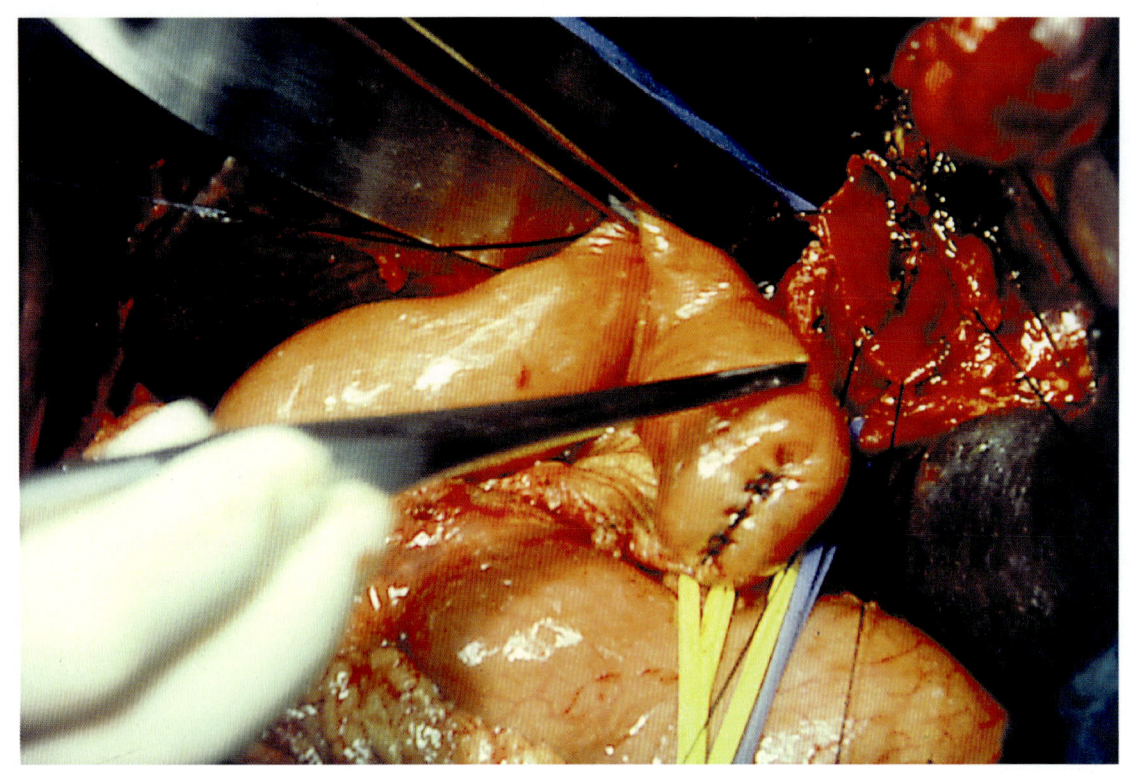

Figure 24.6 – *Preparation of the anastomosis between both right and left hepatic ducts and of a Roux-en-Y loop after resection of the biliary confluence.*

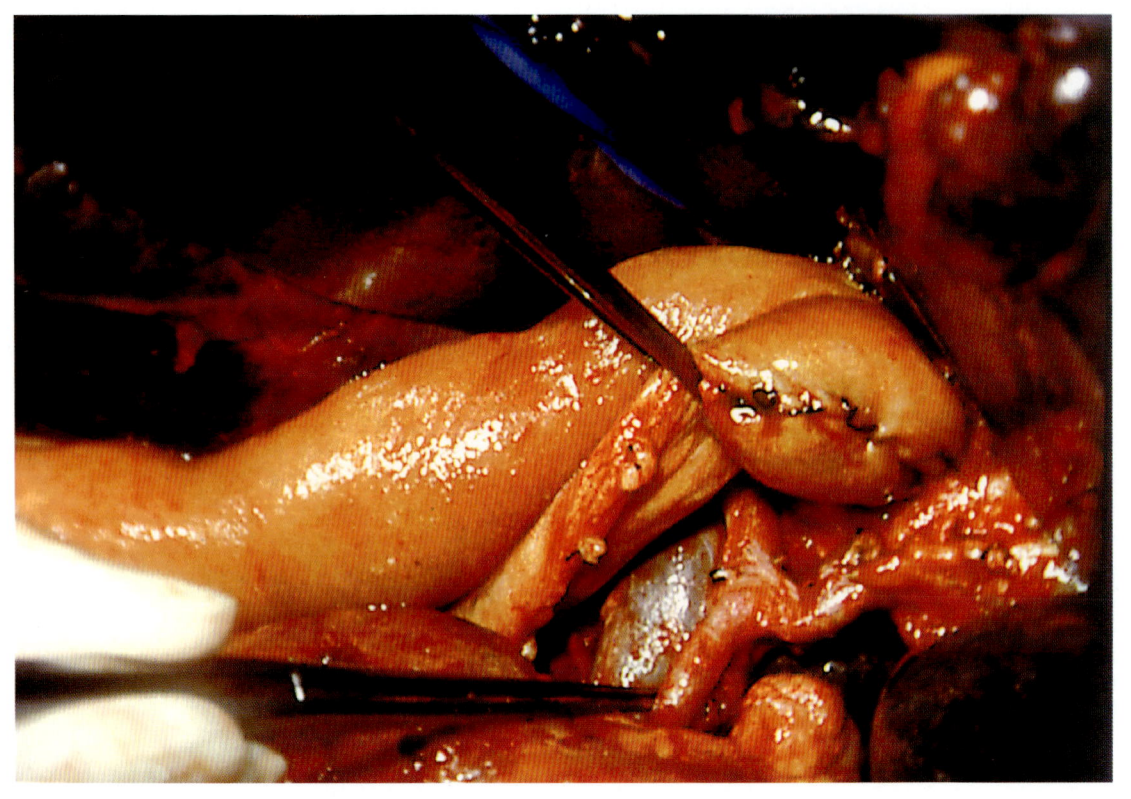

Figure 24.7 – *Same case as Figure 24.6. Anastomosis completed.*

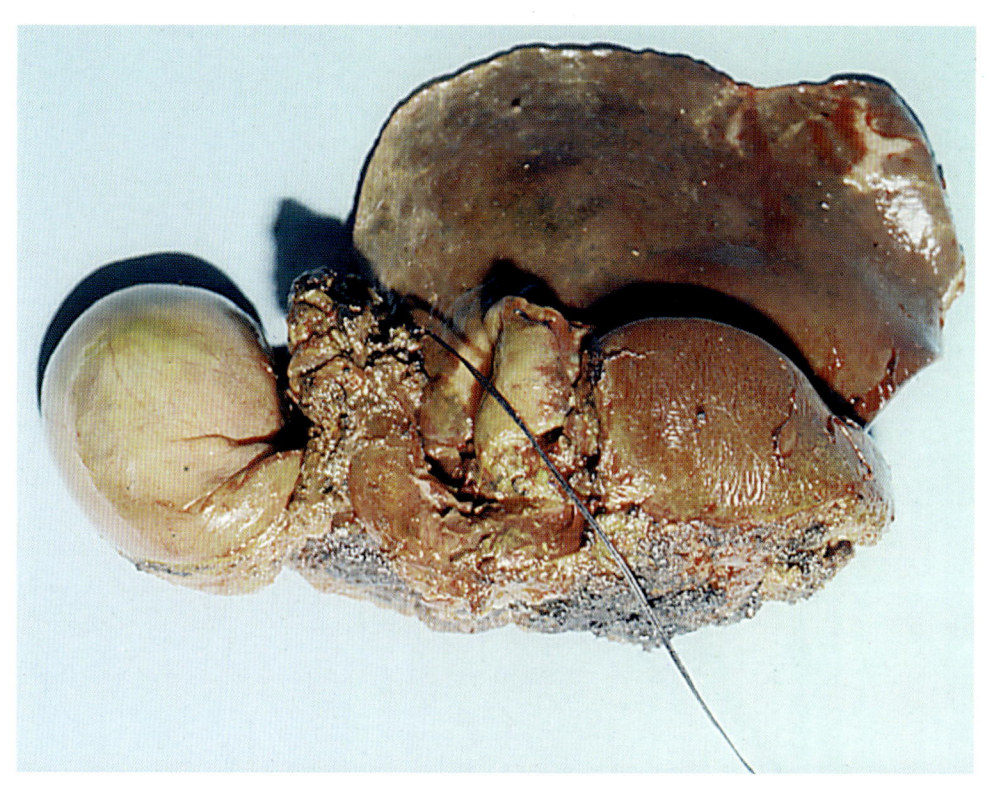

Figure 24.8 – *Resection specimen, which includes the common bile duct and gall bladder as well as the left hepatic lobe including Segment 1.*

ing the retrohepatic vena cava is sectioned at the level of the medial edge of Segment 1. Its posterior face is dissected, separating it from the anterior surface of the vena cava, and using the two or three hepatic veins to help identify, which are occluded and sectioned.

The hepatic parenchyma is then sectioned, following the direction of the Cantlie line, i.e. the longitudinal axis of the middle hepatic vein. In the lower face, the section line follows the medial edge of the bed of the gall bladder, crossing the hepatic hilum very near the sectioned right hepatic duct, bordering its surface to follow the external limit of Segment 1 which partially surrounds the lateral surface of the retrohepatic vena cava. In proximal direction, the section allows the common trunk of the left hepatic vein and the sagittal or middle hepatic vein to be isolated, which is then occluded and sectioned, and excision is performed (*Figure 24.8*)

At times, in order to obtain a sufficient safety margin at the level of the right hepatic duct, it is necessary to make an extended dissection, sectioning the duct corresponding to Segments 5 and 8 and the duct common to Segments 6 and 7, thus leaving two biliary stomae, one anterior and another posterior.

The reconstruction of the biliodigestive continuity is performed by means of a single cholangiojejunal anastomosis between the section surface of the right primary hepatic duct, or by two anastomoses, between the duct of Segments 5 and 8 and Segments 6 and 7 and the jejunal tip, by interrupted suture using reabsorbable material (*Figure 24.9*). If the diameter of the anastomosis is wide enough, there is no need to leave transanastomotic drainage in place. However, if the diameter is smaller, as in the case of pre-operative external biliary drainage, it may be wise to use transhepatic transanastomotic drainage, with outflow through the abdominal wall. If this surgery is performed well, there will be no need for transfusion, and the postoperative stage will be completely benign and tolerable.

TECHNIQUES IN LIVER SURGERY

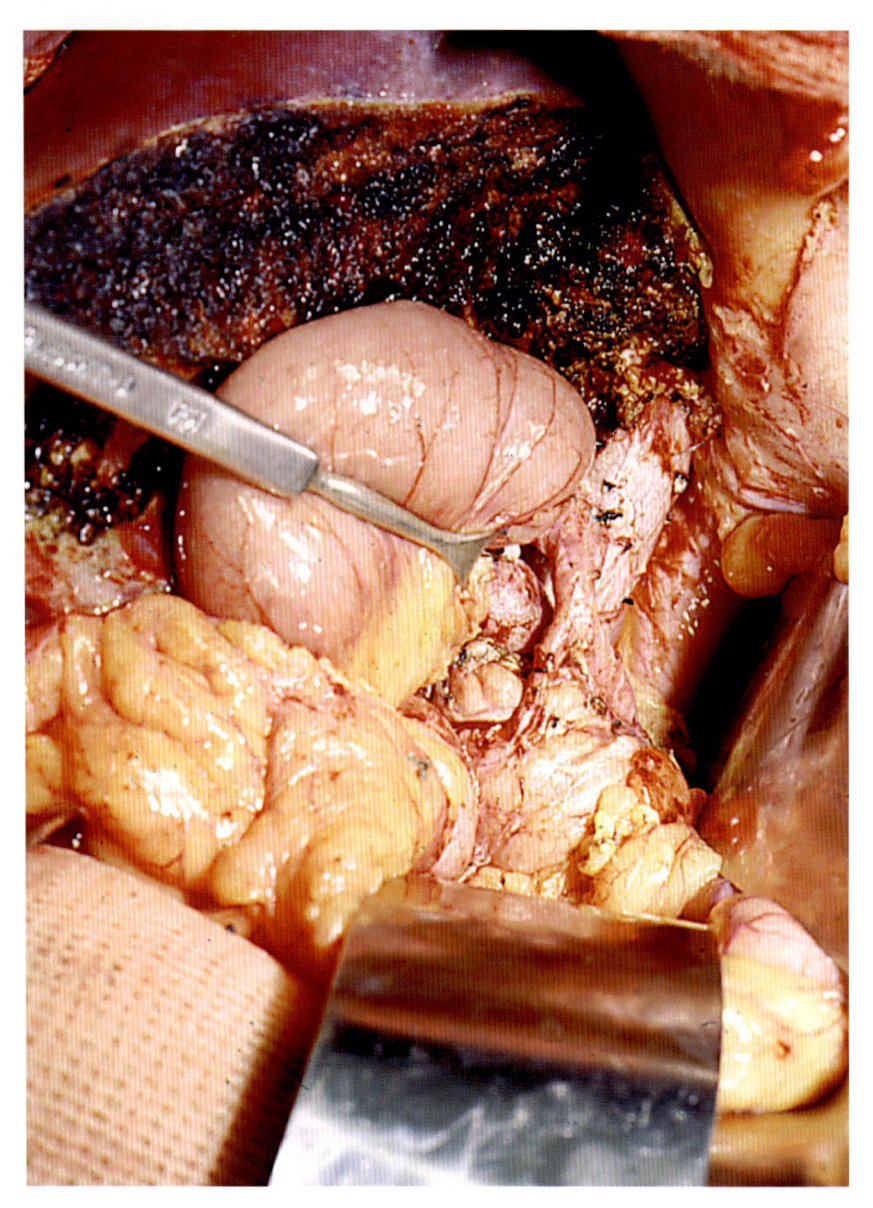

Figure 24.9 – *Resected hepatic surface and hepatic hilum preparation after resection of the accessory common bile duct, biliary confluence and left hepatic lobe. Reconstruction by means of end-to-side cholangio-jejunostomy, on Roux-en-Y loop after resection of the accessory common bile duct enlarged to left hepatic lobectomy including Segment 1.*

Extension of the resection to the right hepatic lobe

It is relatively less common for a tumor in the confluence of the bile duct to extend through the right hepatic duct, without it affecting the left hepatic duct. In this case, after identifying the right hepatic artery, it is occluded and sectioned at the level of its origin on the hepatic artery. The lymphatic tissue is displaced to the right. The gall bladder is left in place. The left hepatic duct is sectioned above the confluence of the branch leading from Segment 1 and, to enable a high calibre stoma to be obtained, the lower surface is sectioned lengthwise to the external edge of the umbilical vein or the middle hepatic artery crossing its anterior surface.

Segment 1 is freed in the same way as in the previous case involving the vena cava. Its anterior-lateral surface then has to be separated from Segments 2, 3 and 4, remaining in continuity with the right hepatic lobe which is surgically removed. The section line of the parenchyma follows the pattern of the previous case along its anterior face (major hepatic incision), the medial edge of the liver and gall bladder bed, and is extended behind the right and left portal vein, separating the anterior face of Segment 1 from Segments 2 and 3 and its medial edge from the retrohepatic vena cava.

Re-establishment of biliodigestive continuity is performed by anastomosis of the left hepatic duct to the tip of the Roux-en-Y loop. As the diameter of the biliary stoma is enlarged by means of a longitudinal section, it is not necessary to install transanastomotic biliary drainage.

Extension of the excision to the external and internal paramedian segments, 4A and 4B

The confluence of the bile duct is limited ventrally by Segments 4 and 5 and at the back by Segment 1. When the growth of tumors in the confluence of the bile duct affects both the right and left ducts symmetrically, and when infiltration of the adjacent hepatic parenchyma in anterior and posterior direction is determined by surgical exploration, the excision of both paramedian segments should be performed in association with Segment 1. The indication for extending the excision is also due to the need to obtain a sufficient safety margin, free from infiltration on both sides.

In the left hepatic lobe, the branch of the internal paramedian segment follows the trajectory of the round ligament from Rex's recess bed and converges on the front surface of the left hepatic duct.

Although two more medial branches also come from the internal paramedian segment, the common trunk of Segments 2 and 3 can be sectioned. If, exceptionally, there was an insufficient safety margin, both segmentary branches should be sectioned separately.

Special care should be taken during dissection of the lateral surface of the round ligament to avoid damaging the umbilical vein and the terminal segment of the left portal vein. The small branches which penetrate from the umbilical vein to the edge of Segment 4 should be occluded and sectioned with great care.

The lateral section is performed through the lower portion of the external hepatic incision, at the edge of Segments 5 and 6. At this level, great caution should be taken, as this line runs parallel to the longitudinal axis of the right hepatic vein, which should not be damaged, or it would jeopardise the venous drainage of Segment 6.

The bile duct of Segment 5 converges with the branch of Segment 8, very close to the limit between Segment 5 and 8. For this reason it can be seen during the transversal section of the hepatic parenchyma, following the edge of Segments 5, 8, 4A and 4B. When a greater extension of the tumor is confirmed along the entire length of right hepatic duct, the common duct to Segments 5 and 8 and the duct leading from Segments 6 and 7 can be resectioned separately through this transversal line, and in this way the excision will comply with the oncological criterion of radicality, although the biliary reconstruction will make it necessary for these two different stomas (*Figure 24.10*) to be taken into consideration. Although they allow sufficient calibre for a precise bilio-intestinal anastomosis to be performed, it would be safer to maintain the anastomoses with transhepatic, transanastomotic, multi-orificed silicone tutors, exteriorzed through the abdominal wall (*Figure 24.11*).

Mobilization of Segment 1 should be performed using the same considerations as those used in the left lobectomy. Care should be taken to keep it in a single block, joined to the paramedian segments, the main gall bladder and hepatoduodenal lymphatic tie. After making the section through the transversal line, the posterior face of Segment 1 of the surface of the vena cava is separated, Displacing the whole block in latero-caudal direction. The proximal end of Segment 1 is freed and thereafter the most lateral end, which, as it is a badly-defined limit, makes it necessary to section the hepatic parenchyma.

Extension of the excision to segment 4 and 1

On mobilizing the internal paramedian segment and progressing in depth, it is seen to have limited surface contact with the biliary tract, while the paramedian segments cover the hepatic hilum like a visor, and the posterior face is the smallest of both segments.

Moreover, the segmentary branches which converge on the convex surface of the left hepatic duct come from the upper half of Segment 4 (4A), whereas the bile duct of the lower half of Segment 4 (4B) is the most distal branch of the left hepatic duct, which

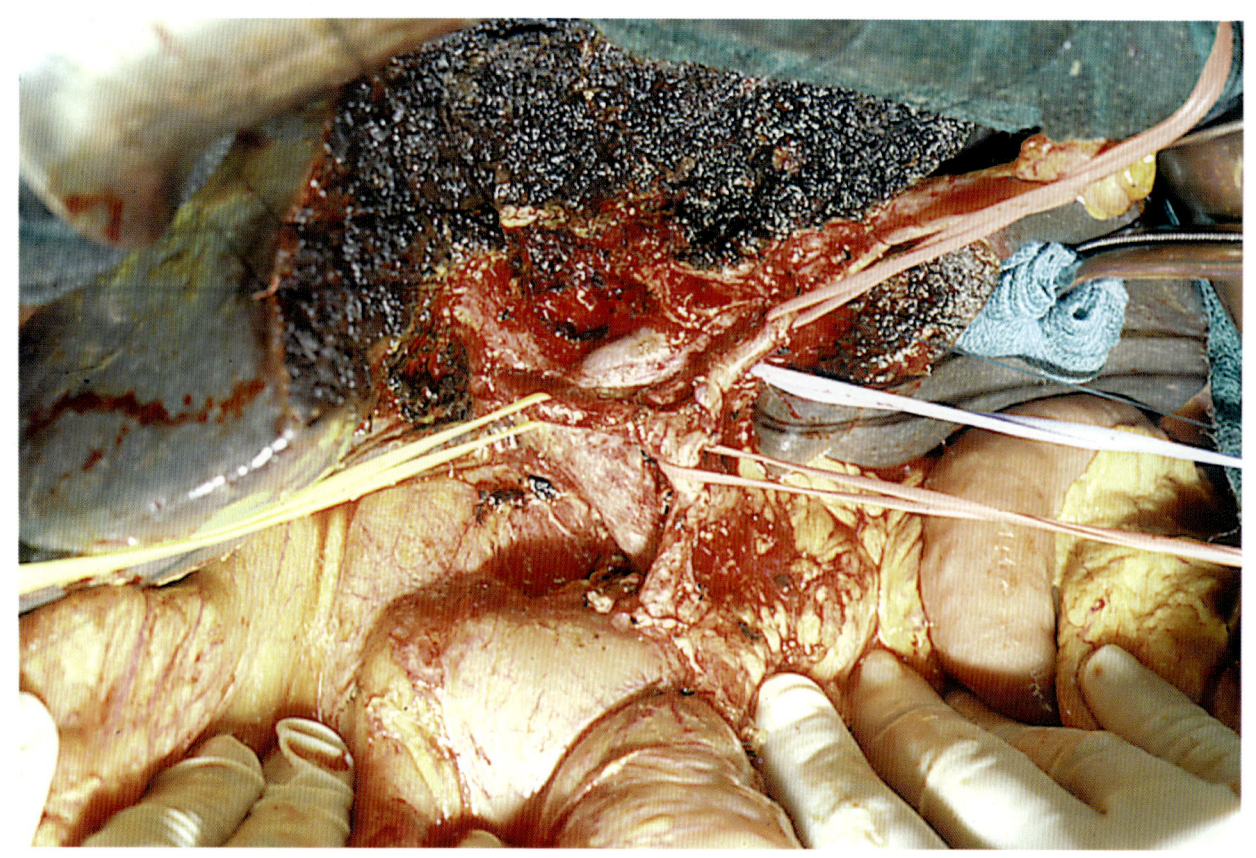

Figure 24.10 – *Surgical field after resection of the common bile duct and paramedian segments.*

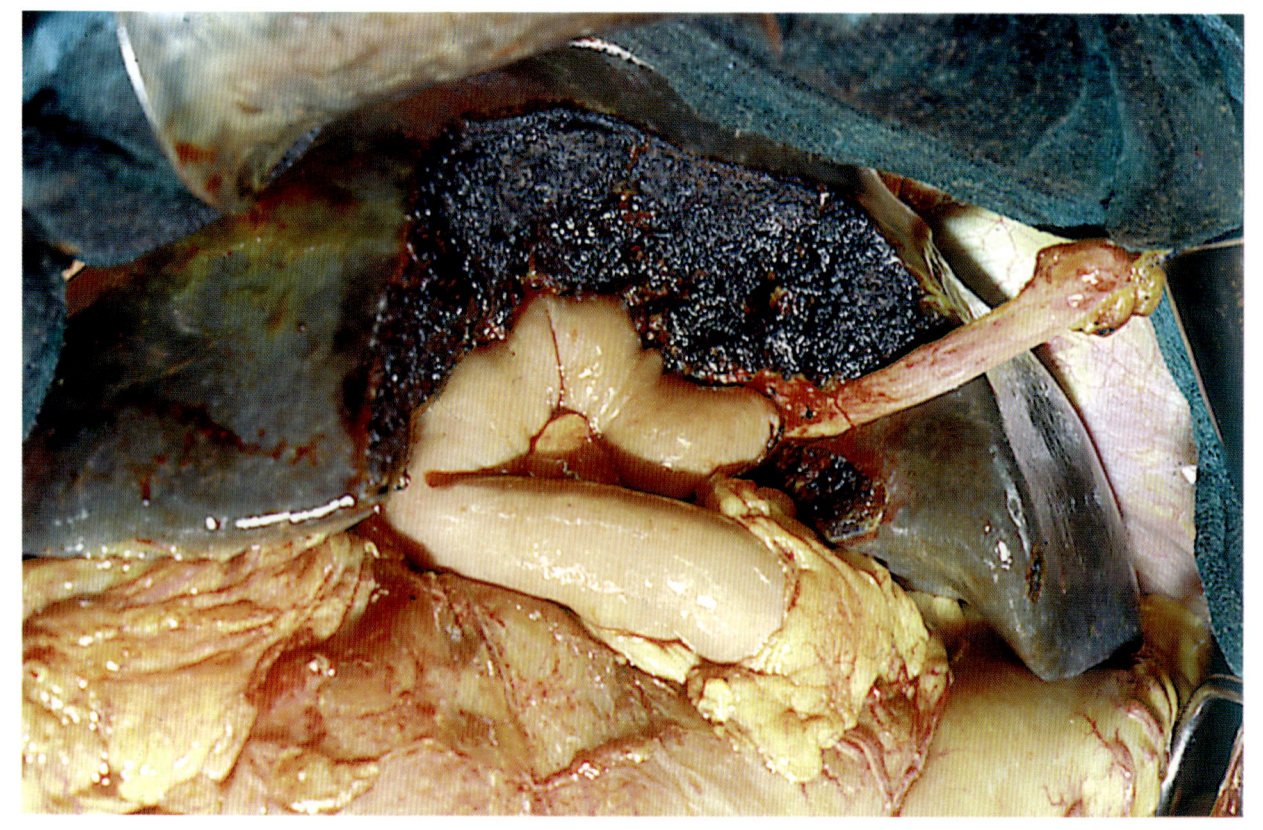

Figure 24.11 – *Reconstruction of the biliary-digestive continuity in the previous patient, by means of Roux-en-Y loop with end-to-side anastomosis of the intrahepatic segmentary branches.*

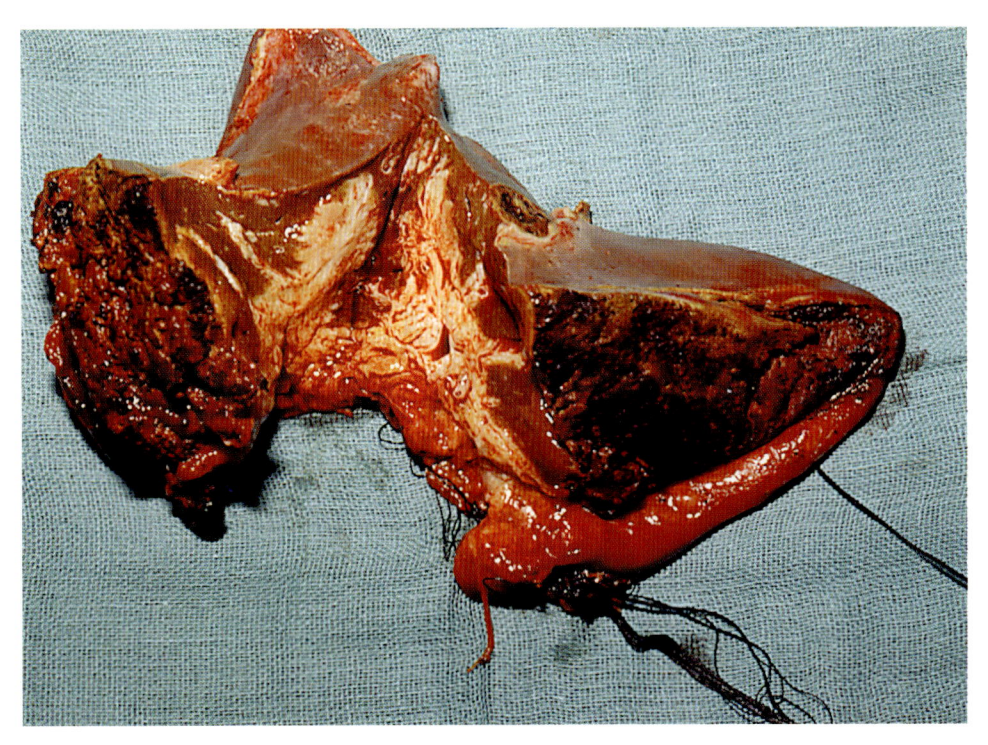

Figure 24.12 – *Resected specimen corresponding to the removal of the accessory common bile duct and Segments 1 and 4.*

converges with the branch of Segment 2 in Rex's recess. It should not be forgotten that a small branch, proximal to it, which converges almost in the same bed, is from the lowest part of Segment 4A.

In view of this, if the left hepatic duct is infiltrated, and in order to provide a sufficient safety margin, the excision should be extended to the internal paramedian segment. The excision of Segment 4A is of even greater importance, and with it the left hepatic duct on which its segmentary branches converge.

Indications are the same as in left hepatic lobectomy, provided that there is no neoplastic obstruction or infiltration of the tumor in the portal vein and left hepatic artery, while Segments 2 and 3 can be left intact.

In the dissection of the hepatoduodenal ligament, the middle hepatic artery and the two branches corresponding to Segment 4, which come from the portal vein, should be occluded and sectioned.

As on previous occasions, extension to Segment 1 is performed in a single block, and it is necessary to identify the external branch of the left portal vein for Segment 1, as well as the two arterial branches which have their origin in the left hepatic artery (***Figure 24.12***).

Biliary reconstruction at the level of the hepatic resection surface at the external limit of Segments 2 and 3 is performed with a single biliary stoma, if the confluence of the branches leading from Segments 2 and 3 is maintained, or with two smaller calibre stomas if the extension of the excision means that the confluence has to be removed. On the right side, reconstruction involves two biliojejunal

Hilar Cholangiocarcinoma
Actuarial Survival: N_0

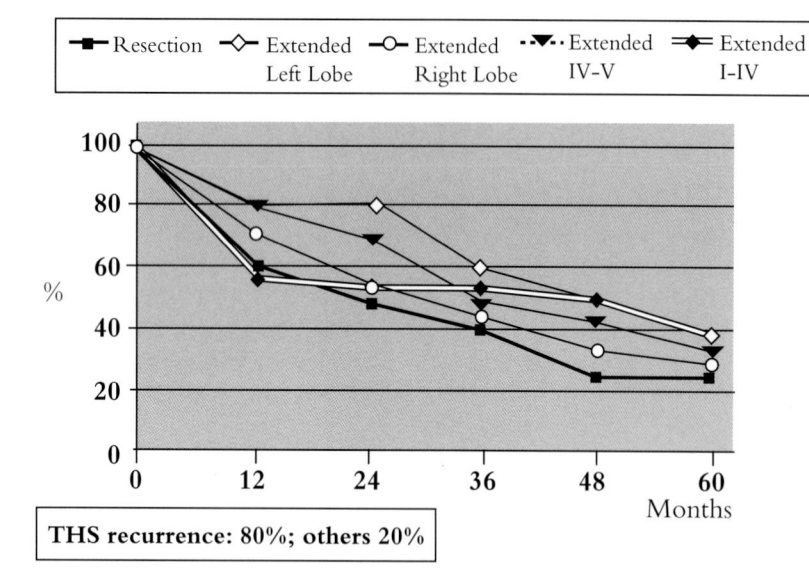

Figure 24.13 – *6-year actuarial survival after resection of cholangiocarcinoma of the biliary confluence without lymphatic metastasis, within the different groups operated on: 1) Resection of the bile duct without extension to the hepatic parenchyma; 2) Resection of the common bile duct with extension to the left hepatic lobe including Segment 1; 3) Resection of the bile duct with extension to segments 4 and 1; 4) Resection of the common bile duct with extension to segments 4 and 5; 5) Resection of the bile duct with extension to the right hepatic lobe and Segment 1.*

THS recurrence: 80%; others 20%

Hilar Cholangiocarcinoma
Actuarial Survival: N_1-N_2

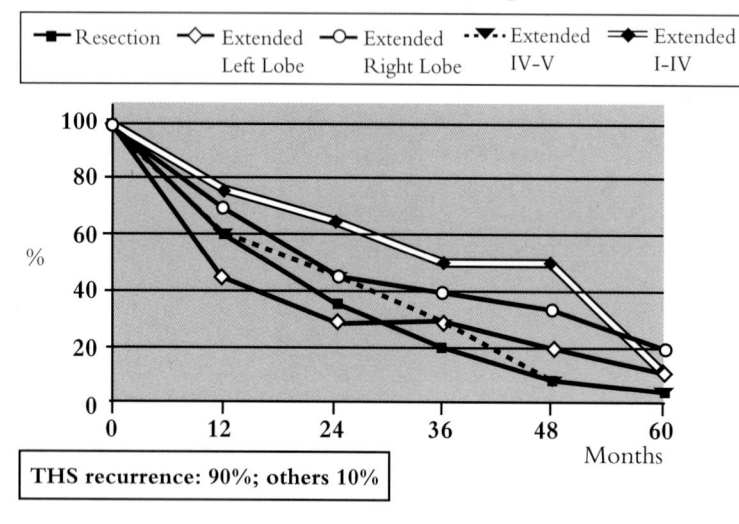

Figure 24.14 – *Actuarial survival in patients with bile duct resection and lymphatic metastasis (NI-N2). The different groups of resection are taken into account. 1) Resection of the bile duct with extension to the left hepatic lobe. 2) Resection of the bile duct with extension to the right hepatic lobe. 3) Enlargement of the bile duct resection to segments 4 and 5. 4) Resection of the bile duct without extension to the hepatic parenchyma. 5) Resection of the bile duct with extension to segments 4 and 1.*

THS recurrence: 90%; others 10%

anastomoses, the foremost corresponding to the drainage conduit of Segments 5 and 8, and the most posterior to that leading from Segments 6 and 7.

The choice of one of these procedures should be based on detailed analysis of the preoperative cholangiography, CT and angiography if complete inspection was performed during surgery, and on the findings observed during surgical dissection.

5 year survival rate has improved noticeably due to the removal of the hepatic parenchyma affected, using anatomical criterion and avoiding resections which lack sufficient anatomical knowledge. Inclusion of Segment 1 is of particular importance in the excision demonstrated, as is logical if the limits and relationships of the biliary tract at the level of the confluence of both primary hepatic ducts are studied (**Figures 24.13 and 24.14**).

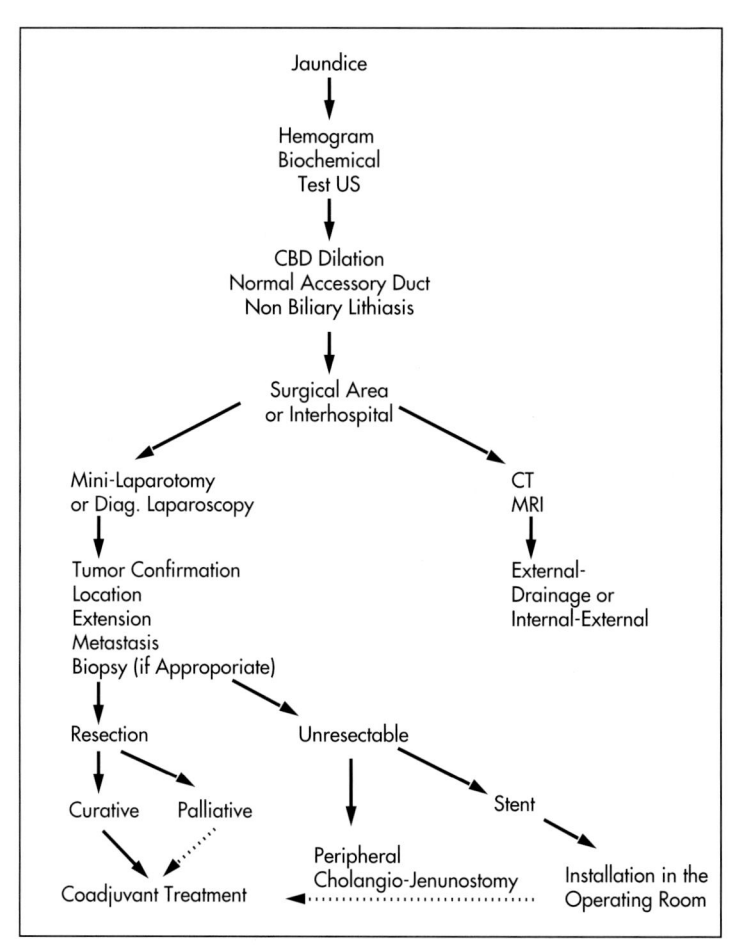

Figure 24.15 – *Diagnosis algorithm.*

Resective surgery in patients previously treated by means of transtumoral wall-stent prosthesis

The utterly beneficial development of interventional radiology has highlighted the importance of multidisciplinary functional units in the treatment of digestive diseases in general, and in carcinoma of the biliary tract in particular. Jaundice is undoubtedly the cardinal symptom in tumors of the biliary confluence and common hepatic duct, and it gives relatively early warning of the existence of a serious, progressive disease, which initially develops into loco-regional extension, and shortly afterwards into extension at a distance. The particular anatomy of the hepatoduodenal ligament and the porta hepatis allows tumor growth to spread rapidly to fundamental elements, such as the portal vein, the distribution branches of the proper hepatic artery, the adjacent hepatic parenchyma and intrahepatic vascular-biliary elements. The tendency towards infiltration in carcinoma of the biliary tract means that there is usually distant transtumoral extension; however, the degree of gravity depends on how much time elapses after its onset until the therapeutic treatment needed is actually applied.

Desquamation from the surface of the tumor in the lumen of the biliary tree can lead to a situation where cells which are not affected by the salts and biliary acids swim across in the biliary juice and become implanted on the internal surface of the proximal or distant intrahepatic biliary tract. These tumoros implants, which are hard to detect at surgery, could be the source of other malignant tumors in the biliary tree, which would eventually affect the proximal hepatic parenchyma and cause metastasis in the hepatic parenchyma itself, which could be confused with focal points of haematogenous dispersion.

When dealing with tumors of the confluence of the bile ducts, the main problems encountered involve confirming the diagnosis (histopathologic confirmation), being able to define the topography of the tumor, identifying its extra-or intrahepatic extension, and establishing the extent to which vascular elements near the surface of the tumor are affected. The onset of rapidly-progressing, painless, silent jaundice is not the most important clinical factor. Thereafter, the absence of biliary lithiasis or of dilation of the accessory biliary tract, together with dilation of the intrahepatic biliary tract, are undoubtely the most relevant data provided by ultrasound scan exploration. Exploration of this kind may make it possible to identify the boundaries of the area of the tumor, although this is unlikely, but will at least indicate how far it has spread, and, if the common and accessory biliary tract are normal, will more often than not diagnose a stone embedded in the common hepatic duct, distal to the biliary confluence, and will describe its clearcut enviromnent and substantially enlarged consistency **(Figure 24.15)**.

Thereafter, abdominal CT will confirm the details of the dilation of the bile duct, the obstruction point, and the absence of distal involvement. However, the information we really need and the information which is of overriding importance, is whether or not there has been extension to one or both main hepatic ducts, or any infiltration of one or both branches of the portal vein or the hepatic artery. Should this prove to be the case, excision would not be contraindicated, as the infiltrated areas can be resected and then

Table 24.3 – *Indications for surgery in patients previously treated by means of transtumoral Wall-stent prosthesis.*

PATIENTS	CHOLANGITIS JAUNDICE	STAGE	CHANGE PROSTHESIS	OBSTRUCTION PROSTHESIS
1	Yes	II	Once	Yes
2	–	I	–	–
3	Yes	III	–	–
4	Yes	II	Twice	Yes
5	–	I	Three	Yes
6	–	II	–	–
7	Yes	II	Once	–
8	Yes	III	Twice	Yes
9	Yes	III	–	–

reconstructed. However, the prognosis would obviously be worse and the risk of morbimortality greater. The characteristics of the disease may be so clearcut that unresectable lesion could be diagnosed simply by carrying out the examination procedures described above. However, before excluding a theoretically curative therapeutic solution, it is absolutely essential to secure the histological diagnosis, either by PEAC, biopsy during laparoscopical exploration, or by means of a small, right subcostal laparotomy. At the same time, it should be remembered that these patients suffer from major haemorrhagic diathesis, which is at times hard to control. Currently, MRI and digital angiography are the two most useful procedures, because of the precision of their definitions and their low morbidity. They also make it possible to detect superficial vascular involvement, complete arterial and/or venous obstruction, and the presence of capillary neoformation, with a high degree of clarity.

As has been explained in the ideas we have put forward about the treatment of tumors such as these, the only efficient procedure is excision, which may, or may not, be followed by complementary treatment. Only then, by associating all these tests, is it possible to confirm that the lesion is untreatable. Thereafter, palliative procedures, aimed only at avoiding dilation of the intrahepatic tract by external or internal-external drainage, should be employed.

There is a risk that the investigation sequence may prove so lengthy in state-run hospitals, university hospitals, or government institutions, that the lesions will have grown more serious and have spread, considerably reducing the resection rate. There is also a growing tendency to perceive surgeons as craftsmen who employ their technical dexterity for the purposes of removal and reconstruction. Nothing could be further from reality. Surgeons are, first and foremost, specialists in surgical diseases, and should therefore be consulted when these are suspected. This is particularly applicable in all cases of obstructive jaundice. Then, depending on their degree of knowledge, surgeons are able to establish the sequence and speed of the diagnostic tests needed, avoiding the risk of biliary infection and, in particular, progressive hepatic insufficiency and the onset of haemorrhagic diathesis. The advent of interventional radiology has led to a treatment route which is being used indiscriminately, with no prior debate, in tumors of the biliary tract. This is done on the assumption that surgery is difficult, on the high mortality rate of the procedures involved, and on the low long-term survival rate. It is for this very reason that patients arriving at departments of surgery with severe jaundice, with Wall-stents, are found to be suffering from frequent episodes of cholangitis caused by repeated obstruction of the stent. Sadly, only then is the appropriateness of performing surgery on the patient given any consideration.

From January, 1994 to December, 1995, surgery was performed on 15 patients. We shall only refer here to the first nine cases (***Table 24.3***), but would stress the gravity of the disease in terms of UICC criteria. The majority were considered to have reached stages 2

Table 24.4 – *Pathological findings in patients previously treated by means of transtumoral Wall-stent.*

PATIENTS	FREE MARGIN	POSITIVE LYMPHONODES	LIVER INFILTRATION	PALLIATIVE TREATMENT	RADICAL TREATMENT
1	1.5 cm	Yes	No	–	Yes
2	2 cm	Yes	Yes	–	Yes
3	Infiltrated	Yes	No	Yes	No
4	2 cm	Yes	Yes	–	Yes
5	2 cm	Yes	Yes	–	Yes
6	Infiltrated	Yes	No	Yes	No
7	1.5 cm	Yes	Yes	–	Yes
8	1.5 cm	Yes	Yes	–	Yes
9	2 cm	Yes	Yes	–	Yes

and 3 and to be unresectable; no surgical criteria whatsoever was taken into consideration. The patients were attended by interventional radiologists, who installed transtumoral expanding Wall-stents. As can be seen from **Table 24.3**, the majority of the patients suffered episodes of cholangitis, which means that they had to be admitted to hospital on several occasions. Mixed antibiotherapy and total parenteral nutrition was used to treat the various episodes, which in one patient lasted for six months after the stent was installed.

After we studied the characteristics of the tumors, no sign of intrahepatic extension of the disease was detected, although in three cases hyperecogenic nodes were detected at the level of the left hepatic lobe, and were considered to be intrahepatic bacterial abscesses. Only in one case was the possibility of the differential diagnosis with metastatic lesions considered. In six of the nine patients, an external-internal catheter was introduced through the stent, unblocking its lumen, and a new stent was installed in four cases. A third stent was subsequently installed in one patient. In three patients, the distal tip of the prosthesis was situated in a 3-4 cm transpapillary, intra-duodenal position. Two patients suffered acute cholecystitis after the stent was installed, possibly as a result of the compression of the cystic-choledocian join, because of the distension caused by the expanding Wall-stent. They were treated by percutaneous puncture and percutaneous "pigtail" drainage.

All the patients underwent surgery involving resection of the whole of the extrahepatic bile duct, from the pancreatic surface to the hepatic hilius. Infiltration of the liver was confirmed in seven patients, as a result of which the excision was extended to the left hepatic lobe in four cases, to the right hepatic lobe in one case, and to the external (5) and internal (4B) paramedian segments in the other two cases. In the four patients who underwent excision of the hepatic lobe, the excisions were extended en bloc to segment 1, and the same occurred in one of the two patients who had undergone excision of segments 4B and 5 (**Table 24.4**). Biliary reconstruction was performed using a 55 cm long Roux-en-Y loop, and three bilio-jejunal anastomoses were performed on the patients treated with paramedian segmentectomy, two of those treated with left hepatic lobectomy, and two on the patients where the excision had been extended to the right hepatic lobe.

Bilio-jejunal anastomosis was performed on a single plane using interrupted suture (reabsorbable, monfilament 5/0 and plaited, reabsorbable monofilament 6/0). In five patients, some multiorificed transanastomotic stent was left to provide greater security for the permeability of the derivation, which had been confirmed in the preoperative stage by HIDA-Tcm99 at six and twelve months.

The pathological study of the resected specimen revealed neoplasic infiltration of the proximal end in two patients, although a biopsy had previously been performed on the distal end of the remaining duct, and had been reported to be free from neoplasic infiltration. This could be interpreted as an

Table 24.5 – *Extension of liver resection and following in patients previously treated by means of transtumoral Wall-stent prosthesis.*

PATIENTS	TUMOR LOCALIZATION	TIME** MONTHS	RESECTION	STAGE DISEASE	FOLLOW-UP MONTHS
1	H.D.*	4	B.D. ***	II	42
2	H.D.Confluence	6 ½	B.D. + 4-5	IV	39
3	H.D.+Cystic D.	4 ½	B.D.	II	31
4	H.D.+Left D.	5	B.D. +1-2-3	IV	30
5	H.D.+Left D.	3	B.D. + 1-4	IV	25
6	H.D.	2 ½	B.D. + I	III	21
7	H. D. + Right D.	4	B.D. + 2-3	III	
8	H.D.Confluence	3	B.D. + 1-4	III	12
9	H.D.Confluence	6	B.D.+1-2-3-4	III	9

*H.D. = Hepatic duct, **Time = form prosthesis insertion, *** B.D. = Bile duct

error in manipulation in the laboratory or be attributed to retraction of the limited margin obtained at surgery (*Table 24.5*).

One patient had a left subphrenic abscess which was drained percutaneously, using ecotomographic control (US-CT scan). Another patient, aged 78, suffered from evisceration, calling for parieto-abdominal closure again. The patient died 38 days after surgery as a result of sepsis and renal insufficiency. The other patients were discharged from hospital in a good state of recovery. Details of the follow-up and the extension are given on *Table 24.5*.

As several different groups of surgeons have already warned, this experience demonstrates that patients with obstructive jaundice, and particularly those showing the first signs of neoplasic disease, should be referred immediately to surgical areas for their cases to be studied and to ensure that the most suitable treatment is administered.

TECHNIQUES IN LIVER SURGERY

SECTION IX

Innovative Techniques

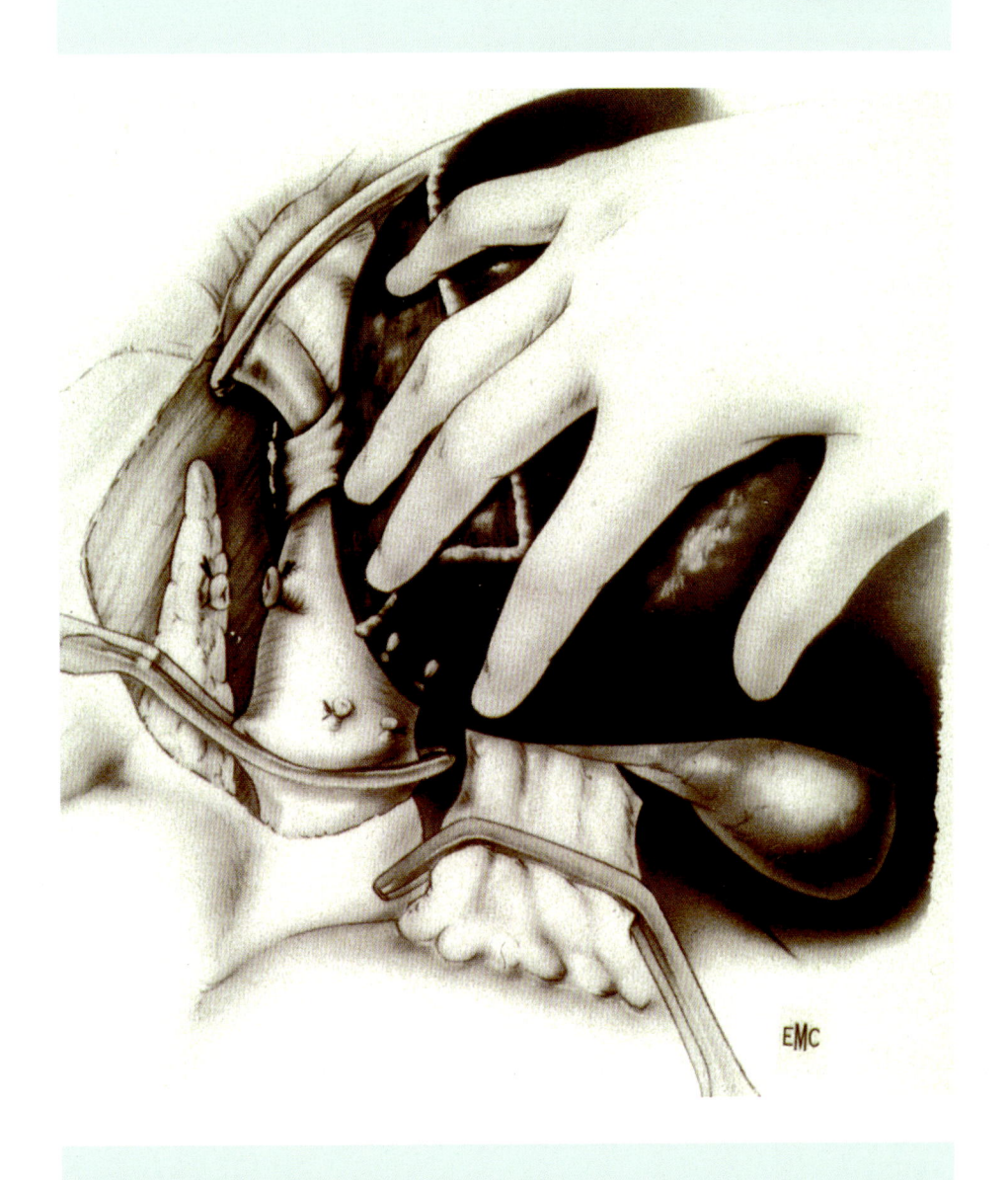

25

Major Liver Resections Using Hypothermic Perfusion

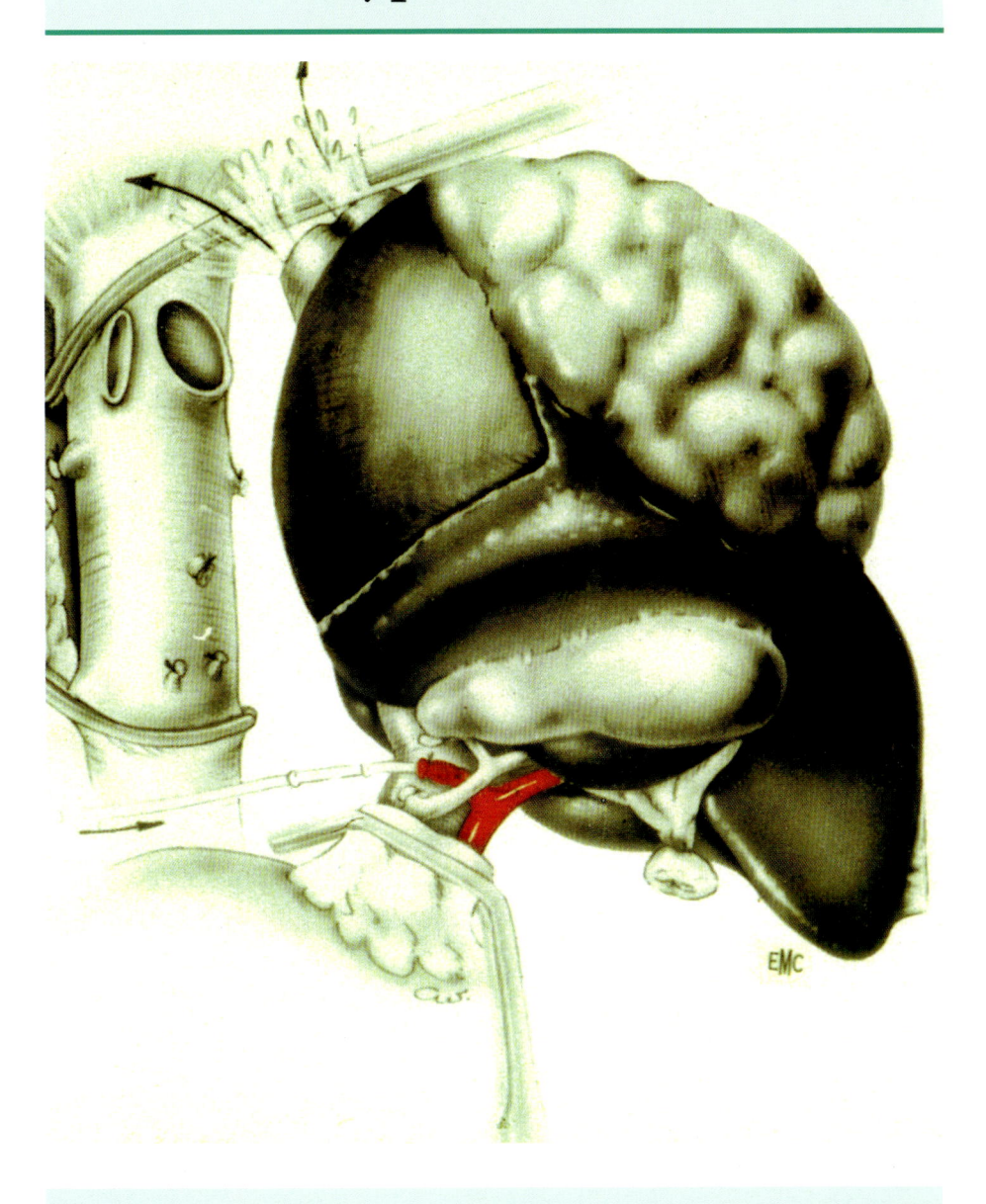

L. Hannoun, D.C. Borie

Normothermic ischemia can be well tolerated for up to 90 minutes in normal livers[7,9] and up to 60 minutes in low severity cirrhotic livers.[3,11,12] Whereas the vast majority of conventional liver resections can be performed within these limits, in very selected cases the period of vascular clamping and resulting ischemia may prove too short to allow major and complex liver resections. Indeed, tumor invasion of either the portal pedicle or the hepatocaval confluence may lead to complex vascular resection and reconstruction that necessitates extensive periods of vascular clamping. As technical skills developed together with orthotopic liver transplantation, the concept of 'extreme liver surgery', consisting of major liver resection with vascular reconstruction of the remaining vessels, was introduced.

To overcome the problem of the limited duration of normothermic ischemia we, and others, hypothesized that cooling the liver with chilled preservation solution, either University of Wisconsin (UW) or HTK Breitschneider solution, routinely used for the preservation of liver grafts, would enhance tolerance of the remnant liver to ischemia. Liver perfusion with 4°C preservation solution was used in three different approaches in major liver resections: *in situ*,[4] *ex situ in vivo* [1,6,8] and *ex vivo* surgery.[10] In *in situ* surgery, the liver, albeit completely mobilized, remains in the right hypochondrium and the integrity of both afferent and efferent vessels is conserved.[4,10] We described *ex situ in vivo* surgery during which the liver is exteriorized from the abdominal cavity (*ex situ*) by transecting efferent vessels, i.e. section of all hepatic veins, without section of the afferent vessels, that is the portal pedicle (*in vivo*).[1,6] In *ex vivo* extracorporeal surgery ('bench procedure'), the liver is completely removed from the abdominal cavity by transection of both afferent and efferent vessels, liver resection and vascular reconstructions are performed on the back-table, and the remnant liver is reimplanted, as would be done for a partial liver graft.[10] All three procedures involve techniques refined as orthotopic liver transplantation developed (hepatic vascular exclusion, venovenous bypass, liver cooling, preservation solution). These techniques are diversely used and combined following analysis of: 1) the estimated duration of ischemia needed to perform the liver resection; 2) the functional reserve of the liver parenchyma; 3) the hemodynamic tolerance to hepatic vascular exclusion; 4) the need for, and site of, potential vascular reconstruction.

Techniques

All three techniques involve hepatic vascular exclusion (HVE), (see Chapter 12).

In situ procedure

The patient is usually placed in a dorsal decubitus position. If a right thoracoabdominal incision is considered, the right hemithorax is slightly raised (3-4 cm) by placing folded towels longitudinally beneath the right half of the patient's back. The arms are left at a right angle to the patient's body and the left axilla and groin areas kept accessible should venovenous extracorporeal bypass become necessary.

A bilateral incision at least 4 cm below the subcostal margins is performed, with midline extension to the xiphoid process. In cases of large tumors of the upper and posterior part of the liver close to the hepatocaval confluence, a right thoracotomy is made. The indications for this incision are rare, however, as it is performed only when tumor invasion of either hepatocaval confluence or diaphragm is present. The incision starts from the upper end of the abdominal medial incision and is centered on the 7th or 8th intercostal space. The cartilaginous part of the rib is split, the thorax entered and the diaphragm split. This incision allows easy access to the intrapericardial inferior vena cava when necessitated by tumor invasion of the hepatocaval confluence.

Preparation for HVE is the same in the three types of liver surgery with hypothermic perfusion. The liver is completely mobilized by dividing the right and left triangular ligaments. The lesser omentum is divided preserving a left hepatic artery if present. The following step where dissection of the right adrenal gland is performed needs to be emphasized. Easy identification of the right adrenal gland with its unique appearance follows careful dissection of the coronary and right triangular ligaments in the appropriate plane. The upper extremity of the gland is dissected free from the right pillar of the diaphragm. The right aspect of the inferior vena cava (IVC) is easily idenitified at this level and separated from the upper part of the gland. This step is usually easy as the right adrenal vein usually joins the IVC at a lower point. Mobilization of the upper part of the gland allows contact with the right side of the IVC and movement of the posterior aspect of the IVC to a safe and avascular site. The infrahepatic IVC above the renal vein is dissected free on its anterior and right aspects. Both these maneuvers give access to the right adrenal vein which may then be divided between stitches. Then, the peritoneum is opened on the left side of the IVC and if encountered, accessory diaphragmatic veins draining into the retrohepatic IVC are divided. Moving upwards, the IVC is completely freed on its left side up to the diaphragm. Posteriorly, dissection encounters the dissection plane used with the right approach. The posterior aspect of the IVC is dissected completely free from the diaphragm to the renal veins.

The portal pedicle is exposed and from now on the dissection technique may vary. Briefly, in the technique described by Fortner,[4] the celiac axis, hepatic artery and gastroduodenal artery must be isolated. The portal vein and common bile duct are isolated and all lymphatic and areolar tissue in the porta hepatis divided between ligatures. Cannulation is through the gastroduodenal artery and the portal vein, the latter being cannulated either through a venotomy or via the branch of the lobe which is to be resected. These cannulae are kept patent with a slow infusion of Ringer lactate at room temperature. The common bile duct is occluded with a small Pott's clamp and the liver is then ready for hypothermic perfusion. The common hepatic artery, portal vein, infrahepatic and suprahepatic vena cava are clamped. A large drain is placed through a cavotomy inferior to the liver and chilled perfusion with Ringer lactate is started. Once resection is complete, blood flow is reestablished and the cannulae are removed except for the gastroduodenal cannula which is preserved for subsequent chemotherapy administration.

In contrast, in our technique,[16,8] pedicle dissection is minimal and restricted to the site where the perfusion is to be performed. The peritoneum of the anterior aspect of the porta hepatis is cut high, at the level of the hilum. The limited dissection of the porta hepatis allows the pedicle clamp to be applied on structures still surrounded by fatty tissue which could prove useful in the prevention of traumatic intimal lesions induced by clamping. Depending upon anatomical conditions, hypothermic perfusion can be performed either through an arterial or a portal branch. The arterial branch supplying the part of the liver to be resected is the preferred access site through which the future remnant liver can be perfused. Access to the artery is usually easier and requires less dissection compared to access through a portal branch. Futhermore, simple proximal ligature of the artery permits closure after the procedure. However, it often proves easier to direct and push the cannula into the branch of the liver to be conserved when the entry point is on the portal branch. Also, it may be that the hepatic artery divides proximally so that the pedicule clamp would be above this division and thus would stop the perfusion from crossing the bifurcation and irrigating the future remnant liver. Whichever vessel is used for perfusion, it is ligated distally to the entry point of the cannula, and it may be divided so that only selective perfusion of the liver to be retained is performed. If the artery has been prepared, the largest catheter possible is introduced through a small incision in the anterior wall and secured with a ligature. If a branch of the portal vein has to be used, the catheter is fixed on the anterior wall using a purse-string suture. We routinely use for perfusion a classical transcystic drain (Porges®) whose caliber matches that of the perfusion vessel (usually 8 or 10 Fr). Due to the small size of this particular drain, it is usually necessary to use a pressure bag to perform the refrigerated perfusion (***Figure 25.1***).

Hepatic vascular exclusion is then tested[2] (see Chapter 12) by successively clamping the porta hepatis, the infrahepatic and the suprahepatic IVC. The pedicule clamp is a 25.5 cm Satinsky Medium Atraugrip® Jaw 4 cm, the infrahepatic IVC is clamped by a Glover clamp (Spoon Shape, 23.5 Atraugrip® Jaw 6.5 cm), and the suprahepatic IVC clamped with a De Bakey

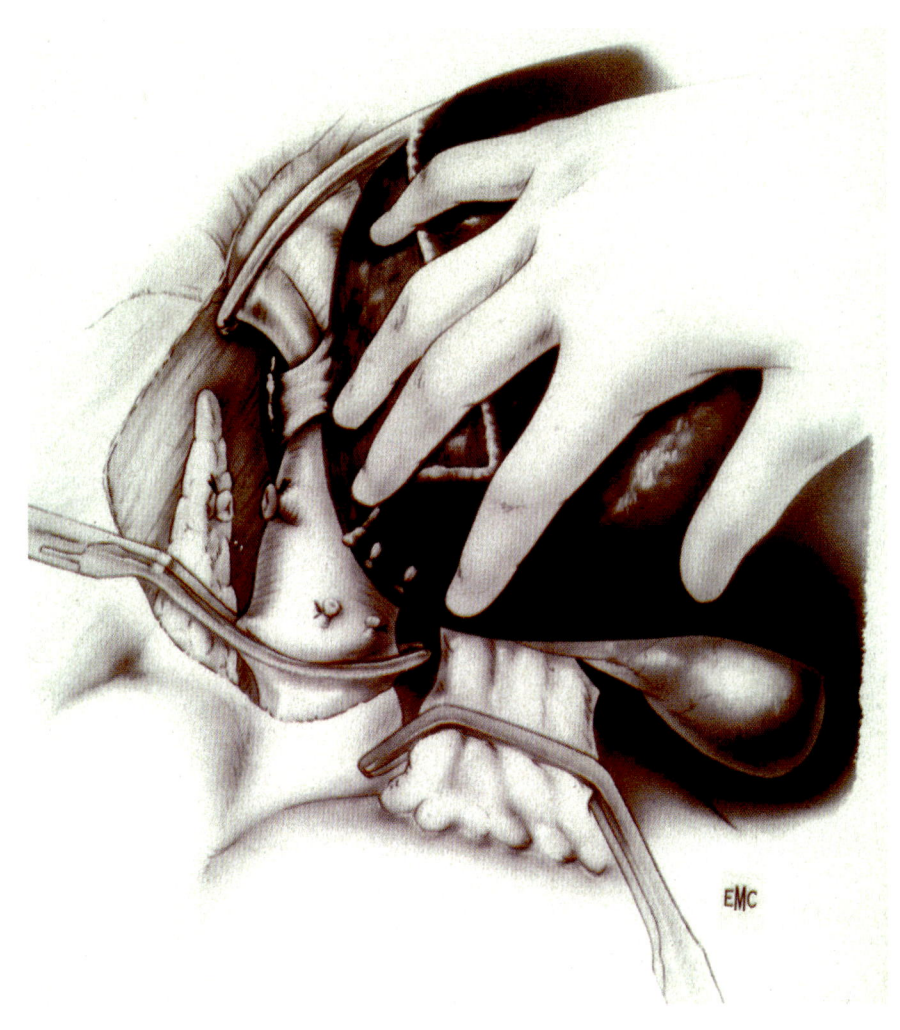

Figure 25.1 – *Hepatic vascular exclusion.*

Reproduced by permission of L. Hannoun and coll. from: 'Technique de l'esclusion vasculaize du foie et des hepatectomies extremes' - Editons Techniques - Encycl. Méd. Chir. (Paris, France), Technique Chirurgcales, App. Dig. 40, 766, 1994

aortic clamp (35 cm Atraugrip® Jaw 12 cm), all three clamps from Pilling®. Good tolerance is shown after a 5-7 minute test period by: 1) a drop of less than 50% of the preciamping cardiac output; 2) a fall in arterial pressure less than 30%, 3) maintenance of the venous oxygen saturation value (SVO_2) above 70%.

Once good tolerance to HVE has been assured, the *in situ* perfusion procedure begins by performing a draining cavotomy either on the infrahepatic IVC or by transecting one of the hepatic veins at its termination on the IVC. The perfusion with 4°C UW solution starts immediately. We perfuse approximately I liter of UW solution but the optimal volume to be perfused and the maximum duration of cold ischemia that can be obtained with this technique is still under investigation. Usually, the perfusion proceeds until the caval effluent becomes clear which can require about 30 minutes considering the small size of the catheter used.

After completion of the resection, the preservation solution is flushed from the remnant parenchyma by perfusing 4°C Ringer lactate. To avoid cardiac arythmias the potassium content of the effluent can be checked before reperfusion. We find that perfusion of 500 ml of Ringer lactate generally gives satisfactory potassium clearance when remnant liver is small and we do not routinely check for potassium content. Hemostasis is completed by occluding leaking points from the raw surface with non-absorbable stitches. The cavotomy is closed with a 4/0 monofilament running suture before unclamping and the perfusion catheter removed. The orifice of the artery is closed with a ligature applied proximally. To prevent the possibility of a stricture of the venous confluence when the perfusion is performed through the vein, this vessel is closed using 5/0 or 6/0 polypropylene stitches.

Hemostasis is secured by cautious and partial unclamping and immediate clamping of the infrahepatic IVC. This allows the most obvious bleeding sites to be easily controlled while the vena cava is still clamped. Unclamping follows this step, starting with the removal of the suprahepatic clamp and then the infrahepatic clamp. Hemostasis is checked and secured at the level of the hepatocaval confluence. Unclamping of the portal pedicle follows. Complete hemostasis is achieved using gentle pressure on the raw surface with a wet sponge. Often additional 5/0 or 6/0 polypropylene stitches are required to secure hemostasis. Once and only once hemostasis is established, hemostatic gauze and fibrin glue are applied to the cut surface.

In the rare instance when the 5-minute clamping test reveals poor tolerance to HVE, venovenous extracorporeal by-pass using a standard heparin-coated circuit with a Biomedicus® pump is performed.[5] The left internal saphenous, inferior mesenteric, and left axillary veins are used as vascular access sites and are cannulated with regular thoracic drains (Argyle®) of the appropriate size. When preoperative liver function is normal, systemic heparinization is usually initiated before starting the extracorporeal perfusion to minimize the risk of intra-shunt clotting. In our experience, this heparinization must be very mild (15-30 mg) and cautious, and may be neutralized after 1 hour to avoid dramatic and uncontrollable hemorrhage on reperfusion of the liver. After the bypass is established, the vascular clamps are applied and hypothermic perfusion of the liver is started. The procedure then continues as described above and the shunt is removed just before restoration of hepatic blood flow.

Ex situ procedures

For very selected and rare cases in which a very long (3-5 hours) ischemia is necessitated by the complexity of the planned resection and vascular reconstructions, *ex situ* procedures have been proposed. The resection may be performed either *in vivo* (*ex situ in vivo*), or *ex vivo* on the back-table.

Ex vivo

In the *ex vivo* technique described by Pichlmayr[10] the principles used are those of liver grafting with some variations. As long vessels and patches are not available, meticulous dissection and re-anastomosis of vessels is mandatory. The suprahepatic vena cava is dissected free from the diaphragm to facilitate clamping and re-anastomosis. Caval branches are dissected and ligated carefully. Hilar neural and lymphatic tissue is removed in most instances in a radical way. The use of bypass is mandatory. Hypothermic liver perfusion is started *in situ* after caval clamping. The liver is removed within 1-2 minutes, given the previous vascular isolation. Extracorporeal perfusion is continued on the back-table after explantation of the liver which avoids cooling of the patient. Perfusion uses HTK Breitschneider solution initially with 6 liters intraportally and 0.5 liters intraarterially and is repeated at intervals of 1 hour with 1 liter and 0.2 liters, respectively. After completion of the liver resection, the remnant liver is brought back into the abdomen and re-anastomosis is carried out.

Ex situ in vivo

The significant advantage of the *ex situ in vivo* procedure over the *ex vivo* technique is that it avoids the need to perform portal, arterial and biliary anastomosis and the subsequent risk of possible complications. Indications for this technique are based on the need for vascular reconstruction due to tumor invasion of either the hepatic vein(s) or the portal vein.

When a large tumor develops close to the hepatocaval confluence the procedure also involves a thoracotomy through the 7th intercostal space and large diaphragmatic splitting. This approach contributes significantly to excellent exposure of the operating field. It facilitates the mobilization of the IVC and intrapericardial IVC can be controlled as dictated by the extent of the tumor.

The dissection of the liver and identification of the vessel to be used for perfusion at the hilum are performed as described previously. The use of the venovenous bypass is essential and is performed through left internal saphenous, inferior mesenteric, and left axillary cannulae. Cautious systemic heparinization (0.25-0.5 mg/kg) is used. Hepatic vascular exclusion is established and the cooling perfusion started.

The technique proceeds in very specific steps. Section of one of the hepatic veins immediately after initiation of the perfusion allows good drainage of the preservation solution. Then, the liver is exteriorized by section at the level of the hepatocaval confluence of each hepatic vein. If the tumor has invaded the termination of one of these veins, part of the IVC is resected and closed with polypropylene sutures or with a vascular patch to avoid stricture of the IVC. The liver is mobilized from the retrohepatic IVC by step-by-step ligation and division of all Spigelian veins. Once complete, the liver remains attached *in vivo* by the porta hepatis, but can be completely exteriorized *ex situ* and placed on heat exchange plates designed for this purpose (**Figures 25.2** and **25.3**). This

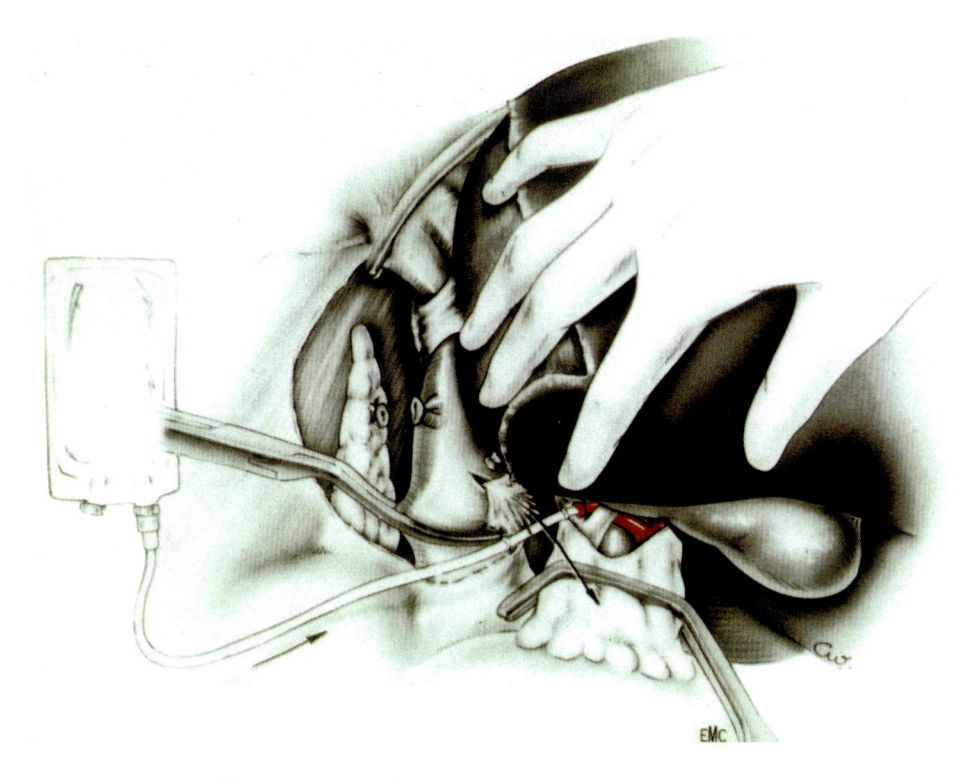

Figure 25.2 –
In the in situ procedure, hilar dissection is minimal and only the artery or the vein used for perfusion is dissected. Drainage is through a short cavotomy. Perfusion is through the right artery to the left liver in order to perform a right hepatectomy.

Reproduced by permission of L. Hannoun and coll. from: 'Technique de l'esclusion vasculaize du foie et des hepatectomies extremes' - Editons Techniques - Encycl. Méd. Chir. (Paris, France), Technique Chirurgcales, App. Dig. 40, 766, 1994

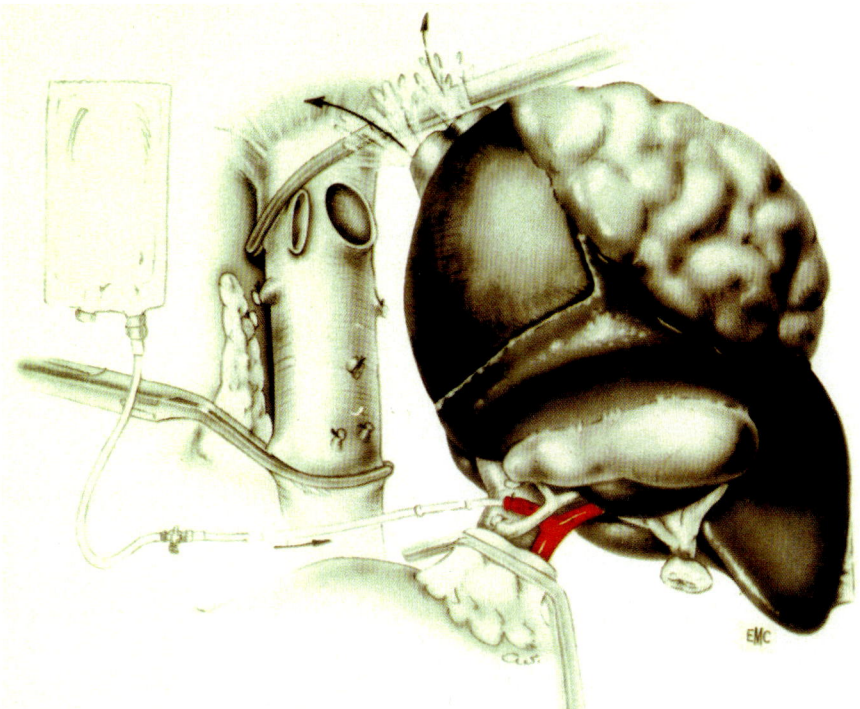

Figure 25.3 –
In the ex situ in vivo procedure, after section of the hepatic veins and ligation of the Spigelian veins, the liver is placed ex situ but remains attached to the porta hepatis. Drainage is through the hepatic veins. Perfusion is through the right artery to the left liver in order to perform a right hepatectomy as again illustrated.

Reproduced by permission of L. Hannoun and coll. from: 'Technique de l'esclusion vasculaize du foie et des hepatectomies extremes' - Editons Techniques - Encycl. Méd. Chir. (Paris, France), Technique Chirurgcales, App. Dig. 40, 766, 1994

apparatus was designed to replace the ice bucket commonly used during back-table procedures. Temperature is controlled on each face and maintained at 4°C and 37°C on the liver and patient sides, respectively. We do not have clear evidence of the efficacy of this device as the core temperature of the organ has not been assessed. Tumor resection and vascular and biliary reconstruction are performed on this refrigerated plane. After completion of liver resection, the cooling system is removed. The hepatic vein of the remnant liver, sometime after having undergone reconstruction, is reimplanted onto its original IVC orifice if possible and, if not, on a cavotomy orifice. The site for reimplantation is actually chosen based on the anatomical situation when the liver is reanastomosed with the IVC. UW solution is rinsed off, the portal line is excluded from the extracorporeal circulation, the perfusion catheter is removed and the cavotomy is closed. In our experience, perfusion of 1-2 liters of UW and 0.5-1 liter of Ringer lactate are usually necessary in this kind of procedure.

Clamps are removed and, after a few minutes, extracorporeal venovenous circulation is interrupted.

In situ perfusion for diseased livers

It is now accepted that non-cirrhotic livers may safely withstand prolonged normothermic ischemia. The tolerance of diseased livers (mainly those with fatty infiltration, chronic hepatitis or cirrhosis) is less clear. When facing these particular situations, we decided to use prospectively *in situ* hypothermic perfusion in the hope that tolerance of the non-tumor parenchyma to ischemia would be improved. Preliminary results from 12 patients treated with this technique have been reported.[8] Patients were considered for inclusion in the study when: 1) there was evidence of severe liver damage on frozen section analysis of a biopsy of the remnant liver taken immediately after entering the abdomen; 2) when hepatic vascular exclusion longer than 1 hour was anticipated because of the technical difficulties of the resection.

In 6 cases with metastatic disease to the liver, non-tumor parenchyma had histological evidence of steatosis greater than 30%. All patients had received several courses of chemotherapy, including intraarterial chemoembolization in 1 patient. Liver cirrhosis classified as Child-Pugh A was present in the remaining cases, either virus C-induced (4 cases), secondary biliary (2 cases), or cryptogenetic (1 case) cirrhosis. If used before resection, chemotherapy was interrupted at least 1 month before hepatectomy.

Major liver resections removing at least 4 segments were performed with an HVE duration of 12 ± 54 minutes and exceeding 2 hours in 5 cases. The volume of UW and Ringer lactate perfused was 1111 ± 553 ml and 700 ± 280 ml, respectively. Vascular reconstructions were performed in 3 patients. The amount of intraoperative blood transfusion ranged from 0 to 9 units of packed red blood cells. Four patients did not require any transfusion.

One patient (8.3%) died from liver failure after reoperation for portal vein thrombosis. Another case of liver failure, this time transient, was noted. Morbidity was low (27%) with I case each of biliary fistula and severe atelectasis necessitating bronchoscopy and lavage. Median ICU stay was 7 days (range 441) and hospital stay 21 days (range 15-26). All 11 patients who left hospital were alive at 1 year, the mean follow-up time being 26.5 ± 6.6 months.

Postoperative course

Postoperative complications of major liver resection under hypothermic perfusion can arise from the technique itself or from the extent of the liver resection.

As a result of multiple vascular access and vascular reconstructions, *vascular complications* can be seen. The occurrence of an outflow block constitutes an emergency diagnosis that has to be made intraoperatively immediately after reperfusion. This may be positional due to a certain degree of kinking of the hepatic vein and may sometimes be completely suppressed, e.g., by repositioning and fixing in a good position a remnant left lobe with a tendency to fall in the right hypochondrium. If the outflow block results from a narrowed anastomosis then the only solution is to redo it after reapplying the clamps. Portal vein thrombosis is also a potentially lethal complication encountered postoperatively. Here again, the diagnosis must be made promptly and for this reason we routinely perform a daily (or twice daily) Doppler examination during the first postoperative week. A positive diagnosis must lead to urgent relaparotomy for portal vein clearance.

Hemorrhage is another potential complication of these procedures. It usually happens after unclamping and blood loss is usually more pronounced than during conventional major liver resection. Different factors are responsible for the occurrence of this complication. Among these, the anhepatic phase, intraoperative hemodilution, and perfusion of the liver may play a role. In our opinion, the most significant factor contributing to hemorrhage is the use of anticoagulants introduced whenever extracorporeal perfusion is used. The results of our early experience prompted the use of heparinization with great caution and neutralization of its effects before unclamping. Protamine sulfate, transfusion of units of fresh frozen plasma, or aprotinin (Antagosan®) infusion may all prove useful to correct hemostasis disorders following unclamping.

Hepatic insufficiency is the most worrying potential complication of major liver resection. It results from the combination of prolonged ischemia, even though it is hypothermic, and extensive liver resection leaving in place an insufficient mass of liver parenchyma. Several ways to assess the risk of such an event have been proposed. None has proved absolutely reliable even though the combination of indocyanine green clearance with results of CT volumetric studies, or the use of arterial ketone body ratio may be helpful. Should hepatic insufficiency occur, no salvage operation apart from liver transplantation is currently available. In the future, this situation may represent an indication for the use of bioartificial liver devices while awaiting liver regeneration.

The techniques described above represent tremendous surgical efforts. From the surgical standpoint, these techniques are often much more technically demanding than conventional orthotopic liver transplantation. Indications are very few and every case must be carefully selected. Indeed, these interventions usually expose the patient to a considerable risk of hepatic insufficiency. The shortage of liver grafts for conventional indications of liver transplantation does not make liver transplantation a potential back-up for these extreme resections should hepatic insufficiency develop. Furthermore, major liver resections are often indicated for large malignant tumors which constitute the poorest indications for liver transplantation.

Considering the indications for major liver resections under hypothermic perfusion, three different situations can be identified. When resection is necessitated by cancer these surgical procedures have the same extrahepatic contraindications as liver transplantation. In brief, extrahepatic dissemination of the disease constitutes, in our opinion, a clear contraindication. On the other hand, major liver resections with hypothermic perfusion can sometimes overcome the intrahepatic contraindications for orthotopic liver transplantation. For resections on a non-tumor normal liver, hypothermic perfusion can be considered when the predicted ischemic time is longer than 2 hours. This situation is very rare, however, as we have shown that normothermic ischemia can be well tolerated by normal parenchyma for longer than 90 minutes.[7] We consider that hepatic vascular exclusion alone can allow the surgeon to perform almost any kind of major liver resection on an otherwise normal liver.

Experience accumulated so far has shown the feasibility of the technique. The surgeon must have at his disposal a large technical 'tool box' including hepatic vascular exclusion, liver perfusion, the use of preservation solutions, external topical cooling of the organ and extracorporeal bypass procedures. A significant factor in the feasibility of the technique is the particular anatomy of the liver which can be completely exteriorized from the abdomen even though afferent vessels are conserved, as in *ex situ in vivo* procedures.

Although we can only report preliminary results, we feel that the application of these new techniques may open up a different strategic approach for the treatment of tumors in diseased livers.

REFERENCES

1. Delriviere L, Hannoun L. *In situ and ex situ in vivo* procedures for complex major liver resections requiring prolonged hepatic vascular exclusion in nonnal and diseased livers. *J Am Coll Surg* 1995; **181**: 272-276.

2. Delva A, Camus Y, Nordlinger B *et al*. Vascular occlusions for liver resections. Operative management and tolerance to hepatic ischemia: 142 cases. *Ann Surg* 1989; **209**: 211-218.

3. Ezaki T, Seo Y, Tomoda H, Furusawa M, Kanematsu T, Sugimachi K. Partial hepatic resection under intermittent hepatic inflow occlusion in patients with chronic liver disease. *Br J Surg* 1992; **79**: 224226.

4. Fortner JG, Shin MH, Kinne DW *et al*. Major hepatic resection using vascular isolation and hypothermic perfusion. *Ann Surg* 1974; **180**: 644-652.

5. Griffith BP, Shaw BW Jr, Hardestyl PL *et al*. Venovenous bypass without systemic anticoagulation for transplantation of the human liver. *Surg Gynecol Obstet* 1985; **160**: 270-272.

6. Hannoun L, Panis Y, Balladur P *et al*. "Ex situ in vivo" liver surgery. Principle and first results. *Lancet* 1991; **337**: 1616-1617.

7. Hannoun L, Borie D, Delva E *et al*. Liver resection with normothermic ischemia exceeding one hour. A ten-year experience. *Br J Surg* 1993; **80**: 1161-1165.

8. Hannoun L, Delriviere L, Gibbs P, Borie D, Vaillant JC, Delva E. Major extended liver resections in diseased livers using hypothermic' protection: preliminary results from the first 12 patients treated with this new technique. *J Am Coll Surg* 1996; **183**: 587-605

9. Huguet C, Gavelli A, Chieco A *et al*. Liver ischemia for hepatic resection: where is the limit? *Surgery* 1992; **ll**: 251-259.

10. Pichlmayr R, Grosse H, Hauss J, Gubematis G, Lamesh P, Bretschneider HK. Technique and preliminary results of extracorporeal liver surgery (bench procedure) and of surgery on the *in situ* perfused liver. *Br J Surg* 1990; **77**: 21-26.

11. Wu CC, Hwang CR, Liu TJ, P'eng FK. Effects and limitations of prolonged intermittent ischaemia for hepatic resection of the cirrhotic liver. *Br J Surg* 1996; **83**: 121-124.

12. Yamaoka Y, Ozawa K, Kumada K *et al*. Total vascular exclusion for hepatic resection in cirrhotic patients. *Arch Surg* 1992; **127**: 276-280.

10 | pro | Rellia = Osteward Leber
10 | — " —   Lunge
42 | Niere

TECHNIQUES IN LIVER SURGERY

SECTION X

Standard Techniques of Liver Transplantation

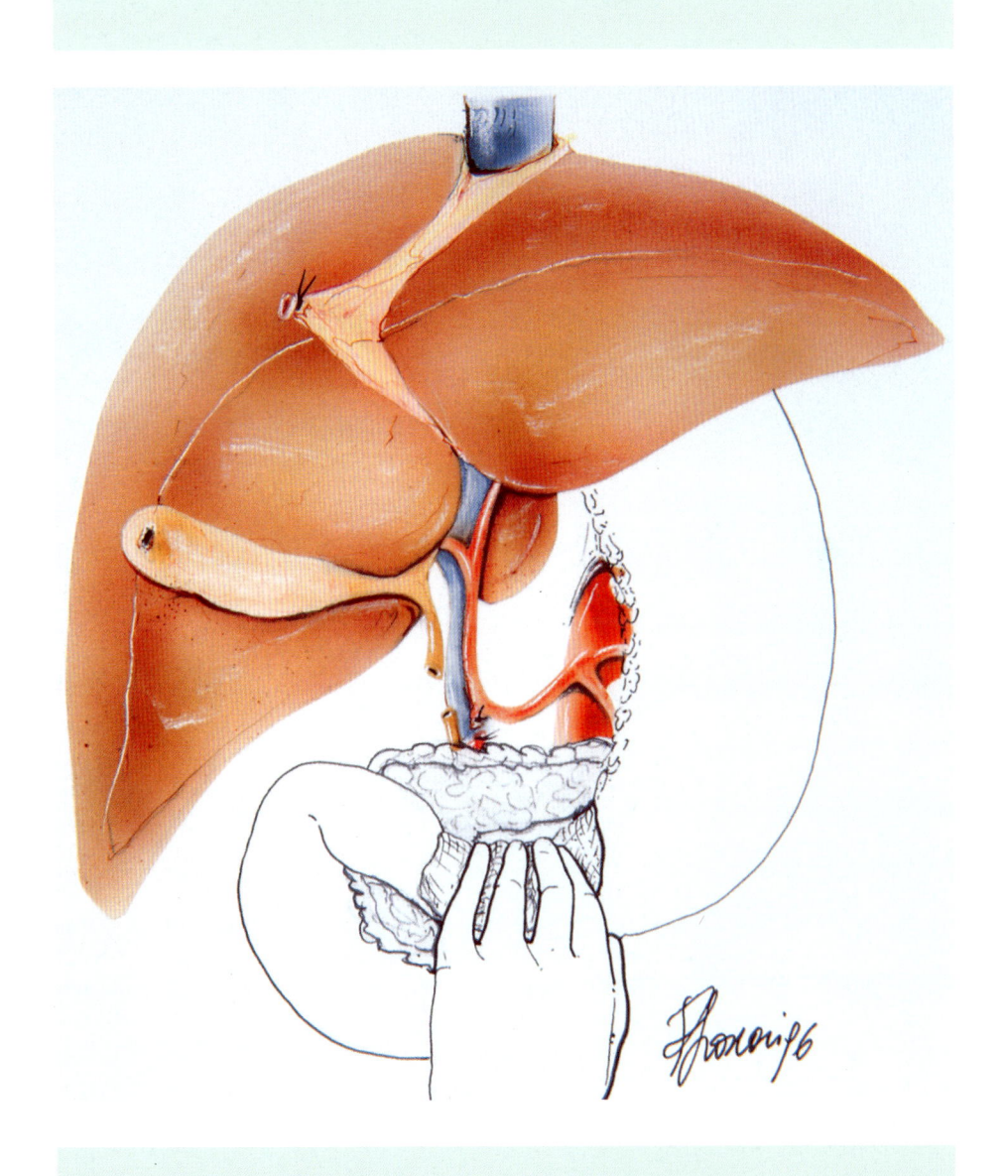

26

Liver Procurement for Transplantation

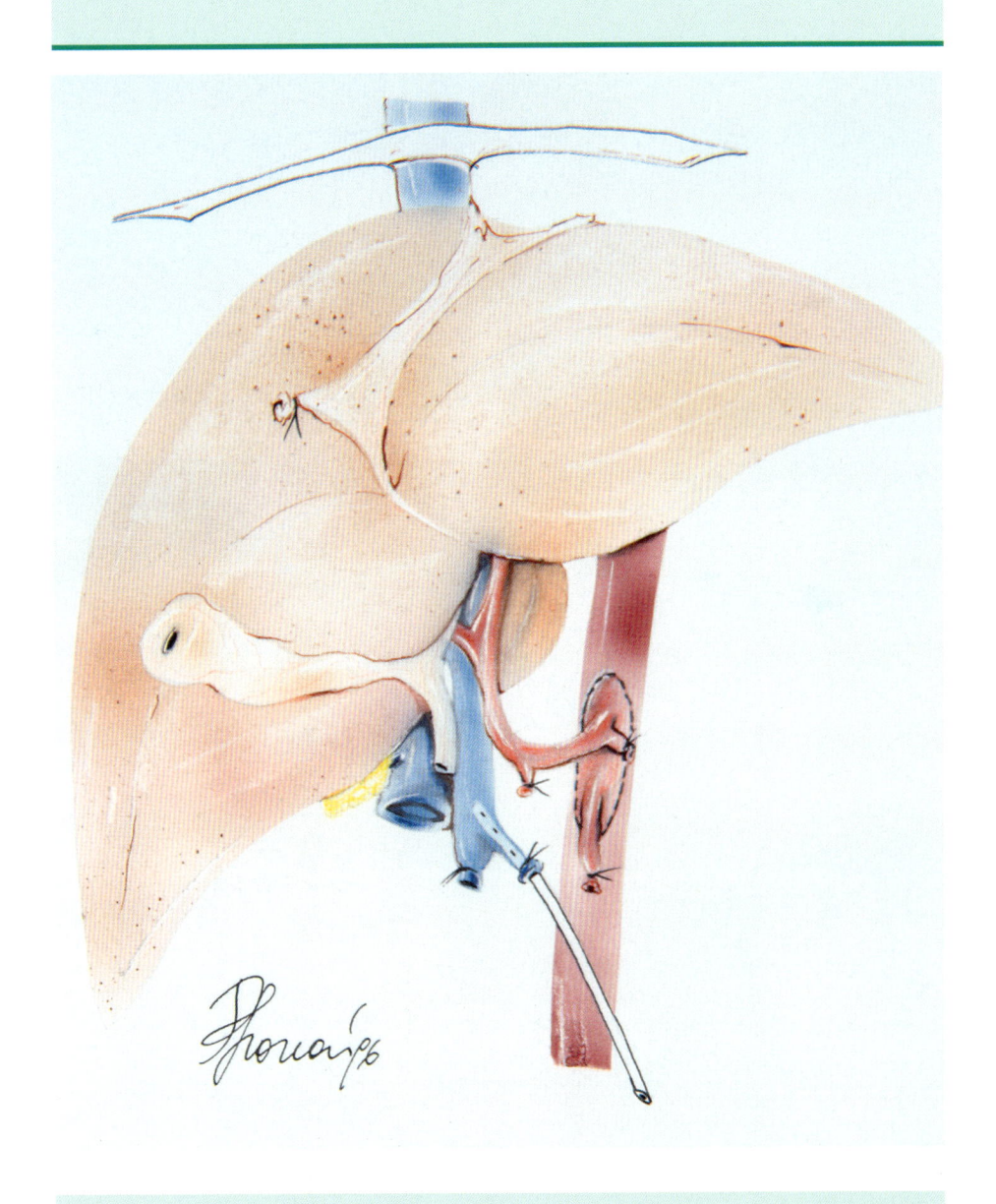

G.L. Grazi, E. Jovine, G. Ercolani, F. Pierangeli

Liver procurement has become a common operation as a result of the increased number of referred organ donors. The operation usually takes place in hospitals far from transplantation centers and sometimes in emergency operating rooms. It is therefore advisable for the surgical unit responsible for liver harvesting to provide basic surgical equipment and suture materials with which it is familiar, in addition to preservation liquids which are the responsibility of the transplant team. The operation is performed with the simultaneous removal of other transplantation organs, usually the heart and kidneys[9,10] and sometimes also the lungs and pancreas.[6] Before starting the operation, if the various teams are not used to working together, they should pre-plan the operation in order to adapt the technique to their own particular procedures.

Technique

The basic technique for liver procurement consists of mobilization of the liver with division of its ligaments, dissection of the bile duct, the portal vein trunk, the hepatic artery as far as the celiac triad and the inferior vena cava above and below the liver. When the heart is perfused with cardioplegic solution, the abdominal organs are washed with a hypothermic preservation solution. The liver is then removed and its vascular pedicles are definitively isolated on the bench and prepared for anastomosis. During liver removal, the dissection maneuvers must respect the anatomical structures of the liver and those of other abdominal organs, with the respective vascular pedicles, which must all be removed during the same operation.

The main difficulty in liver removal is due to the large number of possible anatomical variations of the hepatic artery.[7,11] 'Normal' anatomy, i.e. a hepatic artery arising from the celiac triad, is present in only 60-75% of cases. The most frequent variations encountered are a left hepatic artery arising from the left gastric artery, a right hepatic artery arising from the superior mesenteric artery and a common hepatic artery arising from the superior mesenteric artery. These anomalies can exist individually or in various combinations (see Chapter 23). It is essential that the surgeon responsible for organ removal knows how to recognize these variations and to preserve these vessels during the operation so as not to jeopardize the subsequent transplant.[3,4]

The donor operation, as described below, is the standard technique applied in hemodynamically stable donors.[9,10] The operation can be modified to a 'rapid' or 'super-rapid' technique if the donor becomes unstable before or during removal or in the event of technical accidents which make continuation of the operation problematic.

Multiorgan removal is started by the cardiosurgical team which carries out sternotomy, opens the pericardium and isolates the large intrapericardial vessels. At the end of this first stage, the surgical field is handed over to the surgeon who has to remove the liver. This is followed by median laparotomy as far as the pubis. The umbilical ligament and the falciform ligament are divided. The diaphragm is divided bilaterally by cautery at the anterior insertion points of the muscle in the thoracic wall, in order to widen the exposure of the abdominal cavity which is subsequently kept open with a large Belfour retractor. The transverse bilateral extension (the so-called 'cross' incision) is thus not necessary even if the kidneys are to be removed. Even if the donor is not suitable for removal of the heart, sternotomy is advisable for better access and a better view of the abdomen.

The liver is inspected and palpated to detect any steatosis, oedema or possible focal lesions not revealed by the instrumental examinations. The lesser omentum is inspected to find a left hepatic artery arising from the left gastric artery which must be removed intact together with the liver. Attention now turns to the pedicle, in search of a possible right hepatic artery arising from the superior mesenteric artery. The presence of this artery can be detected by palpating the hepatic pedicle with the left hand, squeezing it between the thumb and the index finger: the presence of a right hepatic artery is revealed by pulsation posterior to the portal vein and to the main bile duct. It should however be remembered that this artery can be masked by the lymph nodes of the hepatic pedicle and its pulsation may not be felt in the event of donor hypotension. It is, therefore, advisable, especially for surgeons without much experience, to proceed as if a right hepatic artery were present, ascertaining whether it does in fact exist during the final stages of removal or during bench surgery.

Due to the frequent hemodynamic alterations of patients with irreversible brain damage, and so as not to lose the organs if these alterations should occur during the operation, the first surgical maneuvers should aim to control the vessels which allow a rapid perfusion of the abdominal organs: the aorta and inferior mesenteric vein. The intestine is retracted cranially to expose the posterior peritoneum. The aorta is identified at the bifurcation with the iliac arteries and the posterior peritoneum is incised by cautery. After reaching the iliac bifurcation, the aorta is isolated as far as the inferior mesenteric artery, which is ligated so that unnecessary organs are not perfused with the preservation solution. Exploration of the aorta for a few centimeters immediately above the inferior mesenteric artery may reveal the presence of accessory renal polar arteries which should be left intact during the subsequent removal of the kidneys. The aorta is encircled immediately above the iliac arteries with two strong ligatures (1 or 2), the most distal of which must ligate the aorta while the proximal one will fix the cannula in the artery for the perfusion. The intestine is rotated towards the patient's right to visualize the inferior mesenteric vein at the level of the ligament of Treitz. The inferior mesenteric vein can be easily identified; it should be isolated and encircled with two 3-0 threads.

The next stage consists of isolation of the aorta below the diaphragm. The left triangular ligament is divided by cautery. The lesser omentum is opened and divided after excluding the presence of a left hepatic artery, which must be respected if present. Moderate traction on the left lobe makes it possible to expose the diaphragmatic crura and the abdominal esophagus. The crura are divided by cautery after retracting the esophagus upwards and towards the patient's left. The aorta is then isolated for a few centimeters and encircled with a tape. The abdominal organs can now be perfused through the aorta and the liver through the portal system in the event of hemodynamic instability or cardiac arrest.

To prevent dispersion of the perfusion liquid, and as subsequent landmarks during dissection, the gastroduodenal artery, the left gastric artery and the splenic artery are usually ligated and divided. The gastroduodenal artery is easily identified above the first portion of the duodenum after dividing the hepatoduodenal ligament and ligating the pyloric veins. Division of this artery does not impair perfusion of the pancreas due to the presence of the collateral circulation provided by the superior mesenteric artery. Division of the thin layer of peritoneum above the upper margin of the pancreas guides the surgeon directly to the celiac triad. This maneuver must be carried out with care to prevent damage to the proper hepatic artery, which runs just above this. The left gastric artery is isolated, ligated and divided a few centimeters above its emergence, where it is clearly visible, so as not to damage the celiac triad. In the presence of an accessory left hepatic artery, division should be distal to the emergence of the artery. A left hepatic artery, either replaced or accessory, can arise from the left gastric artery in about 15% of cases. This vessel is clearly visible where it crosses the upper part of the gastro-hepatic ligament. It is preserved by ligation of the gastric artery branches peripherically at the level of the lesser curvature of the stomach. It is advisable to complete the preparation of the left gastric artery at this time rather than on the back table, in order to facilitate the further dissection of the supraceliac aorta. The splenic artery is identified, isolated and ligated above the upper margin of the pancreas unless the pancreas is to be removed as it is indispensable for perfusion of this organ.

Attention now returns to the hepatic pedicle to wash out the bile tract. The common bile duct is isolated immediately above the head of the pancreas and the most distal part is ligated while the proximal part is left open to allow the bile to drain out. The fundus of the gallbladder is opened by cautery, the bile is aspirated and the gallbladder is irrigated with cold saline solution to completely remove any bile left in the main bile duct. Clear liquid running out of the open common bile duct confirms the efficacy of the lavage (*Figure 26.1*).

These maneuvers complete the dissection for removal of the liver in hemodynamically stable

LIVER PROCUREMENT FOR TRANSPLANTATION

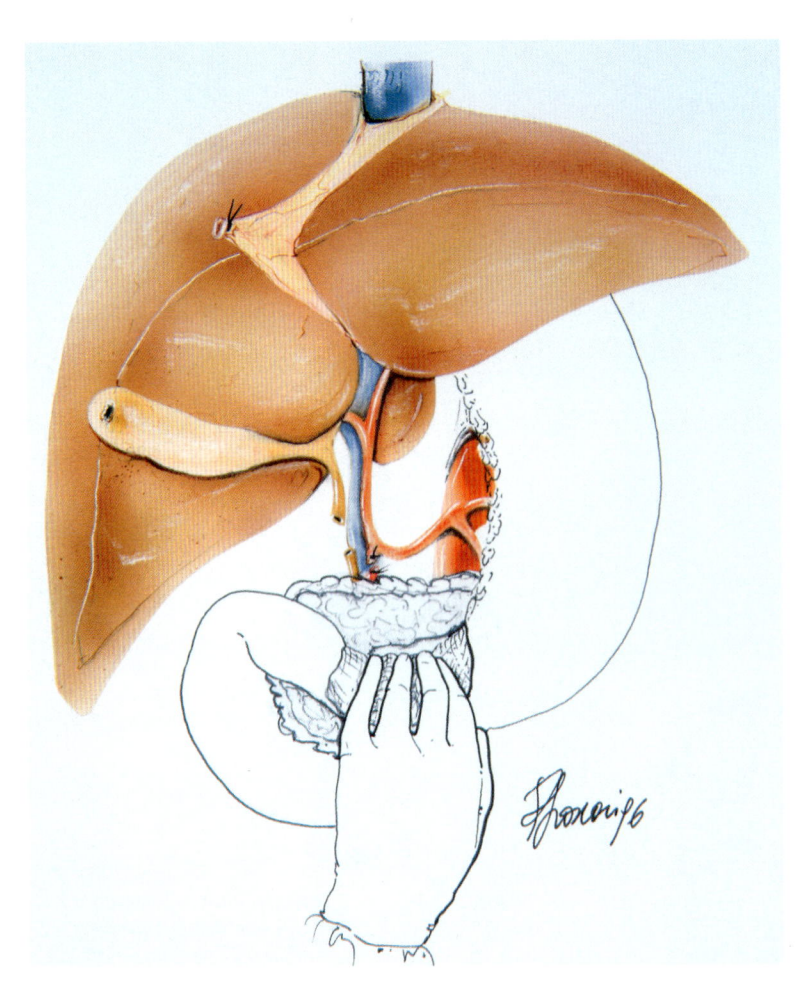

Figure 26.1 –
Liver procurement for transplantation. After isolating the aorta below the diaphragm and distally at the level of the bifurcation, the gastroduodenal artery is ligated and divided and the bile duct is divided.

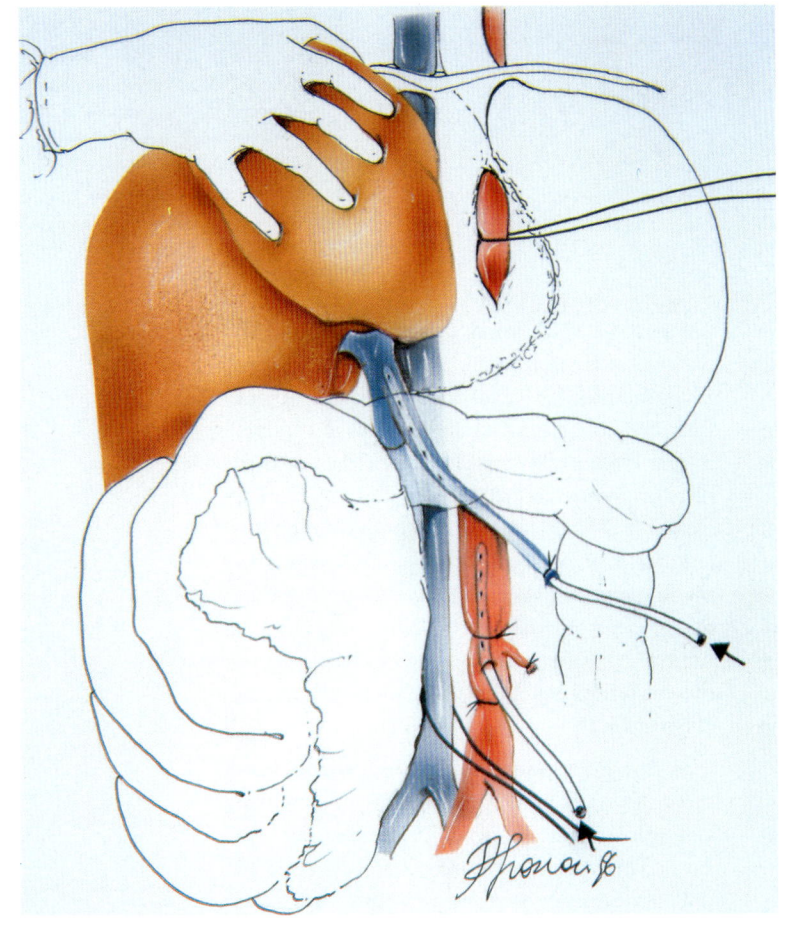

Figure 26.2 – *Cannulation of the aorta and portal vein through the inferior mesenteric vein.*

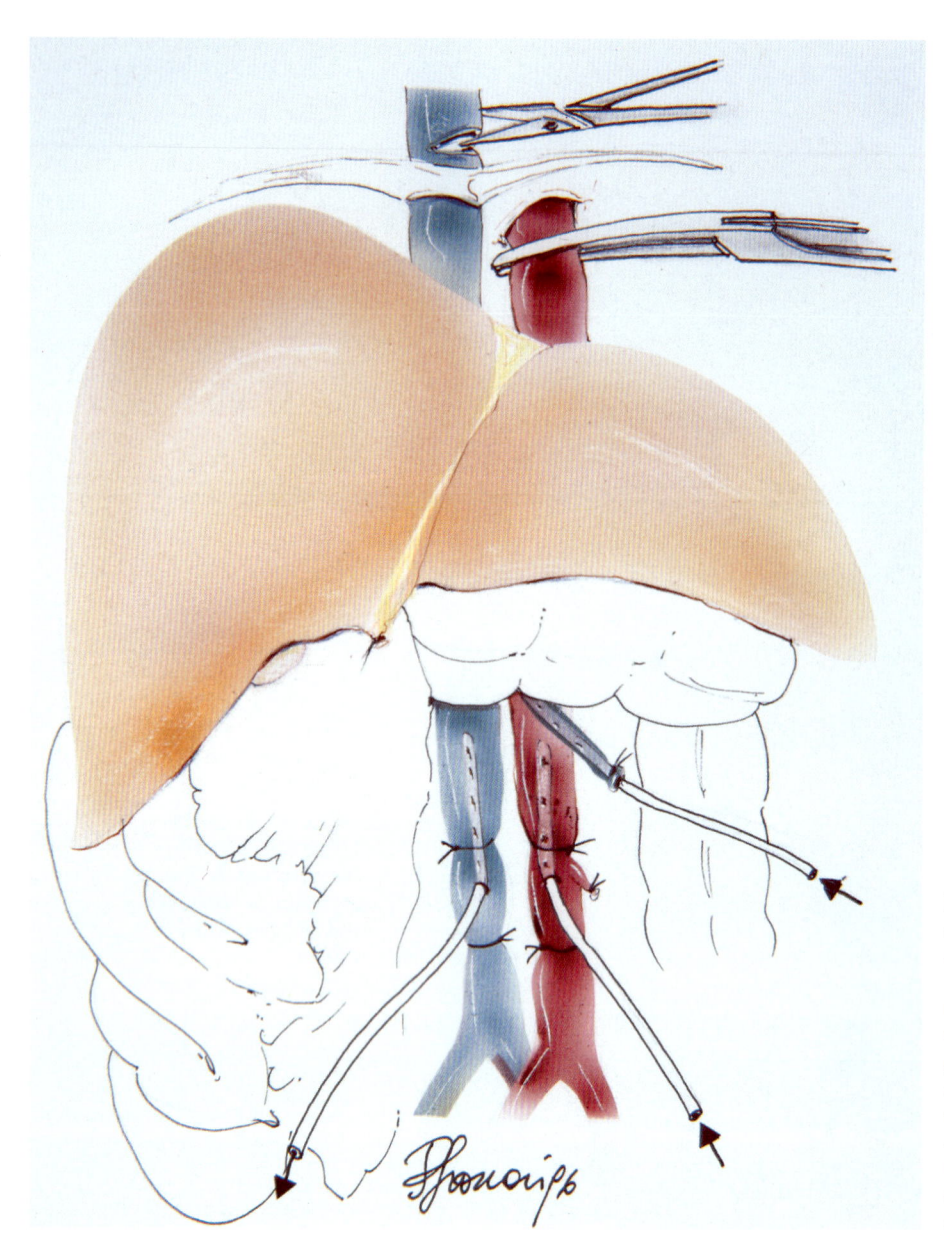

Figure 26.3 – *Flushing of the liver through the aorta and inferior mesenteric vein. The perfusion liquid is flushed through the inferior vena cava which is divided inside the pericardium. The figure shows a cannula inside the subhepatic vena cava for the drainage of the perfusion liquid. Cannulation of the vena cava is in fact no longer carried out in current practice.*

donors. In some cases surgeons who have also to remove the kidneys prefer to carry out a preliminary isolation of the organs and ureters before perfusion. If this is not done, the donor is heparinized and the cannula for portal perfusion is inserted in the inferior mesenteric vein as far as the portal vein; palpation of the hepatic pedicle during this maneuver allows the position of the cannula to be checked in the portal trunk. The aorta is then ligated at the iliac bifurcation, clamped with a De Bakey clamp a few centimeters above and the cannula for aorta perfusion in inserted. The cannula is kept in place by fixing it with the previously positioned ligature (**Figure 26.2**).

The cardiac surgeon then clamps the intrapericardial aorta and infuses the cardioplegic solution. At the same time, the previously isolated part of the aorta, below the diaphragm, is closed with a strong tie or a De Bakey clamp. Hypothermic lavage of the splanchnic organs from the aortic cannula and the portal cannula is simultaneously carried out. The cardiac surgeon now clamps the inferior vena cava intrapericardially for 1 or 2 seconds to open the left atrium in a bloodless zone. This maintains the drainage of the cardioplegic solution and of the blood from the heart. When the clamp is removed, this route is also used for drainage of the perfusion liquid of the abdominal organs (**Figure 26.3**).

The first descriptions of multiorgan procurement foresaw the positioning of a third abdominal cannula inside the inferior vena cava. This cannula permitted the drainage of the abdominal perfusion liquid and was

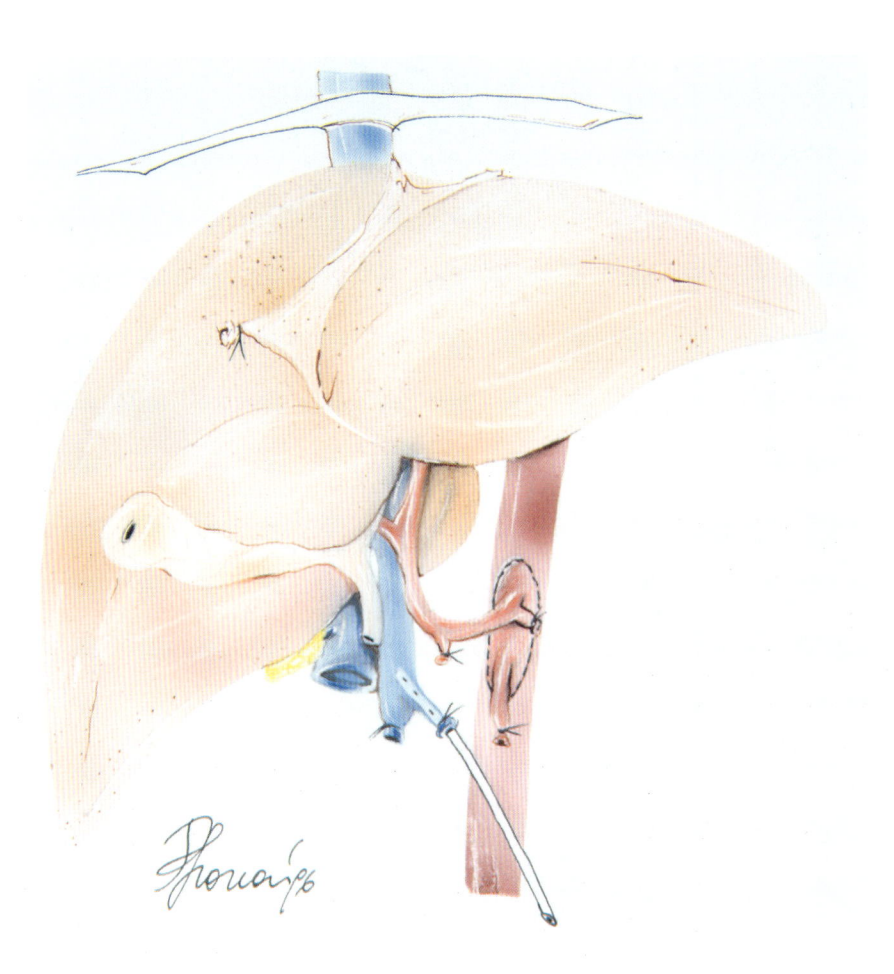

Figure 26.4 – *After flushing the liver, the celiac triad is removed with a Carrell patch.*

necessary since the surgeons kept the inferior vena cava clamped intrapericardially throughout the removal of the heart. The change in approach of cardiac surgeons in the last few years has made positioning of this cannula unnecessary.

The preservation solution used for the abdominal organs is the University of Wisconsin solution (UW, Viaspan®). The use of UW solution allows the graft to be preserved safely for up to 18 hours, although the ideal time acceptable to most transplant teams is less than 13 hours.[12] Three liters of UW solution inserted through the aortic cannula and 1 litre inserted through the inferior mesenteric vein are generally sufficient to achieve good perfusion of all the abdominal organs. During this perfusion, the cardiac surgeon terminates cardioplegia and removes the heart. The abdomen is in the meantime irrigated with a slush of ice and cold water. We prefer not to place the liver in direct contact with the ice, merely washing the organ with a few liters of cold solution.

Once the heart has been removed, attention returns to the abdomen. At this point the abdominal field is completely bloodless. The first maneuver is the repositioning of the portal cannula from the inferior mesenteric vein to the main trunk of the portal vein. Palpation of this cannula inside the pedicle allows easy identification of the trunk of the portal vein, which is clamped as far as the splenomesenteric confluence taking care not to damage the head of the pancreas if this is to be removed. The splenic and superior mesenteric veins are now clamped. The outlet of the inferior mesenteric vein varies: it may arise in an isolated position from the splenic or superior mesenteric vein. The cannula removed from the inferior mesenteric vein is now positioned in the portal vein through the stump of the superior mesenteric vein, taking care to ligate the remaining vessels draining into the portal vein. Brief isolation of the posterior part of the portal vein, by lifting it upwards, allows rapid inspection of the posterior part of the hepatic pedicle where an accessory right hepatic artery may be present arising from the superior mesenteric artery.

The operation continues with mobilization of the celiac triad. If not done previously, the splenic and left gastric arteries are now divided. The left margin of the aorta is isolated starting from the top, taking care to exert slight

TECHNIQUES IN LIVER SURGERY

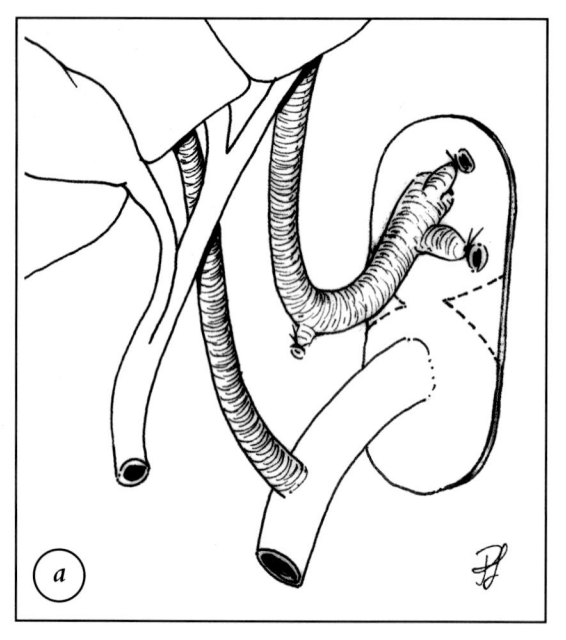

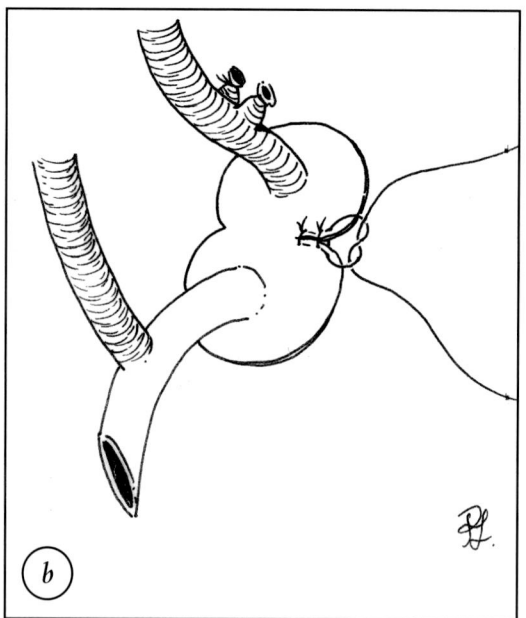

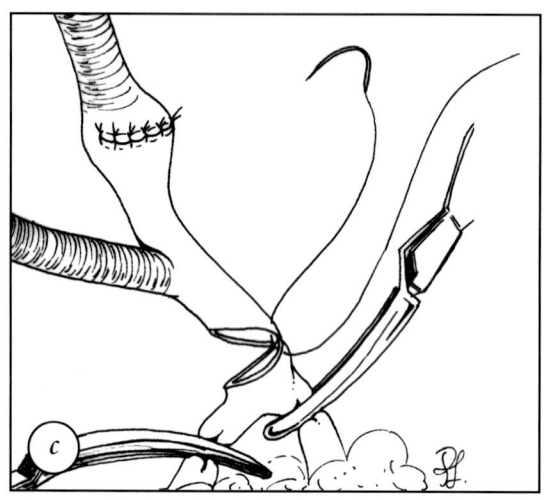

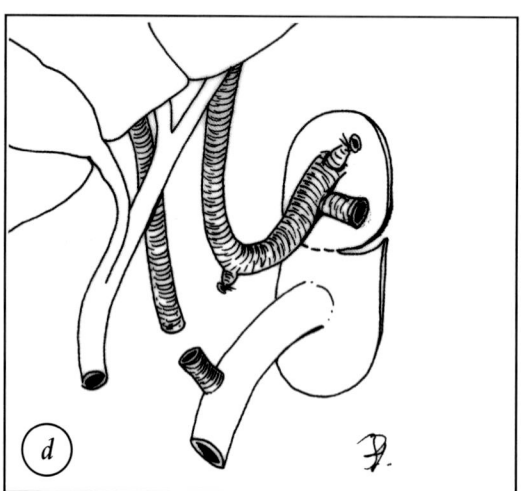

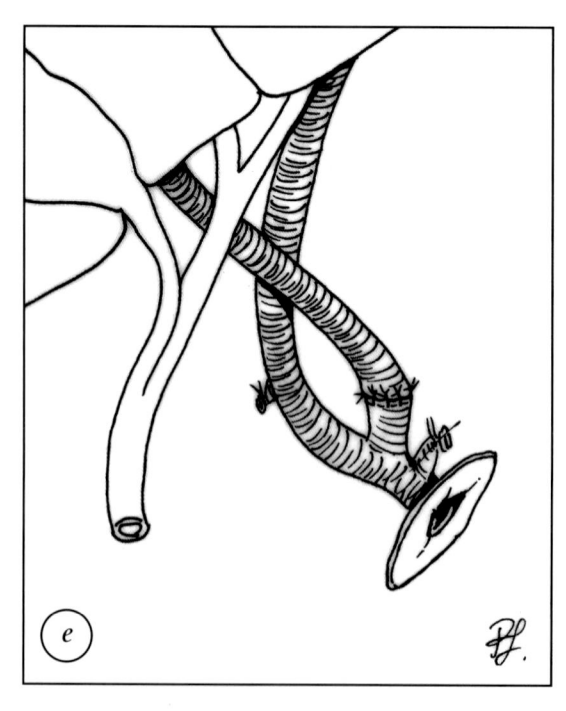

Figure 26.5 – *Arterial reconstruction in the presence of a right hepatic artery arising from the superior mesenteric artery. **a–c)** The most common option is anastomosis of the orifice of the celiac triad with the orifice of the superior mesenteric artery with interrupted Prolene® 5-0 stitches. The distal stump of the superior mesenteric artery will be used for the anastomosis in the recipient. **d–e)** Anastomosis from the right hepatic artery with the stump of the splenic artery. The anastomosis is constructed with interrupted Prolene® 6-0 stitches. This technique is systematically adopted in the event of accidental injury to the right hepatic artery during harvesting or in simultaneous harvesting of the whole pancreas. If there is a discrepancy between the size of the right hepatic artery and the splenic artery, the former can be anastomosed with the gastroduodenal artery.*

pressure on the stumps of the splenic artery and left gastric artery towards the patient's right, dividing the diaphragmatic crura. It is thus easy to reach first the emergence of the celiac triad, which must be left intact and untouched by the instruments, and then the superior mesenteric artery. A short piece of the latter is isolated, exerting slight downward pressure on the pancreas so as not to damage it, for a further check for the presence of an accessory right hepatic artery. The superior mesenteric artery is divided and followed as far as its emergence from the aorta. The anterior wall of the abdominal aorta is then divided obliquely upwards, to respect the emergence of the renal arteries at this point, including the celiac triad with a Carrel patch (*Figure 26.4*).

The subhepatic inferior vena cava is then identified and divided just above the outlet of the renal veins and below the outlet of the suprarenal vein. The liver is finally removed from the abdomen, dissecting a wide part of the diaphragm, which includes both the intrapericardial inferior vena cava (divided previously by the cardiac surgeons) and the insertion of the right triangular ligament, and the retroperitoneal tissues, including the right adrenal gland, without getting too close to the area of the hepatic artery and, if possible, without damaging the pancreas if this has to be removed. The liver is placed in bags for transportation after bench perfusion with another liter of UW, in which it is left immersed. 5 liters of UW solution are therefore sufficient for removal of the liver. Before completing the operation, segments as long as possible of the iliac arteries, including the bifurcation, and of the iliac veins must be removed; these can be used as vascular grafts in the event of anatomical problems during the transplantation stage.[8]

The *rapid procurement technique* is indicated if sharp drops in donor hemodynamics occur during procurement which can compromise the vitality of the liver. The operation requires cannulization of the distal aorta and the inferior mesenteric vein and the preparation of a section of the supraceliac aorta so that clamping can be carried out without further dissection of the hepatic pedicle. Once perfusion of the splanchnic organs is complete, the artery is isolated as far as the triad. The origin of the superior mesenteric artery and a portion of the head of the pancreas are removed *en bloc* in case a right hepatic artery is present. The posterior portion of the diaphragm and the inferior vena cava are then divided.

BACK TABLE PROCEDURE

The final preparation of the graft is carried out in a basin containing the preservation liquid used to perfuse the liver and, separated by a plastic bag, sterile ice slush. At this stage, all the other tissues included in the procurement (diaphragm, lymph nodes, pancreas, right adrenal gland) are removed. The three diaphragmatic veins are sutured, as is the suprarenal vein. The vascular cuffs are prepared for anastomoses with ligation of the portal vein and hepatic artery collaterals.

BENCH RECONSTRUCTION OF A RIGHT HEPATIC ARTERY ARISING FROM THE SUPERIOR MESENTERIC ARTERY

Reconstruction of the right hepatic artery arising from the superior mesenteric artery is carried out during bench surgery. We usually perform anastomosis with interrupted 6-0 stitches of the celiac triad stump with the orifice of the mesenteric artery as described by Gordon and Shaw.[2] Anastomosis on the recipient artery will then be constructed on the distal stump of the donor superior mesenteric artery (*Figure 26.5a-c*). An alternative technique is end-to-end anastomosis with the stump of the splenic artery[1] (*Figure 26.5d,e*).

SIMULTANEOUS LIVER AND PANCREAS PROCUREMENT

When the pancreas is to be used for transplant of the entire organ, it can be removed individually, after removal of the liver, or *en bloc* together with the liver. The problems involved in these two methods are very similar and are therefore discussed together. The surgeons performing the removal operation must decide which technique to use. The problem of procuring both liver and pancreas from the same donor is represented by the vascular pedicles which the organs have in common, and in particular the portal vein, celiac triad and superior mesenteric artery. Drainage of the preservation liquid during perfusion of the abdominal organs is through the portal vein. In order not to over-distend the pancreas during cold perfusion, it is advisable to open the portal vein during this stage so as to discharge this pressure. The technical variation which should therefore be performed during isolation of the liver is isolation of the vena cava, encircling it with tape or a tourniquet and positioning the cannula inside the vein as is usually done through the inferior mesenteric vein. The portal vein can thus be opened after the first liter of aortic perfusion about 1 cm above the upper margin of the pancreas, without modifying the portal perfusion which can continue through the portal cannula interrupted at the portal vein by the tourniquet. The problem of the arteries is different and there is no single technique for their reconstruction. For total pancreatic transplant both the splenic and superior mesenteric arteries are necessary. The Carrel patch of the triad is generally kept for the liver transplant. The arterial pedicle of the pancreas must therefore be reconstructed on the bench, interposing the iliac bifurcation taken from the same donor between the splenic and superior mesenteric arteries, or anastomizing the splenic artery directly to the superior mesenteric artery.[5] Likewise, the portal vein can be lengthened with a segment of iliac vein taken from the same donor.

PITFALLS

The macroscopic aspect is one of the best indicators of liver function. Before starting the removal procedure, a careful visual and manual exploration of the organ is necessary, evaluating consistency and degree of fatty infiltration and fibrosis.

Dissection of the subdiaphragmatic aorta can cause accidental rupture of a diaphragmatic vein. This can be particularly tedious due to the difficulty in achieving satisfactory hemostasis in a usually extremely limited space. In such cases manual packing or the use of sterile dressings is sufficient to successfully complete the removal. The main problem in liver procurement is, however, linked to the recognition and preservation of accessory hepatic arteries, whose presence is very frequent. The surgeon must be extremely familiar with the vascular anatomy of the hepatic pedicle and the main anatomical variations. Accidental division of these arteries is common if they are not correctly recognized and has dramatic consequences on the outcome of the transplant. When an accessory right hepatic artery is divided during the removal procedure and this is recognized before the transplant, it must be reconstructed during preparation of the liver on the back table. The accessory artery can be anastomized either to the stump of the gastroduodenal artery, if this is long enough, or to the stump of the splenic artery with interrupted stitches of 7-0 vascular threads.

Another problem is represented by the suprahepatic inferior vena cava. For this vessel there is a degree of competition between the cardiac and liver surgeons. It is advisable for the liver surgeon always to exert slight pressure downwards on the hepatic dome at clamping of the intrapericardial inferior vena cava, so the portion of the vein removed is as long as possible.

The UW solution leads to bradycardia and cardiac arrest if released into the circulation before clamping of the aorta. During positioning of the cannulas inside the inferior mesenteric vein and the aorta, it is therefore necessary to make sure that the perfusion solution flow routes are completely closed.

Excessive traction during the final stages of organ removal, especially at the level of the right triangular ligament, can cause tearing of the parenchyma.

REFERENCES

1. Casavilla A, Gordon RD, Starzl TE. Techniques of liver transplantation. In: Blumgart L.H. Surgery of the liver and biliary tract, Churchill Livingstone, Edinburgh, 1994, pp. 1863-1888.
2. Gordon RD, Shaw BW, Iwatsuki S, Todo S, Starzl TE. A simplified technique for revascularization of homografts of the liver with a variant right hepatic artery from the superior mesenteric artery. *Surg Gynecol Obstetr* 1985; **160**: 475-476.
3. Hiatt JR, Gabbay J, Busuttil RW. Surgical anatomy of the hepatic arteries in 1000 cases. *Ann Surg* 1994; **220**: 50-52.
4. Mäkisalo H, Chaib E, Krokos N, Calne R. Hepatic arterial variations and liver-related diseases of 100 consecutive donors. *Transplant Internat* 1993; **6**: 325-329.
5. Marsh CL, Perkins JD, Sutherland DER, Corry RJ, Sterioff S. Combined hepatic and pancreaticoduodenal procurement for transplantation. *Surg Gynecol Obstetr* 1989; **168**: 254-258.
6. Mazziotti A, Jovine E, Bellusci R *et al.* Il prelievo multiorgano da cadavere per trapianto. *Chirurgia* 1990; **3**: 135-146.
7. Michels NA. Newer anatomy of the liver and its variant blood supply and collateral circulation. *Am J Surg* 1966; **112**: 337-347.
8. Shaw BW, Iwatsuki S, Bron K, Starzl TE. Portal vein grafts in hepatic tranplantation. *Surg Gynecol Obstetr* 1985; **161**: 67-68.
9. Starzl TE, Hakala TR, Shaw BW *et al.* A flexible procedure for multiple cadaveric organ procurement. *Surg Gynecol Obstetr* 1984; **158**: 223-230.
10. Starzl TE, Miller C, Broznick B, Makowa L. An improved technique for multiple organ harvesting. *Surg Gynecol Obstetr* 1987; **165**: 343-348.
11. Suzuki T, Nakayasu A, Kawabe K. Surgical significance of anatomic variations of the hepatic artery. *Am J Surg* 1971; **112**: 505-512.
12. Vix J, Compagnon Ph, Beller JP, Jack D, Wolf Ph, Boudjema K. Liver grafts can be preserved overnight. *Liver Transpl Surg* 1996; **2**: 105-110.

27
Conventional Transplantation Technique

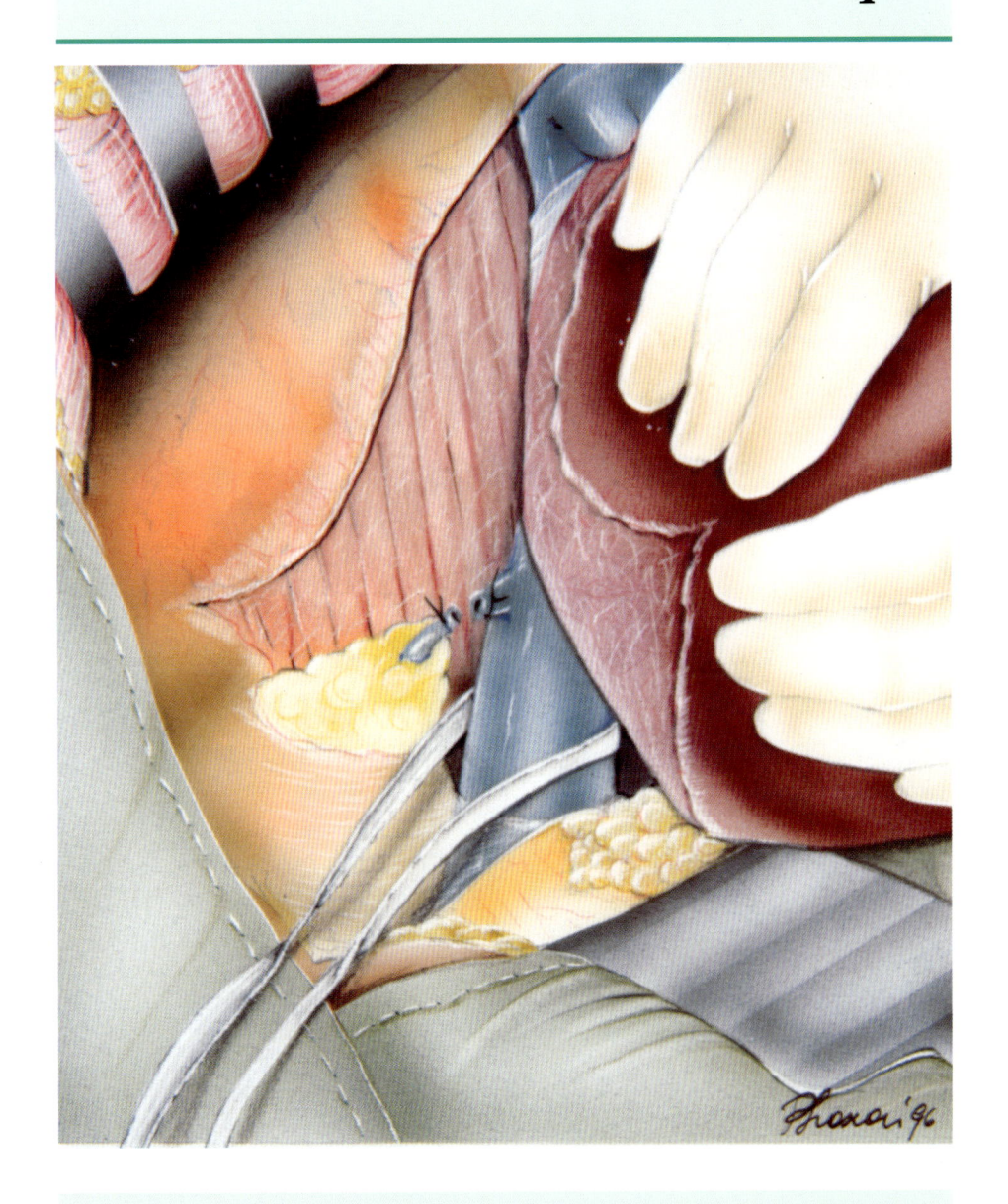

CONVENTIONAL TRANSPLANT TECHNIQUE

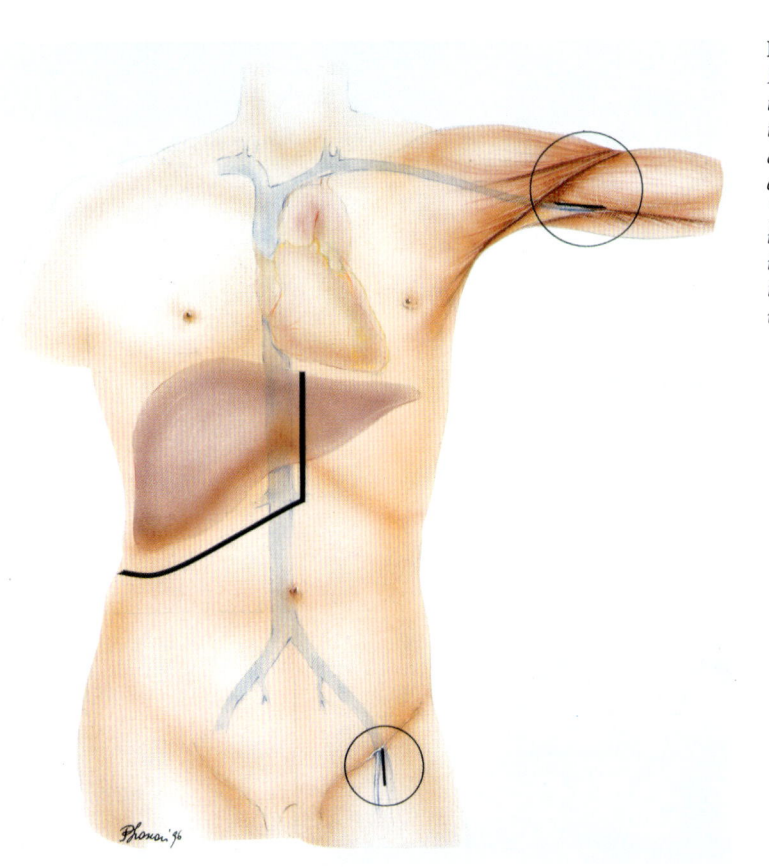

Figure 27.1 –
Incisions for conventional technique of liver transplantation. The abdominal approach in conventional cases is the 'J incision'. The circles indicate the axillary and inguinal incisions for the insertion of the venous bypass.

Liver transplantation has become a common operation in an increasing number of centers and is widely used as a cure for end-stage liver disease. The technique described by Starzl is accepted worldwide and has undergone a few modifications and adaptations for particular circumstances, such as venous grafts for portal thrombosis, reduced-size livers or the 'piggyback' technique which does not interrupt recipient caval flow. From a strictly technical point of view, transplantation has provided important contributions to the entire field of liver surgery and has opened the way to the most advanced techniques of extended hepatectomies and the new frontiers of 'extreme' liver surgery.

Liver transplantation closely follows the technique introduced by Starzl which is the technical foundation of liver transplantation, adopted by the majority of surgical teams throughout the world with minor variations. The stages of the recipient operation and the surgical strategy are modified to take into account the type of disease, prior surgery or other particular conditions such as portal thrombosis or anomalies of the arterial hepatic vascularization.[1]

The following is the description of the basic technique of adult liver transplantation.

Technique

ABDOMINAL INCISION AND EXPOSURE

Before beginning abdominal incision, the access routes for the venous bypass must be prepared: the saphenous vein is isolated at its outlet from the femoral vein, ligating some of its collaterals; the axillary vein is isolated at the apex of the axilla for 3-4 cm. Both these veins are isolated on the left where it is easier to place the bypass circuit and the Bio-Pump.

The abdominal incision most commonly used in adult liver transplantation is the bilateral subcostal incision, extended to the left as far as the mid clavicular line, to the right as far as the mid axillary line and on the median line as far as the xiphoid cartilage. Two wide retractors raise the rib arches. This incision, ('Mercedes' incision) provides complete exposure of the liver and the subdiaphragmatic space. Extension of the incision towards the left is in effect not always necessary and may lead to post-operative respiratory complications such as atelectasis and bilateral pleural effusion. In our department, over the last 2 years 90% of adult transplants have been performed with the subcostal J incision, which extends from the median line about 5 cm from the xiphoid cartilage and deviates to the right 2 cm from the rib margin as far as the posterior axillary line. The Kent retractor is particularly useful in allowing traction on the right costal margin and on the abdominal wall to the left, thus providing the same degree of exposure as the bilateral subcostal incision (**Figure 27.1**). By

TECHNIQUES IN LIVER SURGERY

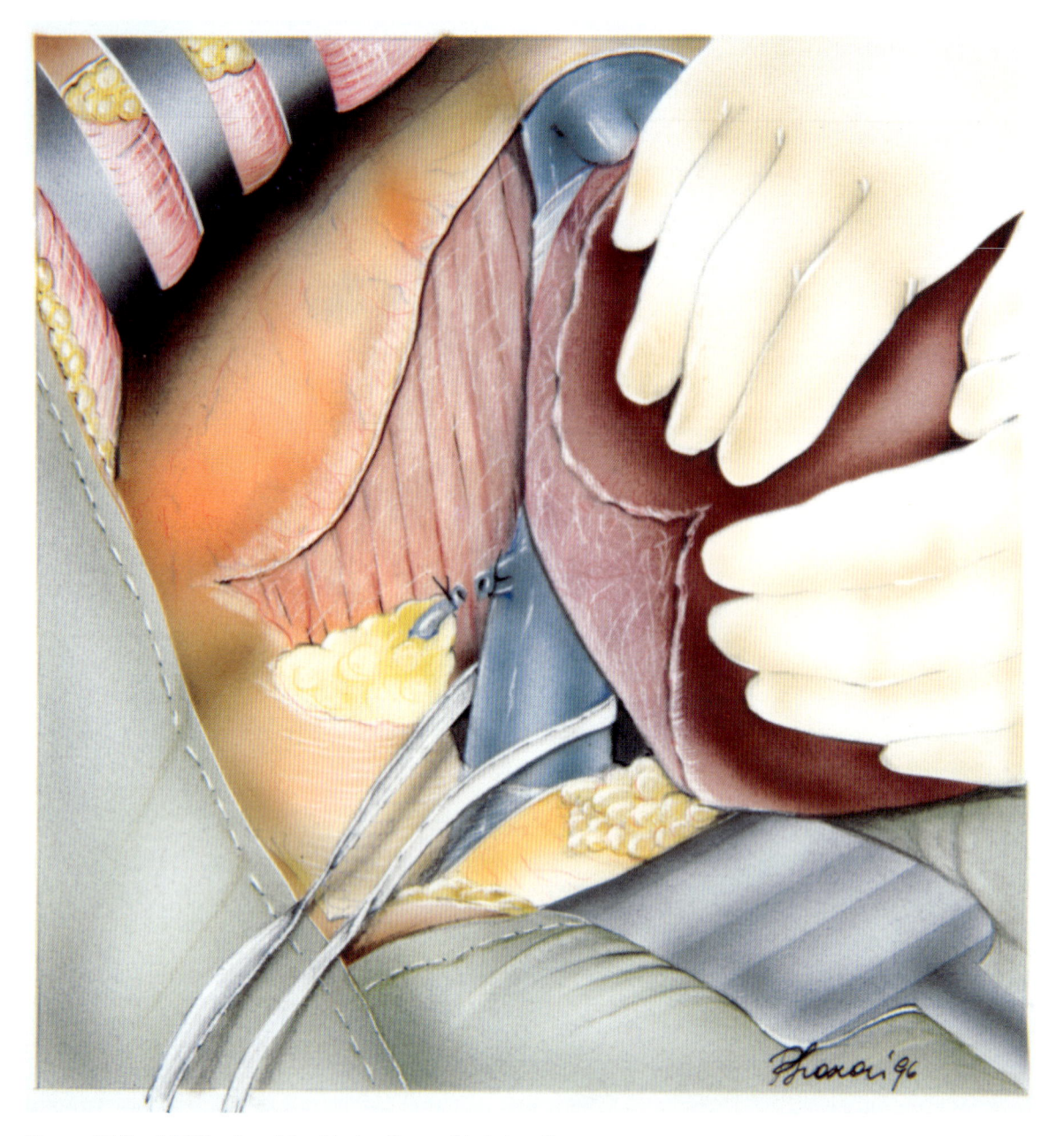

Figure 27.2 – *Mobilization of the right hemiliver and isolation of the lower vena cava. The right adrenal vein is ligated and divided.*

using the J incision we have observed a marked reduction in pulmonary complications and abdominal eventration. In our experience, the bilateral subcostal incision is employed in patients who have already undergone surgery or in the presence of an 'oversized' graft.

The umbilical ligament containing the often greatly dilated vein is ligated and divided. The falciform ligament is divided by cautery, ligating dilated vessels and lymphatics when necessary. Division of the falciform ligament proceeds as far as the two posterior layers, where the loose connective tissue surrounding the upper vena cava is encountered. The lesser omentum is divided, taking care to identify a left hepatic artery which runs along the upper part of the ligament which is generally clearly evident. If this artery exists (20% of cases) it must be ligated and divided.

HILAR DISSECTION

Hilar dissection starts with incision of the anterior peritoneal layer of the hepatoduodenal ligament, staying close to the hepatic margin. The dividing branches of the hepatic artery are ligated, followed by the common bile duct.

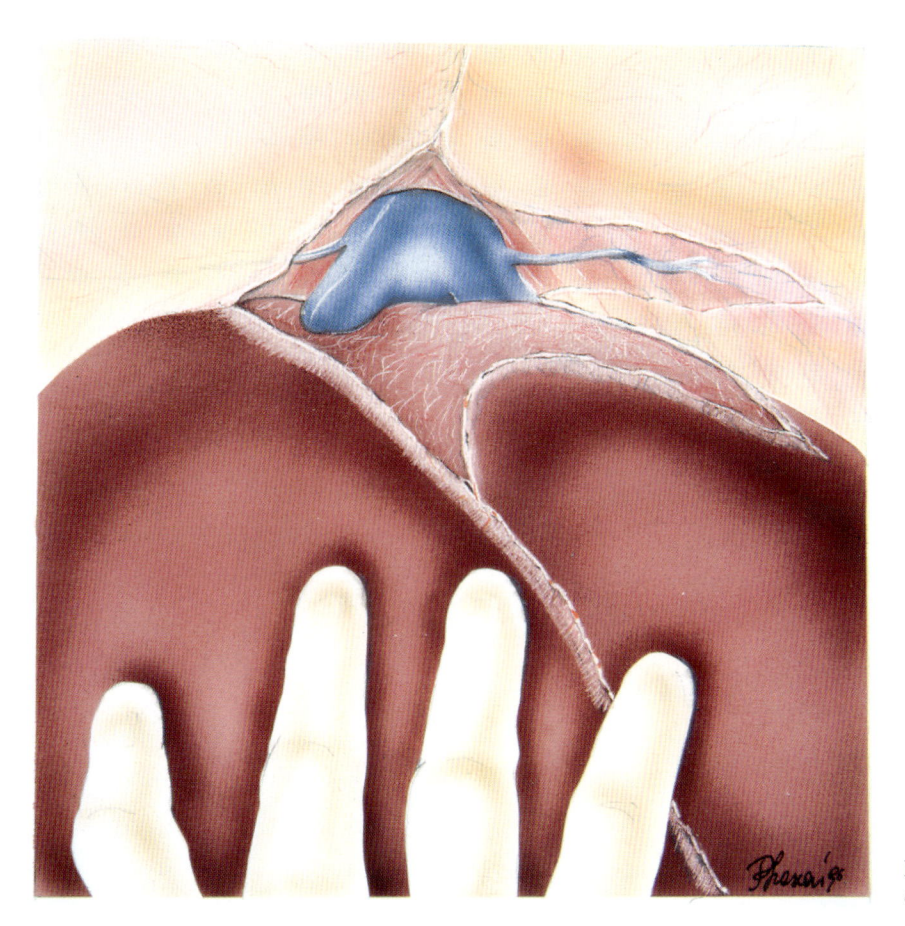

Figure 27.3 – *Detachment of the upper vena cava*

Freeing of the hepatic artery is completed at this stage, ligating the pyloric artery and proceeding proximally until the gastroduodenal artery is encountered. The common hepatic artery is freed for about 2 cm, taking care not to detach the surrounding periadventitial tissue thereby preventing vasospasm. The gastroduodenal artery is also followed for about 1.5 cm, and it is here, at the outlet of the gastroduodenal artery, that the anastomosis will be constructed with the Carrell patch of the donor artery. This preliminary freeing of the hepatic artery will reduce the arterial ischemia time after portal revascularization of the graft and also makes freeing of the portal vein easier. The portal trunk is completely detached from the lymphatic tissue and is followed distally as far as the bifurcation where the vein will be divided and the cannula inserted for the bypass.

DIVISION OF THE TRIANGULAR LIGAMENTS AND PREPARATION OF THE VENA CAVA

Once the hepatoduodenal ligament has been skeletonized, mobilization of the liver continues by dividing the triangular ligaments. The left and right ligaments are incised by cautery, and the posterior aspect of the liver is gradually detached from the diaphragm and the right adrenal gland. Dissection must be carried out very carefully here to avoid penetrating the suprarenal capsule and to avoid hemorrhage which is sometimes a complication. The right adrenal vein is ligated and divided and the posterior aspect of the retrohepatic vena cava can now be detached (***Figure 27.2***). Detachment of the vein above the liver continues in order to obtain as long a segment of vena cava as possible (***Figure 27.3***). To completely encircle the vein its left margin

TECHNIQUES IN LIVER SURGERY

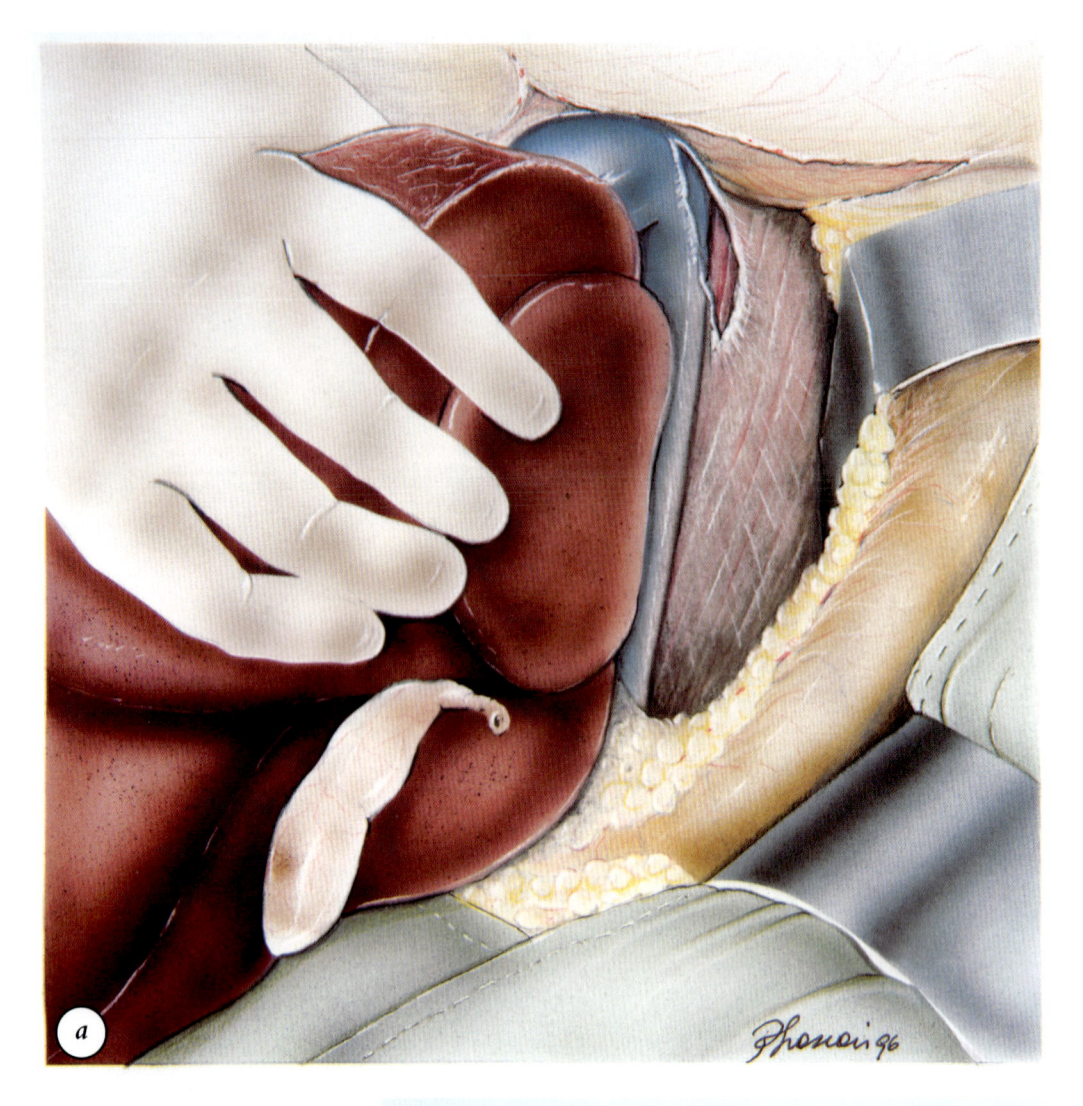

Figure 27.4 – *a) Division of the posterior peritoneum along the left margin of the vena cava. b) The upper vena cava is encircled.*

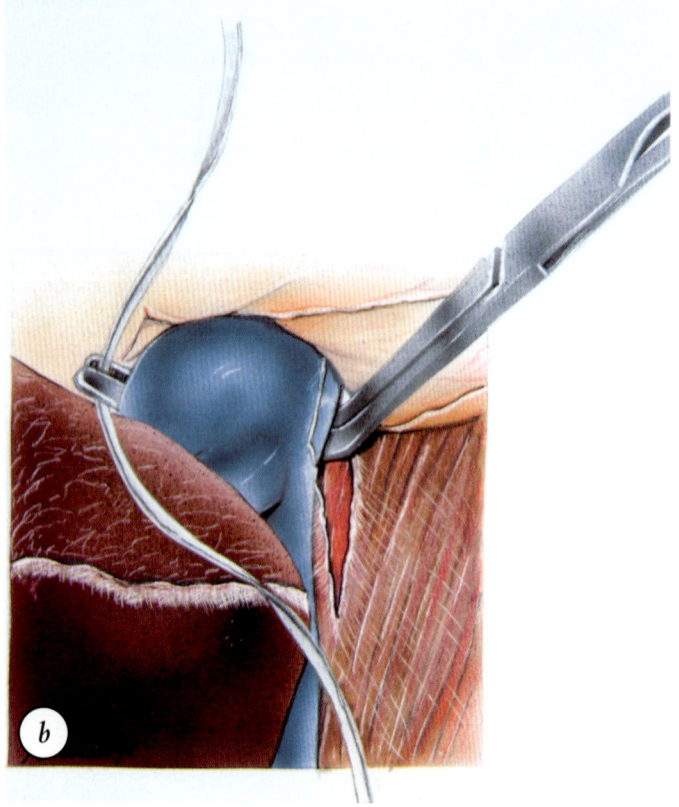

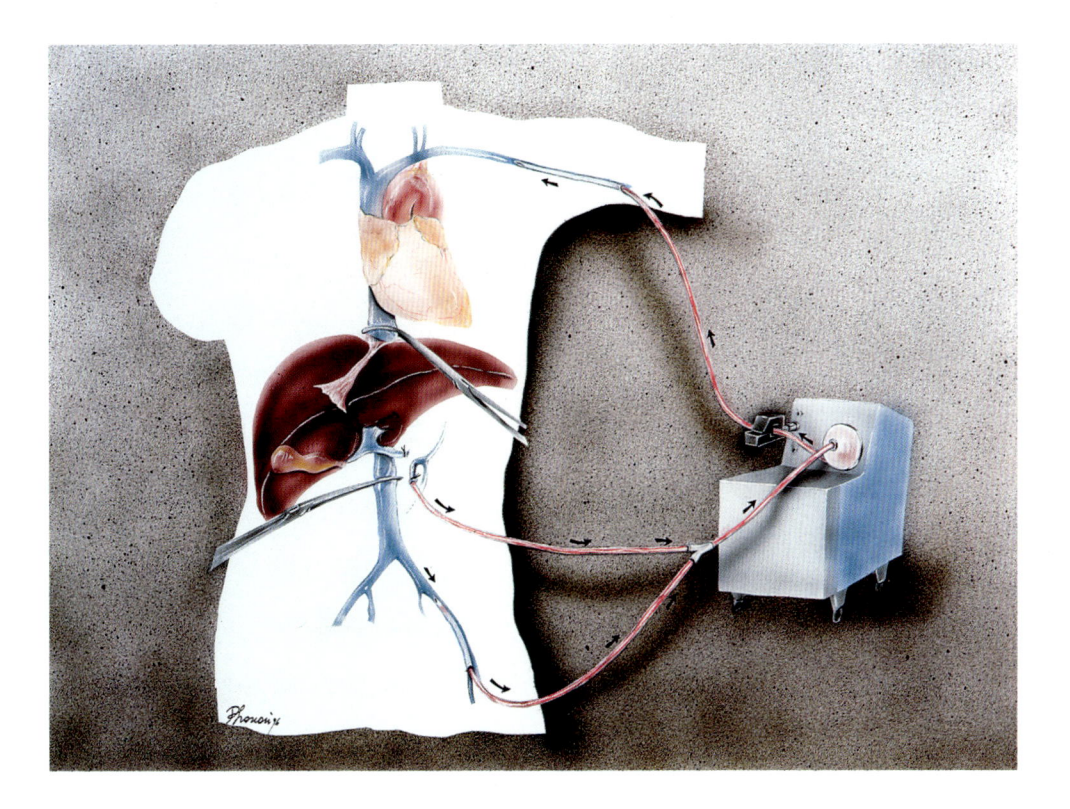

Figure 27.5 – *Diagram of the venous bypass*

must be freed, below the caudate lobe, after dividing the posterior peritoneal layer. It is now possible to pass behind the liver with a wide sling and encircle the upper vena cava (**Figure 27.4**). Distal detachment of the vena cava is easier after division of the posterior peritoneum. At this point it can be useful to ligate the most distal vein of the caudate lobe in order to obtain a longer segment of lower vena cava.

VENOUS BYPASS

Venous bypass is routinely performed in our department for standard adult transplants. The bypass guarantees hemodynamic stability during the anhepatic stage and prevents problems connected with splanchnic and caval sequestration, in particular renal insufficiency due to venous stasis.[3] The bypass constructed with the Griffith circuit is perfectly safe and we have never experienced technical problems or complications with this. The circuit is filled with saline solution and connected to the Bio-Pump. The axillary vein is cannulated, followed by the common iliac vein through the saphenous vein and lastly the portal vein which is interrupted close to the bifurcation. The Bio-Pump is activated only when the absence of air bubbles in the circuit has been confirmed (**Figure 27.5**).

RECIPIENT HEPATECTOMY

The vena cava is clamped below the liver with a De Bakey clamp and above the liver with a specially designed, large, curved vascular clamp which is positioned so as to include a portion of diaphragm and thus block the diaphragmatic veins.

The upper vena cava is divided a few centimeters inside the parenchyma: in this way first the lumen of the hepatic veins and then the caval lumen are encountered. The distal section of the vena cava is then divided at least 1 cm from the clamp and the recipient liver is removed. At this stage, before beginning construction of the vascular anastomoses, hemostasis of the retrohepatic space must be ensured by coagulation or suturing. It is advisable to suture the raw edges of the bare area to complete hemostasis. Before reimplantation of the graft, the orifice of the upper vena cava must be prepared. To obtain a wide

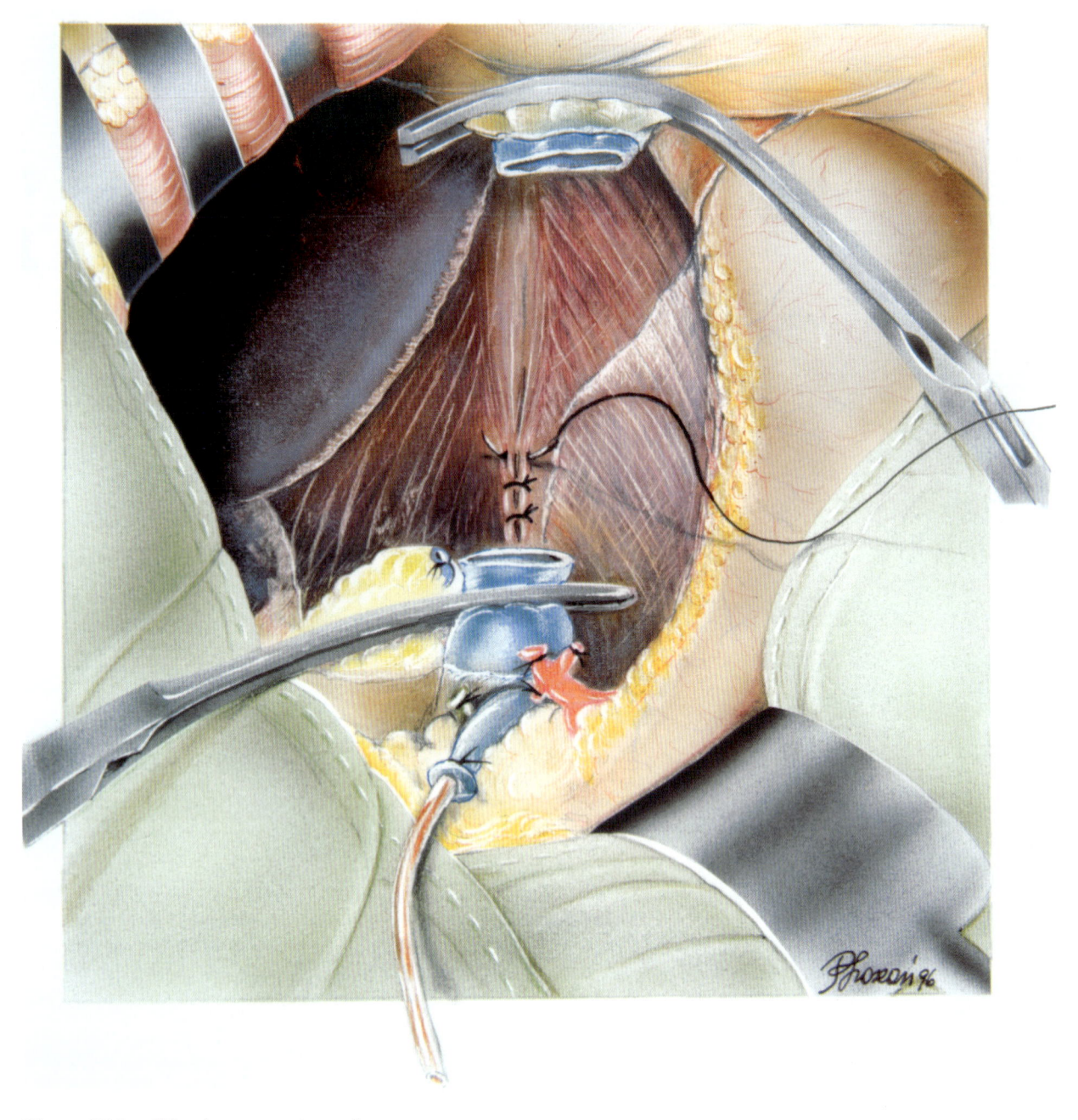

Figure 27.6 – *When hepatectomy is complete, hemostasis of the retrohepatic space must be ensured.*

venous cuff, the outlet of the three hepatic veins is used, encircling the portion of wall between them (**Figure 27.6**).

VASCULAR ANASTOMOSIS

The graft is placed in the operating field and covered with sterile dressings soaked in cold saline solution to keep it cold. The upper caval anastomosis is constructed first, with Prolene® 3-0 stitches. The anastomosis must turn outwards; a traction thread applied at the mid point of the posterior wall makes it easier to assess the anastomosis and align the intima. The caval suture must ensure a perfect seal to prevent hemorrhage at reperfusion which would be difficult to control at this site (**Figure 27.7**). On completion of the upper caval anastomosis, the lower vena cava is anastomosed with Prolene® 4-0 stitches and at the same time the liver is washed through the cannula positioned in the portal vein of the graft, using a 5% albumin solution to

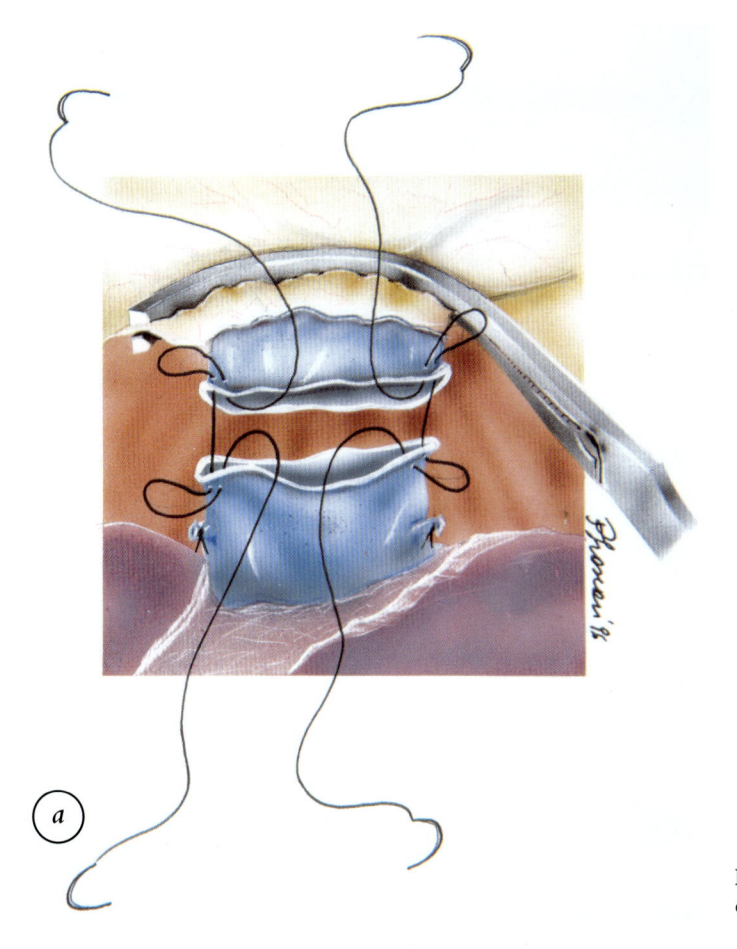

Figure 27.7 – *a,b) Anastomosis of the upper vena cava*

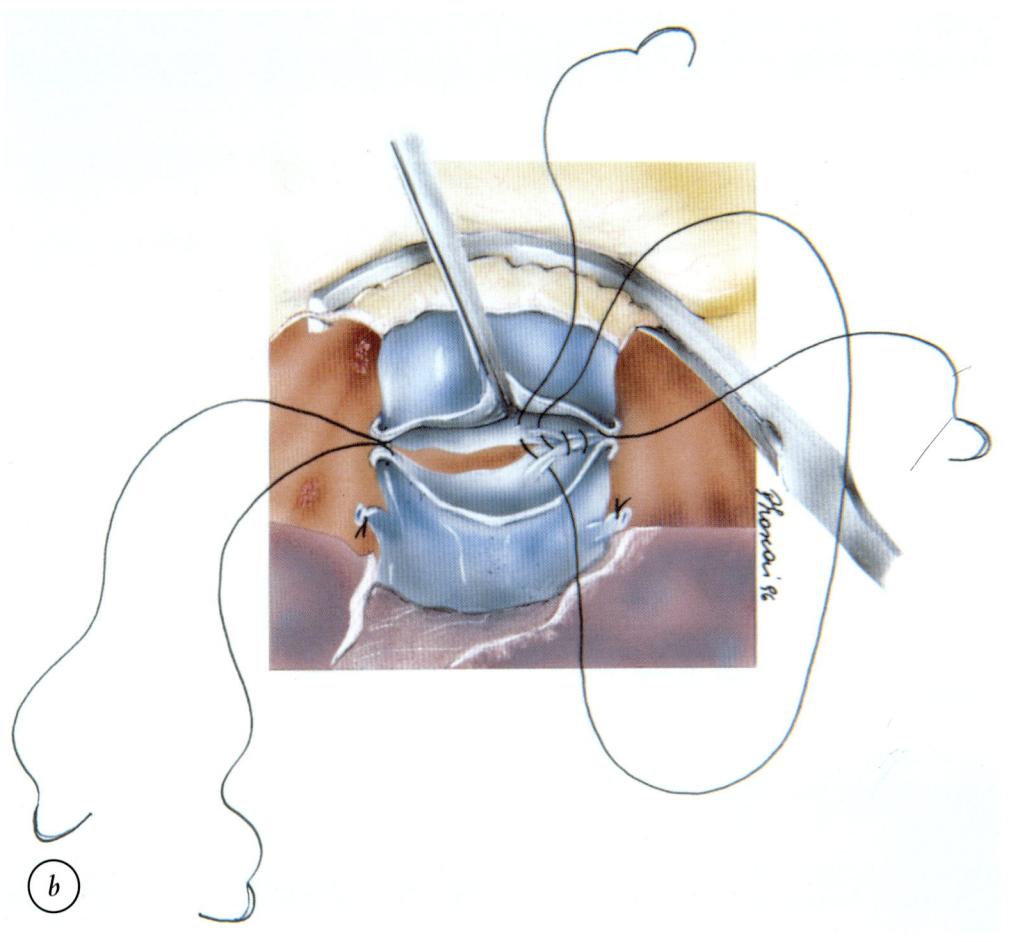

TECHNIQUES IN LIVER SURGERY

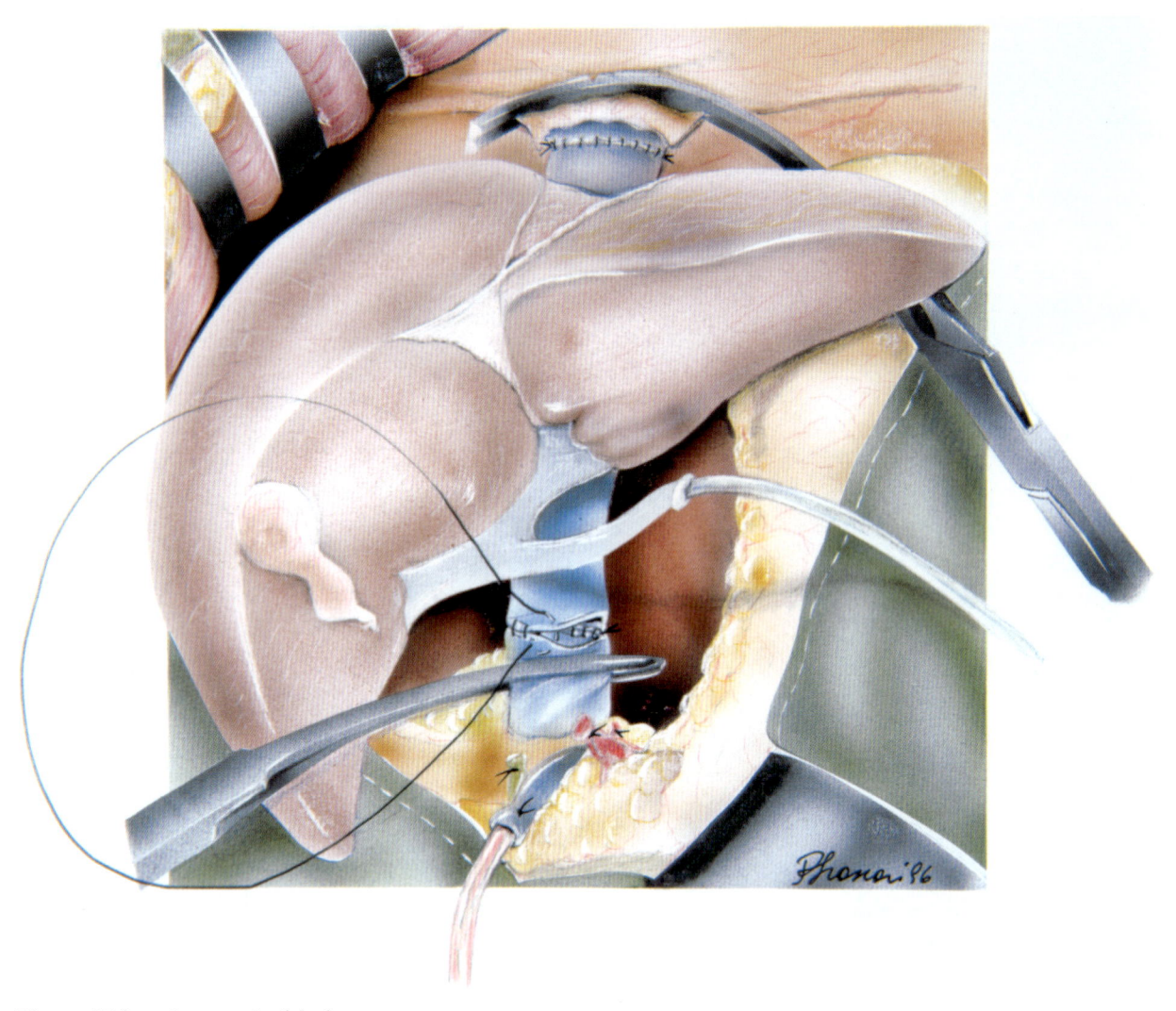

Figure 27.8 – *Anastomosis of the lower vena cava after the graft has been flushed with albumin solution.*

remove the preservation liquid which is rich in potassium and to fill the vascular bed of the graft in order to prevent air embolism (**Figure 27.8**). Generally, 700 cc of solution is used. More flushing solution is required if the graft is very large or if the recipient's kaliaemia is high during the anhepatic stage. Flushing is normally carried out with hypothermic solution at 4°C. At this stage, however, there is often a significant decrease in the recipient's body temperature due to hepatectomy and contact with the hypothermic graft in these circumstances and the graft can be flushed with ambient temperature solution to prevent further decreases in patients whose esophageal temperature is below 33°.

Having removed the venous bypass, the portal anastomosis is constructed after evaluating the distance between the two portal vein stumps of the recipient and the graft and their direction. The anastomosis is constructed with Prolene® 5-0 whipstitches (**Figure 27.9**). The suprahepatic vein is unclamped, then the portal vein and the suture threads are tied after about a minute to allow complete distension of the anastomosis. This has the same purpose as the growth factor described by Starzl.[4] Just before reperfusion, the anesthesiology team must prepare to maintain low central venous pressure to prevent altered venous discharge of the graft.

ARTERIAL ANASTOMOSIS

The usual method for reconstruction of the hepatic artery is a direct anastomosis between the Carrell patch on the donor celiac triad and the recipient common hepatic artery at the level of the gastroduodenal artery outlet. The common hepatic artery and the gastroduodenal

CONVENTIONAL TRANSPLANT TECHNIQUE

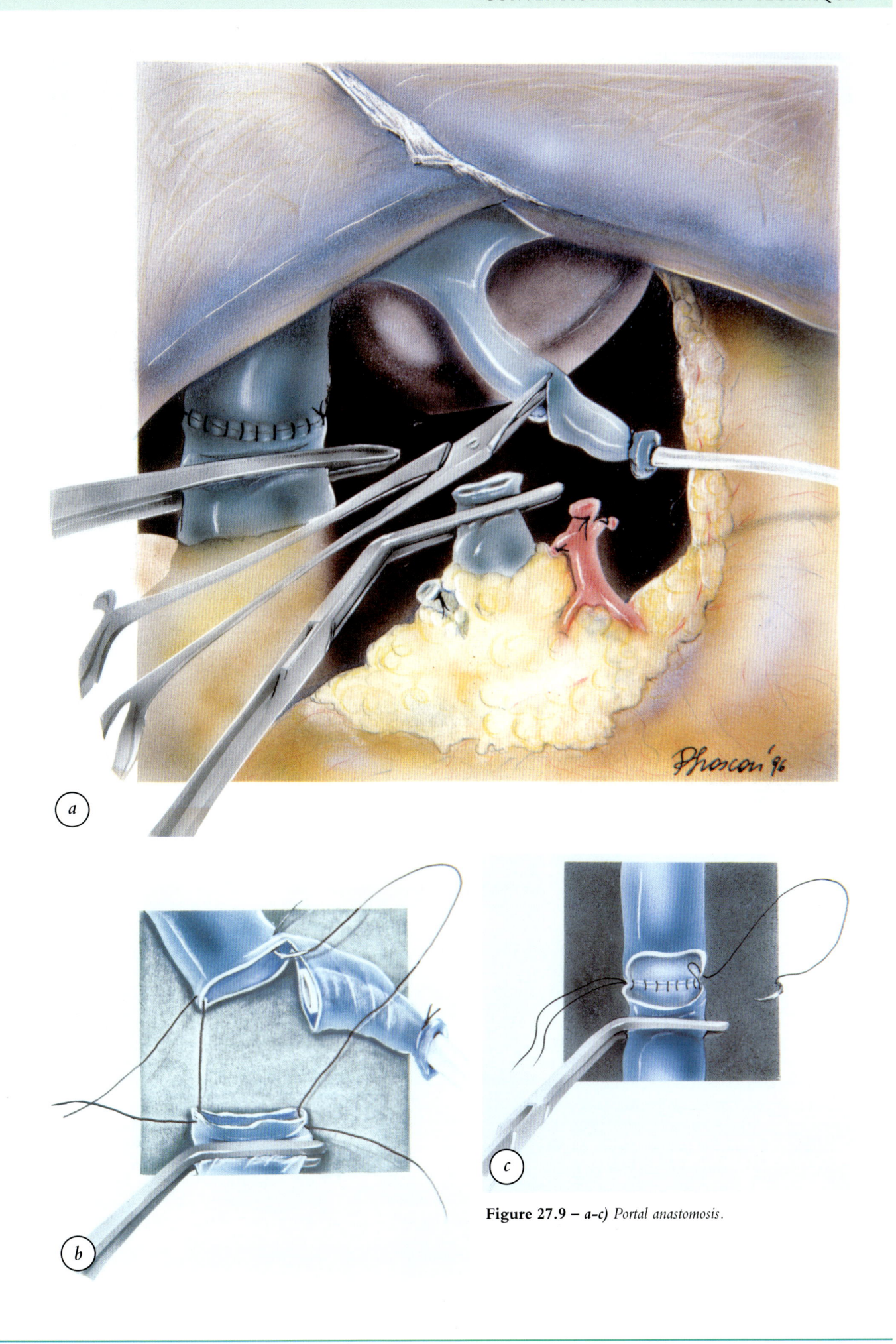

Figure 27.9 – *a-c)* Portal anastomosis.

TECHNIQUES IN LIVER SURGERY

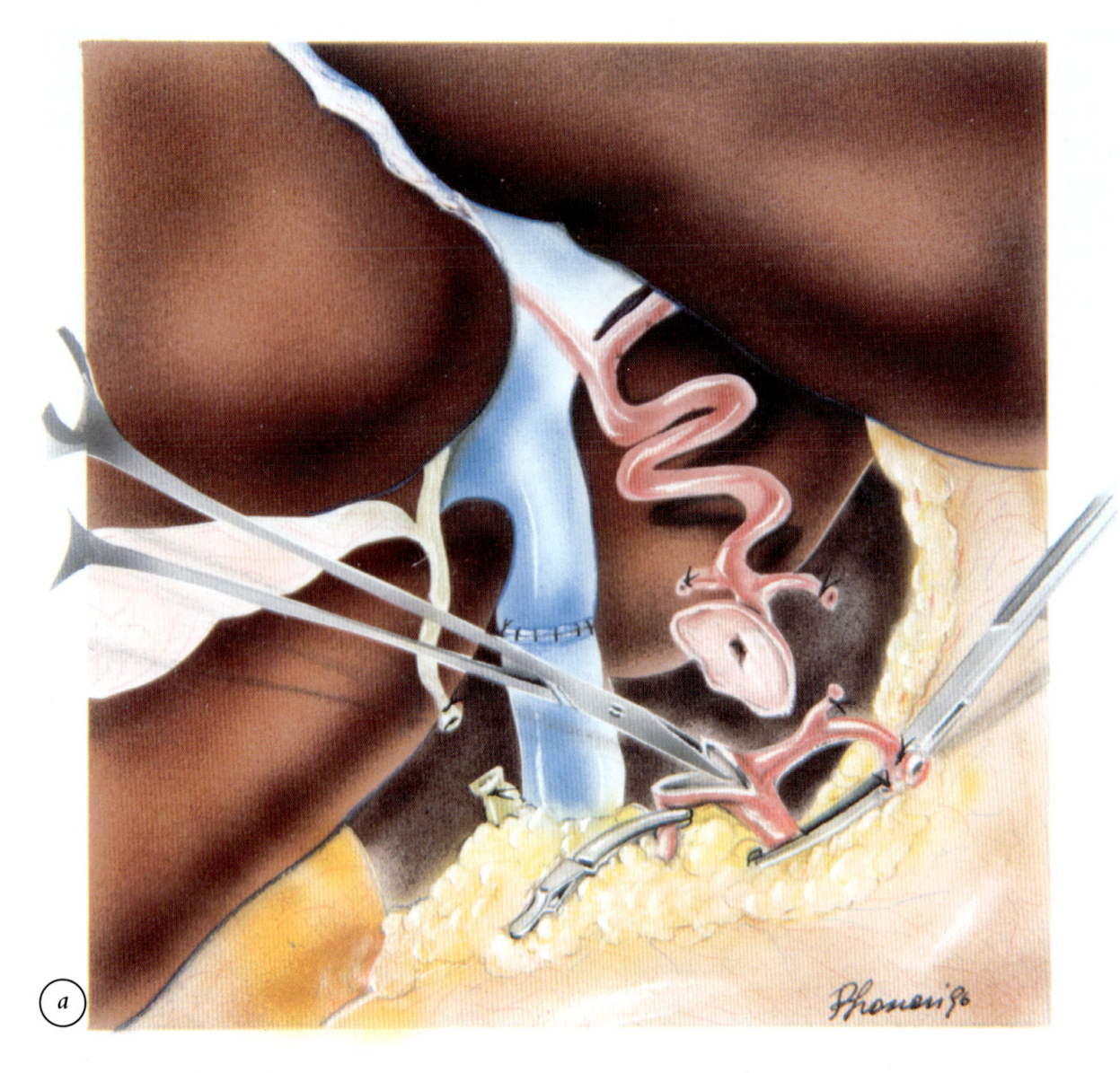

Figure 27.10 – *a,b) Arterial anastomosis.*

artery are clamped separately and the opening of the hepatic artery is enlarged by a few millimeters with a lateral incision of the gastroduodenal artery. The anastomosis is preferably constructed with interrupted sutures, with the assistance of magnifying loops (**Figure 27.10**). Other sites for anastomosis on the recipient artery can be at the level of the bifurcation between the right and left branches of the artery if the diameter is wide enough, or at the level of the splenic artery outlet, isolating the artery as far as the emergence of the celiac triad.[5]

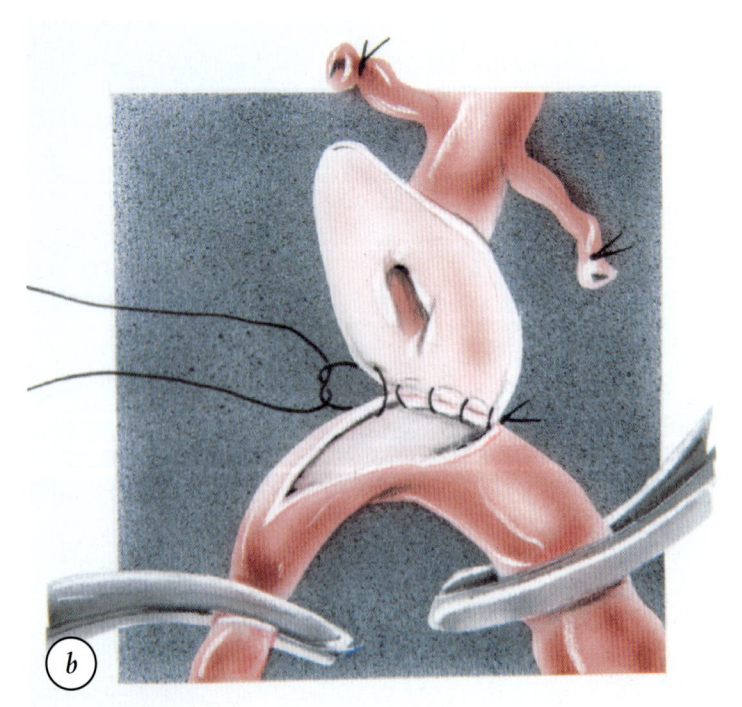

CONVENTIONAL TRANSPLANT TECHNIQUE

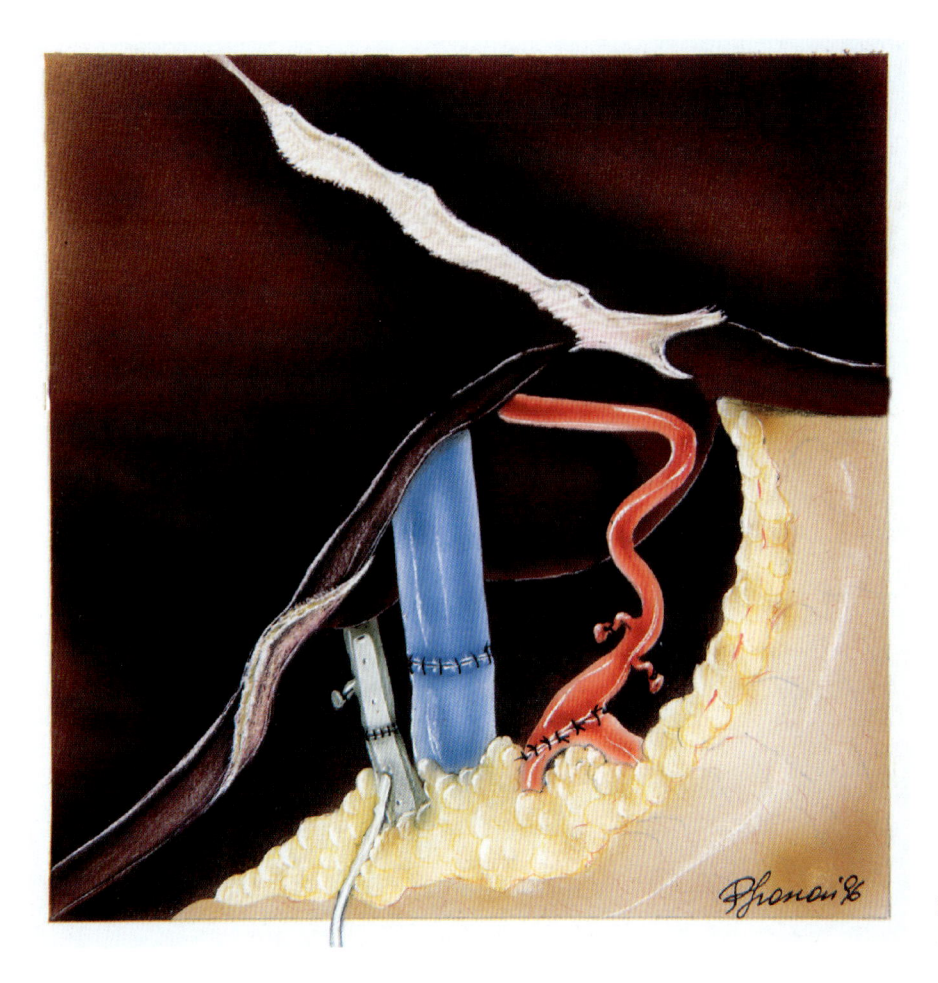

Figure 27.11 –
Biliary anastomosis.

The recipient hepatic artery may not be suitable for direct anastomosis due to size, inadequate flow, or technical problems, such as the dissection of the artery. The common hepatic artery is generally small in diameter when anomalous or aberrant arteries exist, and this is most common in the presence of a right hepatic artery arising from the superior mesenteric artery. When direct anastomosis is not considered feasible or satisfactory, arterial reconstruction is performed with an interposition graft of donor iliac artery. The site of choice for the implant of the graft is the subrenal aorta which is detached for a few centimeters so that the lateral clamp can be positioned. The arterial graft is passed through the transverse mesocolon, behind the stomach and in front of the pancreas, completing the anastomosis with the recipient Carrell patch and with a continuous Prolene® 6-0 suture. This route is certainly the safest and prevents damage to other vascular structures or to the pancreas and has been used in 12% of cases in our unit. An alternative site for anastomosis of the arterial graft is the supraceliac aorta, according to the technique described by Shaked[2] and is more commonly performed in pediatric transplants.

BILIARY ANASTOMOSIS

Biliary reconstruction in adult liver transplantation is usually performed with an end-to-end common bile duct anastomosis over a Kehr tube. The recipient bile duct is followed for more than 1 cm below the initial ligature of the bile duct distal to the emergence of the cystic duct. The graft common bile duct is also detached proximally for about 1 cm, until a well-vascularized zone is reached. As in all biliary surgery, devascularization of the biliary wall during preparation of the two bile duct stumps should be avoided and cautery should be rigorously avoided. The anastomosis is constructed with interrupted PDS® 6-0 stitches. When the posterior wall of the anastomosis is complete, the Kehr tube is brought out through an incision on the anterior wall of the common bile duct, about 2 cm more distally. The arms of the Kehr tube are then positioned and the front wall of the anastomosis is completed (**Figure 27.11**). Suture seal is checked by injecting methylene blue solution in the Kehr tube. Trans Kehr cholangiography is routinely performed. Side-to-side anastomosis is advisable if there is a difference in diameter between the graft and the recipient common ducts, the latter generally being larger. If the recipient common bile duct is inadequate due to previous operations or if the indication for transplantation was sclerosing cholangitis, or in late re-transplants, biliary reconstruction is performed with a choledochojejunostomy on a Roux loop passed by the transmesocolic route. The construction of the Roux en Y loop follows the conventional technique: the jejunum is divided about 20 cm from Treitz's ligament. The proximal stump is closed with a stapler and sewn with Vicryl® 3-0. A very small hole is made in the antimesenteric side of the loop and the anastomosis is constructed with single-layer PDS® 5-0 stitches. A disposable silicone drainage tube is positioned inside the anastomosis, fixed with a stitch to the posterior wall of the jejunal mucosa, or a siliconed drainage tube (urethral tube in 6 or 8 or an infant feeding tube) which is brought out through a separate hole in the bowel loop, about 15 cm more distal to the anastomosis; this drainage tube is Witzel-tunnelled for 5 cm on the intestinal wall to prevent any leakage.

Hemostatic control, when the operation has been completed, must be particularly meticulous, including the vascular anastomoses and the extensive areas of dissection. Two drainage tubes, a posterior one in the retrohepatic space and the other below the liver, behind the biliary anastomosis, are placed routinely.

REFERENCE

1. Casavilla A, Gordon RD, Starzl TE. Techniques of liver transplantation. In: Blumgart LH. *Surgery of the liver and biliary tract,* Churchill Livingstone, New York, 1994, pp. 1870-1888.
2. Shaked A, Takill H, Busuttil RW. The use of supraceliac aorta for hepatic arterial revascularization in transplantation of the liver. *Surg Gynecol Obstetr* 1991; **173:** 198-202.
3. Shaw BW Jr, Martin DJ, Marquez JM *et al.* Venous bypass in clinical liver transplantation. *Ann Surg* 1984; **200:** 524-534.
4. Starzl TE, Iwatsuki S. A growth factor in fine vascular anastomoses. *Surg Gynecol Obstetr* 1984; **159:** 164-166.
5. Todo S, Makowka L, Tzakis AG *et al.* Hepatic artery in liver transplantation. *Transpl Proc* 1987; **19:** 2406-2411.

28

The 'Piggy-Back' Technique

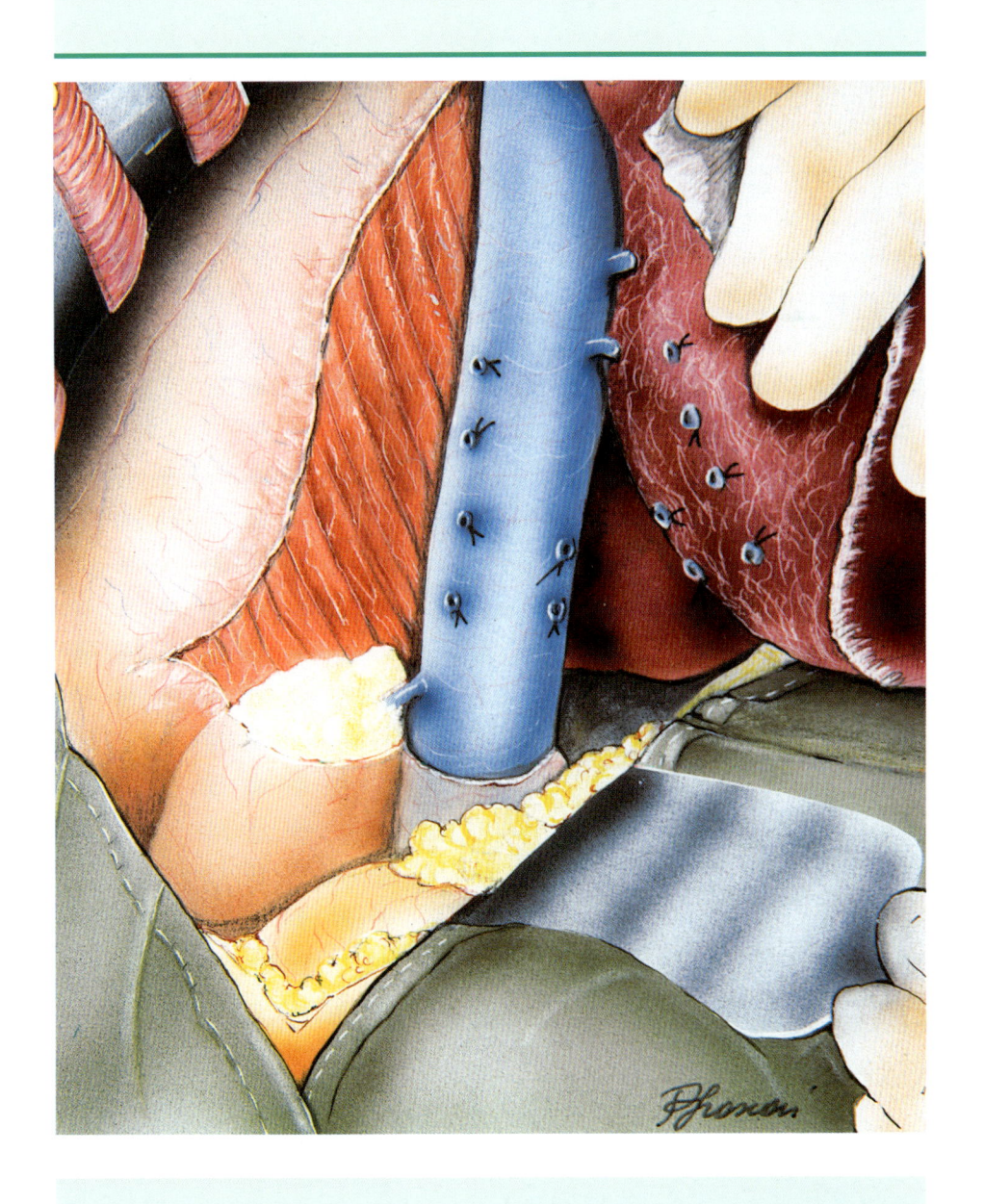

THE 'PIGGY-BACK' TECHNIQUE

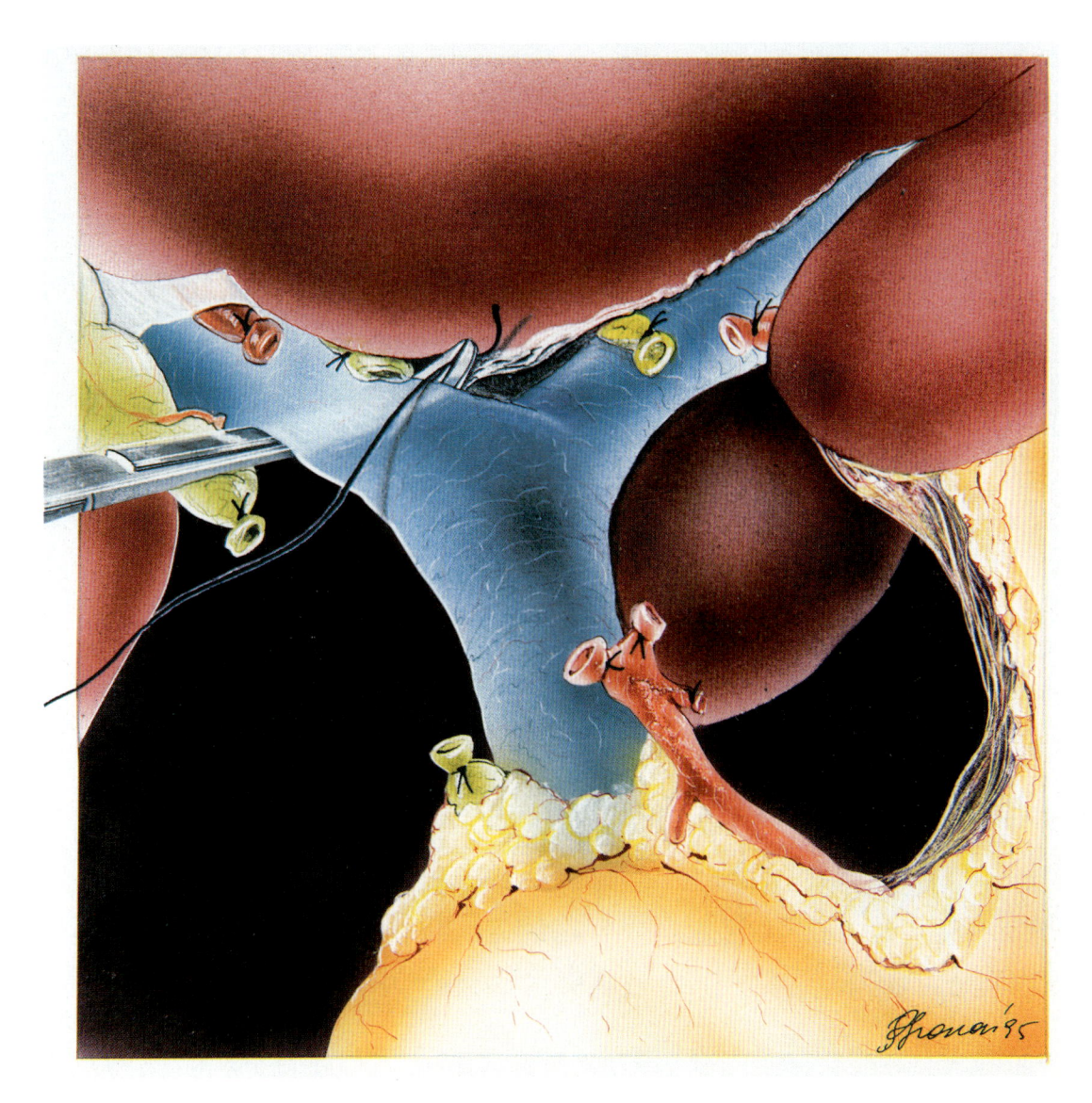

Figure 28.1 – The 'piggy-back' technique for liver transplantation. The bile duct and the hepatic artery are interrupted. The portal vein is skeletonized and the right portal branch is encircled.

Liver transplant with preservation of the recipient vena cava, the 'piggy-back' technique, has been proposed as an alternative to the traditional liver transplant technique in order to maintain caval flow during the anhepatic stage and to avoid the need for venous bypass. The technique involves the progressive detachment of the liver from the retrohepatic vena cava with ligature of the accessory suprahepatic veins and clamping of the main suprahepatic veins without occluding caval flow. A temporary porto-caval anastomosis has been proposed[1] to avoid splanchnic stasis during the anhepatic stage. This anastomosis has, however, rarely proved necessary in the cirrhotic patients treated in our department. Caval anastomosis with grafting may be carried out at the outlet of the three main, appropriately fashioned, hepatic veins, as in the original technique described by Tzakis in children,[6] laterally on the vena cava[1] or on the outlet of the middle and left hepatic veins,[2] as performed in our department. Initially proposed in selected cases,[3] such as reduced-size graft, the 'piggy-back' technique has become increasingly popular with transplant teams. In fact, leaving the retrocaval space untouched prevents hemorrhage in transplants. The problems related to the use of venous bypass are avoided. The non-dissection of the axillary and saphenous veins and the absence of inferior vena caval anastomosis reduce the overall time of the operation.

Technique

The first stage of the operation is identical to the traditional technique, with skeletonization of the hepato-duodenal ligament. The portal vein is isolated as far as the bifurcation and the right branch of the portal vein is encircled with a ligature (**Figure 28.1**). Once division of

TECHNIQUES IN LIVER SURGERY

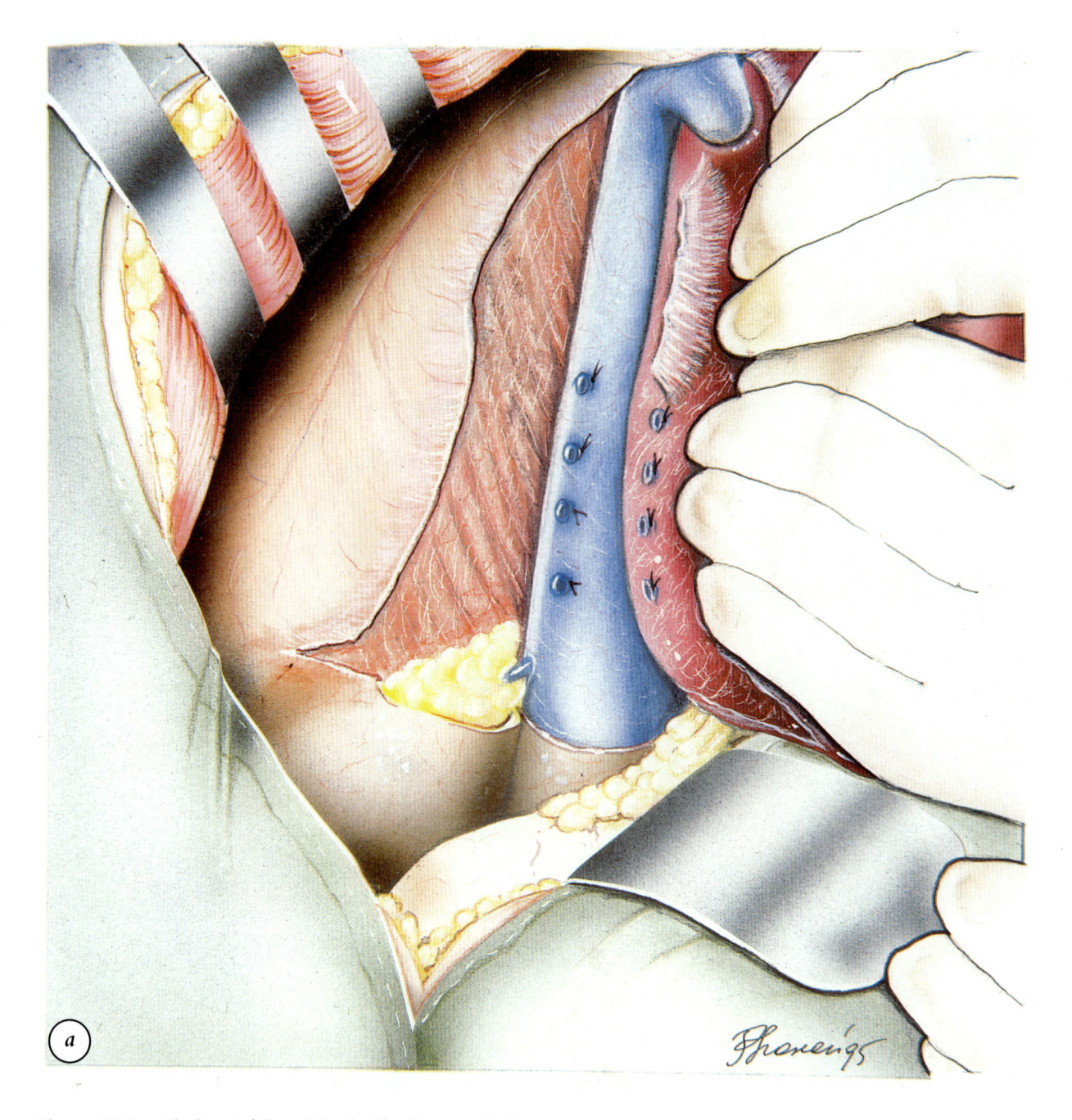

Figure 28.2 – *The liver is fully mobilized. After dissecting the ligament of the vena cava, the right hepatic vein is exposed **a)**. The liver is displaced upwards, exposing the accessory hepatic veins which are ligated and dissected until the anterior aspect of the vena cava is freed **b)**. (Opposite page.)*

the right triangular ligament is complete, the dorsal ligament of the vena cava is divided. The lateral margin of the vena cava is not dissected and the right adrenal vein is not ligated. The liver is raised and the accessory hepatic veins are ligated, proceeding in a caudo-cranial direction and progressively mobilizing the entire anterior facies of the vena cava as far as the outlet of the right hepatic vein (**Figure 28.2**). The collateral vessels on the caval side

THE 'PIGGY-BACK' TECHNIQUE

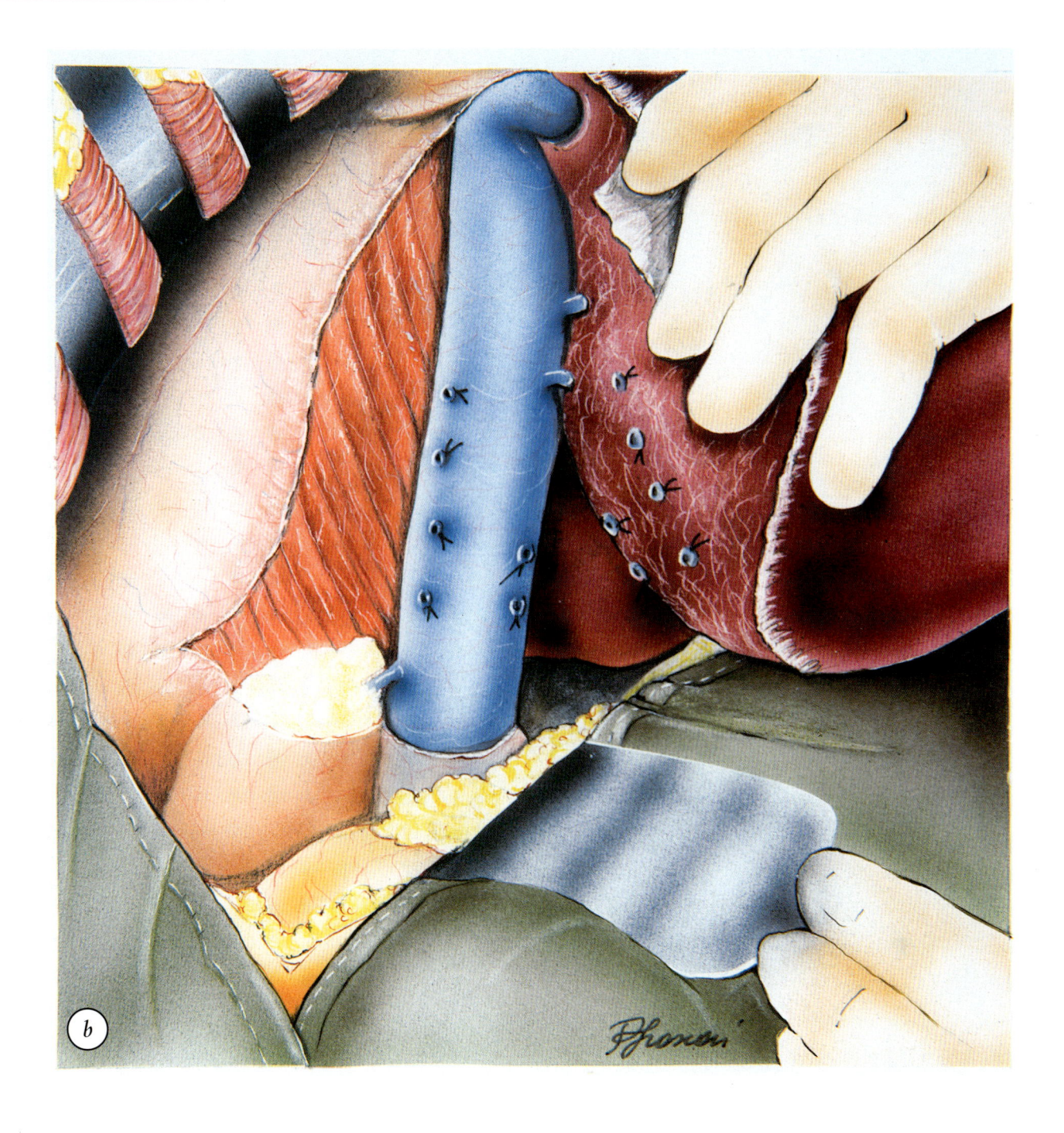

are closed with transfixed Prolene® 4-0 sutures, while on the hepatic side they are ligated or simply closed with clips.

At this point, before isolating the hepatic veins, the left edge of the caudate lobe must be completely detached from the vena cava. Dissection proceeds from the left, raising the left lobe completely freed of its ligaments and dividing the peritoneum which covers the left edge of the caudate lobe. In cirrhotic subjects this peri-

TECHNIQUES IN LIVER SURGERY

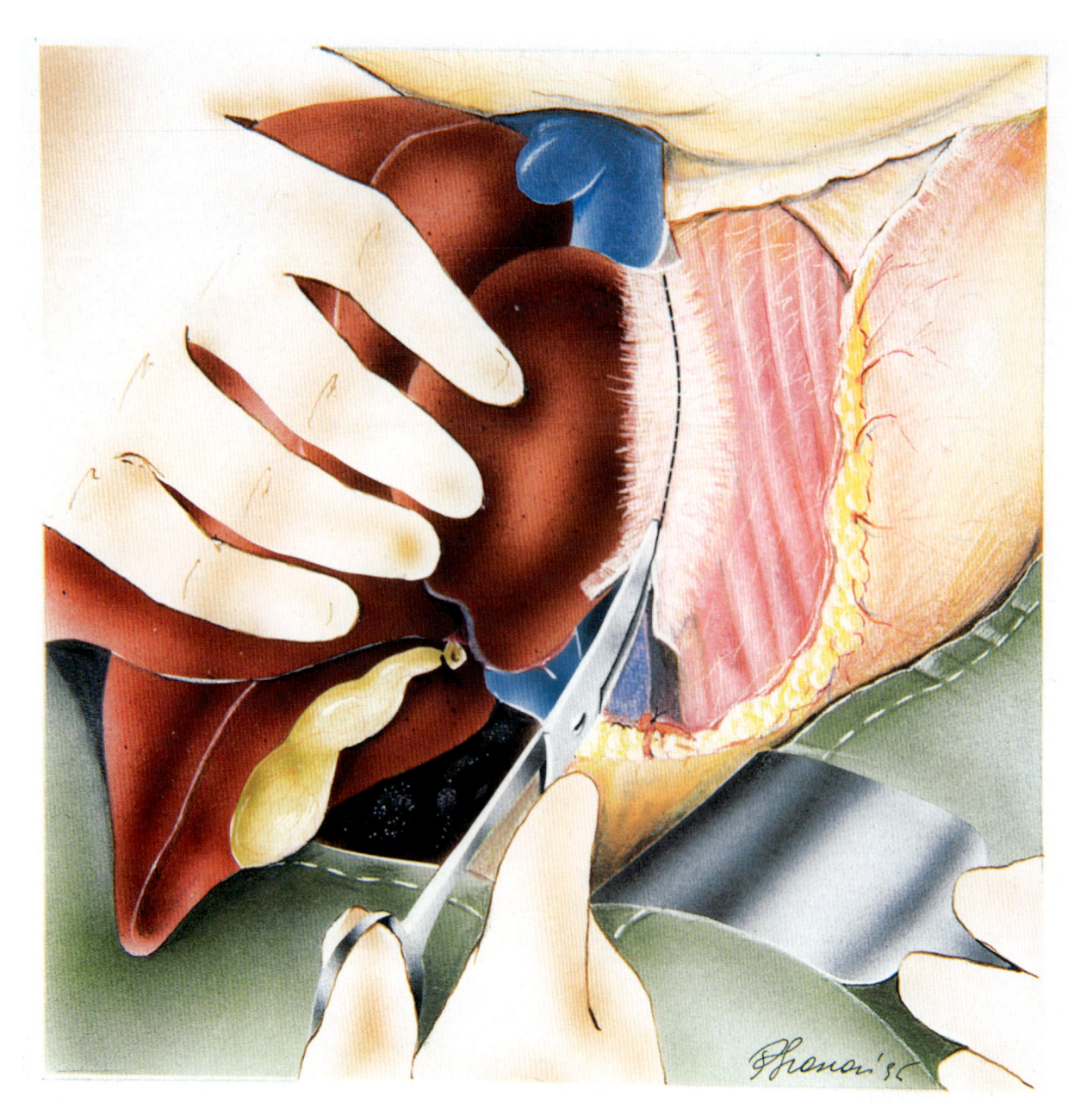

Figure 28.3 – *Mobilization of the caudate lobe with incision of the posterior peritoneal layer and exposure of the left edge of the vena cava.*

toneal layer, which extends from the liver to the posterior aspect of the retrocavity, contains small veins which are simply coagulated. The left part of the caudate lobe can thus be raised, exposing the vena cava and ligating some of the collateral veins on this side too (**Figure 28.3**).

Once the anterior aspect of the vena cava is freed, the liver is only attached to the trunk of the three hepatic veins. Before clamping the trunk of the right hepatic vein, the right branch of the portal vein is first isolated to prevent venous congestion in the right part of the liver and then ligated. The portal vein should not be fully clamped as it is used to drain the portal blood, reducing splanchnic stasis time in the anhepatic stage. This technique reduces portal clamping time to less than an hour. The trunk of the right hepatic vein is clamped with an angled clamp on the caval side, sutured on the hepatic side and divided. The stump of the suprahepatic vena cava is sutured with a Prolene® 4-0 whipstitch (**Figure 28.4**).

At this point, the portal trunk and the common trunk of the middle hepatic vein can be clamped on the left and the liver removed (**Figure 28.5**). The clamp on the hepatic vein is positioned laterally so that it also includes a portion of vena cava, giving a wider orifice.

THE 'PIGGY-BACK' TECHNIQUE

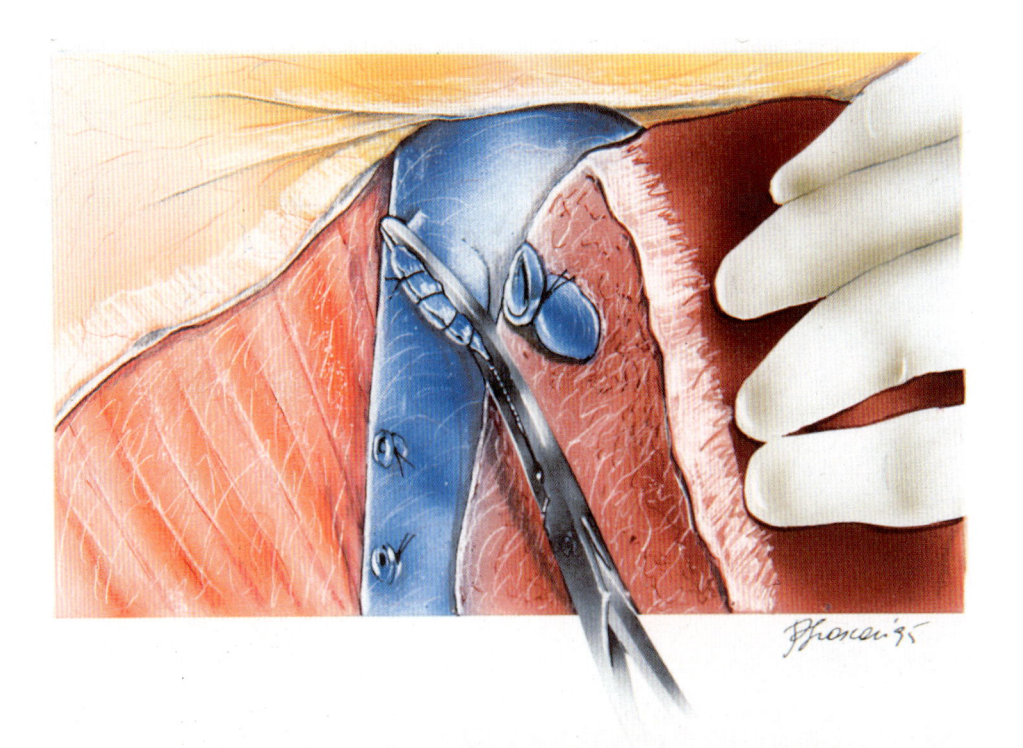

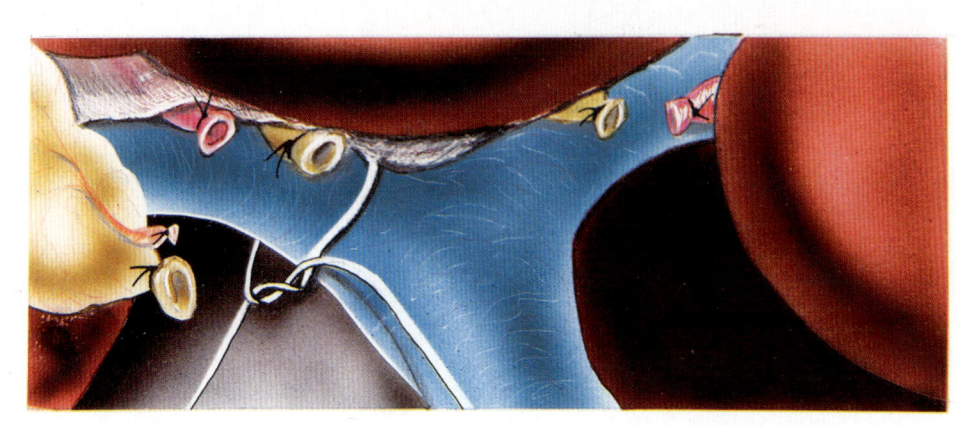

Figure 28.4 – *Clamping of the right hepatic vein trunk and simultaneous ligation of the right portal branch*

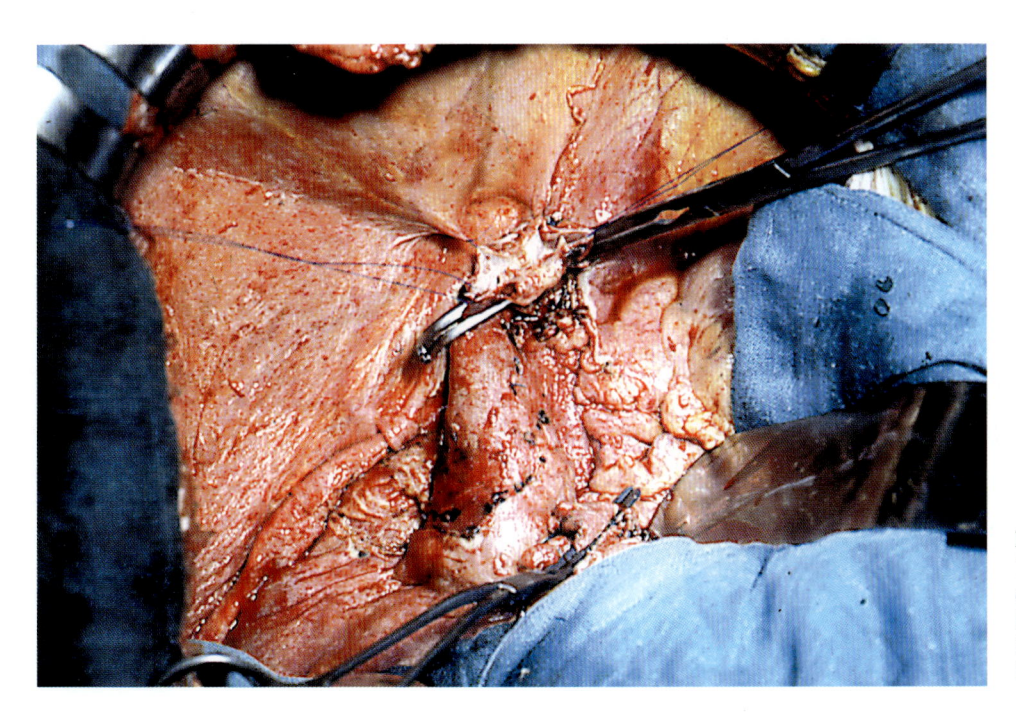

Figure 28.5 – *The common trunk of the middle and left hepatic vein is clamped and the liver removed.*

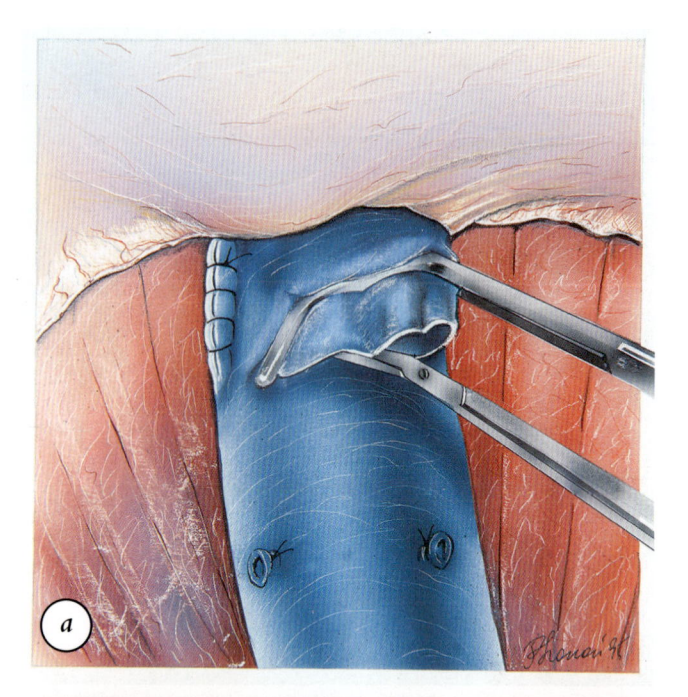

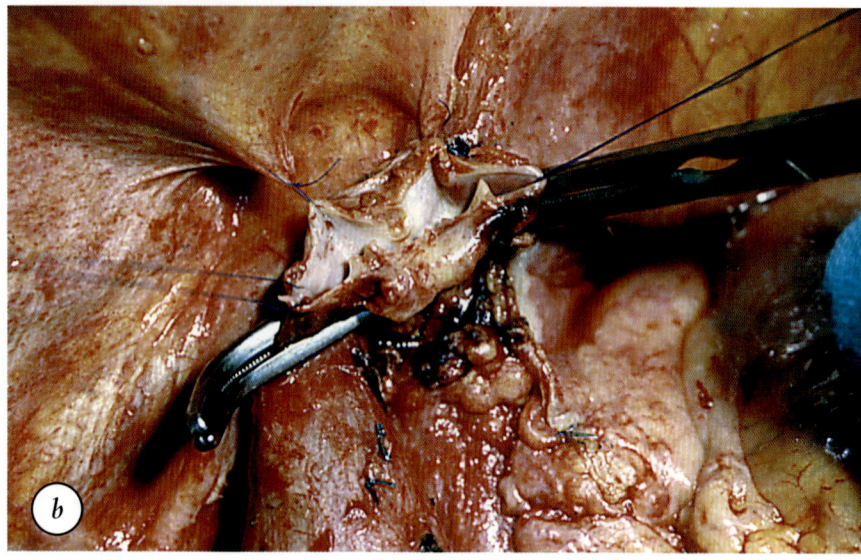

Figure 28.6 –
*The orifice of two hepatic veins is enlarged by dissecting the septa and also incising a portion of caval wall **a)** until a wide common orifice is obtained, appropriate for correct caval anastomosis **b)**.*

The orifice on the hepatic veins is modeled by dividing the septa and widening the incision on the vena cava by around 1 cm (**Figure 28.6**).

Caval anastomosis is performed with an evaginated Prolene® 3-0 whipstitch, according to the technique described for conventional transplantation in Chapter 27 (**Figure 28.7a**). Liver flushing should be started with albumin solution during caval anastomosis. When the graft is irrigated with about 600-800 cc of solution, the subhepatic stump of the vena cava is closed with a vascular stapler (**Figure 28.7b**).

The rest of the transplant follows exactly the traditional transplant stages, with portal anastomosis followed by revascularization of the graft, arterial and biliary anastomosis.

THE 'PIGGY-BACK' TECHNIQUE

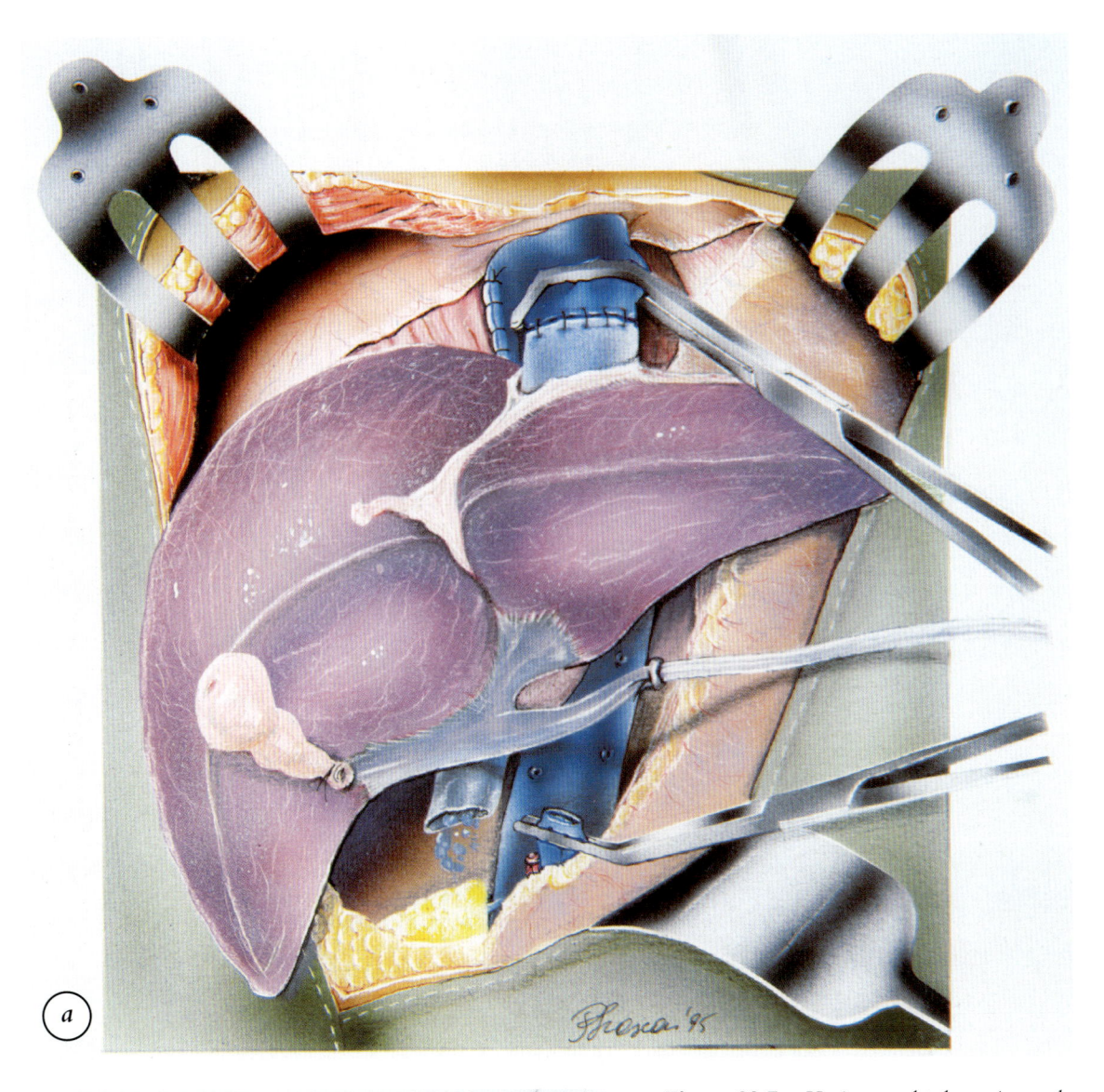

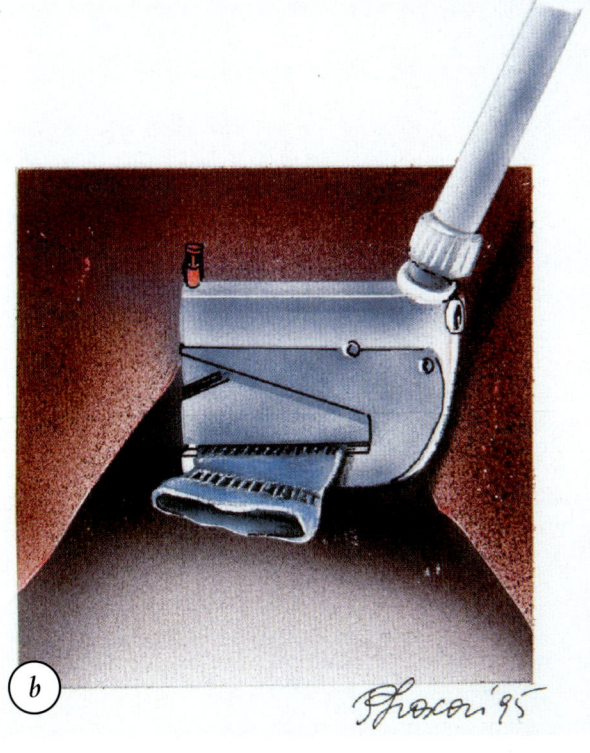

Figure 28.7 – *Having completed superior caval anastomosis, the graft is flushed with 600-800 cc of albumin solution **a)**. The subhepatic caval stump is then closed with a vascular stapler **b)**.*

283

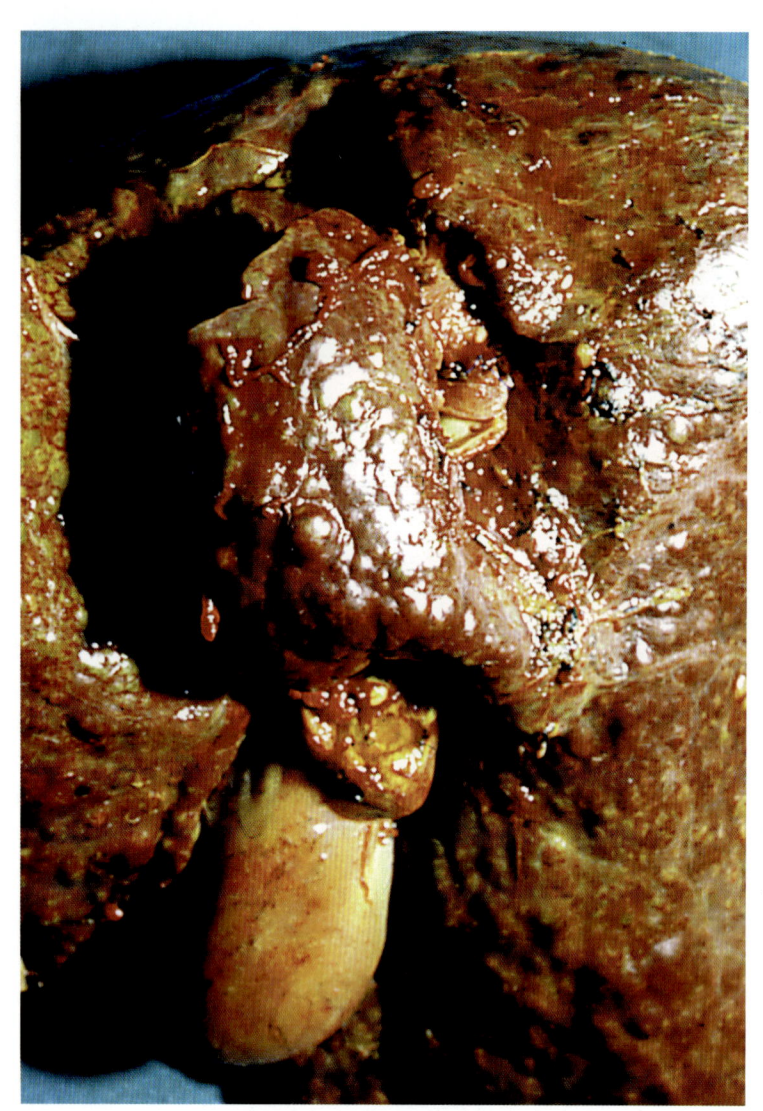

Figure 28.8 –
Parenchyma bridge joining the caudate lobe to the right lobe of the liver, completely encircling the vena cava. In this case, the transplant had begun with the 'piggy-back' technique but was switched to the conventional technique.

Problems and complications

The 'piggy-back' technique is feasible in most, if not all, cases.[1,2] In our experience technical problems are rarely encountered in the presence of a caudate lobe totally surrounding the retrohepatic vena cava (**Figure 28.8**) and in cases of notable recipient hepatomegaly. In a randomized study in our unit between 'piggy-back' and conventional technique, involving 50 consecutive cirrhotic patients, it was necessary to switch to the traditional technique only in two cases. In 1 case this was due to the presence of a parenchymal bridge joining segment 7 to the caudate lobe, making dissection tedious and potentially hemorrhagic, and in the second due to a lesion of the caval vein during dissection (**Figure 28.8**) due to the presence of a hypertrophic caudate lobe.[4] A crucial stage of the technique is the positioning of the suprahepatic caval clamp: to ensure sufficiently extensive anastomosis the clamp must include not only the trunk of the middle and left hepatic veins but also a portion of the vena cava. Care should be taken during these maneuvers so as not to occlude the caval lumen completely. Adequate hemodynamic monitoring makes it easy to recognize this occurrence. It is, however, advisable to perform a clamping test before widening the incision in the vena cava and beginning caval anastomosis. One case of stenotic suprahepatic anastomosis

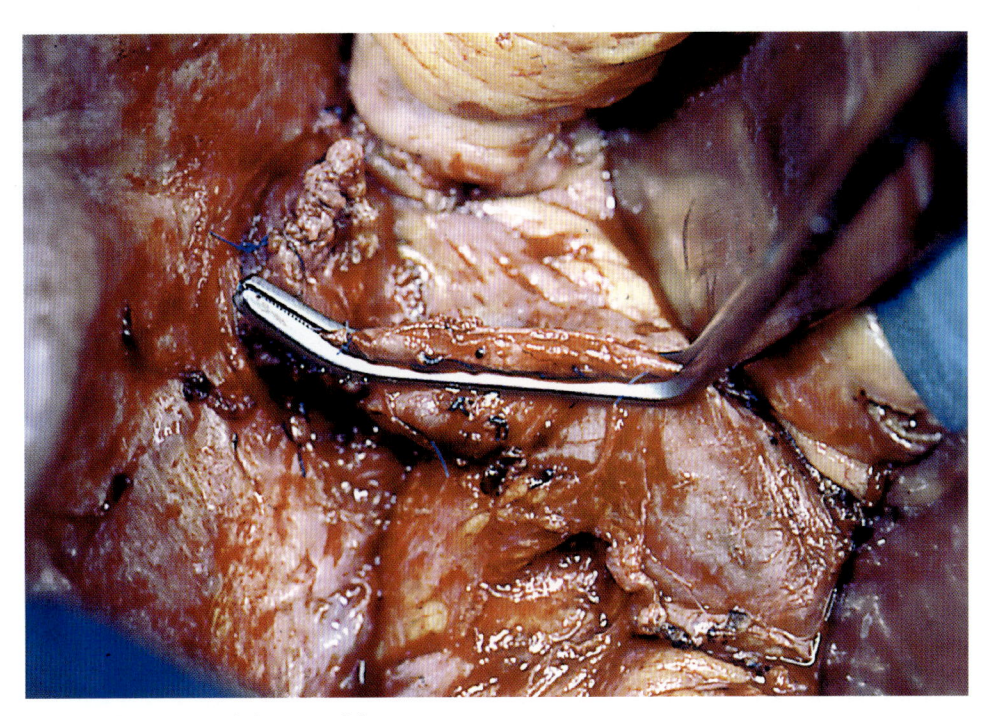

Figure 28.9 – *Lateral clamping of the recipient vena cava for a side-to-side anastomosis with the graft vena cava. The orifice of the hepatic veins has been sutured.*

which required a re-transplant has been reported.[2] If clamping at the level of the hepatic veins is somewhat difficult, it is possible to resort to the alternative technique of side-to-side anastomosis between the recipient vena cava and the retrohepatic vena cava of the graft (**Figure 28.9**). The superior and distal caval stumps of the graft are closed with a vascular stapler after graft flushing has been performed. This latter technique can prove useful for large grafts.

Temporary porto-caval anastomosis to prevent splanchnic stasis during the anhepatic stage was performed in only 10% of our transplants using the 'piggy-back' technique. In our technique, clamping of the portal trunk is begun only after dividing and suturing the right hepatic vein immediately before removing the native liver. The mean time of the anhepatic stage, until revascularization of the graft, is 40 minutes and this period of portal clamping is well tolerated by the cirrhotic liver. If the liver is non-cirrhotic, periods of splanchnic congestion with hypotension can occur with clamping lasting as long. In one case of transplantation for familial amyloid polyneuropathy, massive splanchnic sequestration occurred during the clamping stage with severe hypotension, requiring emergency porto-caval anastomosis. Temporary porto-caval anastomosis is systematically performed in cases of transplantation for fulminant hepatitis so the native liver can be removed early, while the donor liver is being harvested.

We greatly favor the 'piggy-back' technique in liver transplants. A randomized study in our center demonstrated a reduction in the warm ischemic period due to the absence of the inferior caval anastomosis and a minor incidence of post-operative renal insufficiency.[4] The technique avoids the need for venous bypass and thus gives an economic advantage. Any re-transplant is much easier since it is sufficient to remove the diseased liver, place a lateral clamp on the vena cava, divide the vena cava of the graft adjacent to the parenchyma and repeat the 'piggy-back' technique with the new liver. The technique is almost always feasible except in the presence of a huge recipient liver and large caudate lobe, or rare cases in which the caudate lobe completely surrounds the vena cava, displacing it posteriorly and laterally towards the right. In such cases, the lengthy and hazardous dissection of the vena cava does not, in our opinion, justify the choice of this type of operation. The 'piggy-back' method is an advantageous alternative to the traditional technique if the team is technically experienced. This technique seems to be the preferable elective choice if there is a great discrepancy between recipient graft and native liver, in reduced-size liver, or in contraindications to venous bypass due to bilateral saphenectomy or thrombosis of the subclavian vein.

This method also seems to us to be advisable in two particular situations: in the presence of a previous portocaval anastomosis or fulminant hepatitis. In the first case the anastomosis is left in place, the other components of the hepatic pedicle near the liver are closed and the anterior aspect of the vena cava is dissected, avoiding the risk of hemorrhage with dissection of the retrocaval space (the vena cava is generally dilated in the presence of a surgical shunt). In transplants for fulminant hepatitis, the 'piggy-back' technique minimizes hemodynamic alterations. It is also possible - once a suitable donor has been found - to remove the necrotic liver (a source of toxins and aromatic amino acids - 5) before the transplant operation, and to construct a temporary portocaval shunt while the transplant is being completed.

REFERENCES

1. Belghiti J, Panis Y, Sauvanet A, Gayet B, Fekete F. A new technique of side to side anastomosis during orthotopic hepatic transplantation without inferior vena cava occlusion. *Surg Gynecol Obstet* 1992; **175:** 271-273.

2. Fleitas MG, Casanova D, Martino E *et al*. Could the piggy-back operation in liver transplantation be routinely used? *Arch Surg* 1994; **129:** 842-845.

3. Jones R, Harky KJ, Fletcher DR, Michell I, McNicol PL, Angus PW. Preservation of the inferior vena cava in orthotopic liver transplantation with selective use of veno-venous bypass. *Transpl Proc* 1991; **24:** 189-191.

4. Jovine E, Mazziotti A, Grazi GL *et al*. Piggy back vs conventional technique for liver transplantation. *Transpl Intern*, 1997;**10:**109-112.

5. Mazziotti A, Bernardi M, Antonini L *et al*. Plasma amino acid pattern in experimental acute hepatic failure: comparison between hepatectomy and liver devascularization in pigs. *Surgery* 1981; **90:** 527-534.

6. Tzakis A, Todo S, Starzl TE. Orthotopic liver transplantation with presevation of the inferior vena cava. *Ann Surg* 1989; **210:** 649-652.

29

Technical Problems and Complications of Liver Transplantation

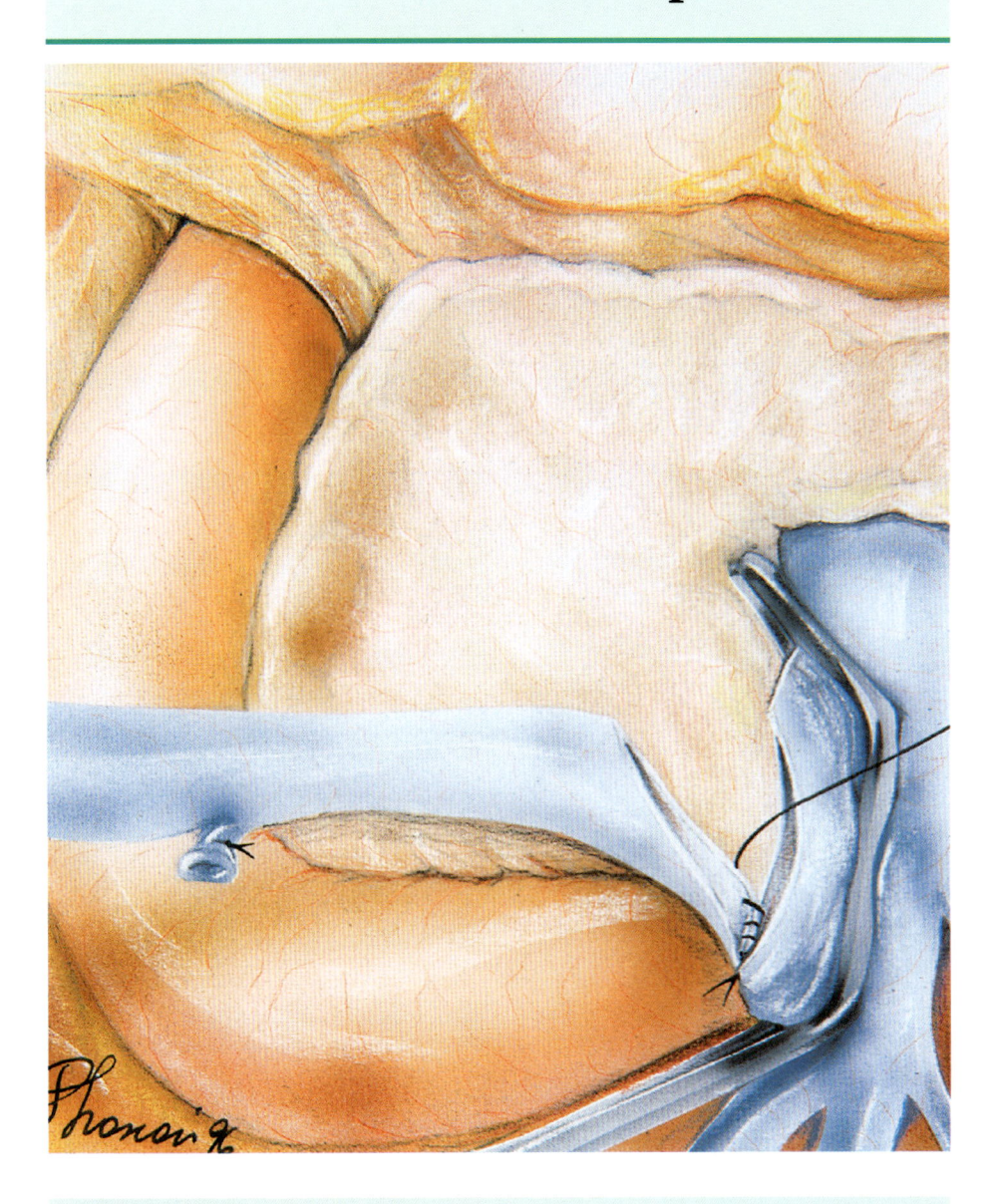

Despite the advances in patient selection and surgical technique, which have led to a drastic reduction in operative mortality and a net improvement in the long-term results of transplantation, a significant percentage (around 10%) of technical complications still exists which can necessitate reoperation or retransplantation. The great majority of technical complications occur within the first month after transplantation. The problems and complications can be defined as immediate or intra-operative, early or late post-operative.

Intra-operative problems and complications

INTRA-OPERATIVE HEMORRHAGE

Liver transplants are performed more and more often without the need for blood transfusions. Patients with severe coagulopathies, or who have previously undergone abdominal surgery, may nevertheless have a marked tendency to hemorrhage and present difficulties in achieving hemostasis. In the presence of coagulopathies, the infusion of fresh frozen plasma and antifibrinolytic agents[17] is indicated. Meticulous surgical hemostasis is, however, the key point.

Previous abdominal surgery, especially bilioenteric anastomosis or operations on the stomach (gastrectomy or esophageal transection) cause multiple, firm hemorrhagic adherences with Glisson's capsule. The problems associated with previous portacaval anastomosis will be discussed separately. Various technical solutions can be employed according to individual circumstances. In our department, when the supramesocolic space is not easily accessible, we prefer to first carry out a venous bypass which makes recipient hepatectomy easier. The portal catheter of the bypass is placed in the inferior mesenteric vein. In some special circumstances, when it is not possible to isolate the structures, of the hepatic pedicle, a long clamp is applied to include all the hilar structures with the venous bypass in operation, and the liver is then quickly removed.

In certain conditions with massive hepatomegaly, clamping of the vena cava below the liver has been proposed, with the bypass functioning, and dissection of the liver along the sagittal fissure as far as the anterior aspect of the vena cava; the two hemi-livers are then removed after clamping the right and left hepatic veins.[9]

PROBLEMS WITH ARTERIAL ANASTOMOSIS

Arterial anastomosis is a particularly delicate stage in transplantation. Obstruction of the arterial anastomosis compromises the result of a transplant irreversibly. The complications involved in an arterial anastomosis may not only be technical (stenosis, torsion, intimal flap) but may also depend on an unsuitable recipient hepatic artery, due to arterial hypoplasia generally in relation to the presence of two or more hepatic arteries. There may also be problems connected with the graft, such as intimal dissection during removal, or arterial reconstruction on the graft due to the presence of an arterial anatomical variation, or to technical errors made during the donor operation.

The anatomical variations of the recipient, especially in the presence of a large right hepatic artery arising from the superior mesenteric artery, can suggest hypoplasia or a reduced flow in the common hepatic artery, unsuitable for a direct anastomosis. In these cases, an anastomosis on the aorta with a donor iliac artery conduit is highly advisable.[8,19,26] The site of choice for the graft placement is the subrenal aorta: this is clamped laterally and the graft anastomosed end-to-side with Prolene® 5-0 whipstitching. The graft is then tunnelled through the transverse mesocolon, passed in front of the pancreas and behind the stomach and anastomosed end-to-end with the donor hepatic artery (*Figure 29.1*). Retropancreatic tunnels or anastomosis with the supraceliac artery are less frequently used. The splenic artery may exceptionally be used if the diameter is large enough, (*Figure 29.2*).

Stenosis or torsion of the arterial anastomosis must be recognized and repaired. Intra-

TECHNIQUES IN LIVER SURGERY

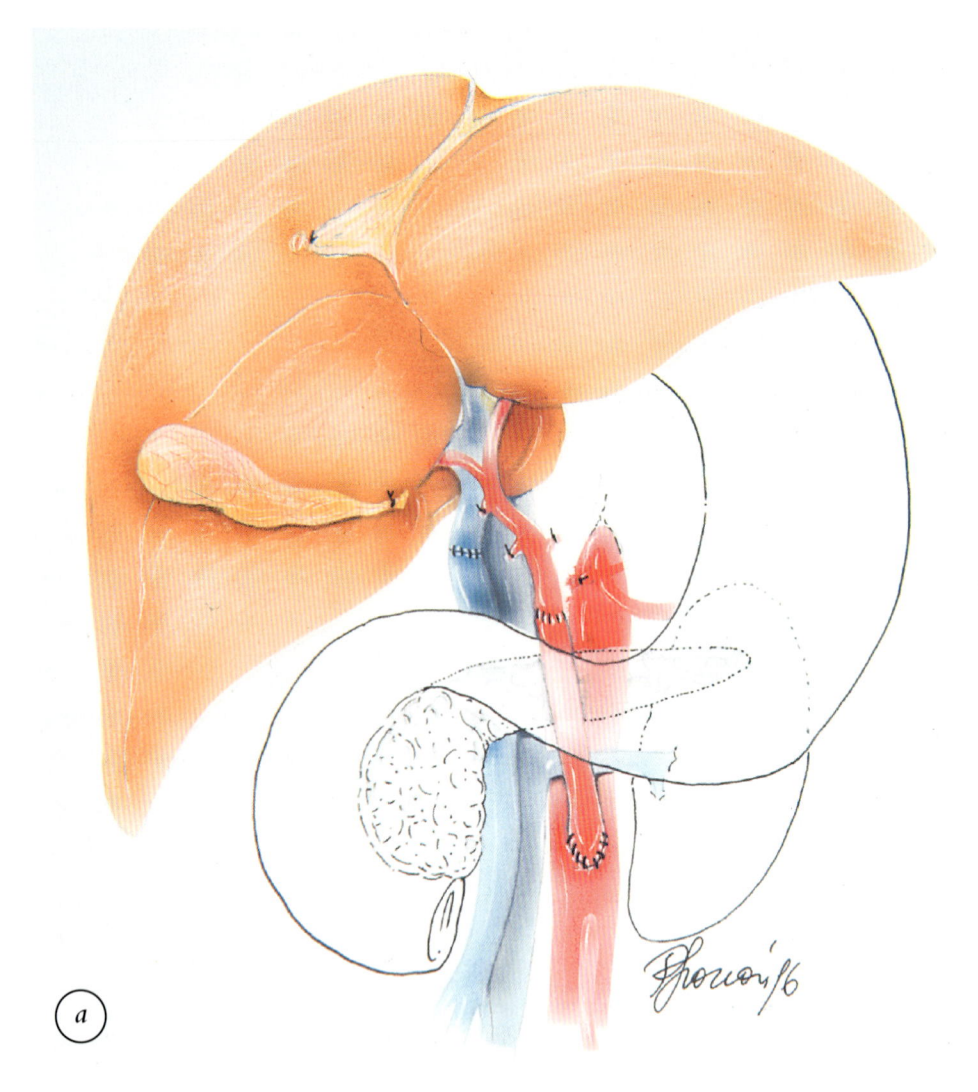

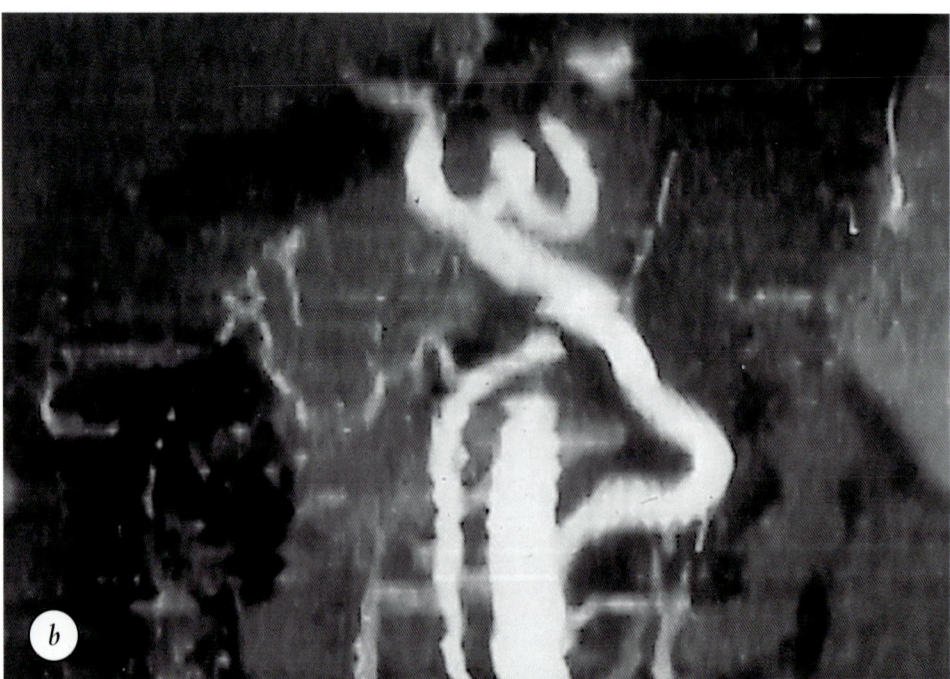

Figure 29.1 –
a) Arterial jumping graft using the donor iliac artery. The artery is anastomosed with the subrenal aorta, tunneled through the transverse mesocolon behind the stomach and anastomosed with the donor hepatic artery. **b)** Post-operative angiographic control of an arterial jumping graft using a Gore-Tex® prosthesis. In this case the donor arterial graft was not available due to widespread atherosclerosis. The prosthesis graft is patent 2 years after the transplant.

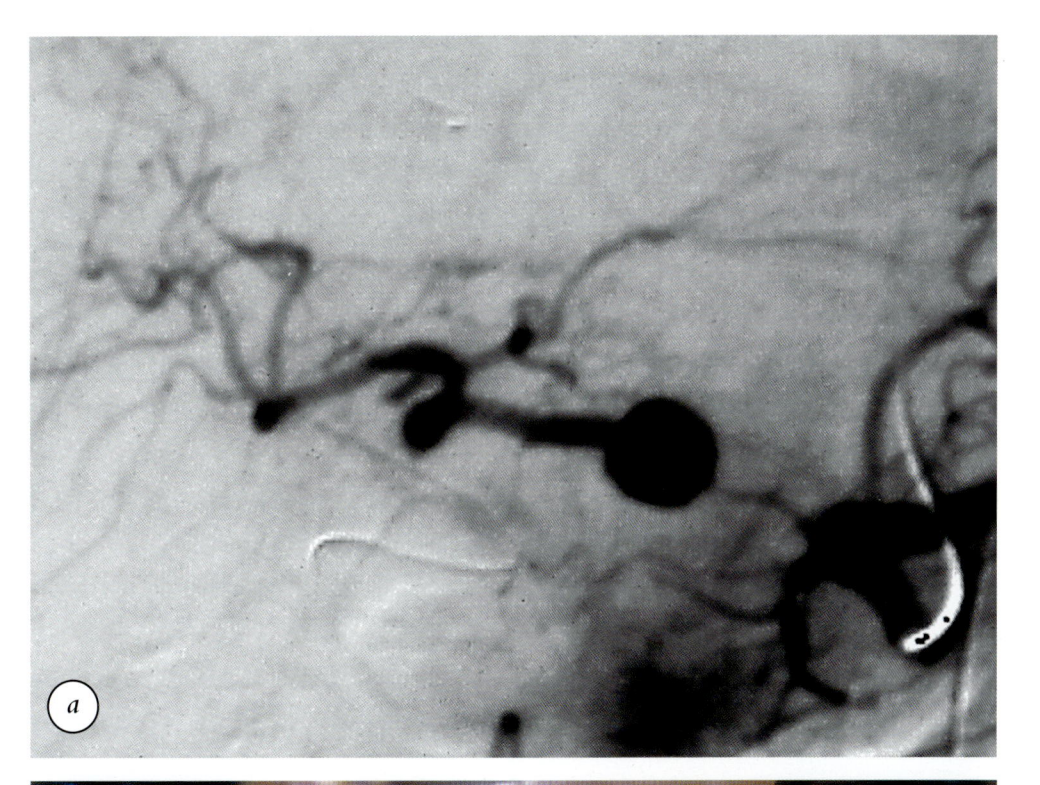

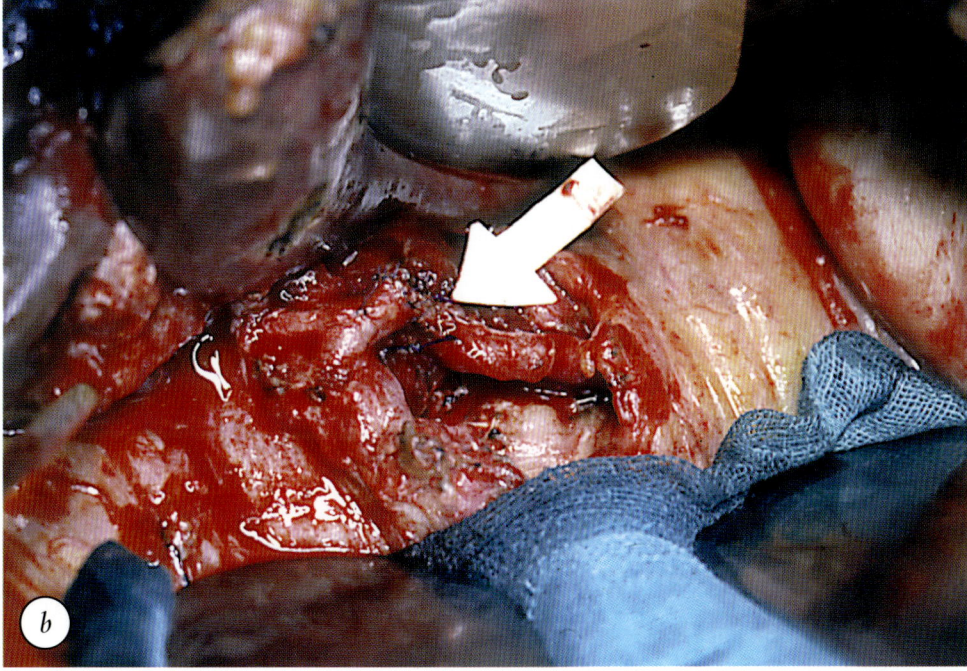

Figure 29.2 –
a) Arterial anastomosis using the recipient splenic artery. The patient had developed an aneurysm of the hepatic artery nine months after the transplant. *b)* After resection of the aneurysm, the splenic artery was divided about 5 cm from the triad, detached from the upper border of the pancreas, and anastomosed end-to-end with the hepatic artery of the graft, which had been isolated downstream from the aneurysm.

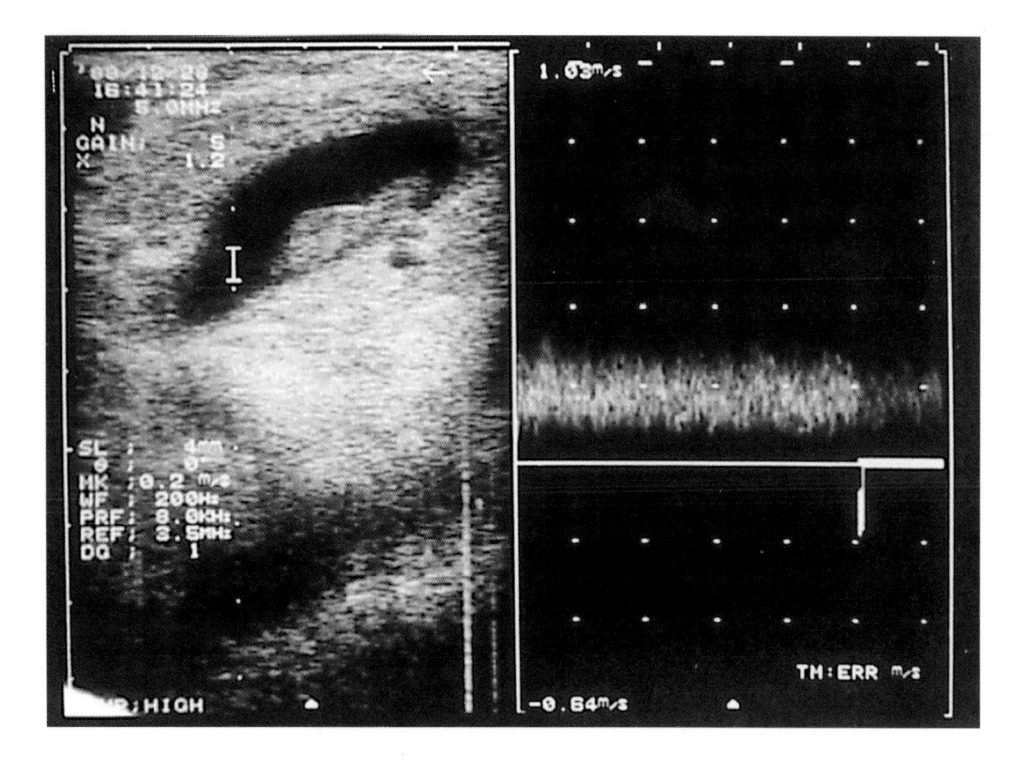

Figure 29.3 – *Recipient portal vein thrombosis. Intra-operative Doppler. The thrombus takes up ⅓ of the vessel lumen in the middle section of the portal trunk.*

operative Doppler may be useful in detecting these complications which may lead to thrombosis.[10] Periarterial injection of papaverin may be useful in the event of a spasm of the artery after declamping. The direct infusion of heparin and anti-coagulant treatment can prevent the onset of a secondary thrombosis in the event of problems arising during aterial anastomosis.

RECIPIENT PORTAL VEIN THROMBOSIS

Partial or total thrombosis of the portal vein may be observed with a frequency of 4 to 13%[16,18,24] in cirrhotic patients. Coagulopathies and stasis are responsible for this problem. It is, however, necessary to exclude the presence of hepatocarcinoma, which can spread inside the portal branches with a neoplastic thrombosis, and is a contraindication to transplantation. Apart from limited parietal thromboses, which do not cause particular technical problems when carrying out the transplantation, the presence of a portal thrombosis detected at pre-operative Doppler assessment requires angiography and, if necessary, a CT to establish the extent of the thrombosis and the involvement of the splenic and superior mesenteric veins which may be used for portal flow conduit. The presence of a complete portal spleno-mesenteric thrombosis with cavernomatous transformation is a serious limitation. (see below).

Isolated thrombosis of the portal vein can be treated with thrombectomy or by construction of the anastomosis distal to the spleno-portal confluence, or with a 'jumping graft' on the mesenteric vein. Portal thrombectomy is indicated in the presence of a thrombosis which occupies the portal lumen without structural alterations of the vessel lumen. Intra-

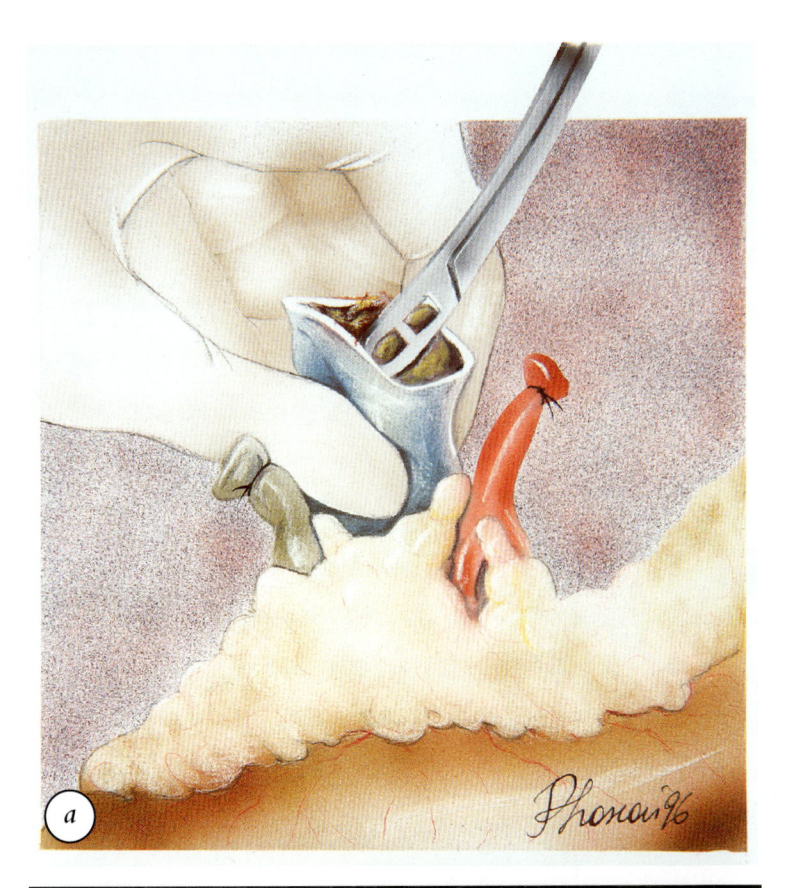

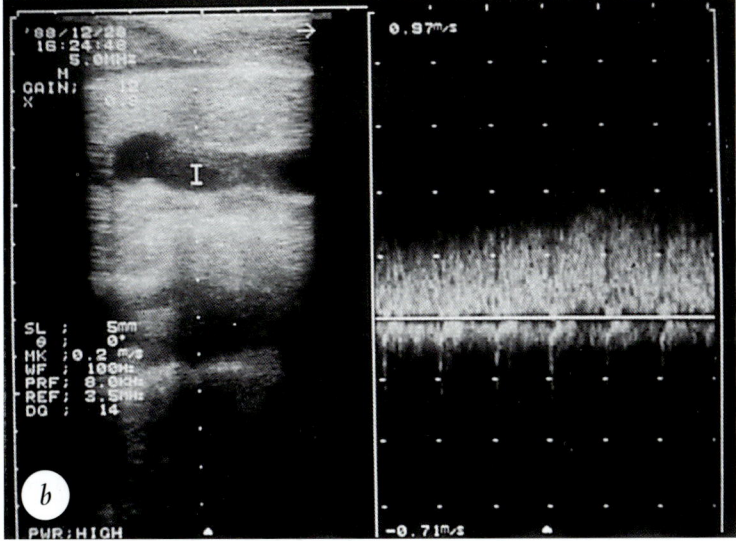

Figure 29.4 – **a)** *Portal vein thrombectomy.* **b)** *Intrao-perative Doppler control after the anastomosis with the graft portal vein.*

operative Doppler can be useful in establishing the exact intraluminal extension of the thrombus (**Figure 29.3**). After skeletonizing the hepatic pedicle and dividing the portal vein, the thrombus can be removed with a smooth clamp or a Fogarty catheter (**Figure 29.4**). The vein must then be washed with heparin and post-operative anticoagulant treatment is advisable. Anastomosis may be performed on the spleno-portal confluence if the thrombus adheres closely to the wall of the portal vein, altering the walls and making the vessel unsuitable for direct anastomosis. The portal vein is dissected distally after dividing the artery and the common bile duct. After removing the lymph node situated on the left aspect of the portal vein, above the common hepatic artery, the portal trunk is detached from the pancreas as far as the spleno-portal confluence in a zone free from thrombotic deposits. Anastomosis can be constructed at this level, or directly with the portal vein of the graft, if it is long enough, or with the interposition of a donor iliac vein graft. (**Figure 29.5**).

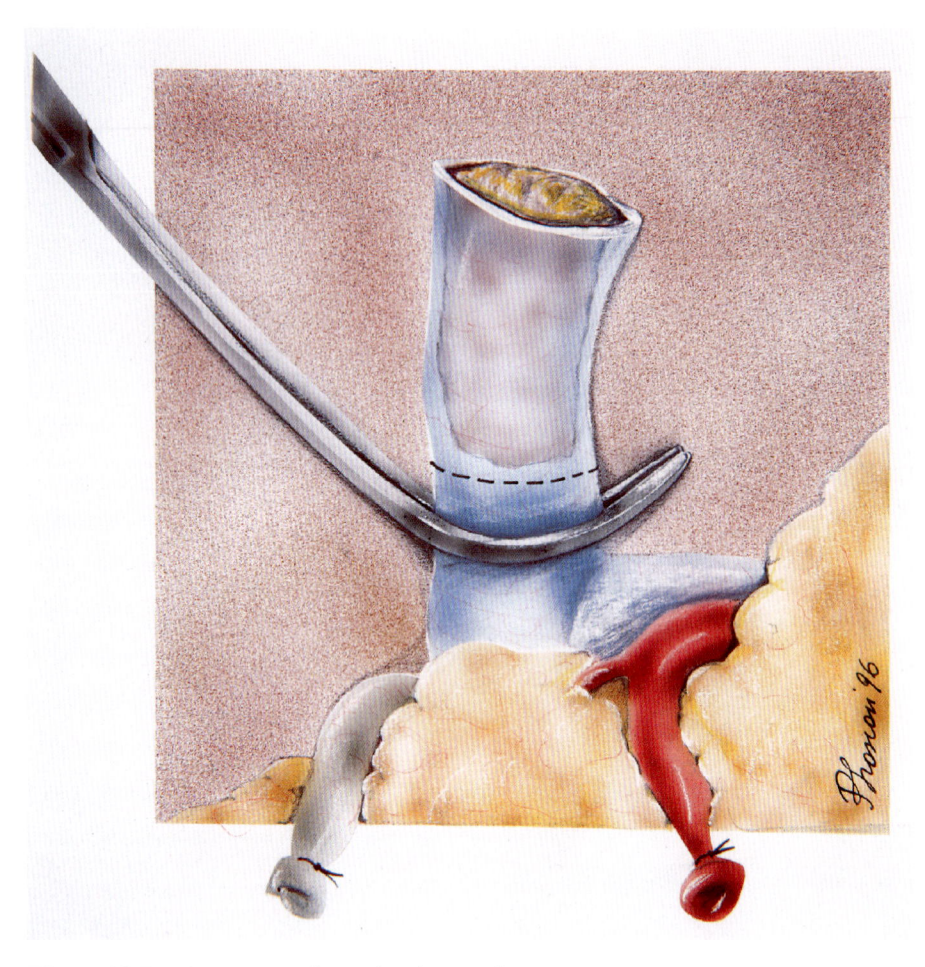

Figure 29.5 – *Recipient portal vein thrombosis. Isolation of the spleno-mesenteric confluence after mobilization of the pancreatic head.*

If neither the portal trunk nor the spleno-portal confluence can be used (as occurs in the cavernomatous transformation of the vein, e.g., after splenectomy) the anastomosis can be constructed on the superior mesenteric vein with interposition of a donor iliac graft.[3,11,20,22,25] This 'jumping graft' is an end-to-side anastomosis to the superior mesenteric vein. It is then tunneled through the transverse mesocolon anterior to the pancreas to reach the hepatic hilum for end-to-end anastomosis to the graft portal vein (**Figure 29.6**).

A review of the major reported series showed that thrombosis of the recipient portal vein was observed in 135 (6%) out of 2,230 transplants. Treatment consisted mainly of thrombectomy (95/135) and only in 40 cases was a venous graft performed. The incidence of rethrombosis varied from 6 to 29%.[4-6,11,12,15,18,24]

HYPOPLASTIC PORTAL VEIN
OR LOW PORTAL FLOW

Low portal flow in the recipient may be the consequence of hypoplasia of the portal vein or, more often, of a wide spontaneous collateral circulation. Pre-operative Doppler investigation, completed by angiography, reveals the site of these collateral circulations. Low portal flow can lead to hypoperfusion of the graft or be the consequence of a late thrombosis of the portal anastomosis.

In the event of a hypoplastic portal vein, the anastomosis can be constructed at the level of the spleno-portal confluence or with a jumping graft on the mesenteric vein. If the reduction in flow is due to a wide spontaneous anastomosis, this must be identified and closed. The most frequent spontaneous shunts are at the level of the left gastric vein, which is

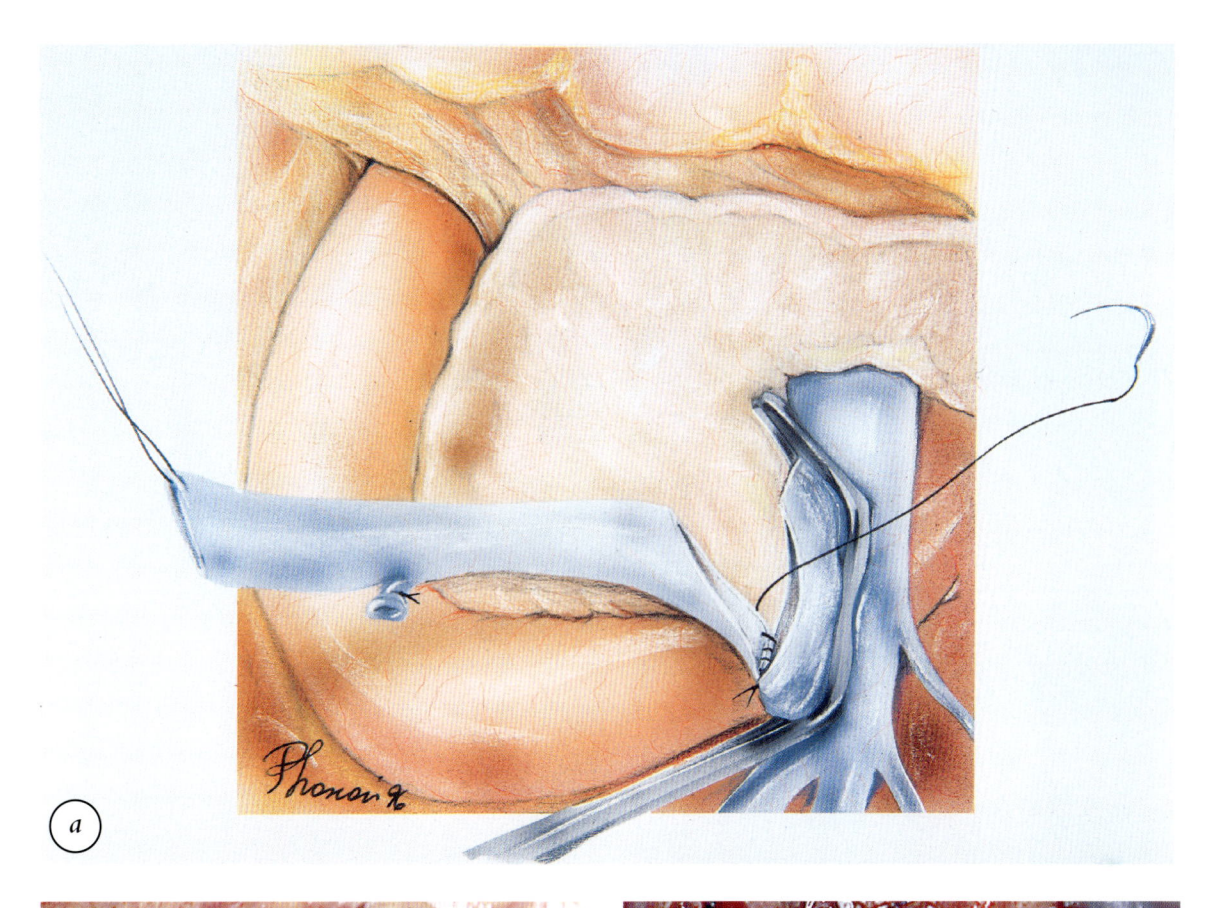

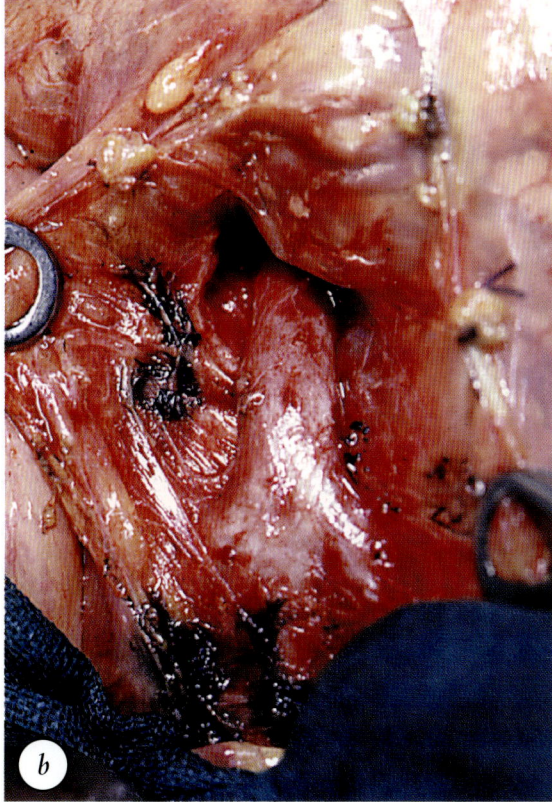

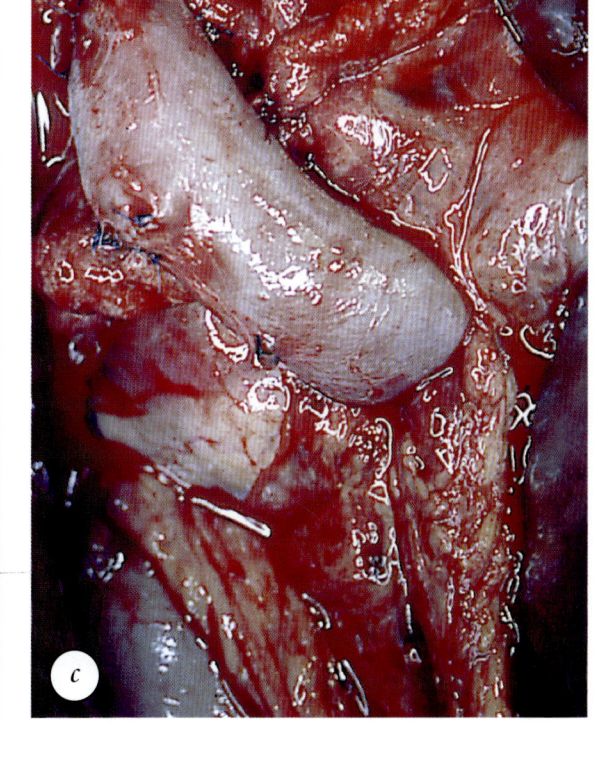

TECHNICAL PROBLEMS AND COMPLICATIONS OF LIVER TRANSPLANTATION

Figure 29.6 – *a)* Portal vein thrombosis. Venous jumping graft with the donor iliac vein anastomosed with the recipient mesenteric vein. The venous graft is tunneled through the transverse mesocolon, in front of the duodenum, and anastomosed with the donor portal vein. *b)* Isolation of the superior mesenteric vein. *c)* The intra-operative field after declamping.

TECHNIQUES IN LIVER SURGERY

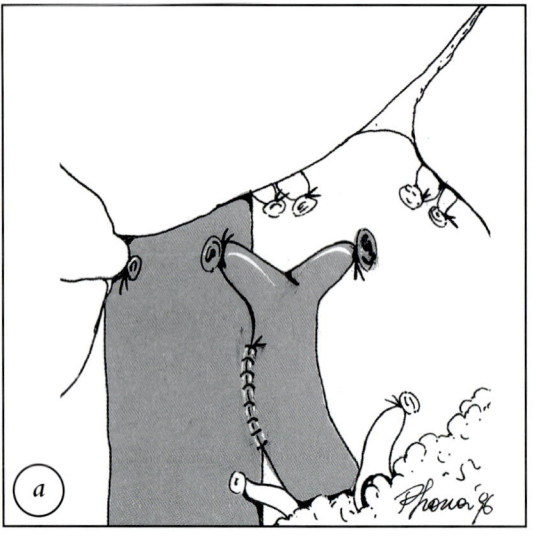

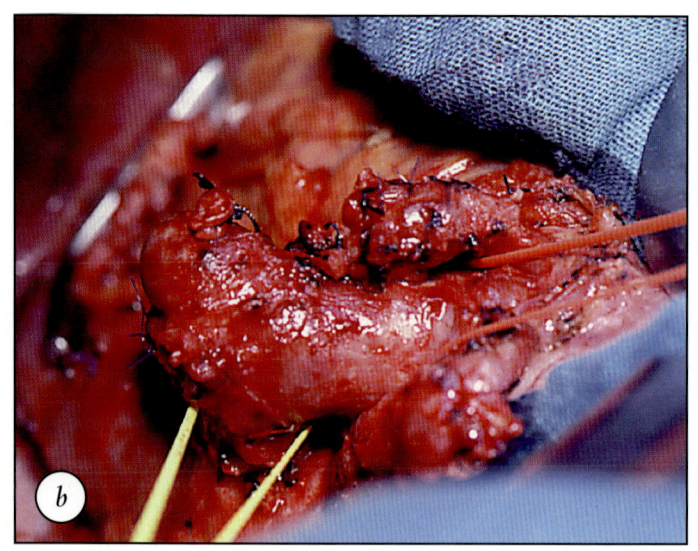

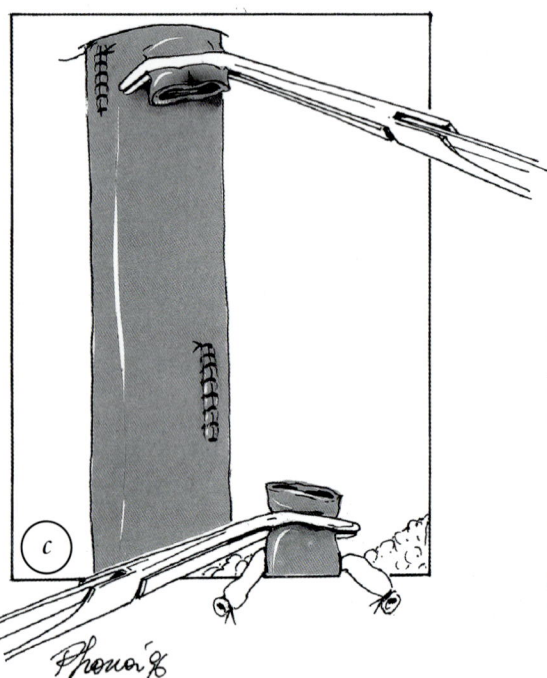

Figure 29.7 – *Transplantation techniques used in patients with previous side-to-side portocaval anatomosis.* ***a)*** *The hepatic pedicle is skeletonized, ligating the bile duct, the hepatic artery and the portal vein distally to the anastomosis. The liver is removed, detaching the vena cava progressively with the 'piggy-back' technique. The right hepatic vein is sutured and the common trunk of the middle and left hepatic veins is clamped.* ***b)*** *The intra-operative field after completion of the hepatectomy. The portal vein was ligated at the level of the bifurcation, a few centimetres above the anastomosis. The portal trunk is encircled with a red tape, the anastomosis with a yellow tape.* ***c)*** *The portocaval anastomosis is closed, the vena cava is sutured and the portal vein is clamped proximally to the previous anastomosis. The graft is then implanted using the 'piggy-back' technique.*

clearly visible on the superior margin of the pancreas, or between the splenic vein and the left renal vein. A spontaneous spleno-renal shunt is more difficult to detect, being situated in the retroperitoneal space between the lower tip of the spleen and the adrenal loggia, in an area where dissection is particularly difficult. If portal flow is reduced, it is advisable to reperfuse the liver first through the artery.

HEMATOMAS OR RUPTURE OF THE GRAFT

Capsular rupture of the graft can be caused by tearing of the ligaments during removal of the donor liver or by trauma during transplantation. If the lesion is detected during graft branch surgery, it must be treated with fibrin glue or with careful suturing if the lesion is deeper. After reperfusion, suturing is more hazardous and can enlarge the wound due to the great fragility of the graft. More extensive lesions may require the use of a Vicryl® mesh (**Figrue 22.3**). SubGlissonian hematomas of the graft should not be opened.

OVERSIZED ALLOGRAFTS AND DIFFICULTY IN CLOSING THE ABDOMINAL WALL

The use of oversized grafts can involve serious technical difficulties in constructing caval anastomoses. The pressure exerted by the abdominal wall and the rib arch on closure of the abdomen may cause ischemia of the peripheral segments of the liver with irreversible impairment of the graft. An increase in abdominal pressure can also lead to an obstruction of the portal vein or of the hepatic veins. It is inadvisable to use donors weighing over

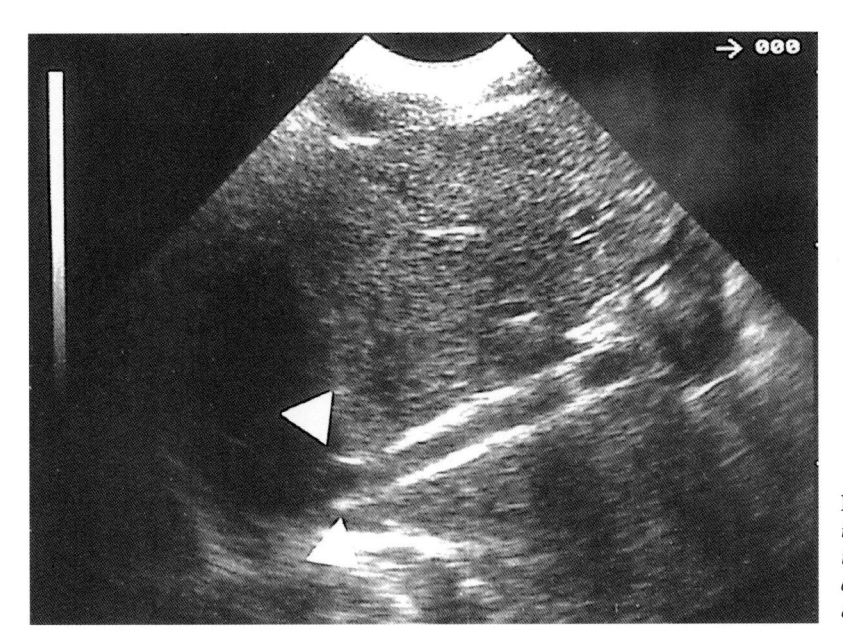

Figure 29.8 – *Dislocation of a TIPS inserted for portal hypertension in a liver transplant candidate. IOU showed the cephalad end of the TIPS (arrow) situated at the level of the right atrium.*

20 kg more than the recipient unless the graft is reduced before transplantation. At times, edema of the graft at reperfusion, or of the intestine, may make it difficult to close the abdominal wall. In these conditions, the wall is closed with a Dacron mesh or the skin may be closed only temporarily, delaying final closure of the abdominal wall until the edema of the liver or the intestine has resolved.

PROBLEMS CONSEQUENT TO A PREVIOUS PORTOSYSTEMIC ANASTOMOSIS

The application of transjugular intrahepatic portosystemic shunts (TIPS) has now resolved many of the problems of gastrointestinal hemorrhage not controlled by sclerotherapy in liver transplant candidate cirrhotic patients. Portosystemic anastomosis is required less and less frequently. Surgical shunts can, however, be used in patients with good liver function and long life expectancy in the event of repeated digestive hemorrhages refractory to sclerotherapy. The presence of a surgical shunt causes particular technical problems depending on the type of anastomosis. The best procedure when transplantation is anticipated is the interposition of a mesocaval graft. In this case, the interposed prosthetic or venous graft is quite simply ligated before reperfusion. Warren's operation causes the most difficult problems. A distal splenorenal shunt leads to a progressive reduction in flow and diameter of the portal vein, and sometimes to portal thrombosis.[1] Suppression of the shunt at transplantation involves splenectomy.

Adoption of the 'piggy-back' technique (see Chapter 28) simplifies many of the technical problems in the presence of a portocaval anastomosis, which was previously considered a particularly problematic condition for liver transplantation. The anastomosis can function throughout the hepatectomy, thus preventing intra-operative hemorrhage. The hepatic pedicle is skeletonized and, after ligating the artery or the bile duct, the portal vein is isolated at the hepatic hilum beyond the anastomosis, ligating and dividing the right and left branches at the bifurcation. The liver is then removed, preserving the recipient vena cava. The portal vein is clamped upstream from the anastomosis, which is then closed on the caval aspect with a vascular TEA (***Figrue 29.7***).

PROBLEMS RESULTING FROM A PREVIOUS TIPS INSERTION

TIPS have been recommended in liver transplant candidates with severe portal hypertension as a palliative procedure while awaiting a suitable donor. However, as the number of cases treated with this technique has increased, a series of complications or technical problems have been reported. The latter include the dislocation of TIPS proximally into the vena cava, right atrium or distally into the portal trunk, which can seriously hinder liver transplantation.[7,13,14] The most complex occurrence is proximal dislocation of the cephalad end of the TIPS (***Figure 29.8***). Decubitus of the TIPS on the caval wall makes this very fragile and the caval wall can easily rupture during attempts to clamp it.[7,14]

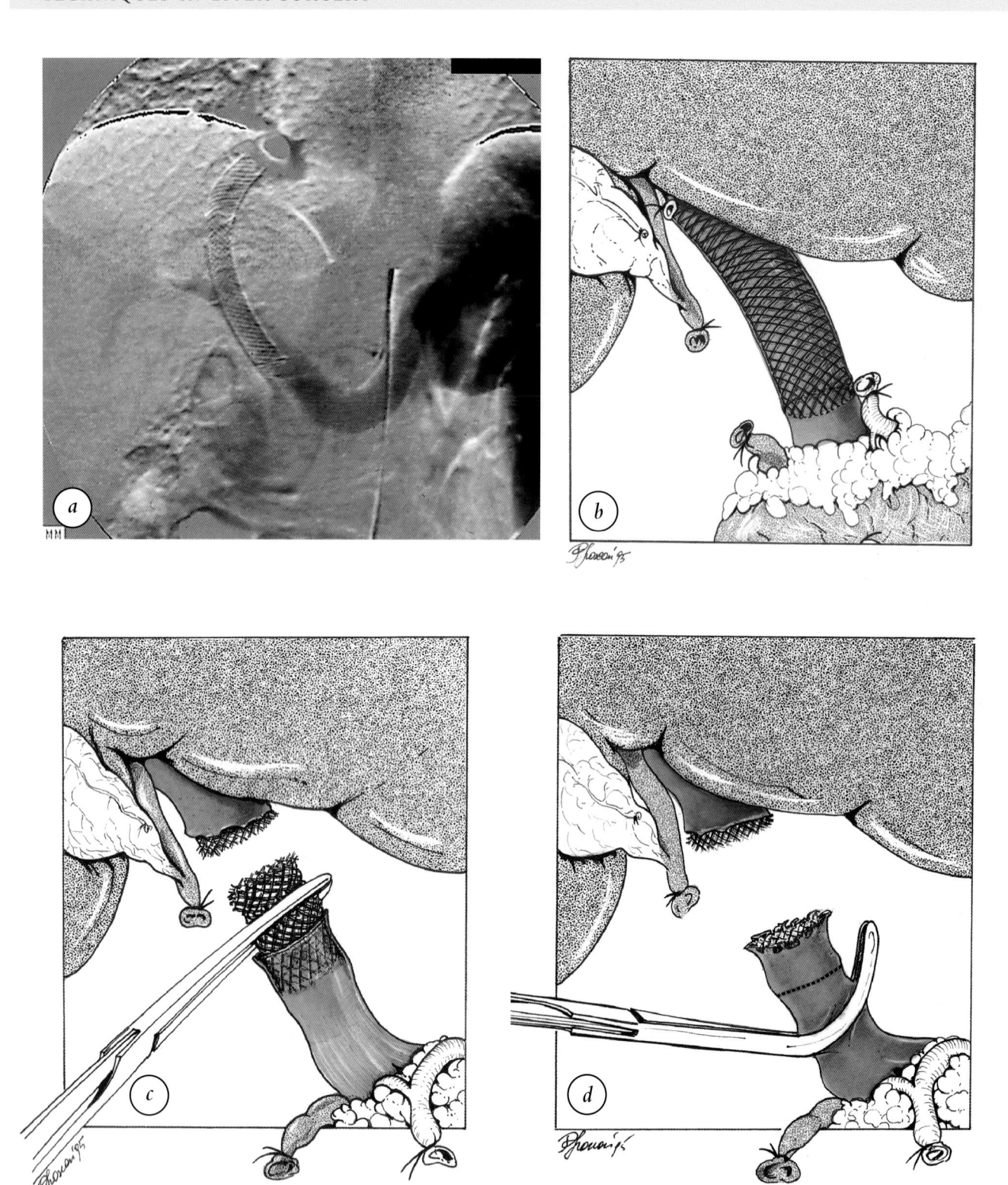

Figure 29.9 – *Dislocation of a TIPS inside the portal trunk. a) Preoperative arteriography. b) The hepatic pedicle is skeletonized and the hepatic artery and the common bile duct are divided. c) The portal vein is detached from the posterior aspect of the pancreas until the splenomesenteric convergence is exposed. Before recipient hepatectomy is performed ('piggyback' technique) the portal trunk containing the TIPS is clamped and divided. d) The portal vein is clamped close to the splenomesenteric convergence. Anastomosis with the graft is constructed distally at the end of the TIPS, in an area of undamaged endothelium.*

The upper vena cava must be isolated higher up than the end of the TIPS, if necessary by opening the diaphragm immediately around the orifice of the vena cava. In the event of dislocation of the distal end of the TIPS in the portal trunk, this should be managed as for portal thrombosis, detaching the portal vein as far as the posterior aspect of the pancreas after displacing the hepatic artery and exposing the spleno-portal confluence (**Figure 29.9**). The portal clamp is positioned in this distal site so that an anastomosis can be fashioned with the portal vein of the graft in a safe area.

Patients who have undergone TIPS need careful radiological evaluation before transplantation, in order to ascertain the correct position of the stent. If ultrasound suggests malpositioning of the TIPS, then a CT or angiography must be performed to avoid any unexpected, catastrophic consequences during transplantation. In cirrhotic transplant candidates, the stents should be as short as possible to prevent the ends of the TIPS protruding outside the liver, due to the generally reduced dimensions of the liver in advanced cirrhosis.

Cavoportal transposition for complete porto-splenic-mesenteric thrombosis

Total occlusion of the portal trunk, the splenic and superior mesenteric veins with cavernomatous transformation was considered a contraindication for liver transplantation. In 1996, Tzakis from the University of Miami (personal communication) performed two successful liver transplantations in such conditions, introducing a new technique using the retrohepatic recipient vena cava as a conduit for graft portal reconstruction.

We performed this cavoportal transposition early in 1997 in a 62-year-old cirrhotic patient with refractory ascites and marked liver insufficiency. The patient had never presented gastro-esophageal bleeding. An attempt at portal and mesenteric disobstruction failed due to massive thrombosis. The retrohepatic vena cava was prepared, dividing the accessory hepatic veins, the right adrenal and the posterior diaphragmatic veins (**Figure 29.10a**). A cavo-axillary by-pass by means of a Bio-pump was inserted through the left saphenous vein. The inferior vena cava was clamped above and below the liver and sectioned at the level of the confluence of the main hepatic veins, removing the native liver and leaving an 8 cm segment of vena cava above the renal veins (**Figure 29.10b**). The upper vena cava of the graft was anastomosed end-to-end with the recipient sub-diaphragmatic cava. The lower vena cava of the graft was stapled after flushing the graft with albumin solution (**Figure 29.10c**). The recipient vena cava was then turned anteriorly and anastomosed with the graft portal vein, this latter was fashioned to balance the difference in diameter between the two vessels,(**Figure 29.10d**). The venous by-pass was stopped, the clamp released and the graft revascularised. The remaining part of the operation followed the routine technique. The early postoperative period was uneventful with a transient ascites treated with diuretics, albumin infusion and paracentesis. The patient was discharged in good condition 32 days after the operation. Cavography shows the patency of the cavo-portal anastomosis (**Figure 29.10e**).

This technique will allow transplantation in certain patients formerly considered unsuitable. The ascites which occurred in the early postoperative period in our patient gradually disappeared, confirming that portal thrombosis does not lead to ascites if the liver is healthy. Nevertheless, the indication for this technique must be carefully considered in patients with esophageal varices refractory to scierotherapy. In such patients a complementary technique must be contemplated to prevent the risk of recurrent hemorrhage (esophageal transection, embolization of the spienic artery).

Late complications

HEMORRHAGE

Post-operative hemorrhage can originate from the surgical dissection zones or from the vascular anastomoses. Extensive hemorrhage can also be the result of coagulation disorders. Relaparotomy must allow examination of the entire supramesocolic space, the vascular anastomoses and the graft in order to detect a capsular rupture or small venous branches, such as a diaphragmatic vein, which have been badly sutured during bench preparation.

SEPTIC COMPLICATIONS

Subphrenic abscesses are generally the result of biliary leakage and must be treated primarily with ultrasound and CT-guided percutaneous drainage. Intestinal perforations have rarely been described and can be the consequence of a serosal defect produced during the dissection of previous adherences. Ileal perforation must be recognized immediately and treated with direct suture or intestinal resection.

TECHNIQUES IN LIVER SURGERY

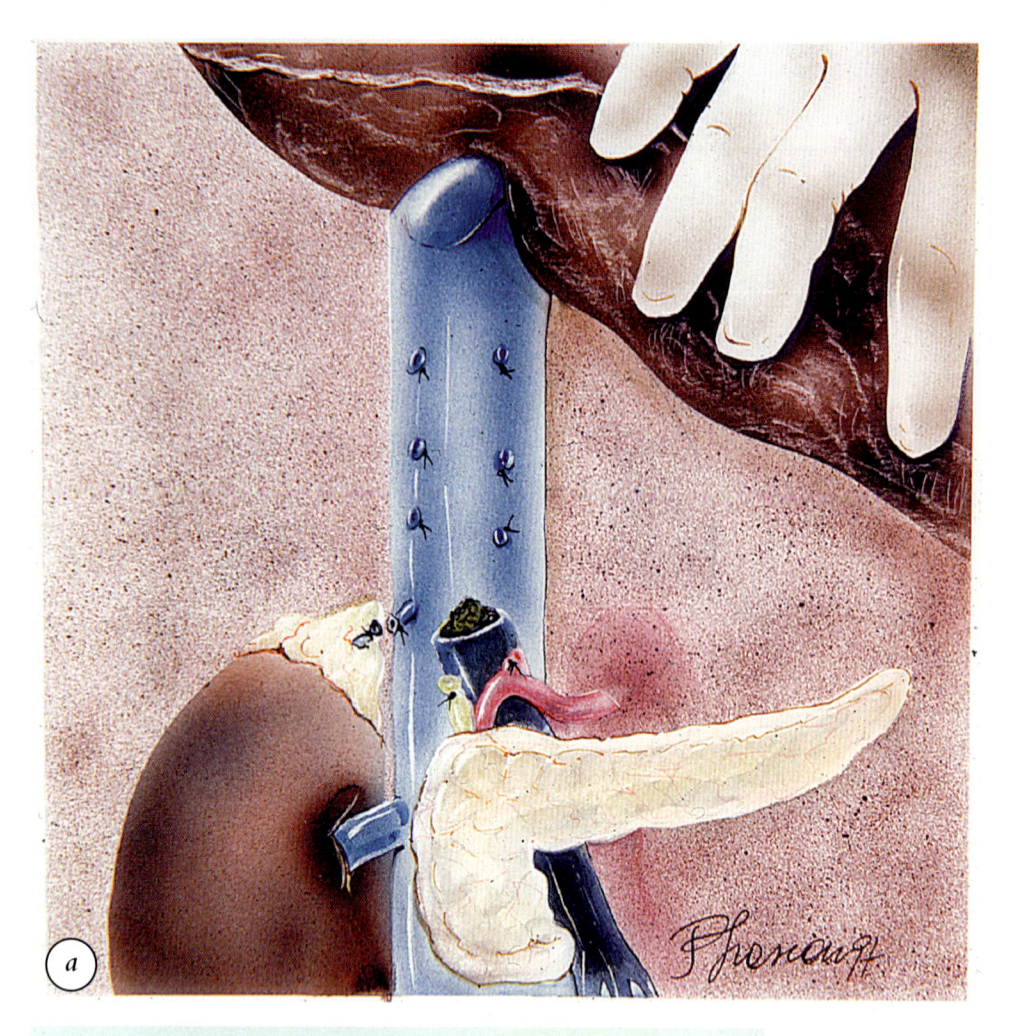

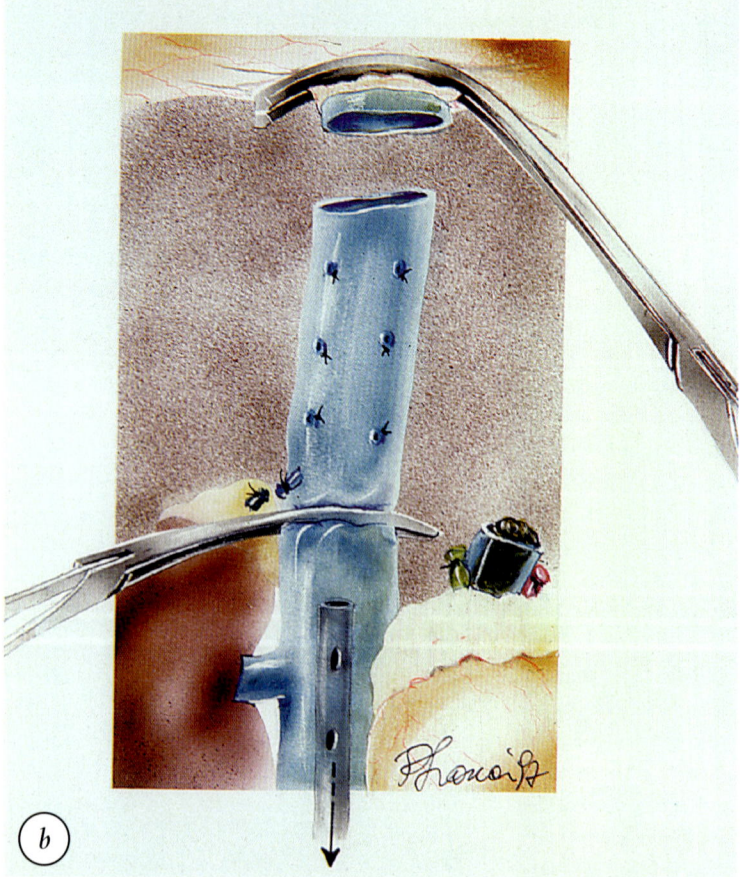

Figure. 29.10 – *Cavo-portal transposition for complete porto-splenic-mesenteric thrombosis.*
a) *The hepatic pedicle is scheletonized. Portal trunk, hepatic artery and bile duct are sectioned. The liver is pulled up and the accessories hepatic veins are interrupted. The right adrenal vein is also sectioned in order to free completely the retrohepatic vena cava.* ***b)*** *Patient is placed on cavo-axillary by-pass. The inferior vena cava is clamped below and above the liver and the hepatectomy is completed leaving in place a long segment of distal vena cava.*
c-e) *Opposite page.*

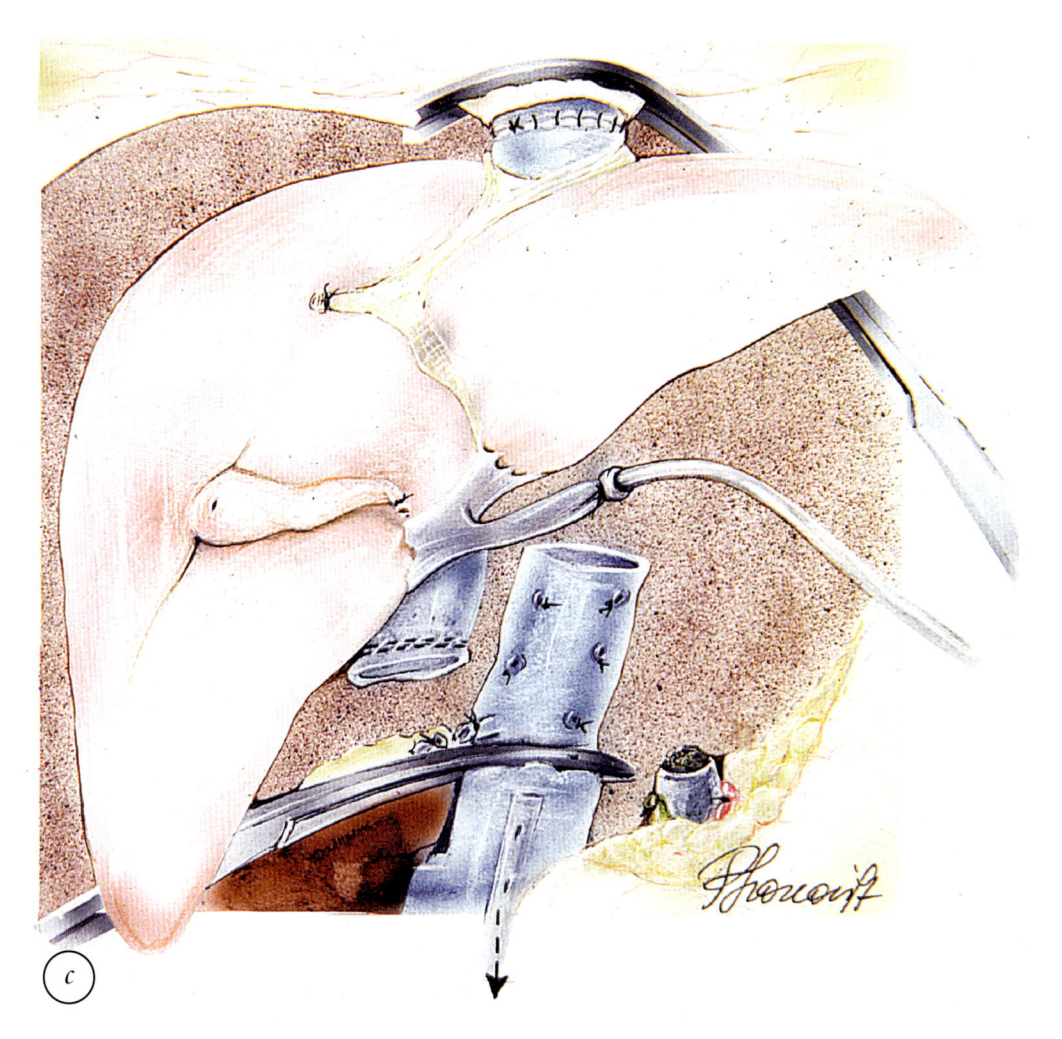

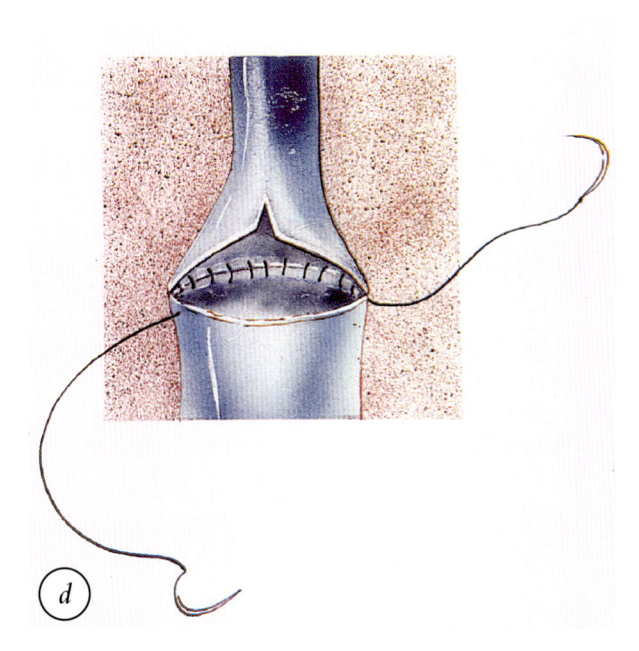

Figure. 29.10 – *Cavo-portal transposition for complete porto-splenic-mesenteric thrombosis. (continued)*

c) The upper vena cava anastomosis is accomplished, the graft flushed and the lower vena cava of the graft stapled.
d) Anastomosis between the recipient vena cava and the graft portal vein.
e) Cavography performed on the 10th post-operative day.

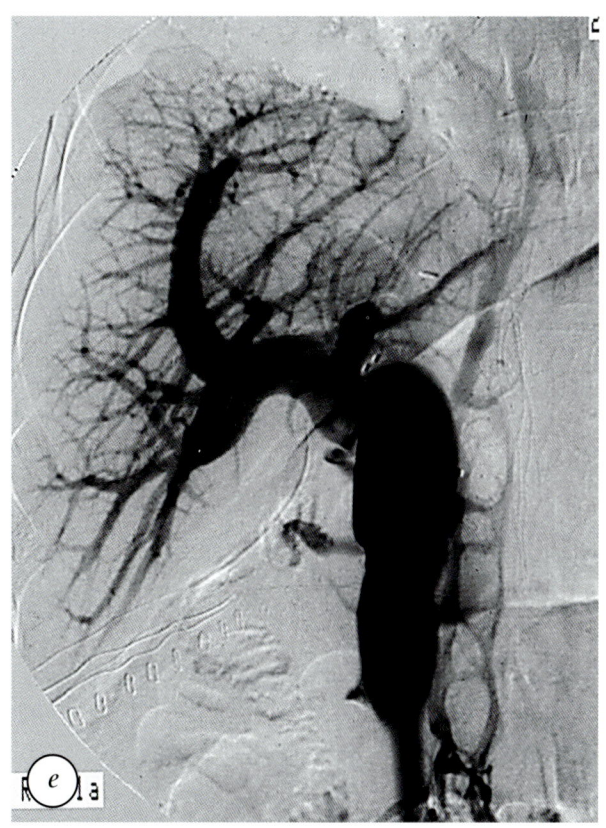

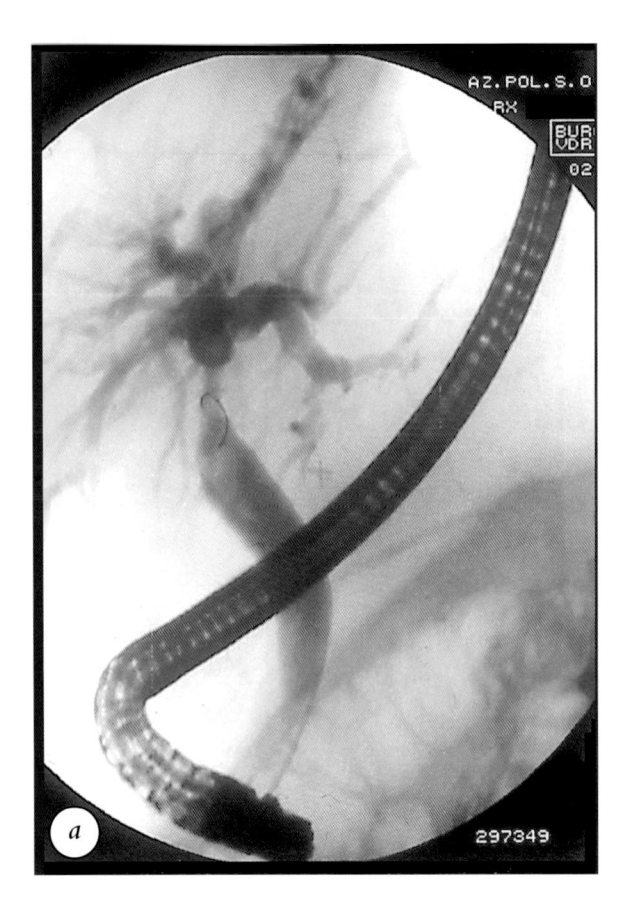

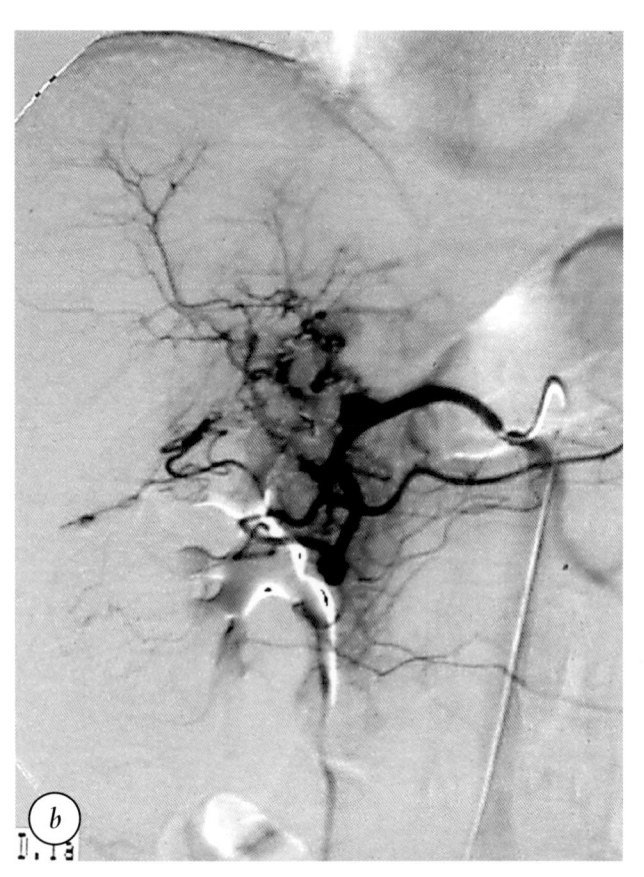

Figure 29.11 – *Stenosis of the biliary anastomosis due to a late thrombosis of the hepatic artery, nine months after transplantation. The cytolytic enzymes were within the normal range and the hepatic biopsy did not show ischemic lesions. The patient underwent bilioenteric anastomosis with Roux loop and presented no problems 2 years after the operation.* **a)** *Retrograde cholangiography showing the stenosis of the commom hepatic duct above the anastomosis.* **b)** *Hepatic arteriography showing the thrombosis of the anastomosis and the partial revascularisation of the graft through collateral vascular beds. During the hepatojejunostomy great care was taken to respect these arterial collaterals and the entire posterior wall of the bile duct was, therefore, left intact.* **c)** *Postoperative cholangiographic control before removing the transanastomotic stent, 3 weeks after the hepatojejunostomy.*

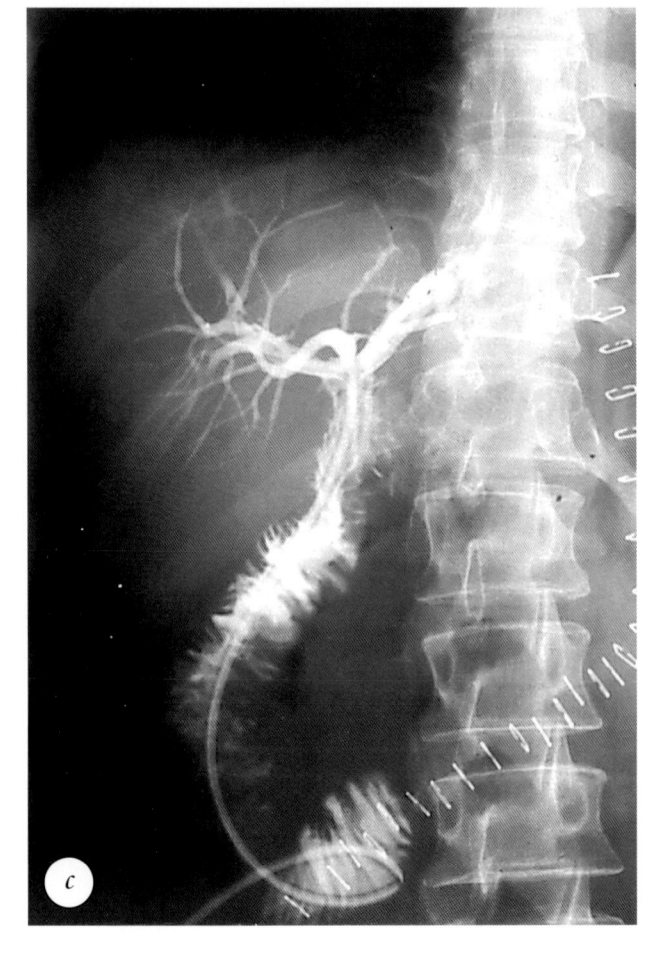

BILIARY COMPLICATIONS

Biliary anastomosis complications are the most frequently encountered surgical problems after transplantation. They include biliary leakage, stenosis of the anastomosis and late complications. These problems may be caused by an error at biliary anastomosis or by vascular problems, such as ischemia of the common bile duct stumps or thrombosis of the hepatic artery. Cholangiography through the Kehr tube at the end of the operation can detect the tightness of the common bile duct anastomosis, technical problems or malpositioning of the Kehr tube itself. Post-operatively, cholangiography through the T-tube should be performed if there is an increase in bilirubinemia or cholestatic enzymes. In the event of stenosis of the biliary anastomosis or biliary leakage, Doppler investigation of the hepatic artery should always be carried out, since these complications could be the result of an ischemic problem arising from thrombosis of the arterial anastomosis. Minor biliary leaks heal spontaneously by means of the abdominal drainages, but taking care to keep the T-tube open. More persistent leaks require perendoscopic intubation.[2,21] Stenoses of the anastomosis must also be treated, first transendoscopically, or with dilation and percutaneous catheterization. Bilioenteric anastomosis on a Roux loop is the definitive treatment for this complication, which has an incidence of 1 to 4% in the various series.

THROMBOSIS OF ARTERIAL ANASTOMOSIS

Clinical presentation of a thrombosis of arterial anastomosis can be massive necrosis of the graft, biliary complications, or stenoses of the biliary anastomosis due to late thrombosis. Early thrombosis of the artery leads to necrosis of the graft a halt in bile production, fever and a dramatic increase in the cytonecrosis enzymes. Doppler allows immediate diagnosis which should be confirmed at arteriography. In late thromboses, a few months after transplantation, biliary sepsis prevails, with stenosis of the biliary anastomosis and the formation of intrahepatic abscesses with biliospetic crises. Re-transplant is the only solution in these situations. Thrombosis of the artery can, occasionally, lead to an isolated stenosis of the bile tract without signs of cytolysis and without septic complications. This is a late thrombosis with gradual onset and formation of collateral circulations. This occurrence was observed in our department in two cases out of more than 300 transplants, and was successfully treated with a bilioenteric anastomosis (*Figure 29.11*).

REFERENCES

1. Bolondi L, Gaiani S, Mazziotti A, Casanova P, Cavallari A, Gozzetti G. Morphological and hemodynamic changes in the portal venous system after distal splenorenal shunt: an ultrasound and pulsed Doppler study. *Hepatology* 1988; **8**: 652-657.

2. Born P, Bruhl K, Rosch T, Ungeheuer A, Neuhaus N, Classen M. Long term follow up of endoscopic therapy in patients with post surgical biliary leakage. *Hepato-Gastroenterol* 1996; **43**: 477-482.

3. Burdock JK, Pitt HA, Colombani PM *et al*. Superior mesenteric vein inflow for liver transplantation when portal vein is occluded. *Surgery* 1990; **107**: 342-345.

4. Busuttil RW, Shaked A, Millis JM *et al*. One thousand liver transplants. The lesson learned. *Ann Surg* 1994; **219**: 490-499.

5. Busuttil RW, Klintman GB. Transplantation of the liver. WB Saunders, Philadelphia, 1996.

6. Davidson BR, Gibson M, Dick R *et al*. Incidence, risk factors, management and outcome of portal vein abnormalities in liver transplantation. *Transplantation* 1994;**57**:1174-1177.

7. Freeman RB, Fitz-Maurice SE, Greenfield AE, Halin N, Hang CE, Roher RJ. Is the transjugular intrahepatic portosystemic shunt procedure beneficial for liver transplant recipients? *Transplantation* 1994; **58**: 297-302.

8. Goldstein RM, Secrest CL, Klinturalm BB, Husberg BS. Problematic vascular reconstruction in liver transplantation. Part 1: *Arterial. Surgery* 1990; **107**: 540-543.

9. Gordon RD, Van Thiel D, Starzl TE. Liver Transplantation. In Schiff L, Schiff ER *Diseases of the Liver*, Lippincott, Phildalphia, 1993.

10. Gozzetti G, Mazziotti A, Bolondi L, Barbara L. *Intraoperative ultrasonography in hepato-biliary and pancreatic surgery*. Kluwer, Dortrecht, 1989.

11. Kirsch JP, Howard TK, Klintman GB *et al*. Problematic vascular reconstruction in liver transplantation. Part II. Portovenous conduits. *Surgery* 1990; **107**: 544-548.

12. Langnas AN, Maruso WC, Stratta RJ, *et al*. A selective approach to pre-existing portal vein thrombosis in patients undergoing liver transplantation. *Am J Surg* 1992; **163**: 132-136.

13. Mazziotti A, Morelli MC, Grazi GL, Jovine E, Cavallari A. Beware of TIPS in liver transplant candidates. *Hepato-Gastroenterol* 1996; **43: 1606-1010**.

14. Millis MJ, Martin P, Gomes A *et al*. Transjugular intrahepatic portosystemic shunt: impact on liver transplantation. *Liver Transpl Surg* 1995; **1**: 229-233.

15. Moreno Gonzales E, Garcia IG, Sanz RG *et al*. Liver transplantation in patients with thrombosis of the portal-splenic or superior mesenteric vein. *Br J Surg* 1993; **80**: 81-85.

16. Nonami T, Yokoyama I, Iwatsuki S, Starzl TE. The incidence of portal vein thrombosis at liver transplantation. *Hepatology* 1992; **16**: 1195-1198.

17. Palareti G, Legnani C, Maccaferri M, Gozzetti G, Mazziotti A. Coagulation and fibrinolysis in

orthotopic liver transplantation: role of the recipient's disease and use of antithrombin III concentrates. *Hemostasis* 1992; **21**: 68-76.

18. Shaked H, Busuttil RW. Liver transplantation in patients with portal vein thrombosis and portacaval shunt. *Ann Surg* 1992;**214**:690-672.
19. Shaw BW Jr, Iwatsuki S, Starzl TE. Alternative methods of arterialization of the hepatic graft. *Surg Gynecol Obstetr* 1984; **164**: 491-194.
20. Shaw BW Jr, Iwatsuki S, Bron K *et al*. Portal vein graft in hepatic transplantation. *Surg Gynecol Obstetr* 1985; **161**: 65-69.
21. Sherman S, Shaked S, Goldstein LI, Busuttil RW. Endoscopic management of biliary fistulas complicating liver transplantation and other hepatobiliary operations. *Ann Surg* 1993; **218**: 167-175.
22. Shiel AGR, Thompson JF, Stewens MS *et al*. Mesoportal graft from thrombosed portal vein in liver transplantation. *Clinical Transplant* 1987; **1**: 18-20.
23. Starzl TE, Putnam CW, Hansbrough JF *et al*. Biliary complications after liver transplantation with special reference to the biliary cast syndrome and technique of secondary duct repair. *Surgery* 1986; **81**: 212-221.
24. Stieber AC, Zetti R, Todo S *et al*. The spectrum of portal vein thrombosis in liver transplantation. *Ann Surg* 1991; **213**: 199-203.
25. Tzakis AG, Todo S. Stieber A, Starzl TE. Venous jump grafts for liver transplantation in patients with portal vein thrombosis. *Transplantation* 1989; **46**: 530-531.
26. Tzakis AG, Todo S, Starzl TE. The anterior route for arterial graft conduits in liver transplantation. *Transplant Intern* 1989; **2**: 121-124.

TECHNIQUES IN LIVER SURGERY

SECTION XI

Advanced Techniques of Liver Transplantation

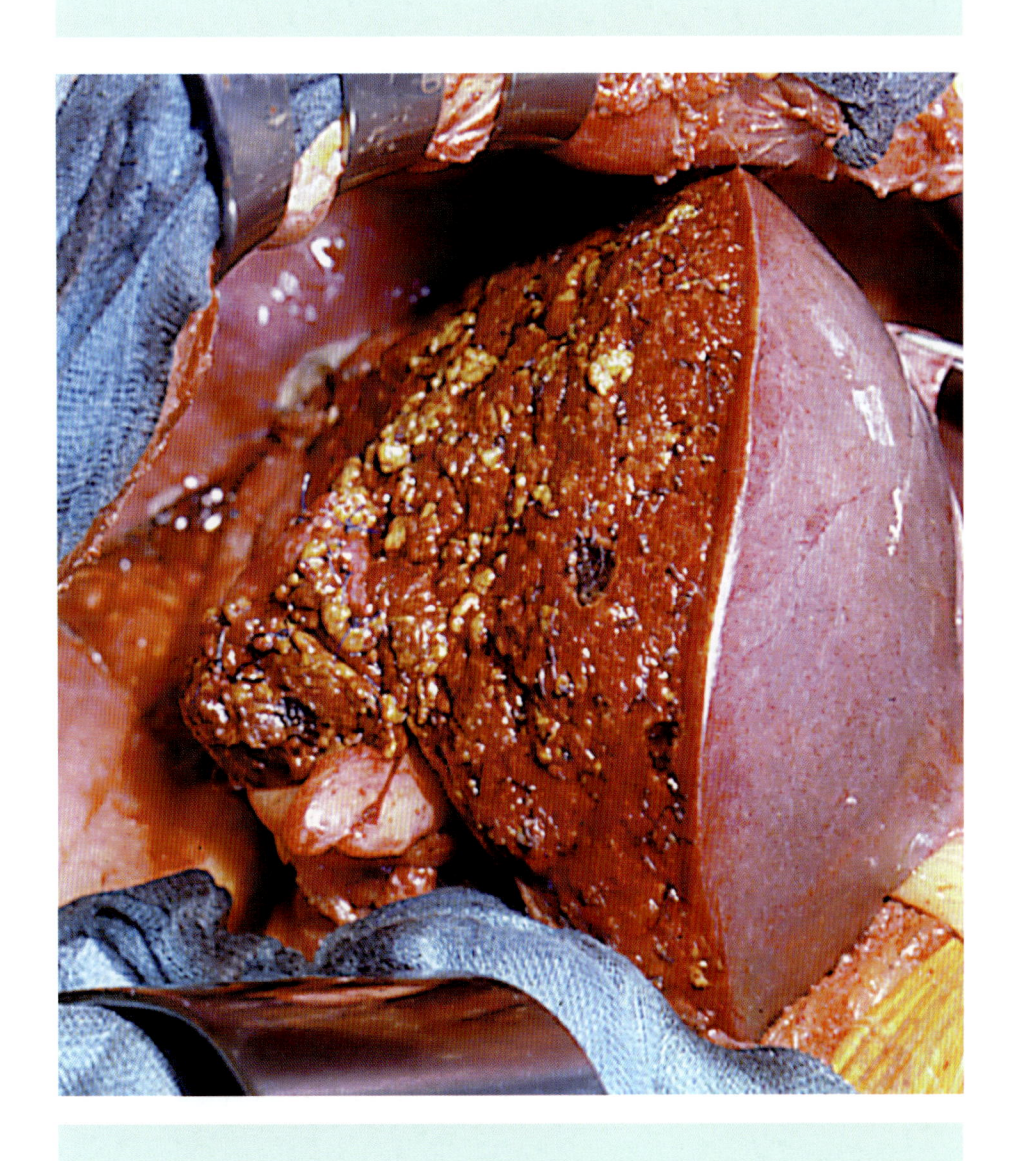

30

Reduced Grafts and Split Liver Transplantation

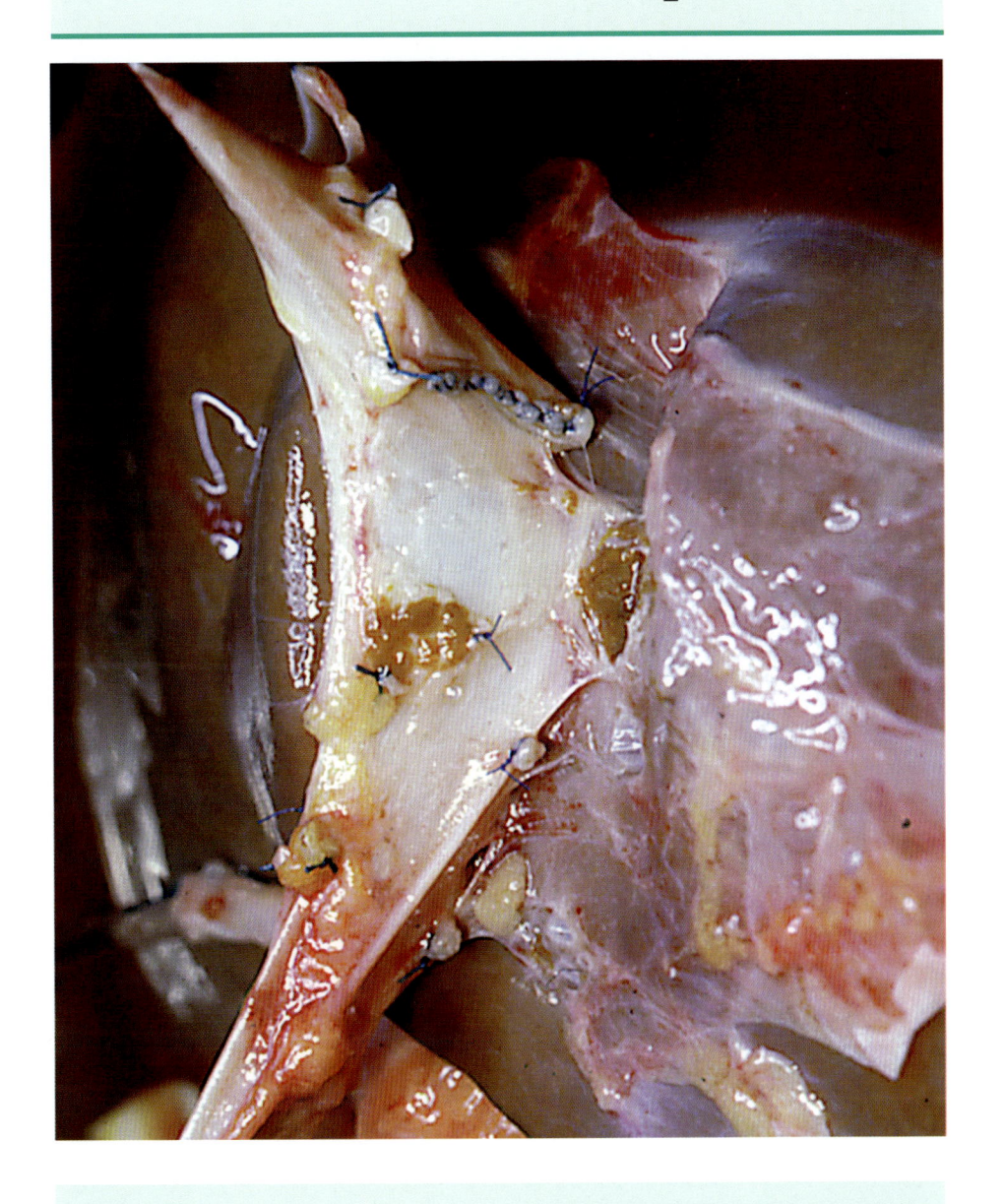

G.L. Grazi

The rapid improvement in results achieved with liver transplantation has led to an extension of its indications. There has not, however, been a parallel increase in organ donations, with the result that the waiting time to obtain a graft has grown. A number of patients consequently die while awaiting donor livers.[4,5,8] This problem is particularly acute in the pediatric population, for whom the pool of compatible donors in terms of body size is extremely limited. One possible solution is the transplant of reduced size grafts for small recipients: infants, children or very small adults. The possibility of such a procedure is based on the segmentary anatomy of the liver (see Chapter 1). The same consideration has permitted further development of the reduction technique, making it possible to transplant two patients with the same graft, previously divided on the bench.

The technical problems, both for reduced size organ transplants and more so for split transplants, are due to the large number of vascular and biliary anatomical variations. Many of the technical considerations and the possible pitfalls involved in performing reduced size grafts or split liver transplants are similar to those for major liver resections. The initial results of reduced size and split liver transplants from the pioneering centers were disappointing. This was due, at least in part, to the critical clinical condition of the patients undergoing transplantation. The improvements in technique and growing experience have led to satisfactory results, comparable to those obtained with whole organs,[1] and add these procedures to the list of techniques carried out by the liver transplant surgeon. Two surgical teams are required for reduced size grafts and split transplants, the first to carry out the harvesting and preparation of the organ on the bench and the second to perform the transplant, so as to reduce the hypothermic ischemia time.

Reduced size liver transplantation

Indications

When a patient can benefit from transplantation of a whole liver, this is always the operation of choice. However, in small adults or in critically ill children, it is possible to consider the use of an organ from a donor with different characteristics, after the liver has been reduced in size on the bench. There are a number of criteria to be considered in deciding which segment of the liver to transplant[12] and the choice is not always easy in view of the difference in weight and volume of the various segments in different individuals. In children, the weight of the donor should not be more than 10 times the weight of the recipient.[4] However, left lateral segment size does not correlate with donor weight. It is the actual size of the segment used that is the important factor. A higher donor/recipient weight ratio can be incompatible with adequate perfusion of the graft.[16] Reduction in size, carried out on the bench, was initially described by Bismuth[2] and Broelsch.[3] Three different types of reduced livers are used: the whole right hemiliver (S5,6,7,8), the whole left hemiliver (S2,3,4) or just the left lateral segments (S2,3), according to Couinaud's description.

Technique

The initial preparation of the liver is performed according to the technique commonly employed for whole organs. On the bench, immersed in the preservation solution in a bag and surrounded by a slush of cold water and ice, the liver is freed from the diaphragm and parts of the peritoneum included in the harvesting. As for whole organs, the arterial, portal and biliary structures of the hepatic hilum are isolated, but dissection is carried out until the arterial and portal bifurcations and the convergence of the left and right hepatic ducts

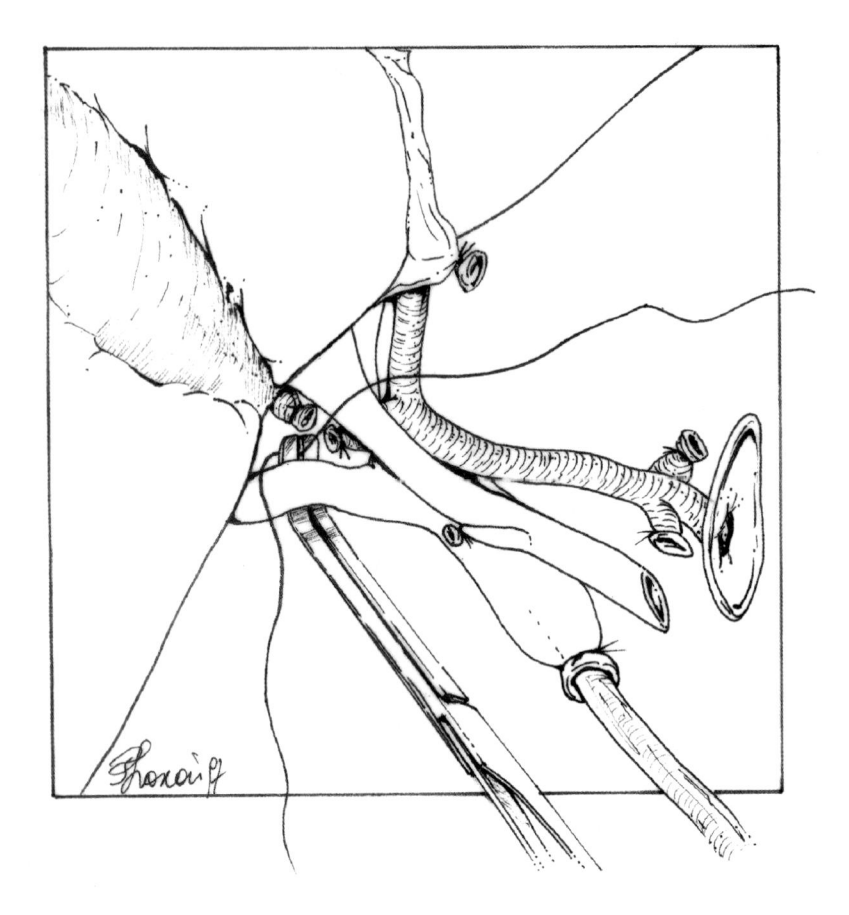

Figure 30.1 – *Reduced size liver transplantation. Hilar dissection.*

can be seen. Once they have been identified, these structures are encircled with a vessel loop before proceeding further. Exploration with a blunt probe which does not damage the vascular and biliary endothelium can help to establish possible anatomical anomalies. Another consideration, regardless of the segments to be transplanted, is that the dissection of the biliary tract must be sufficient to allow the isolation of the duct of the hemiliver to be removed, but not so extensive as to risk impairing the vascularization of the duct to be transplanted, with possible ischemic necrosis. Finally, great care must be taken to identify possible anatomical variations of the hepatic artery: any accessory arteries afferent to the graft must be recognised and preserved. An accessory right hepatic artery arising from the superior mesenteric artery must be reconstructed according to the conventional 'folding' technique or anastomosed end-to-end on the stumps of the splenic artery or the gastroduodenal artery.

Our preferred resection technique is very similar to the procedure adopted during hepatic resections performed transparenchymally in vivo. After dividing Glisson's capsule with a scalpel blade, the parenchyma is divided by gently crushing it with a Kelly clamp. The intraparenchymal vessels are generally easy to identify with this method. Small vessels are ligated with Vicryl® 4-0 only on the liver to be transplanted, and then divided. The Glissonian pedicles and the peripheral branches of the hepatic veins are sutured with Vicryl® or Prolene®. Once division of the parenchyma is complete, the organ is perfused through the portal vein and the celiac trunk with the same preservation solution used during procurement: this allows detection of leakage of liquid from the resected surface. The use of magnifying loops is extremely useful. In view of the leakage after revascularisation with reduced grafts, it is advisable to treat the resected surface with biological glues before implantation.

REDUCED GRAFTS AND SPLIT LIVER TRANSPLANTATION

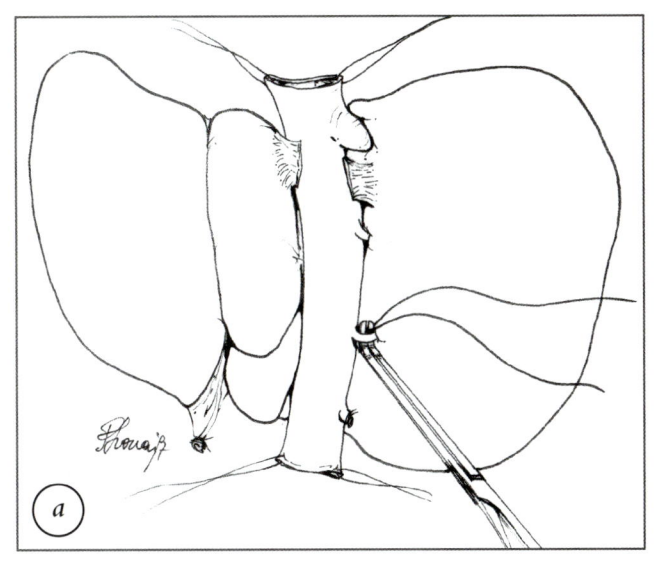

Figure 30.2 – *Reduced size liver transplantation. **a)** Ligation of accessory hepatic veins. **b)** Suture of the right hepatic vein.*

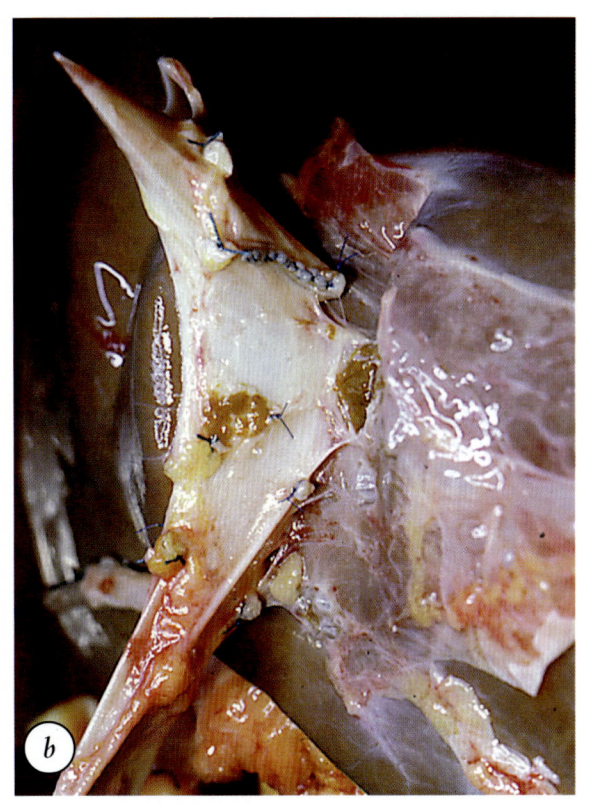

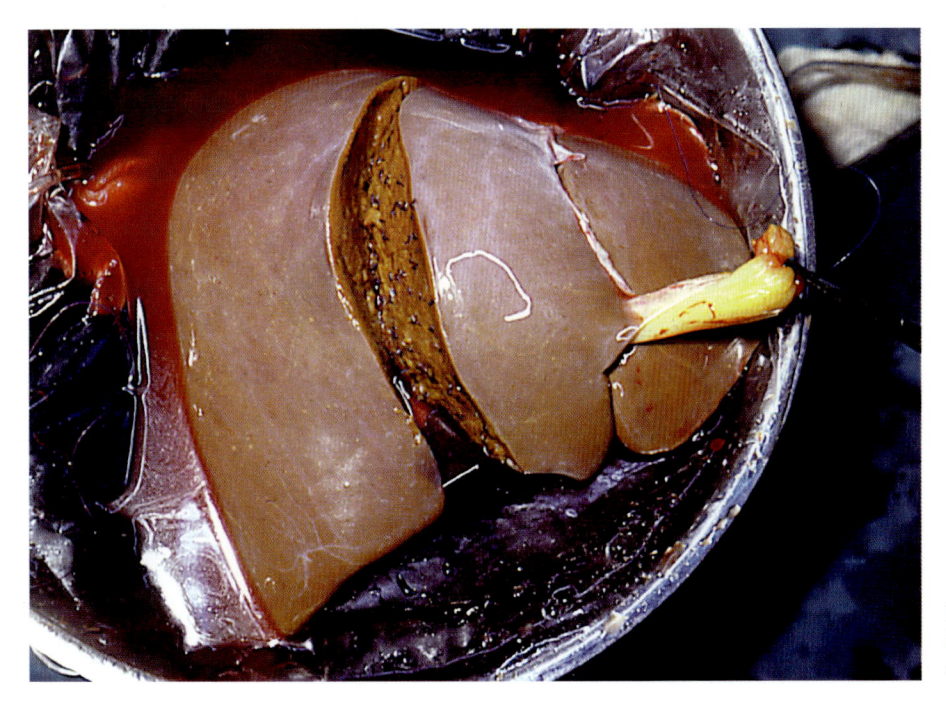

Figure 30.3 – *Division of the graft along the Cantlie line*

Preparation of the left hemiliver

The gallbladder is removed, ligating and dividing the cystic artery and the cystic duct. After minimal dissection of the hilum, the right hepatic artery and the right hepatic duct are ligated and divided (**Figure 30.1**). The right branch of the portal vein is divided and sutured with a running Prolene® 5-0 stitch. Preparation of the vena cava includes logation of accessory hepatic veins (**Figure 30.2a**). The removal of the caudate lobe is not mandatory when the entire hemiliver is used.[9] The right hepatic vein is divided and sutured with a running single-thread stitch with Prolene® 4-0 (**Figure 30.2b**). Resection of the parenchyma starts from the gallbladder fossa to the right margin of the vena cava (**Figure 30.3**) along a

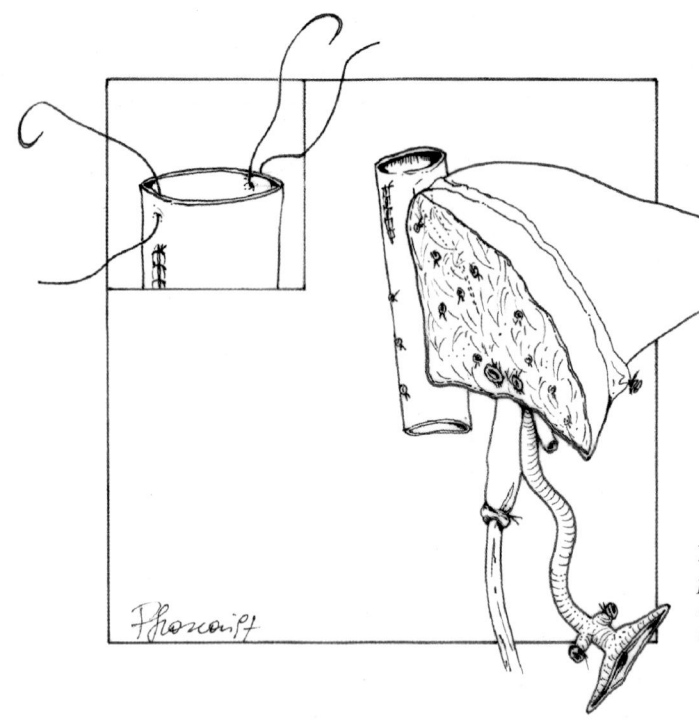

Figure 30.4 – *The reduced left hemiliver graft after parenchymal transection performed on the bench. Note that part of the parenchyma has been left on the right of the middle hepatic vein to prevent tearing of the vein wall.*

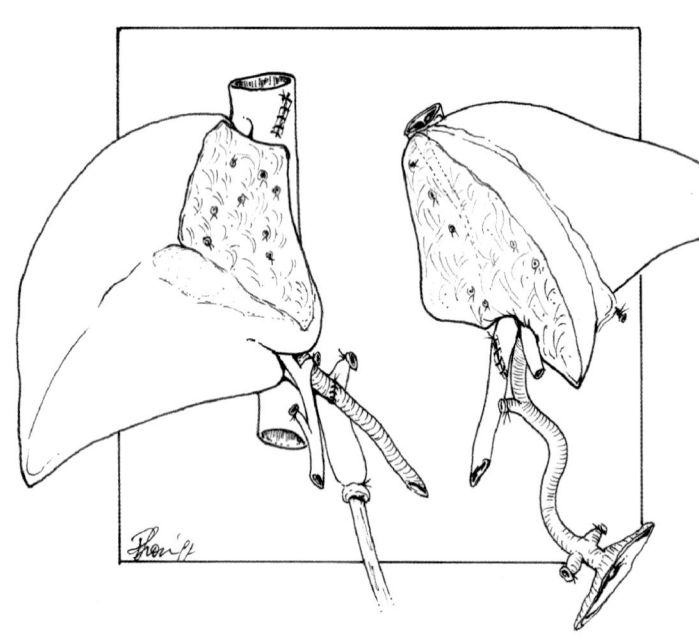

Figure 30.5 – *Split liver transplantation. The right hemiliver retains the vena cava, the common bile duct and the portal trunk. The right branch of the hepatic artery has been anastomozed with Prolene® 7-0 sutures to the donor iliac artery. The left hemiliver retains the common hepatic artery with the celiac trunk. The left branch of the portal vein has been anastomozed with a segment of donor iliac vein. The left hepatic duct will be anastomozed to a jejunal loop. Note the junction of the middle and left hepatic veins fashioned to obtain a wide single trunk, as described in Chapter 31.*

plane passing 1 cm to the right of the middle hepatic vein so as not to tear its wall, thus causing bleeding that is difficult to control at the time of revascularisation during the transplant (*Figure 30.4*). It is important to stress that when implanting the reduced graft the vena cava must be anastomosed by turning it on its sagittal axis toward the right to favor the positioning of the graft in the right hypochondrium without torsion (*Figure 30.4 -insert*).

Preparation of the left lobe

Preparation of the left lobe includes a bench resection comparable to a right hepatectomy extended to segment 4. After removal of the gallbladder, resection starts with division and ligation of the right bile duct and the biliary branches which drain segment 4. The right hepatic artery is ligated and divided. The left hepatic artery is isolated until the arterial branches for segment 4 are visible; these are also ligated and divided. The right branch of the portal vein is divided and sutured with a running single-thread stitch; the portal branches for segment 4 and the caudate lobe are ligated and divided. The vena cava is isolated from the caudate lobe and from the posterior wall of the right lobe. The junction of the left and middle hepatic veins should now be visible; care must be taken not to skeletonize the end of the left vein too much, in order to prevent bleeding during the transplant. The middle hepatic vein is then divided and sutured to allow preparation of a wide caval cuff to be used during the transplant: it may be necessary to divide this vein transparenchymally so as not to risk damaging the left one. The parenchyma is resected along a line parallel to the falciform ligament, keeping 1 cm to the right.

Preparation of the right hemi-liver

This is the most rarely used reduced graft. Removal of the gallbladder is the first step. The Glissonian structures for the left part of the liver are divided and sutured. The vena cava is detached from the caudate lobe and the collaterals are ligated. The anterior wall of the vena cava is detached from the left lobe. The confluence of the left and middle hepatic veins into the vena cava, generally a common one, is sutured after the veins have been divided. Resection then begins, incising Glisson's capsule along the line extending from the gallbladder fossa to the vena cava.

Split liver transplantation

The further development of the concept of size reduction has led to the possibility of using the same liver for two different recipients. The technique was introduced in 1988 by Pichlmayr[14] and subsequently applied in several centers with satisfactory results.[1,5,8,11,13,15,16] The possibility of using the same liver for two different recipients was initially motivated by the patients' need for urgency, when the clinical conditions would not have permitted either of them to wait for a whole organ to be available. The indications for the split liver technique have currently been extended to include semi-urgent or elective situations. It should in fact be stressed that, especially if one of the two recipients is a child, the long-term results reported in the more recent series with split graft transplantation are identical to those achieved with whole liver transplants.[1] The preparation of the two grafts on the bench retains the retrohepatic vena cava with the right graft, due to the large number of possible anatomical variations for venous drainage of the right hemi-liver. The left graft therefore consists of the left hemi-liver, which can be transplanted as such or, in the case of smaller recipients, reduced in size to segments 2 and 3 (left lobe) only. In the latter case, division of the parenchyma can be carried out from the beginning at the level of the falciform ligament. The left liver is kept for the smaller recipient and the right for the larger. The first 100 transplants reported in the European Register confirm that the donor/recipient weight ratio was 4.8 ± 2.3 for the left liver and only 1.5 ± 0.8 for the right.[8]

Technique

The anterior wall of the retrohepatic vena cava is detached from the left lobe. Dissection proceeds superiorly to isolate the confluence of the hepatic veins into the inferior vena cava. There is generally a single orifice for the right hepatic vein and a common one for the left and middle hepatic veins; each orifice stays with the respective hemi-liver. Dissection of the hepatic hilar structures must be very limited, especially for the left liver, to prevent ischemia of the bile ducts. Identification of the anatomical structures is easier if a blunt probe is used to explore the Glissonian pedicle from inside, without damaging the vascular endothelium. The use of contrast medium, preferably diluted with UW solution, for bench angiography and cholangiography in order to study the intraparenchymal anatomy was common during the first cases, but is now carried out less often thanks to the experience acquired.[9,11]

Division starts from the posterior wall of the portal trunk which is first isolated to prevent damage to the arterial and biliary structures in front of the portal vein. The main portal trunk generally remains with the right lobe, since the left branch of the portal vein is longer. Anatomical anomalies may be encountered in the portal system, less frequently than the arterial ones, and must be recognized and dealt with appropriately. Among the most frequent is the possibility of a 'trifurcation' of the portal vein that includes the presence of a 'medial' branch to the contralateral hemi-liver, originating from the right or left branch. In such cases, it is necessary to overcome the anomaly by anastomozing this middle branch to the portal branch for to the same hemiliver. The

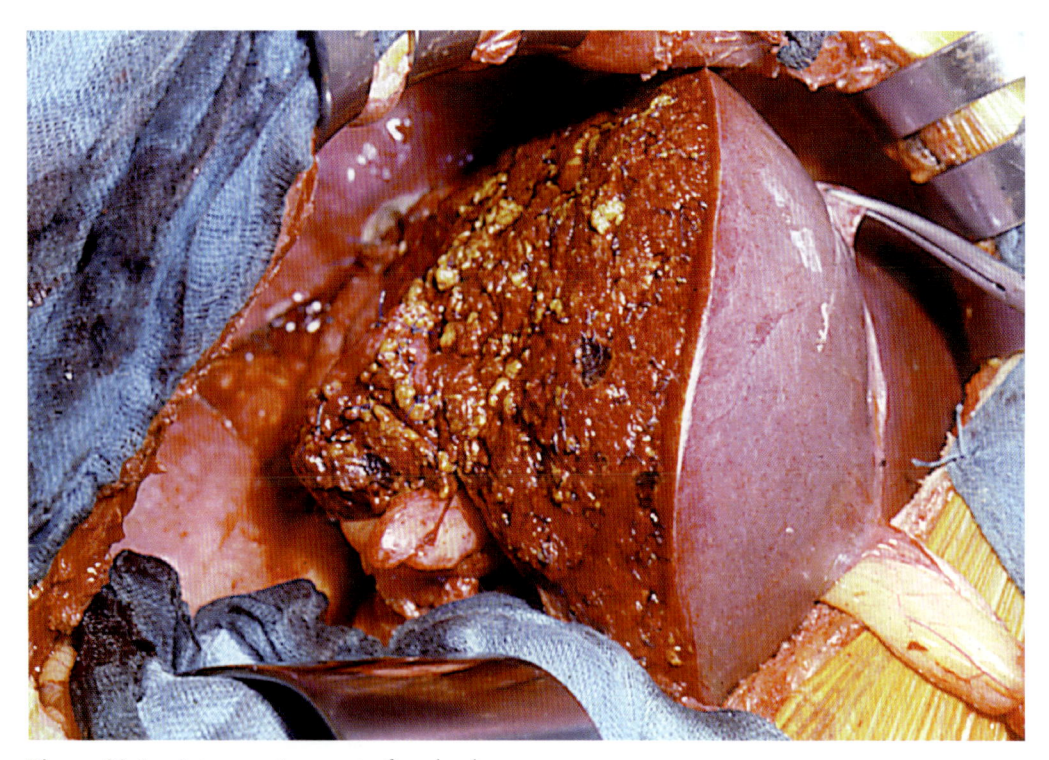

Figure 30.6 – *Intra-operative aspects of a reduced graft (left hemiliver) after revascularization. The graft was implanted retaining the donor vena cava according to the conventional techniques.*

celiac trunk generally remains with the left graft and this must always be the case if an accessory left hepatic artery arising from the left gastric artery is present. In the presence of an accessory right hepatic artery arising from the superior mesenteric artery, it is necessary to ascertain, during bench preparation, whether a hepatic artery is present for the paramedian segments (5 and 8) arising from the common hepatic artery. If this artery is present, a bench reconstruction is necessary: the celiac triad stays with the right graft and the accessory right hepatic artery is anastomozed to the stump of the splenic artery[16] or of the gastroduodenal artery. If the artery for the paramedian segments arises directly from the anomalous right hepatic artery, it is sufficient to preserve the proximal part of the superior mesenteric artery with the right lobe, to be used for the anastomosis during the transplant. The main bile duct remains with the right graft (**Figure 30.5**). The anatomy of the biliary tract may also present a wide range of anomalies, which must nevertheless be dealt with according to the principles of hepatic segmentary distribution. Hilar dissection for recognition of the anomalous anatomical structures must not be excessive and it is inadvisable to proceed as far as the secondary bifurcations.

When the two recipients are similar in body size, the two hemi-livers are transplanted: division of the graft starts from the line of the main portal scissure, separating the right and left hemi-livers. When one of the recipients is much smaller than the other, the parenchyma is divided at the level of the falciform ligament so that the left lobe can be used (segments 2 and 3). In this case the main technical problem concerns segment 4. This segment is anatomically a part of the left hemi-liver, as already described in Chapter 5. The preparation of a right liver graft when only the left lobe (segments 2 and 3) is to be transplanted, would thus assume systematic resection of segment 4, to be carried out after the left lobectomy for construction of the left graft.[6,7] The first papers published did in fact seriously doubt whether this segment could be used as part of the right graft.[5,10] However, vascularisation of segment 4, particularly the arterial one, can originate from the right Glissonian pedicles in at least 10% of cases and the outlet of the bile duct of segment 4 is also subject to numerous variations, including the possibility of flowing directly into the main bile duct in at least 12% of the cases. Subsequently, some centres included this segment in the right graft in order to obtain a larger mass of parenchyma.[11] In the first 100 transplants reported in the European Register, segment 4 was removed on the bench in only half the cases.[8] Moreover, the experience acquired dividing the graft in situ, i.e. during organ procurement with the donor's heart still beating, showed that the perfusion of segment 4 is not impaired when this segment remains with the right liver.[15] The caudate lobe is, on the other hand, systematically removed.

Transplant procedure

All the grafts obtained from reduced size livers, both left and right, can retain the vena cava and can therefore be transplanted according to the conventional technique (**Figure 30.6**) or using the 'piggy-back' technique. In grafts obtained by the split liver technique, the vena cava remains with the right hemi-liver; in this case it is still possible to choose the technique preferred for caval anastomosis. On the other hand, when transplanting left grafts, which lack the retrohepatic vena cava, the 'piggy-back' or similar techniques must be used, anastomozing the orifice of the hepatic veins laterally to the recipient vena cava, as already described. Anastomosis of the portal vein and the hepatic artery is performed as usual. Using the vessels of a reduced size liver for a transplant should not create technical problems as far as length is concerned. It is, on the other hand, generally necessary to resort to vascular grafts when transplanting split liver left grafts. The caliber of the biliary tract, especially in very small pediatric recipients, and the particular anatomical arrangement make the construction of a Roux-en-Y hepaticojejunostomy preferable. It is important to keep the length of the biliary tract to be used for the anastomosis as short as possible, in order to limit the risk of ischemic stenosis due to devascularization of the distal biliary margin.

Pitfalls

Patients transplanted with reduced size organs or with split livers are subject to the same complications described for whole liver transplantation: rejection, infections, etc. There are, however, a series of complications specific to these two techniques, which are discussed together as they have common aspects. Due to the time necessary for bench resection, the cold ischemia time is often much longer than with whole organ grafts. Organs with longer ischemia times present more conspicuous hemorrhage on revascularization.[11]

It has been pointed out above that removal of the caudate lobe is undertaken during bench preparation. This is due both to the devascularisation caused by ligation of the vascular pedicles during bench resection and to the possible onset of problems of difficult venous return caused by compression of the caudate lobe on the inferior vena cava.[13] The vena cava of the recipient is generally smaller than the donor vena cava and in some cases the difference may be considerable. This problem can be overcome if the transplant is performed with the 'piggy-back' technique or with any other technique which consists of direct anastomosis of the hepatic veins in the inferior vena cava. If, instead, the transplant is carried out with the conventional interposition of the graft vena cava and two end-to-end vascular anastomoses, it may be necessary to modify the graft vena cava in order to reduce the diameter.[12] In left graft transplants the end-to-end anastomosis between the donor and recipient hepatic veins involves the construction of a very long and mobile conduit which can hinder blood flow.[5,10] It is therefore preferable to use short hepatic vein cuffs for the anastomosis, to be calibrated during construction of the anastomosis.

Thrombosis of the hepatic artery now represents an event with a similar frequency to that reported for whole organs.[13] Portal vein thrombosis has also been described above, notably in the first series. The first etiological factor for this is the difference between the diameter of the reduced graft portal vein and the diameter of vascular grafts, generally iliac veins, that need to be interposed in the anastomosis to overcome the problem of short vessels. The second factor, a peculiarity of left anatomical lobe grafts (segments 2 and 3) and only in some left hemi-liver transplants (segments 2, 3 and 4), and because the right liver is absent, the graft may rotate to the right, around the sagittal axis of the vena cava, and occupy the empty right hypochondrium. The stretching of the Glissonian pedicle vessels caused by this rotation leads to thrombosis of the vessels. To overcome this problem, implantation of the graft in an anticlockwise direction, up to an angle of 180°, has been proposed. This complication can, nevertheless, be avoided by simply positioning the omentum or the transverse colon in the same space. Particularly severe rejection episodes can lead to a significant increase in intraparenchymal resistance, favouring the onset of thrombosis.

Biliary complications include fistulas or stenosis of the biliary-enteric anastomosis in small pediatric patients. In the majority of cases these are due to ischemic lesions secondary to the thrombosis of the hepatic artery, but can also be caused by devascularisation of the biliary tract during excessive bench dissection carried out in order to identify the first bifurcation.

One serious difficulty which may occur during transplantation of reduced size grafts is bleeding from the resected surface. It is therefore necessary to ensure that any leakages of preservation liquid injected through the celiac trunk and the portal vein are identified during bench preparation. The resected surface can be treated with biological glues before implantation. After revascularization the Argon beam coagulator is particularly useful, but in some cases it may also be necessary to close the abdomen of the patient after having packed it, due to the onset of multifactorial and uncontrollable coagulopathies.

No exact formula exists for calculating how much liver can be transplanted. A reduced size graft may still be larger than the removed portion, particularly if edema occurs after reperfusion. Closure of the abdomen under tension may cause compression on the abdominal organs, including the graft which may thus become ischemic. The interposition of an abdominal prosthesis (Gore-Tex® or Prolene Mesh®) may thus be necessary for temporary closure of the abdomen, delaying the definitive procedure until later.

REFERENCES

1. Azoulay D, Astarcioglu I, Johann M, Adam R, Castaing D, Bismuth H. The split liver in liver transplantation: a recent experience. *HPB Surgery* 1996; **9 (suppl 2):** 3-7.

2. Bismuth H, Houssin D. Reduced-size orthotopic liver graft in hepatic transplantation. *Surgery* 1984; **95:** 367-372.

3. Broelsch CE, Neuhaus P, Burdelski M. Orthotope Transplantation von Lebersegmenten bei Kleinkindern mit Gallengangsatresien. Orthotopic transplantation of hepatic segments in infants with biliary artesia. *Langenbeck Archiv Chir Forum* 1984; **(Suppl):** 105-109.

4. Broelsch CE, Emond JC, Thistlethwaite JR *et al*. Liver transplantation, including the concept of reduced-size liver transplants in children. *Ann Surg* 1988; **208:** 410-420.

5. Broelsch CE, Emond JC, Whitington PF, Thistlethwaite JR, Baker AL, Lichtor JL. Application of reduced-size liver transplants as split grafts, auxiliary orthotopic grafts and living related segmental transplants. *Ann Surg* 1990; **212:** 368-373.

6. Couinaud C, Houssin D. Partition réglée du foie pour transplantation. Contraintes anatomiques. C. Couinaud, Paris, 1991.

7. Couinaud C. Un scandal: segment IV et transplantation du foie. *J Chir* 1993; 130: 443-446.

8. de Ville de Goyet J. Split liver transplantation in Europe - 1988 to 1993. *Transplantation* 1995; **59:** 1371-1376.

9. de Ville de Goyet J, Otte JB. Cut-down and split liver transplantation. In: Busuttil LW, Klintman GB *Transplantation of the liver*. WB Saunders, Phildaelphia, 1996, pp.481-496.

10. Emond JC, Whitington PF, Thistlethwaite JR *et al*. Transplantation of two patients with one liver. *Ann Surg* 1990; **212:** 14-22.

11. Houssin D, Boillot O, Soubrane O *et al*. Controlled liver splitting for transplantation in two recipients: technique, results and perspectives. *Br J Surg* 1993; **80:** 75-80.

12. Kalayoglu M, D'Alessandro AM, Sollinger HW, Hoffman RM, Pirsch JD, Belzer FO. Experience with reduced-size liver transplantation. *Surg Gynecol Obstet* 1990; **171:** 139-147.

13. Langnas AN, Marujo WC, Inagaki, Stratta RJ, Wood RP, Shaw BW. The results of reduced-size liver transplantation, including split livers, in patients with end-stage liver disease. *Transplantation* 1992; **53:** 387-391.

14. Pichlmayr R, Ringe B, Gubernatis G, Hauss J, Bunzendahl H. Transplantation einer Spenderleber auf zwei Empfänger (Splitting-Transplantation): Eine neue Methode in der Weiterentwicklung der Lebersegmenttransplantation. *Langenbecks Arch Chir* 1988; **373:** 127-130.

15. Rogiers X, Malago M, Habib N *et al*. In situ splitting of the liver in the heart-beating cadaveric organ donor for transplantation in two recipients. *Transplantation* 1995; **59:**1081-1083.

16. Shaw BW, Wood RP, Stratta RJ *et al*. Management of arterial anomalies encountered in split-liver transplantation. *Transplantation Proceedings* 1990; **22:** 420-422.

31

Transplantation from Living Related Donors

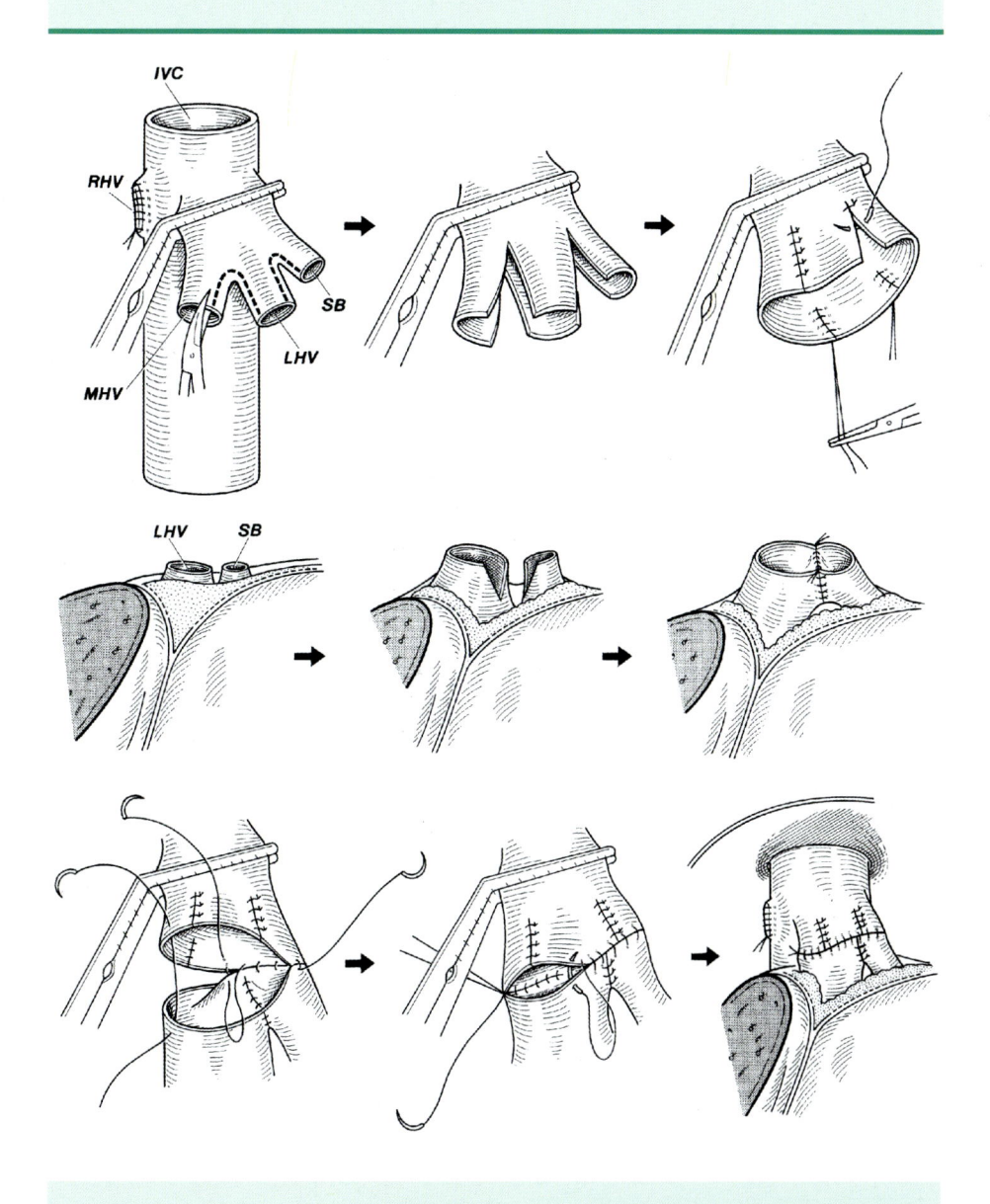

M. Makuuchi, S. Kawasaki, T. Takayama

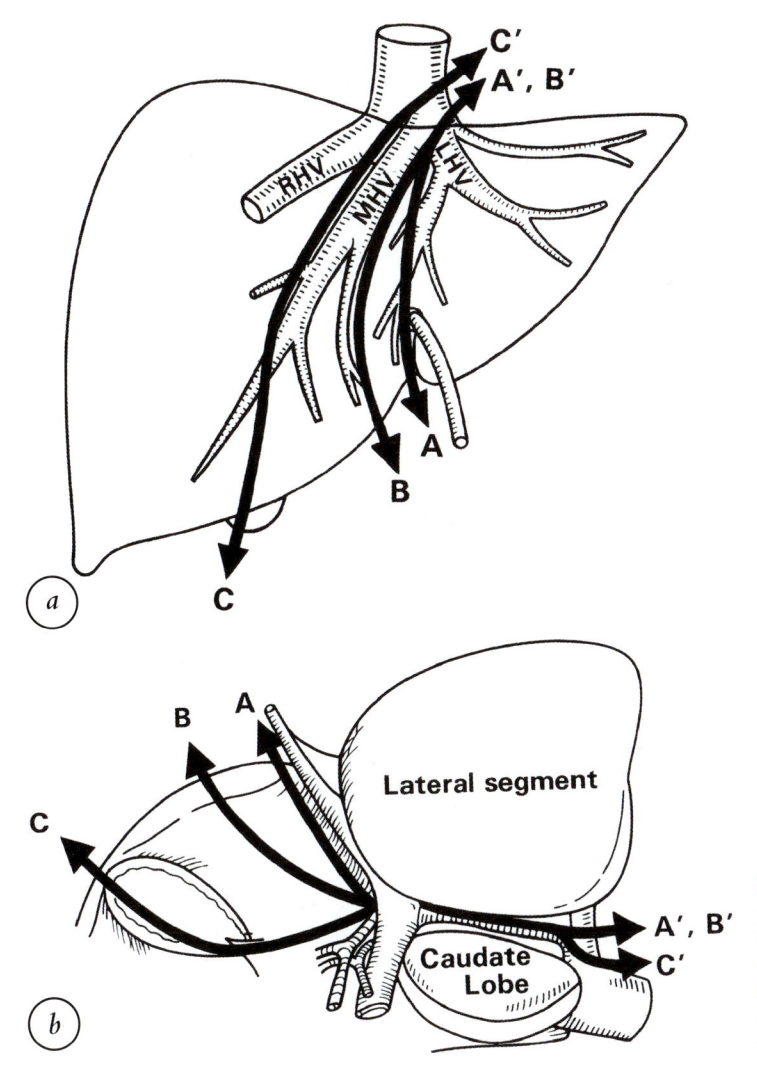

Figure 31.1 – *Three types of donor hepatectomy (from Kawasaki et al.[7] with permission). **a)** Anterior view; **b)** left caudal view. A-A', B-B', C-C': transection lines to perform lateral segmentectomy, extended lateral segmentectomy and whole left hemihepatectomy, respectively. RHV, MHV, LHV: right, middle and left hepatic veins, respectively.*

Living related liver transplantation (LRLT) represents one of the most important innovations in transplant surgery and is being performed by a growing number of experienced surgeons.[1,10,13,16] In Western countries, LRLT has been used to overcome cadaveric graft shortage for children,[1,13] whereas in Japan it is, for legal, social and religious reasons, the only transplant procedure available.[10,16] The LRLT operation presents a dilemma in that the graft removed should be as small as possible to prevent donor complications, but needs to be large enough to meet the recipient's requirements. Safety for the living donor has to be guaranteed and a successful transplant remains a priority in recipients for whom retransplantation is seldom indicated.[11] In the last 6 years, we have performed 56 LRLTs with successful outcomes, with a recipient 5-year survival rate of 88% and no donor mortality or morbidity.[8] Our accumulated experience has enabled us to expand the indications for LRLT to include selected adult recipients.[3]

Donor operation

A prerequisite for LRLT is left-sided hepatectomy in living donors performed with minimal risk while preserving graft viability. Our experience with hepatic resections for cancer comprises 637 patients in the last 6 years, 68 of whom underwent left-sided hepatectomy with an average blood loss of 770 ml and no operative mortality.[11] This clinical background enabled us to start the LRLT program in Japan where no cadaveric donor organs are available. After obtaining informed consent and permission from the ethical committee of our university, a volunteer donor is selected from the recipient's parents or relatives on the basis of ABO blood group, liver function and graft size matching. One of three types of partial hepatectomy - lateral segmentectomy, extended lateral segmentectomy and whole left hemihepatectomy together with the middle hepatic vein (***Figure 31.1***), is selected according to the relationship between the

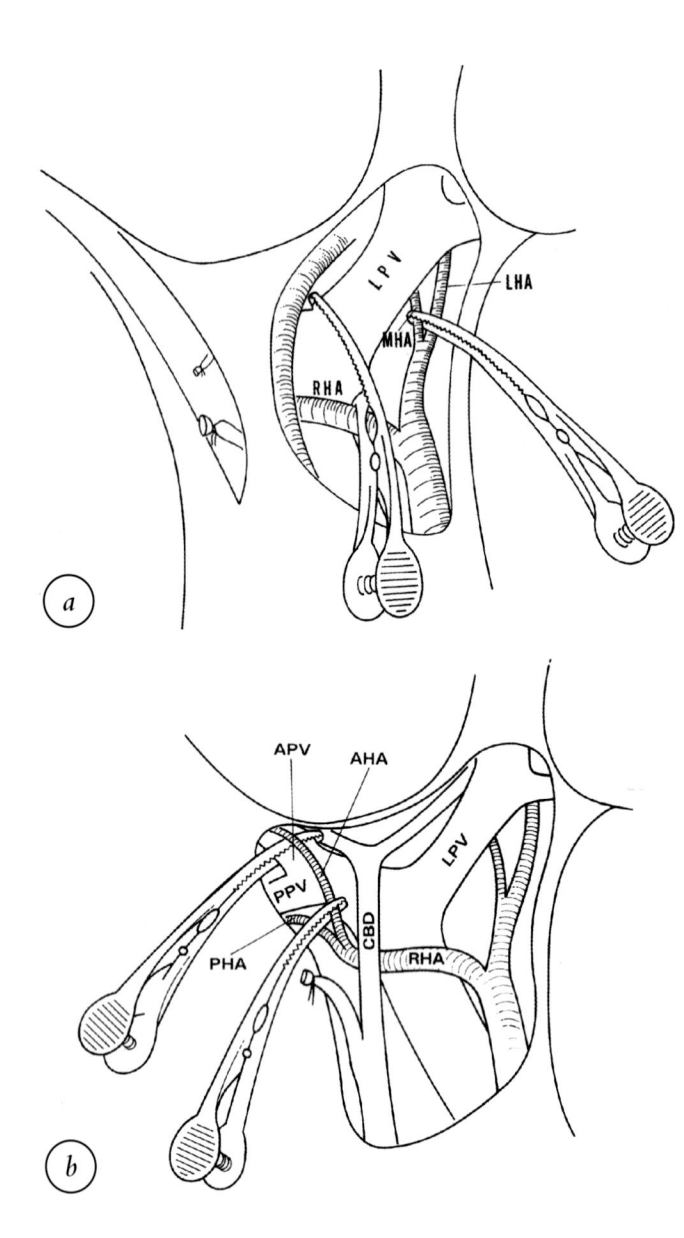

Figure 31.2 – *Selective vascular occlusion (from Makuuchi et al [1,11] with permission).* ***a)*** *Occlusion for extended lateral segmentectomy;* ***b)*** *occlusion for whole left hemihepatectomy. LPV, APV, PPV: left, anterior and portal veins, respectively. MHA, LHA, RHA, AHA, PHA: middle, left, right, anterior and posterior hepatic arteries, respectively. CBD: common bile duct.*

recipient's body size and segmental donor liver volume. The segmental graft liver volume can be estimated with acceptable accuracy preoperatively using CT scanning.[7] Although the minimum graft volume needed for successful LRLT remains unknown, our experience suggests that LRLT can be performed safely using a small-for-size graft when the actual graft to recipient standard liver volume ratio is > 0.34.[7]

To harvest a left-sided liver graft from a living donor,[9,11] an inverted T-shaped incision is made into the abdominal cavity. We use operative ultrasound to demonstrate the intrahepatic vascular structure, especially the ramification pattern of the hepatic venous tributaries around the caval insertions. When performing extended lateral segmentectomy, the tributary draining the left part of the medial segment needs to be identified to determine the transection plane and avoid inadvertent injury.[9] After cholecystectomy, the left and middle hepatic arteries and the left portal vein are dissected and encircled at the hepatic hilum. The transverse portion of the left portal vein is completely freed by ligating and dividing the small falciform, left coronary and triangular ligaments, followed by division of Arantius' ligament. Dissection is performed around the suprahepatic vena cava to expose the origins of the major hepatic veins with the cava. Whole left hemihepatectomy requires extrahepatic isolation of the middle and left hepatic veins at their common trunk.

After these preparations, transection of the hepatic parenchyma is carried out under selective vascular occlusion to minimize donor blood loss.[11] Intermittent occlusion of the middle hepatic artery and left portal vein (**Figure 31.2a**), which produces ischemia in segment 4, is applied during parenchymal transection of donors who undergo extended lateral segmentectomy. In those undergoing whole left hemihepatectomy, the right anterior branches of the hepatic artery and portal vein are occluded to make the anterior segment ischemic (**Figure 31.2b**). The 15 minute occlusion of the left side or the 30 minute occlusion of the right, followed by 5 minutes' reperfusion, are repeated until transection is complete. We have adopted this warm ischemia as previous experimental study indicated that short-term ischemia produced little damage to grafts in monkeys.[11] In fact, these procedures have resulted in excellent graft viability and insignificant donor blood loss in all our transplant pairs (see below). The forceps fracture method is used to transect the liver parenchyma without damaging the vessels and ducts, which are subsequently ligated on both sides and divided between the ligatures. The Glissonian triads to the caudate lobe are divided just beneath the connective tissues of the hepatic hilum. After total parenchymal division, whilst maintaining the blood supply, operative cholangiography is carried out to confirm the site of the bile duct division. Finally, the partial liver graft is removed with division of the left hepatic duct, left (and middle) hepatic artery, left portal vein and left (and middle) hepatic vein. On the donor's backtable, University of Wisconsi (UW) solution is infused through a portal pedicle and hepatic artery. The proximal part of the left (and middle) hepatic vein is dissected free from the parenchyma to obtain a piece long enough for future anastomosis. The left hepatic vein and its superficial branch are linked together to eliminate graft congestion as far as possible. The graft is then preserved in UW solution until required for recipient hepatectomy.

Recipient operation

Extensive division of the adhesions is carried out to free the whole liver, the vessels at the hepatic hilum are separated and taped, and the diseased liver is then mobilized from the vena cava followed by extrahepatic isolation of the right hepatic vein. We have not used a venous bypass system in patients undergoing LRLT, but in patients with no portal hypertension, a temporary portocaval shunt is placed using the right portal venous branch.[8]

An outflow tract is reconstructed by anastomozing the left hepatic vein of the graft end-to-side to the recipient's vena cava, because a graft from a living donor must be implanted with the cava.[13] However, the risk of outflow obstruction remains an issue in LRLT, because anastomotic kinking due to inappropriate positioning or sizing of the graft can occur.[1] Among our early LRLT series using the standard technique, 1 patient had hepatic venous obstruction, necessitating, revascularization.[14] For all subsequent patients, we have used a new technique of outflow Y-reconstruction by hepatic vein end-to-end anastomosis after venoplasty.[15] Just after completion of hepatectomy with vena caval preservation, recipient hepatic venoplasty is performed *in situ* to obtain a wider anastomotic ostium. Under cross-clamping, the middle and left hepatic veins are made confluent to form a common venous trunk. This technique has been used for relatively large children, whereas for infants, the right hepatic vein is also included in the common trunk.[12] The venous trunk is anastomosed end-to-end to the left hepatic vein of the graft with a continuous everted mattress or over-and-over sutures, achieving a Y-shaped reconstruciton of both hepatic veins (**Figure 31.3**). Using this technique, no patient has shown any evidence of anastomotic stricture or thrombosis in the outflow tract. Broelsch[1] preferred a triangulation method, which necessitates total clamping of the vena cava; our technique does not require such clamping because the trunk of the recipient hepatic veins after venoplasty is longer.

Hepatic arterial reconstruction is also critical in LRLT because the arterial branches of the graft are thinner and shorter than those of whole or reduced-size cadaveric liver transplants. We carried out arterial reconstruction with the naked eye in the first 10 patients, but thereafter performed it with the aid of an operating microscope.[4] In cases where there is only one graft hepatic artery, it is anastomosed to the recipient hepatic artery in an end-to-end manner by interrupted sutures with 8-0 or 9-0 monofilament. When there are two graft arteries, both are anastomosed if their diameters are almost the same. When there are multiple arteries, the thickest one is reconstructed first and the others are ligated after confirming pulsatile back bleeding from their cut stumps and intrahepatic arterial blood flow signals by Doppler ultrasound. The 10 patients who underwent single arterial reconstruction have had neither arterial thrombosis nor liver dysfunction that could be related to the arterial blood supply.[4] Hepatic arterial blood flow and caliber of the single reconstructed branch will increase in due time. Based on the success and simplicity of this technique we believe it is

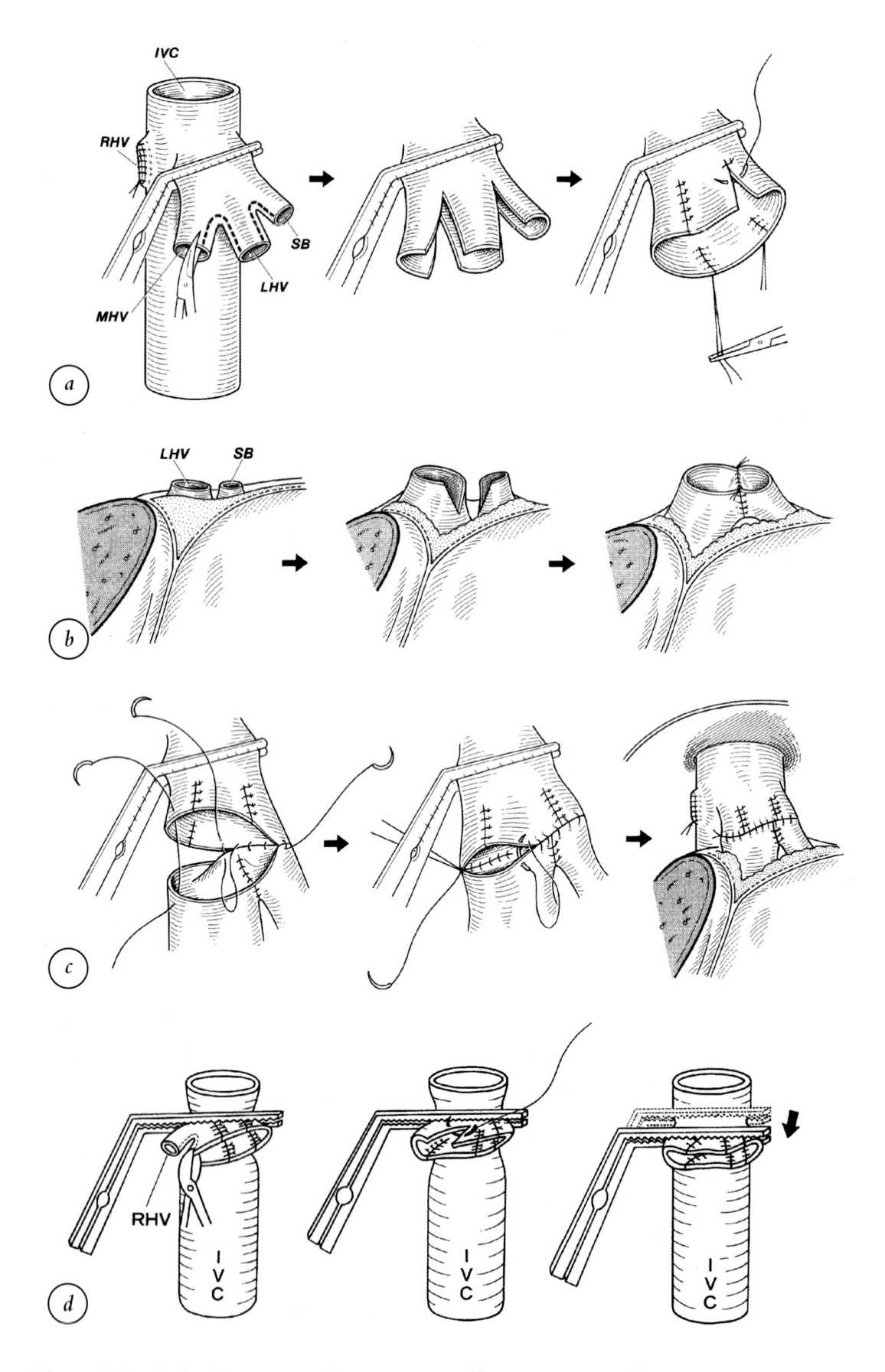

Figure 31.3 – *Outflow Y-reconstruction (from Takayama et al[15] and Matsunami et al[12] with permission).* **a)** *Recipient venoplasty;* **b)** *graft venoplasty;* **c)** *Y-shaped end-to-end anastomosis;* **d)** *recipient venoplasty using the major three hepatic veins. IVC: inferior vena cava; RHV, MHV, LHV: right, middle and left hepatic veins, respectively. AB: superficial branch of the LHV.*

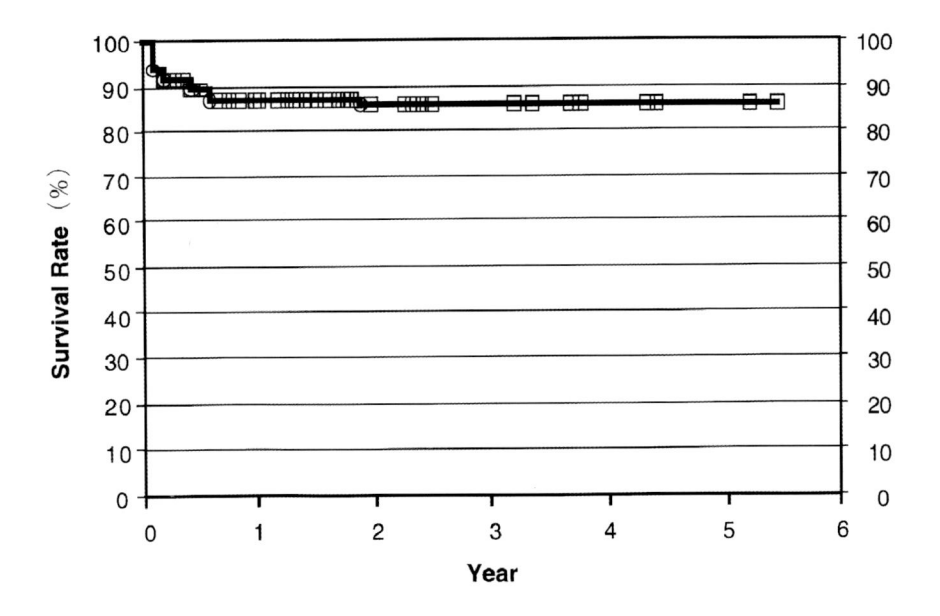

Figure 31.4 – *Cumulative overall survival rates after LRLT in 56 patients.*

better to reconstruct only one of the graft hepatic arteries in LRLT. Portal venous reconstruction is performed in an end-to-end manner by continuous sutures with an adequate growth factor, and the bile duct is anastomosed end-to-side to a Roux-en-Y loop of the jejunum.

Immunosuppressive treatment consists of cyclosporin with azathioprine and steroids, or tacrolimus with steroids. We administer intensive anticoagulant therapy comprising heparin, anti-thrombin 11, prostaglandin El, protease inhibitors, and fresh frozen plasma for several weeks after LRLT,[2] and routinely carry out daily Doppler ultrasound examination to confirm the patency of the intrahepatic vessels.[5]

Surgical outcome

The results below are based on the analysis of 56 LRLTS, including 12 adult recipients and 4 ABO-incompatible cases. The primary diseases necessitating urgent liver transplantation were biliary atresia (n=34, including 1 adult), acute liver failure (n=6), familial amyloid neuropathy (n=5, all adults), primary biliary cirrhosis (n=4, all adults), neonatal hepatitis or liver cirrhosis with hepatocellular carcinoma (n=3), Alagille's syndrome (n=1), Byler disease (n=1), citrullinemia (n=1, adult), and cholestatic disease of unknown cause (n=1, adult). The living related donors consisted of recipients' fathers (n=25), mothers (n=22), husbands (n=4), siblings (n=3), and sons (n=2).

During the donor hepatectomies, the blood loss was 660 ± 180 (mean ± SD) ml (lateral segmentectomy, 519 ± 282 ml; extended lateral segmentectomy, 515 ± 150 ml; left hemihepatectomy, 850 ± 438 ml), for which only autotransfusion was needed. Postoperative donor complications included mild liver enzyme elevations (n=5), stress ulcer (n=3), bile leakage (n=2), and wound infection (n=2). All these minor complications were cured and all the donors are now living normal lives.

The graft volumes ranged from 245 to 530 ml, which corresponded to actual graft to standard liver volume ratios of 0.34-1.54. Functional insufficiency due to small-for-size grafts was not observed in any recipient, including the adults. No thrombosis of either the hepatic artery or portal vein was encountered in any patient. Of the 56 recipients, 49 are currently alive after LRLT. Causes of recipient mortality were posttransplant lymphoproliferative disorders (n=2), systemic cytomegalovirus infection (n=1), respiratory failure (n=1), aspergillosis (n=1), sudden cardiac arrest (n=1), and thrombotic thrombocytopenic purpura (n=1). The cumulative overall patient survival rate (and graft survival rate) was 88% 5 years after LRLT (***Figure 31.4***).

REFERENCES

1. Broelsch CE, Emond JC, Vv'hitington PF et al. Application of reduced-size liver transplants as split grafts, auxiliary orthotopic grafts, and living related segmental transplants. *Ann Surg* 1990; **212**: 368.
2. Hashikura Y, Kawasaki S, Okumura N et al. Prevention of hepatic artery thrombosis in pediatric liver transplantation. *Transplantation* 1995; **60**: 1109.
3. Hashikura Y, Makuuchi M, Kawasaki S et al. Successful living-related partial liver transplantation to an adult patient. *Lancet* 1994; **343**: 1233.
4. lkegami T, Kawasaki S, Matsunami H et al. Should all hepatic arterial branches be reconstructed in living-related liver transplantation? *Surgery* (in press).
5. Kasai H, Makuuchi M, Kawasaki S et al. Intraoperative color Doppler ultrasonography for partial-liver transplantation from the living donor in pediatric patients. *Transplantation* 1992; **54**: 173.
6. Kawasaki S, Hashikura Y, Matsunami H et al. Temporary shunt between right portal vein and vena cava in livina related liver transplantation. *J Am Coll Surg* (in press).
7. Kawasaki, S, Makuuchi M, Matsunami H et al. Preoperative measurement of segmental liver volume of donors for living related liver transplantation. *Hepatology* 1993; **15**: 1115.
8. Kawasaki S, Makuuchi M, Matsunami H et al. Living related liver transplantation: a wider application. *Transpl Proc* 1995; **27**: 1170.
9. Kawasaki S, Makuuchi M, Miyagawa S et al. Extended lateral segmentectomy using intraoperative ultrasound to obtain a partial liver graft. *Am J Surg* 1996; **171**: 286.
10. Makuuchi M, Kawarasaki H, lwanaka T et al. Living related liver transplantation. *Surg Today* 1992; **22**: 297.
11. Makuuchi M, Kawasaki S, Noguchi T et al. Donor hepatectomy for living related partial liver transplantation. *Surgery* 1993; **113**: 395.
12. Matsunami H, Makuuchi M, Kawasaki S et al. Venous reconstruction using three recipient hepatic veins in living related liver transplantation. *Transplantation* 1995; **59**: 917.
13. Strong RW, Lynch SV, Ong TH et al. Successful liver transplantation from a living donor to her son. *N Engl J Med* 1990; **332**: 1505.
14. Takayama T, Makuuchi M, Kawarasaki H et al. Venacavaplasty to overcome outflow block in living related liver transplantation. *Transplantation* 1994a; **58**: 116.
15. Takayama T, Makuuchi M, Kawasaki S et al. Outflow Y-reconstruction for living related patial liver transplantation. *J Am Coll Surg* 1994b; **179**: 226.
16. Tanaka K, Uemoto S, Tokunaga Y et al. Surgical techniques and innovations in living related liver transplantation. *Ann Surg* 1993; **217**: 82.

32

Auxiliary Liver Transplantation

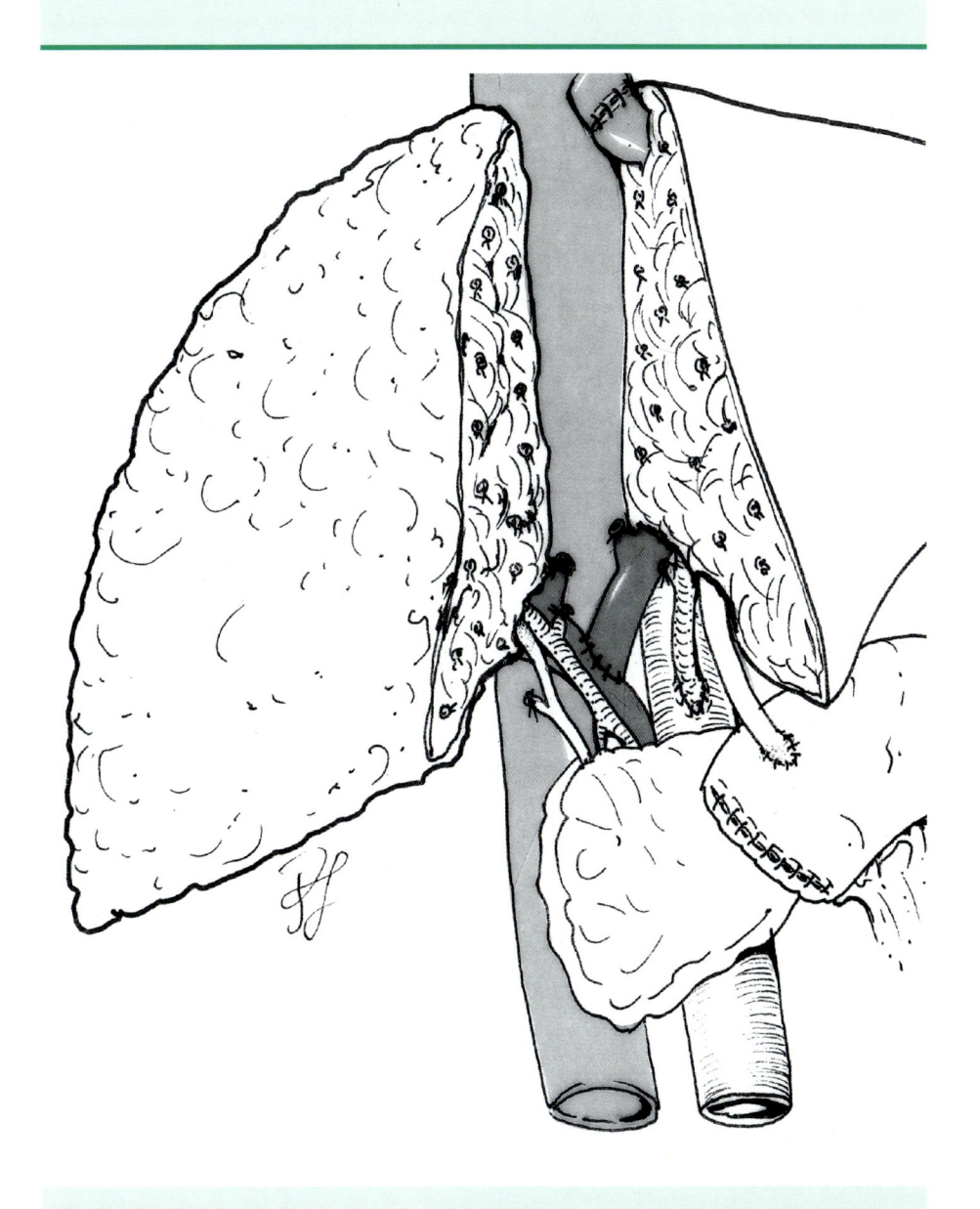

J. Belghiti, A. Sauvanet, O. Farges

Orthotopic liver transplantation (OLT) was validated in 1983 as a therapeutic modality for end-stage acute or chronic liver disease and has, since then, become extremely popular with 6 to 7,000 transplants performed every year world-wide. It has simultaneously become very successful, with an overall 1-year patient survival rate averaging 80%, both in Europe and in the United-States.

Steps initially considered as critical in OLT included the hemodynamic and metabolic changes associated with the anhepatic phase, the risk of initial graft poor function during the first few postoperative days and the risk of acute rejection. These were the initial rationale for attempting, as early as 1965, to perform auxiliary transplantations. In this technique, a liver graft is placed in the abdominal cavity but the recipient's liver is left in situ. Consequently, hepatectomy is avoided, and the consequences of the graft's failure, should it occur, are limited, the native liver being still able to support some hepatic functions. Although very attractive, this procedure did not gain wide acceptance due to very poor initial clinical results.[19] In addition, there were justified doubts that liver malignancies could occur within the native liver or that in patients with viral related cirrhosis, the persistence of the native liver could favour viral recurrence within the graft.[14] Simultaneously, innovative techniques have been developed to limit the consequences of the recipient's hepatectomy, such as the preservation of portal and caval blood flow,[1] the requirements for good initial graft function have been better defined and powerful immunosuppressive agents have been developed that are very effective in preventing acute rejection. Hence, the initial rationale for auxiliary transplantation have become less crucial.

There has been, however, over the past 5 years or so, a renewed interest in the use of auxiliary liver transplantation (ALT) in patients with fulminant or sub-fulminant liver failure, for the following reasons. First, it clearly became obvious that while immunosuppressive agents had became very effective in preventing rejection, they had also became very hazardous because of their lack of specificity. Currently, the most frequent cause of death after transplantation is from sepsis due to over-immunosuppression and every effort is therefore made to reduce as much as possible, if not discontinue, immunosuppression.[7] Secondly, reports appeared in the literature of complete regeneration without histological or functional sequel of the native liver of patients transplanted with an auxiliary graft for acute liver failure.[4,8,15] In addition, in patients with HBV related fulminant liver failure, there was a frequent disappearance of viral infection. Finally, the technical requirements for an auxiliary graft to function have become better understood. The current rationale for auxiliary liver transplantations is, therefore, not so much to simplify the transplantation procedure as to allow the native liver to recover from the acute injury, so as to be able, in the long term, to discontinue immunosuppression. The aim of this chapter is to focus on the various techniques of auxiliary liver transplantation, to report our results as well as those available from the literature and to try to summarise what may be anticipated from this technique in the future.

Lessons learned from animal models

The predominant technical difficulties associated with auxiliary liver transplantation result from the lack of space in the abdominal cavity and from the physiological inflow and outflow requirements for a liver to function optimally. Failure to create a sufficient amount of space in the abdominal cavity may result in compression of the graft, of the recipient's organ or major vessels, or simply in a rise in abdominal pressure. The latter is associated with increased inferior vena cava (IVC) pressure that is detrimental to the graft's venous outflow (see below). Although not directly addressed in the setting of ALT, experimental studies in rodents have shown a poorer outcome after OLT of grafts larger than the

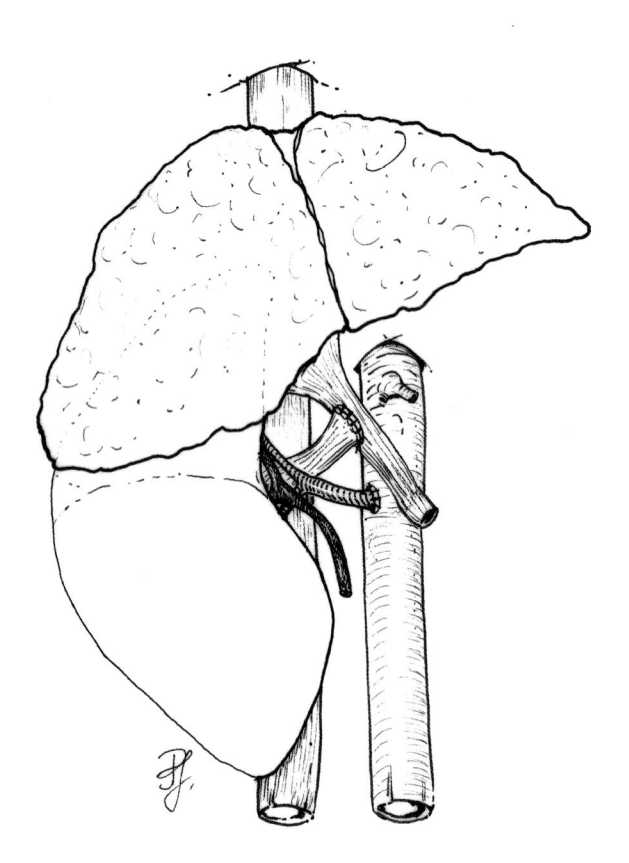

Figure 32.1 – *Technique of heterotopic liver transplantation. The graft's portal vein is anastomosed to the recipient portal vein. The graft's artery is anastomosed to the recipient's infrarenal aorta. The graft's suprahepatic vena cava is anastomosed to the recipient's infrarenal vena cava.*

native liver probably as a result of this rise in abdominal pressure.[22]

The arterial supply to the graft is the easiest to perform and any major branch can be used. The venous inflow and outflow are more problematic for several reasons. The liver in its physiological position drains into the IVC close to the right atrium. At this level, the pressure is low and pulsatile, two features that facilitate liver drainage. These favourable conditions do not exist in other areas of the sub diaphragmatic venous bed, especially in the orthostatic position when the pressure in the inferior vena cava increases by 0.77 mmHg per centimetre below the right atrium. An increase in central venous pressure is transmitted almost quantitatively back to the sinusoids. For a 1 mmHg rise in hepatic venous pressure, the intrahepatic blood volume may increase by as much as 4 ml/100 g liver and in cardiac failure, it may increase up to 60 ml/100 g. This increase is attributed to passive distension of the capacitance vessels and may result in cytolysis, reduced portal blood perfusion, liver failure and severe fibrous sequel in the long term. This is the rationale for performing the outflow anastomosis on the recipient's vena cava as close as possible to the right atrium. Experimental models have even used intrathoracic grafts to fulfil this requirement.[11]

Portal vein inflow has unique characteristics, the most important of which are a relatively high pressure of 6-10 mmHg and a high concentration of substances originating from the intestine and the pancreas thought to have an important role in liver function and regeneration as evidenced by the progressive atrophy of livers deprived of portal blood. Nevertheless, liver regeneration has been demonstrated both experimentally and in the clinical situation in the absence of direct portal blood supply (although it is delayed), OLT may be successful when the inferior vena cava is anastomosed to the portal vein (as described in patients with diffuse thrombosis of the splanchnic bed), and experimental heterotopic transplantations may be successful when a systemic vein is anastomosed to the portal vein. This is probably related to the fact that these hepatotrophic factors may reach the graft through the arterial circulation. The latter situation is however not optimal, yielding inconsistent experimental results and may become even worse in the clinical setting should an increase in the graft's resistance occur as a result of preservation injury of rejection. For all of these reasons, the graft's portal vein should be anastomosed somewhere on the recipient's splanchnic bed (*Figure. 32.1*).

This situation raises the, as yet, unresolved problem of the competition between the

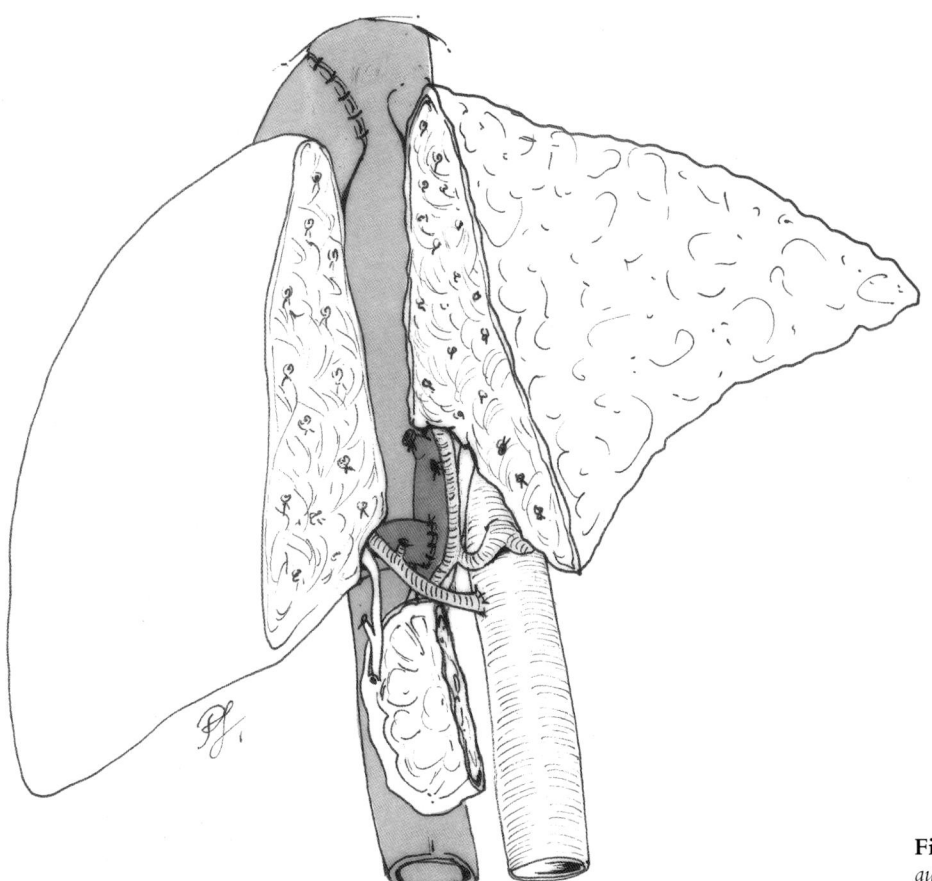

Figure 32.2 – *Technique of auxiliary liver transplantation of a right graft.*

native liver's and the graft's portal supply. An adequate portal blood flow must indeed be provided to both the graft (so as to allow good initial function) and the native liver (so as to allow regeneration to occur). If the graft only receives portal blood flow, the native liver undergoes atrophy.[9] If, on the contrary, the portal blood flow is maintained to the native liver and the graft only receives venous perfusion by the IVC, then this graft undergoes rapid atrophy.[23] Similarly, graft atrophy resulting from either rejection, chronic cholestasis or low portal perfusion is associated with a progressive hypertrophy of the native liver.[10,12] In fact, both flow and content of portal blood are probably crucial in regulating the size and function of the native and grafted livers. An increase in the graft's resistance (as a result of preservation injury or rejection) or in the recipient's liver (as a result of the underlying liver disease) will be associated with a preferential perfusion of the recipient's liver or of the graft respectively. Devices have therefore been proposed to mechanically control portal flow. An alternative approach has been to dissociate the splanchnic bed so as to perfuse auxiliary liver grafts with mesenteric blood, and perfuse the native liver with the spleno-gastro-pancreatic blood.[23,10] Further experimental studies based on this approach are in progress aiming at improving the regeneration of the native liver.[17]

Heterotopic auxiliary liver transplantation for end-stage chronic disease

Since 1964, approximately 50 cases of auxiliary liver transplantation for end-stage chronic liver disease have been published. The majority of these auxiliary grafts were placed in an heterotopic position, in the right sub hepatic region, according to the technique developed by Terpstra *et al*.[20] In this technique, the graft is turned 90° counter clockwise so that its hilum faces the recipient aorta, the large right liver is placed in the right lower abdominal quadrant and the smaller segment 2 and 3 are removed. The graft's inferior vena cava is anastomosed into the recipient's vena cava (***Figure 32.2***). An end-to-side anastomosis is created between the graft's and the recipient's portal veins, followed by an anastomosis between the graft's celiac trunk and the recipient's infrarenal aorta. Bile drainage is restored by an hepatico-jejunal

Roux-en-Y anastomosis. Several points are crucial to the success of this technique.

First, the graft should not be too large, so as to prevent compression, by the graft of the major blood vessels or to prevent compression of the graft at the time of abdominal closure. Patients with massive ascites usually have enough space, provided the graft is not too large.

Second, the caval anastomosis must be performed as close as possible to the heart. As indicated above, the normal entrance of the hepatic veins close to the right atrium where the pressure of the vena cava is low and pulsatile is probably very important in facilitating normal liver drainage. Removing the left lateral segment therefore allows implantation of the heterotopic graft to be performed at least on the recipient's suprarenal vena cava. In addition, the suprahepatic vena cava of the graft must be as short as possible to allow for optimal venous outflow. Failure to do so will otherwise result in a compression of the cavo-caval anastomosis and hence in a very detrimental congestion of the graft.

Third, the graft's portal vein should not be too long as this may otherwise result in kinking. This may prove somewhat difficult to judge at the time of anastomosis as segments 4 to 6 have to be retracted upwards to expose the graft's portal vein. On the other hand, there is a risk, if the liver enlarges as a result of preservation damage, rejection or venous outflow obstruction, that the hilum is displaced towards the median line and hence that a portal vein of initially correct length becomes too long. This is particularly crucial in patients who do not have portal hypertension or who have important porto-systemic shunts.

Another technique of heterotopic ALT is to place the graft in the left hypochondrium after having removed the spleen.[18] The graft's infrahepatic vena cava is anastomosed end-to-side to the recipient's left renal vein, the graft's portal vein is anastomosed end-to-end to the recipient's splenic vein and the graft's hepatic artery is anastomosed end-to-end to the recipient's splenic artery. Biliary drainage is achieved by means of a Roux-en-Y jejunal loop. This technique was initially described in a patient with portal vein thrombosis and it is probably in this setting that this technique is most useful.

As indicated earlier, heterotopic ALT for end stage chronic liver disease was initially thought of as a means to reduce the surgical risk of transplantation by avoiding the recipient's hepatectomy. Indeed, a number of patients having undergone this procedure had been rejected for orthotopic liver transplantation because they were considered too great a surgical risk due to the extent of liver failure. Although some initial satisfactory results were published[1] and a retrospective study showed comparable results of orthotopic and heterotopic grafts,[2] the high rate of postoperative complications with disappointing long-term results and the dramatic simultaneous improvement of conventional orthotopic liver transplantation led to almost abandoning this technique.

Othotopic auxiliary liver transplantation for fulminant hepatic failure

The possibility of spontaneous liver regeneration in some patients with fulminant hepatic failure without functional or histological sequel as well as the lessons from split liver transplantations and from living related donors have revived interest in this approach. Recent reports of successful ALT in patients with fulminant hepatic failure showed that total or partial liver grafts implanted either heterotopically or orthopically have immediately restored liver function and normal consciousness.[2,5] Moreover, in some cases, native liver regeneration, even several months after transplantation, allowed permanent interruption of immunosuppression.

TECHNICAL CONSIDERATIONS

Auxiliary orthotopic liver transplantation requires that both the graft and the recipient's liver are reduced.[5] Although early in our experience, we used, full-size grafts in 4 recipients, this is associated with a high incidence of vascular complications, due to difficulties in correctly orienting the graft and compression by the abdominal wall, and we no longer use or advocate this technique.[2] Size reductions are performed on opposite sites (removing left segments of the recipients liver and of right segments of the graft or the other way round) so that after transplantation, the recipient approximately has an overall normal liver. The surgical team has technically the choice of the topography and extent of the resections provided an anatomical transsection of the liver is performed. In practice, this is governed by the size of the graft and by the severity of the recipient's encephalopathy.

DONOR PROCEDURE

The graft is harvested using a standard technique of multiorgan procurement and is preserved in the UW solution. The initial back-table graft preparation is similar to that used for conventional OLT, and includes dissection of the portal vein and hepatic arteries up to their bifurcation and dissection of the suprahepatic vena cava, so as to clearly identify the number and terminal anatomy of the hepatic veins. Graft reduction is performed while the organ is immersed in ice-cold solution and continuously perfused through a portal canula with preservation solution. Although no rules can yet be established, it is usually agreed that large (as opposed to small) grafts will speed up the recovery from fulminant liver failure but may, at the same time, jeopardise the chance of recovery of the native liver. In practice, a left graft may be used unless this is too small (i.e. less than 0.5 - 1% of the recipient's body weight) or if there is a very severe encephalopathy. In these latter cases, we would tend to use the larger right segments.

Preparation of the right liver consists in an anatomical left hepatectomy with a supra-hilar approach, so that the risk of vascular damage to the common bile duct is minimal. The hepatic artery is dissected, beginning at the celiac trunk, followed along the common hepatic artery and the proper hepatic artery to the bifurcation, and the branches going to the left liver are ligated. The portal vein is isolated until the left portal branch is identified and divided. The site of the excision is closed with a 6-0 running suture to maximise the length of the vessel. The inferior vena cava is isolated from the caudate lobe by sharp dissection with ligation of individual small hepatic veins entering the IVC until the major hepatic veins are isolated. The left hepatic vein is divided, and sutured. The transection of the parenchyma is started at the gallbladder fossa and is directed toward the hilum. On the liver surface, the line of division is directed to the left edge of the IVC to preserve the middle hepatic vein with the graft. The incision is progressively deepened using either a thin clamp or an ultrasound dissector. Each vascular or biliary structure on the right side is suture-ligated. The left hepatic duct is divided-sutured without dissection a few millimetres from the hilar bifurcation. The cut surface is inspected by flushing the portal vein and the biliary tree. Fibrin glue is applied on the transected area.

Preparation of the left liver follows the same initial steps. A cholecystectomy is performed first and a cannula is inserted in the cystic duct. After isolation of the hepatic artery (including the celiac trunk, the common hepatic artery, and the proper hepatic artery), the right branch of the hepatic artery is ligated and divided. Finally, the portal vein is isolated, the right portal vein is divided, and the site of bifurcation oversewn with 6-0 running suture. The right hepatic vein is divided, and the site is closed with 4-0 running suture. Parenchyma dissection preserves the middle hepatic vein and all vascular structures on the transected surface are suture-ligated. The right biliary duct is divided without dissection, a few millimetres from the hilar bifurcation.

RECIPIENT PROCEDURE

It is particularly important to have good access to the suprahepatic IVC, and this is achieved successfully by a bilateral subcostal incision close to the lower rib with an inverted T-shaped median incision along the xyphoid process. A frozen section biopsy of the native liver is usually sampled (see below) in order to assess the absence of fibrosis (that would otherwise suggest that this is not a fulminant or sub-fulminant liver failure) and the presence of viable hepatocytes. Because the resistance in the native liver is usually greater (due to extensive necrosis) than in the graft, no attempt is initially made to partially interrupt portal flow.

Right liver transplantation

Both the right and left lobe should be completely mobilized. The falciform ligament is incised using diathermy up to the suprahepatic vena cava. Incision of the left triangular ligament will help in mobilizing the right lobe and will give access to the supra hepatic vena cava should this be controlled in emergency. The right lobe is mobilised using diathermy to incise the anterior leaf of the coronary ligament and the right triangular ligament. In this way, the right lobe can progressively be displaced inferiorly and across to the left of the abdomen. Adhesions between the right adrenal gland and the bare area of the right lobe are freed, allowing the right side of the IVC to be exposed. The liver is subsequently lifted upwards and all the short accessory veins between the anterior surface of the IVC and segment 1 are secured between fine ties, proceeding cranially. We avoid using clips because they tend to fall off, a possible source

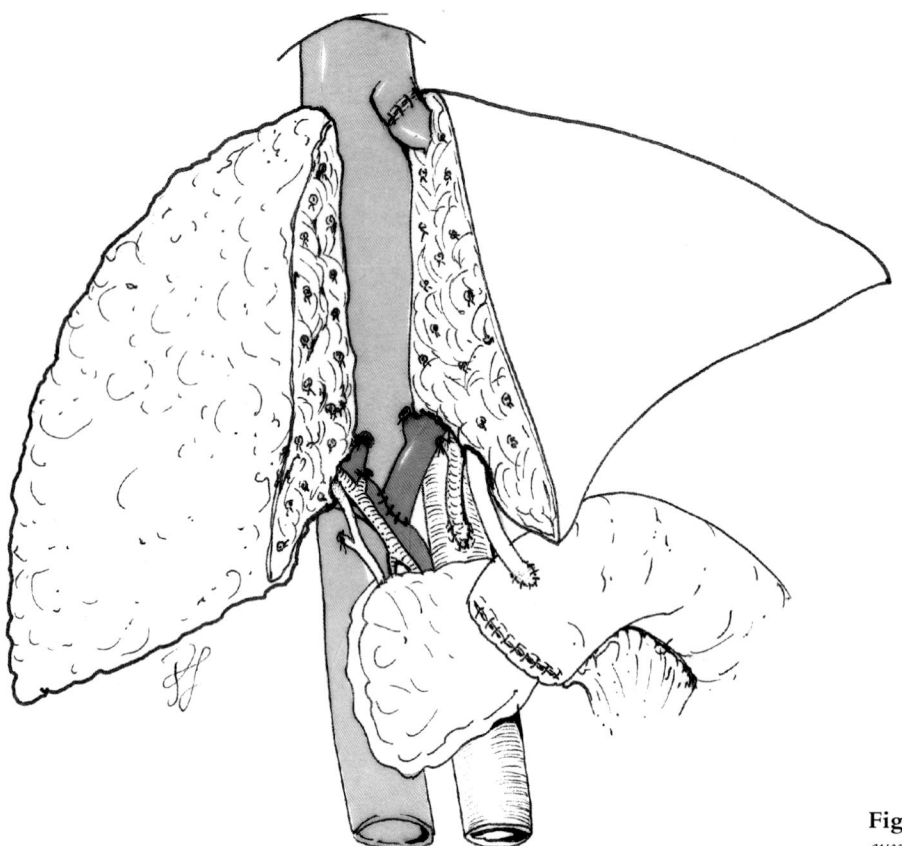

Figure 32.3 – *Technique of auxiliary liver transplantation of a left graft.*

of postoperative bleeding. This maneuvre facilitates exposition of the right lateral side of the inferior vena cava and division of the IVC ligament which runs between the dorsal edge of the caudate lobe and the right lobe. This ligament should be ligated before division since it may contain large hepatic veins. After this step, the right hepatic vein is easily exposed and controlled. The right liver resection is performed with an extra hepatic dissection of the right pedicle. A cholecystectomy is first performed and a transcystic drain secured. This facilitates exposure of the right portal vein and allows for injection of methylene blue in the cystic duct after the hepatectomy to ensure that no biliary leakage is present on the cut surface (see below). The first structure to be ligated is the right hepatic artery as distally as possible in order to preserve blood supply to the common bile duct. The main portal vein is dissected free from the surrounding adventitial tissue by blunt dissection and controlled. Proceeding cranially, its bifurcation is identified and the right branch controlled with a vessel loop. Care should be taken to avoid injury of small caudate branches passing posteriorly. The right branch of the portal vein is transected between vascular clamps and the proximal stump is closed with 5-0 running suture taking care not to narrow the portal bifurcation. A clear line of demarcation develops on the liver surface, running from the gallbladder fossa to the middle of the IVC in the principle vascular plane. The right hepatic vein is clamped and divided without suture of its caval stump, taking care to leave a 1-2 cm long stump on the cava side. Parenchyma transection is performed using either a thin clamp or an ultrasound dissector. Clamping of the hepatic pedicle should be avoided to prevent hemodynamic disturbances and additional injury to the left liver. This step tends to be easier in patients with fulminant liver failure because the liver is usually atrophic. Each vascular or biliary structure is sutured-ligated on the left side. The right hepatic duct is ligated with the hilar plate and transected a few millimetres from the biliary bifurcation. The cut surface is inspected for bile leakage after flushing methylene blue through the cystic duct, and subsequently sealed with fibrin glue. The vena cava around the stump of the right hepatic vein is gently mobilised from the diaphragm and the surrounding hepatic parenchyma and clamped laterally; the caval wall is incised caudally along 1-2 cm from the inferior edge of the right hepatic stump.

The graft is placed in the right hypochondrium so that both cut surfaces of the graft and of the native liver are face-to-face (**Figure 32.3**). The graft is slightly rolled to the right to allow completion of an end-to-side caval anastomosis between the suprahepatic stump of the graft's IVC and the recipient's right hepatic vein. During completion of this anastomosis, the graft is flushed through the portal vein with Ringer's solution at 4°C. This anastomosis can be invetigated endoluminally through the infrahepatic stump of the graft's IVC which is subsequently closed with a TA 30 vascular stapler. The caval clamp can be gently displaced to the right and applied to the anastomosis to relieve any obstruction of the caval flow. The right side of the recipient's portal vein is clamped laterally just above the head of the pancreas and opened. An end-to-side anastomosis is performed between the graft and the recipient's portal veins using running sutures of the posterior wall and interrupted sutures of the anterior wall of 5/0 polypropylene. The graft is subsequently revascularized and the cut surface of the graft is explored to ensure that no hemorrhage is present. The graft's celiac axis is anastomosed to the recipient's infrarenal aorta. Bile flow is restored through a Roux-en-Y hepatico-jejunostomy. Intraoperative ultrasound is essential in assessing the patency of all vascular anastomoses. The right subphrenic space is drained. A primary abdominal closure is almost always possible. Should this result in a compression of the graft, only the skin is closed after extensive undermining on an absorbable mesh sutured to the musculofascial walls, full abdominal closure being performed some days or weeks later. The drain placed in the recipient's cystic duct may be retained to allow for the monitoring of the native liver's bile and clearance function.

Left liver transplantation

The falciform and left triangular ligaments are divided to completely mobilise the left lateral segments (segment 2 and 3). We advocate extensive resection to segment 1 and 4 inorder to increase the space. Left hepatectomy is performed using a standard technique. In brief, all portal, arterial and biliary branches arising from the right of the umbilical fissure are ligated and divided following division of the overlying bridge of hepatic parenchyma if this is present. The extra-parenchymal segment of the left hepatic vein is controlled and a tap is placed around it. The liver is then transsected along the line of colour demarcation observed to the left of the falciform ligament using either a thin clamp or an ultrasound dissector. Vascular clamping of the portal pedicle is not necessary and should be avoided so as to prevent any changes in the patient's haemodynamics or additional injury of the liver remnant. Small vascular or biliary pedicles along this usually bloodless plane of transection are secured by fine ligatures. The left hepatic vein is clamped as close as possible to the IVC and is divided intraparenchymally leaving a stump of 2 cm. The transsected liver surface is examined for bile leakage by injecting diluted methylene blue in the cystic duct and is then sealed with fibrin glue. In order to prepare for a safe lateral clamping of the IVC during caval anastomosis, we also perform a complete dissection of the anterior surface of the IVC up to the left and middle hepatic veins, dividing between fine ties the small accessory caudate veins. The left part of the caudate lobe is subsequently resected. At that stage, it is possible to precisely determine the optimal site of implantation of the graft's suprahepatic vein. If the middle and left hepatic veins of the recipient drain separately in the IVC, the clamp is placed so as to include the ostium of the left hepatic vein and a short segment of IVC below which it is opened. If, on the contrary, left and middle hepatic veins drain through a common channel, the stump of the left hepatic vein is oversewn and the IVC is clamped laterally.

The graft is put in the subphrenic space so that both cut surfaces of the graft and of the native liver are face-to-face. The graft is slightly rolled to the left to allow completion of an end-to-side caval anastomosis between the stump of the left and median hepatic veins and the left side of the recipient IVC. During this step, the graft is flushed through the portal vein with 4°C Ringer solution. The caval clamp can be gently displaced to the left and applied on the anastomosis to ensure optimal caval flow in the recipient. The left side of the recipient portal vein is laterally clamped just above the head of the pancreas and opened. This is necessary to ensure that no twisting occurs at the origin of the graft's portal vein. The graft's portal vein is anastomosed end-to-side by a continuous running suture of the posterior wall and interrupted sutures of the anterior wall using 5/0 polypropylene. The graft is subsequently revascularized. The graft's artery is anastomosed either to the recipient's aorta or splenic artery. Biliary reconstruction is performed using a Roux-en-Y anastomosis. It may be useful to secure the graft in position with interrupted sutures between its falciform ligament and the diaphragm.

It should be remembered that the risk of parenchymal or vascular compression at the time of abdominal closure is greater with these left grafts. Intraoperative Doppler ultrasound is required to ensure that blood flow in the arterial, portal and hepatic branches is normal. If there is any risk of compression, the skin only is closed over an absorbable mesh, full abdominal wall closure being undertaken once the graft has regained a normal size. The drain placed in the recipient's cystic duct may be retained to allow for the monitoring of the native liver's bile and clearance function.

Immunosuppressive therapy and postoperative follow-up

There is no rationale for administering an immunosuppressive regimen distinct from that used for OLT, at least during the initial postoperative period. This is currently based on cyclosporine, or FK 506, in association with steroids and azathioprine if kidney function is normal. The incidence of acute rejection within auxiliary grafts is comparable to that reported for non-auxiliary grafts. There is in addition experimental evidence that both cyclosporine and FK 506 enhance liver regeneration.[13]

Neurological status is monitored clinically, electrically or by means of the cerebral perfusion pressure. Overall liver function is assessed by daily assays of serum transaminases, bilirubin, prothrombin time (PT) and proconvertin (factor V). Separate assessment of the graft and of the native liver is based on Doppler ultrasound, histology, volumetry and hepatobiliary scintigraphy.

Indications, results and prospects

The ability of the liver to regenerate following fulminant or subfulminant liver failure is currently based on clinical and biological parameters known as the Child-Paul Brousse or the King's College criteria.[3,16]. These include the etiology of liver injury, the severity of the encephalopathy, the age of the patient, the factor V plasma level, the serum creatinine level and the pH. Using these well-defined and validated criteria, it is possible to identify patients who are at high risk of death and in whom, therefore, transplantation is indicated.

This method is, however, not infallible, and it is usually agreed that 5-20% of patients transplanted with these criteria would have survived without transplantation. This is obviously the first group of patients in whom auxiliary liver transplantation is most advantageous. Another group of patients in whom auxiliary liver transplantation will also prove useful are those patients in whom liver regeneration will occur but is delayed. Auxiliary liver transplantation will allow these patients to safely await regeneration and avoid the consequences of liver failure and cerebral edema. Cerebral edema and liver failure do not always have parallel evolutions. Approximately 10% of patients undergoing an OLT for fulminant or subfulminant liver failure will die of cerebral edema, even though their graft functions perfectly.[3] The timing of auxiliary liver transplantations should, therefore, as for OLT, be performed as quickly as possible once the patient fullfills the criteria for transplantation. There is, however, a third group of patients in whom regeneration will not occur. In these patients, ALT is of no benefit over OLT. The main difficulty, therefore, is to preoperatively identify those patients in whom regeneration will occur (even with a delay time) without irreversible damage, i.e. those patients in whom immunosuppression may eventually be discontinued. In addressing this issue, one should bare in mind that full recovery of the native liver may require up to 2 years.[5,15]

To address this issue, a workshop was held in Strasbourg (France) in October 1994 on the joint experience of twelve European centres totalling 30 auxiliary liver transplantations for fulminant or subfulminant liver failure. Overall, complete regeneration of the native liver was observed in 68% of the patients, while incomplete regeneration with areas of obvious fibrosis or extensive fibrosis were observed in 14% and 18% of the patients respectively. Hence, 13 of the 19 survivors (representing 43% of the transplanted patients) had been withdrawn from all immunosuppressive regimen at the time of evaluation. The best clinical variables predictive of this favourable development were, aged less than 40 years, a delay between the onset of jaundice and encephalopathy less than 7 days, and an injury related to viral hepatitis or paracetamol overdose. In contrast, the percentage of surviving hepatocytes at the time of transplantation was not predictive.[6]

Based on these preliminary observations and on the fact that recipients of auxiliary partial liver grafts are undoubtely at increased risk of early postoperative complications than recipients of an OLT, we believe that this procedure should not be performed earlier than standard OLT, i.e. it should be indicated using the same criteria as those in use for conventional OLT, and should only be indicated in patients aged under 40 years, without evidence of chronic liver disease and without hemodynamic instability (as this has been shown to be improved by total hepatectomy of the native liver). In addition, because the amount of hepatocytes generated by this technique is lower than what would be anticipated using the standard technique, we believe that only ABO compatible, non steatotic grafts, harvested from young donors with normal liver function tests, should be used.

It is possible, although yet unproven, that the presence of the auxiliary graft may favor the regeneration of the native liver through the release of hepatotrophic factors, or the clearance of detrimental toxins or biological mediators. There is on the other hand, a risk that the presence of the auxiliary grafts prompts the development of cirrhosis in the native liver after fulminant HBV infection, in contrast to what is observed in patients who spontaneously recover from this injury. We do not believe, however, that fulminant hepatis B is a contraindication to auxiliary liver transplantation.

It is somewhat paradoxical that auxiliary liver transplantations, initially advocated to avoid hepatectomy in the recipient, have proved successful when associated with a partial resection of the native liver, an operation that would have been thought 'formidable' some years ago, since patients with fulminant or subfulminant liver failure are particularly sensitive to hemodynamic variations and have disastrous hemostasis. This development is the result of considerable improvement in both liver resection and graft reduction. Orthotopic partial auxiliary grafts have, to date, predominantly been performed in patients with fulminant liver failure but have also been successful in patients with metabolic disorders.[21] This may prove useful in the future in adult patients with chronic liver diseases to overcome the shortage of organ donors or even as an adjunct for gene therapy.

REFERENCES

1. Belghiti J, Noun R, Sauvanet A. Temporary portocaval anastomosis with preservation of caval flow during orthotopic liver transplantation. *Am J Surg* 1995; **169**: 277 - 279.
2. Belghiti J, Zinzindohoue F, Durand F, Noun R, Sauvanet A, Bernuau J. Auxiliary liver transplantation for fulminant liver failure: limits of an attractive concept. *Hepatology* 1995; **22**: 153A (abstract).
3. Bismuth H, Samuel D, Castaing D et al. Orthotopic liver transplantation in fulminant and subfulminant hepatitis. The Paul Brousse experience. *Ann Surg* 1995;**222**:109-119.
4. Boudjema K. Jaeck D. Siméoni U. et al. Temporary auxiliary liver transplantation for subacute liver failure in a child. *Lancet* 1993;**342**:778-779.
5. Boudjema K, Cherqui D, Jaeck D et al. Auxiliary liver transplantation for fulminant and subfulminant hepatic failure. *Transplantation* 1995; **59**: 218 - 223.
6. Chenard-Neu MP, Boudjema K, Bernuau J, et al. Auxiliary liver transplantation: regeneration of tha native liver and outcome in 30 patients with fulminant hepatic failure. A multicenter european study. *Hepatology* 1996;**23**:1119-1127.
7. Farges O, Saliba F, Farhamant H et al. Incidence of acute and chronic rejection after liver transplantation as a function of the primary disease : possible influence of alcohol and polyclonal immunoglobulins. *Hepatology* 1996; **23**: 240-248.
8. Gubernatis G, Pichlmayr R, Kemnitz J et al. Auxiliary partial orthotopic liver transplantation (APOLT) for fulminant hepatic failure: first successful case report. *World J Surg* 1991;**15**:660-666.
9. Hess F, Willemen A, Jerusalem C. Auxiliary liver transplantation in the rat: influence of the condition of the recipient's liver on the fate of the graft. *Eur Surg Res* 1977; **9**: 270-9.
10. Hess F, Willemen A, Jerusalem C. Survival of auxiliary rat liver grafts with decreased portal blood flow. *Eur Surg Res* 1978; **10**: 444-55.
11. Lecompte Y, deRiberolles C, Grange D, Brunet AM, Bismuth H. Canine intrathoracic hepatic homograft. A life-supporting procedure. *Arch Surg* 1974; **109**: 809 - 811.
12. Lorente L, Arias J, Aller MA, Ispizua JI, Rodiguez J, Duran H. Heterotopic auxiliary liver transplantation with portal flow: gradual development of the collateral circulation. *HPB Surgery* 1990; **2**: 281-93.
13. Mazzaferro V, Porter KA, Scotti-Foglieni CL, Venkataramanan R, Makowka L, Rossaro L, Francavilla A, Todo S, Van Thiel DH, Starzl TE. The hepatotrophic influence of cyclosporine. *Surgery* 1990; **107**: 533-9.
14. Metselaar H.J, Hesselink E.J, De Rave S et al. A comparison between heterotopic and orthotopic liver transplantation in patients with end-stage chronic liver disease. *Transplant Proc* 1991; **23**: 1531-1532.
15. Moritz MJ, Jarrell BE, Munoz SJ, Maddrey W.C. Regeneration of the native liver after heterotopic liver transplantation for fulminant hepatic failure. *Transplantation* 1993;**55**: 952-954.
16. O'Grady JG, Alexander GJ, Hayllar KM, Williams R. Early indicators of prognosis in fulminant hepatic failure. *Gastroenterology* 1989; **97**: 439 - 445.
17. Sauvanet A, Yang S, Bernuau J et al. How to improve native liver regeneration in auxiliary liver transplantation. *HPB Surgery* 1996; **9**: 28.

18. Suc B, Fourtanier G, Lloveras JJ, Dubois G, Gonzales N. Heterotopic liver transplantation in the left hypochondrium after splenectomy: long-term follow-up of two cases. *Transplant Proc* 1994; **26:** 263-264.
19. Terpstra OT, Reuvers CB, Schalm SW. Auxiliary heterotopic liver transplantation. *Transplantation* 1988; **45:** 1003-1007
20. Terpstra OT, Schalm S, Weimar W *et al*. Auxiliary partial liver transplantation for end-stage chronic liver disease. *N Engl J Med* 1988; **319:** 1507-1511.
21. Whitington PF, Emond JC, Heffron T, Thistlethwaite JR. Orthotopic auxiliary liver transplantation for Crigler-Najjar syndrome type 1. *Lancet* 1993; **342:** 779-780.
22. Xu HS, Pruett TL, Jones RS. Study of donor-recipient liver size match for transplantation. *Ann Surg* 1994; **219:** 46-50.
23. Yu W, Wan X, Wright IR, Coddington D, Bitter-Suermann H. Heterotopic liver transplantation in rats: effects of intrahepatic islet isografts and split portal blood flow on liver integrity after auxiliary liver isotransplantation. *Surgery* 1994; **115:**108-17.

33

Intestinal and Multiorgan Transplantation

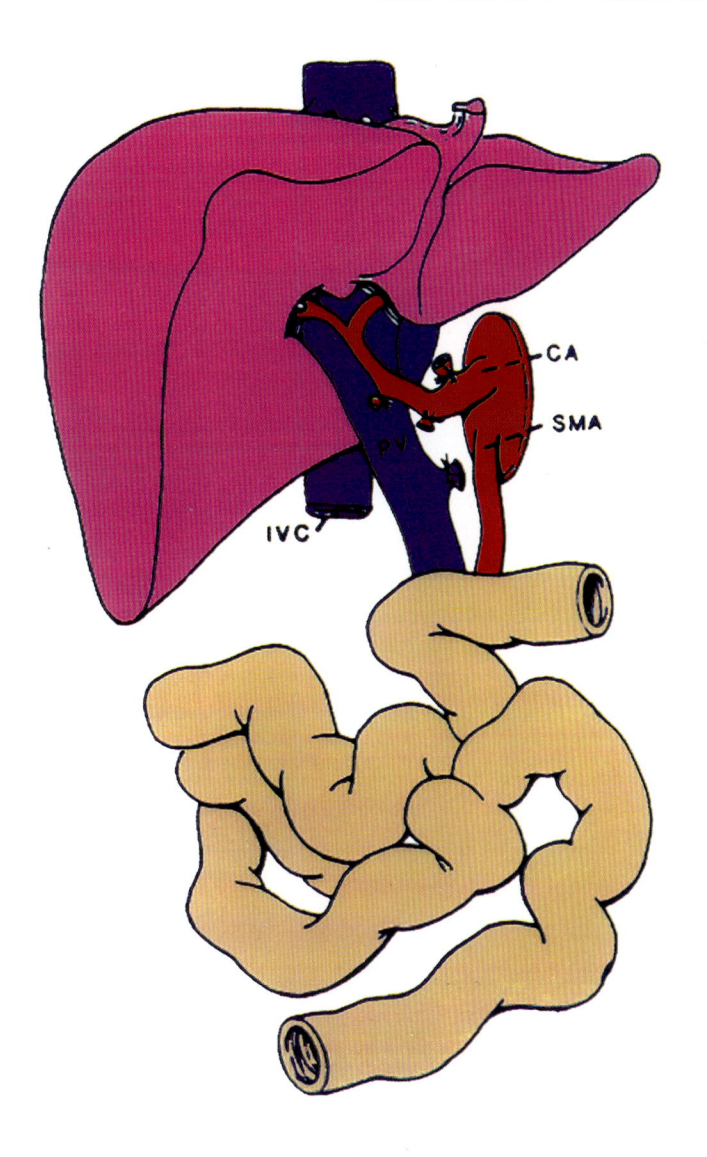

A.G. Tzakis et al

CAUSES OF INTESTINAL FAILURE
In the adult
Thrombosis/Vascular injury to superior mesenteric pedicle
Crohn's disease
Desmoid tumors
Traumatic mesenteric transection
Pseudo-obstruction
Radiation enteritis
Severe secretory diarrhea
Malabsorption syndrome
Volvulus
In the child
Volvulus
Gastroschisis
Necrotizing enterocolitis
Intestinal atresia
Pseudo-obstruction
Microvillus atrophy
Intestinal polyposis
Aganglionic syndrome

Table 33.1 – *Causes of intestinal failure.*

Lillehei described in 1959 experimental, and later clinical, intestinal transplantation for patients with intestinal failure as a life saving procedure.[1,12] Although the operation was technically feasible, the immunosuppressive agents available at that time were unable to prevent or control graft rejection. Major improvements in immunosuppressive therapy after introduction of Cyclosporine and later Tacrolimus (Prograf/FK506) have reintroduced intestinal and multivisceral transplantation to clinical practice with encouraging results.[18,20] Isolated intestinal transplantation successes were reported by Deltz, (Kiel, 1988) and Goulet, (Paris, 1991).[2,5] Two patients underwent multivisceral transplantation and had a stormy postoperative course and succumbed to tumor recurrence one year after transplantation, and lymphoproliferative disease six months after transplantation respectively.[13,16] The first successful combined liver intestinal transplant was performed by Grant et al. in 1988 under Cyclosporine immunosuppression.[7] The introduction of FK 506 (Prograf) at the University of Pittsburgh marked the beginning of a new era for intestinal transplantation with persistent, though not yet satisfactory, long term success. More recently (1993) the addition of contemporaneous bone marrow infusions from the same donor, by inducing donor specific tolerance and introduction of Mycophenolate Mofetil, (CellCept, MMF, 1995) are promising to further improve the results.

Indications

Intestinal transplantation is indicated in patients with intestinal failure who are depleted of intravenous access or are suffering severe complications from total parenteral nutrition (TPN) or their disease. Intestinal failure is defined as the chronic and irreversible inability of the intestine to provide the nutritional needs of the patient. The incidence of intestinal failure is estimated to be 2 patients per million of population per year.[3]

Patients with intestinal failure are dependent on TPN for their survival. Introduced by Dudrick[3] in 1968, TPN revolutionized the prognosis of patients suffering from intestinal failure. TPN allowed them long term survival and acceptable quality of life. Nevertheless, it is expensive (estimated cost of uncomplicated home TPN $100,000 - $200,000 per year) and imposes social and work restrictions which are intolerable to some patients. In addition, TPN can result in severe, and at times, life-threatening complications, such as central vein thrombosis, line sepsis and progressive liver disease.

In the adult patient, the most frequent causes of Short bowel syndrome (SBS), leading to intestinal failure, include injury with or without thrombosis of the superior mesenteric pedicle, Crohn's disease, unresectable benign tumors of the intestine, and congenital or other acquired causes that lead to anatomical or physiological loss of the small intestine. In pediatric patients the most common causes are due to congenital abnormalities such as volvulus, gastroschisis, intestinal atresia and necrotizing enterocolitis. (***Table 33.1***).[4,8,11,22]

TECHNIQUES IN LIVER SURGERY

Figure 33.1 – *Multivisceral transplantation (including the ascending and right transverse colon)*

(Reproduce with permission of Waverly, Williams and Wilkins from Intestinal Transplantation in Composite Visceral Grafts or Alone. Annals of Surgery Vol 216, No 3, September 1992.)

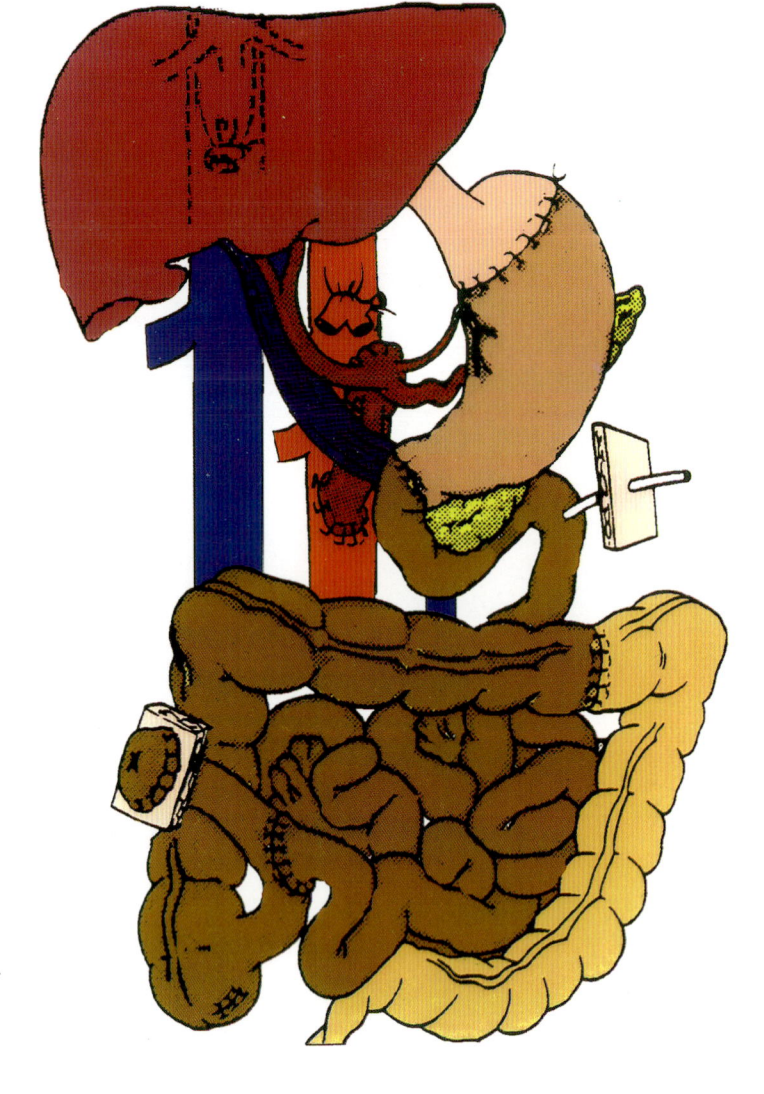

The evaluation process for small intestine transplantation is individualized for each patient based on the original disease process and current medical condition. The main goals of the preoperative evaluation process is to assess the technical feasibility and associated risk factors that may modulate the type of graft to be transplanted, i.e. isolated intestine, liver-intestine or multivisceral. Most commonly, an isolated intestinal graft is used when there is no irreversible damage to the liver because of intravenous nutrition. An intestinal/liver graft is used when there is irreversible damage to the liver. A multivisceral graft may be performed when all intra-abdominal organs need to be replaced. The latter may be secondary to diffuse thrombosis, tumors involving all intra-abdominal organs or generalized motility disorder.

Although in the early experience the liver was included with the graft in some centers for its immunoprotective effect, currently it is replaced only if it is irreversibly damaged. Liver replacement is also indicated in the event of natural anticoagulant deficiencies. Transplantation with a phenotypically normal liver will correct the deficiency and prevent future visceral thromboses.

CONTRAINDICATIONS

As with any other organ transplantation, uncontrolled sepsis, AIDS and unresectable malignancies are absolute contraindications to intestinal transplantation. Cardiovascular and respiratory compromise, cerebral edema and multiorgan failure, severely degrade the prognosis.

Organ donation and preservation

Prospective donors are identified and selected based upon ABO compatibility, and in size equal to, or less than that of the potential recipient. Potential donors must be free of active infection and have a negative history of intestinal disease. Normal liver function tests are required in donors whose organs are selected for use in recipients undergoing either liver/small intestine or multivisceral transplantation. Decontamination of the donor's intestine is accomplished by administering, via a nasogastric tube, a mixture of polymixin B, gentamicin and nystatin or amphotericin B. Prophylactic antibiotic agents are also given intravenously. The donor operation consists of an *en bloc* dissection of the entire abdominal contents. The gastrointestinal tract from the

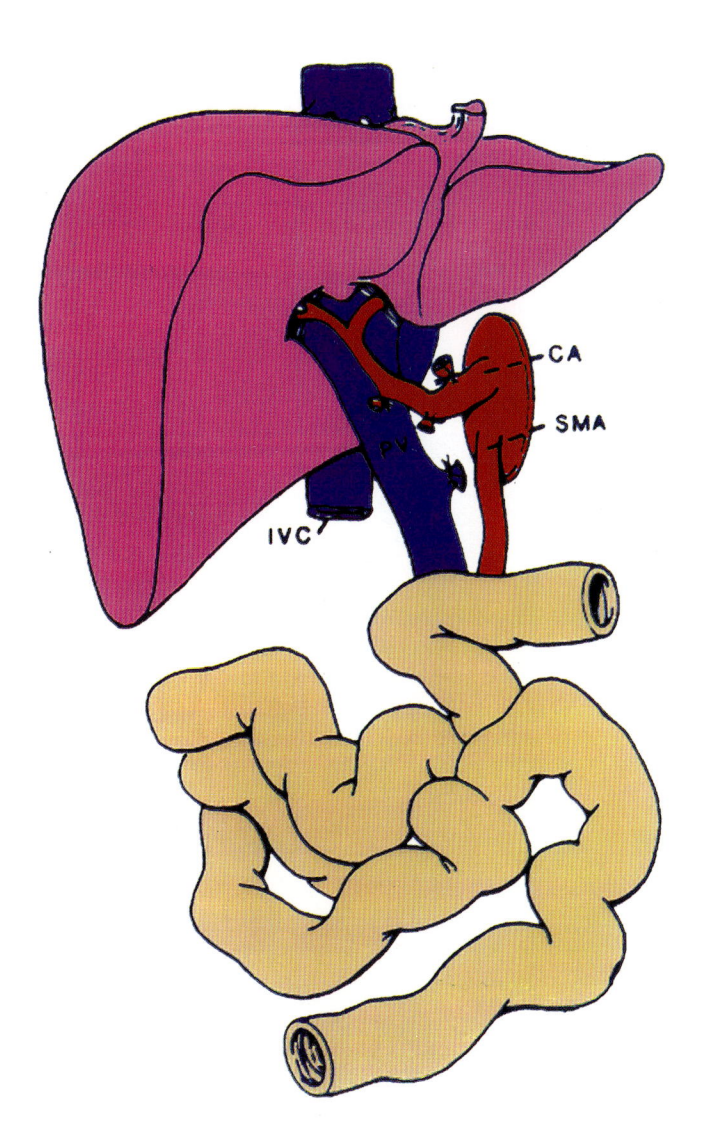

Figure 33.2 – *Small bowel liver allograft, with the Carrel patch containing the origin of the SMA and the celiac axis.*
IVC = Inferior vena cava;
PV = Portal vein;
CA = Celiac artery;
SMA = Superior mesenteric artery

(Reproduced with permission of Waverly, Williams and Wilkins from Intestinal Transplantation in Composite Visceral Grafts or Alone. Annals of Surgery Vol 216, No 3, September 1992.)

gastroesophageal junction to the descending colon (including liver, pancreas and spleen) is transected from its attachments and mobilized *en bloc*. The inferior mesenteric artery (IMA) is identified and divided, and the diaphragm is split to have access to the suprahepatic inferior vena cava (IVC). The thoracic aorta is cross-clamped and the cold preservation solution infusion is started. The IVC is transected at the level of the right atrium to vent the flushing solution. The esophagus and descending colon are divided and the abdomen is filled with ice slush for surface cooling. The aorta is cut below the origins of the celiac axis and SMA, leaving a cuff of aorta (Carrel's patch) for both vessels. The infrahepatic IVC is cut just above the junction of the left renal vein. The gastrointestinal tract (stomach, duodenum, small and large bowel) as well as the liver, pancreas and spleen are removed *en bloc* and secured in a sterile bag with cold preservation solution. The iliac vessels and thoracic aorta are removed also in order to be used as interposition grafts. The University of Wisconsin (UW) solution is used as a preservation solution during the retrieval.

OPERATIVE TECHNIQUE

The surgical procedure begins with a midline incision from the xiphoid process to the symphysis pubis with transverse extensions, but may vary according to pathology and previous surgeries. After appropriate exposure, the remnant native intestine is removed. The distal duodenum and proximal jejunum are preserved for anastomosis to the graft (in case of liver/intestinal or isolated intestinal grafts). If a multivisceral transplant is needed, the stomach, duodenum and pancreas are also removed. In the multivisceral procedure the graft consists of all of the intra-abdominal organs, except for the spleen (**Figure 33.1**). The graft is envisioned as a grape cluster (proposed by Starzl) with a double central stem consisting of the celiac axis and superior mesenteric artery.[15,17] A Carrel patch with the origins of these arteries is anastomosed directly to the recipient aorta or via an interposition graft. Outflow of the graft is accomplished by anastomosing the donor suprahepatic cava to the host hepatic vein ostia with the 'piggyback' technique. In the hepatic-intestinal graft transplant procedure the small bowel and the liver are retained in continuity (**Figure 33.2**) and removal of the other viscera from the stem vascular structures can be done

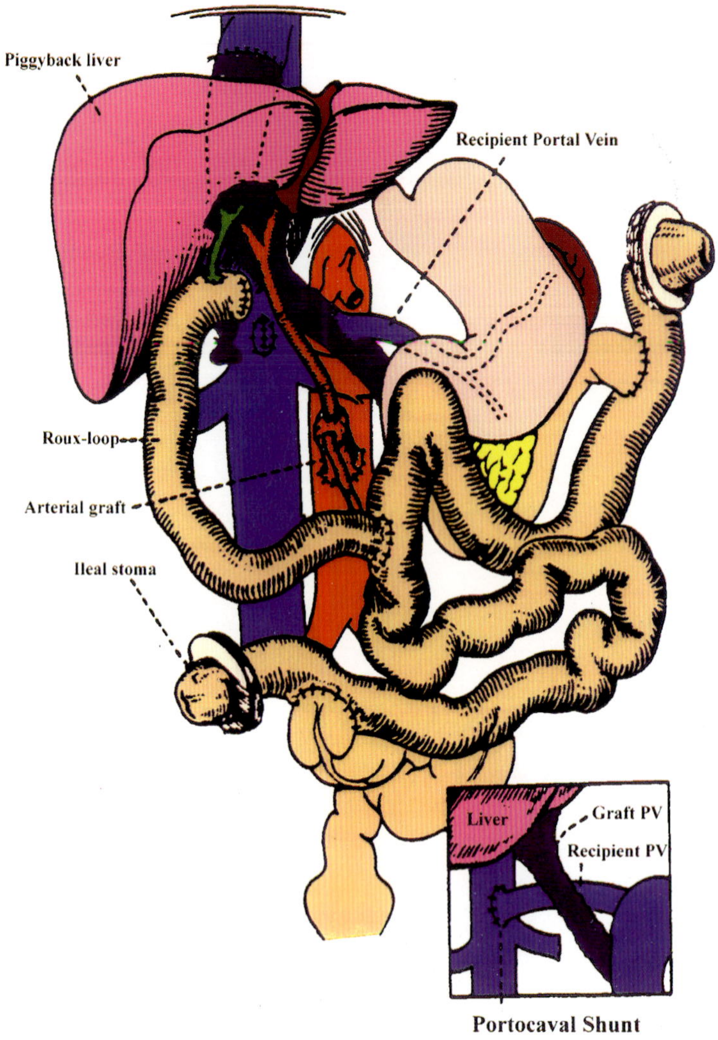

TECHNIQUES IN LIVER SURGERY

Figure 33.3 – *Liver-small bowel transplantation. Native liver is replaced by the 'piggy-back' technique. The recipient's portal vein is drained into the graft portal vein or into the inferior vena cava (inset). Two ends of the intestinal graft are exteriorized by enterostomy (at the left upper and right lower quadrant of the abdomen).*

(Reproduced with permission of Waverly, Williams and Wilkins from Intestinal Transplantation in Composite Visceral Grafts or Alone. Annals of Surgery Vol 216, No 3, September 1992.)

on the back table.[15,19] In this procedure (**Figure 33.3**) an end-to-side portocaval shunt is performed to drain the retained host splanchnic organs via the native portal vein during surgery when the venous outflow is blocked. After the graft is revascularized, the recipient portal vein is then reanastomosed to the side of the donor portal vein to maintain hepatopetal flow. This porto-portal anastomosis cannot be performed in some cases (size discrepancy) and the constructed portocaval shunt drains the native organs that are left in place. If the intestine is to be transplanted alone, the liver can be separated from the intestine on the back table and given to another recipient along with the celiac axis and upper portal vein, while the distal portal vein and complete superior mesenteric artery are retained with the intestine. The infrarenal abdominal aorta is usually the source of arterialization of solitary intestinal grafts and the venous outflow of the isolated graft is directed into the native portal system (**Figure 33.4**).

Gastrointestinal continuity is established with conventional techniques. Proximally, the donor graft jejunum is anastomosed to the native residual jejunum or duodenum. A proximal jejunostomy is performed for graft decompression and early tube feeding. Distally, the ileum is connected to the native colon (if present) in a side-to-side fashion, bringing out the ileostomy for drainage and early decompression of the transplanted intestine. (A Bishop-Koop ileostomy is performed.) (**Figure 33.3**). The stoma constructed using the graft allows physician easy access when performing endoscopies and biopsies. In the combined liver intestinal transplant the donor bile duct is drained into a Roux-en-Y loop which is constructed using donor jejunum (**Figure 33.3**), while in the multivisceral transplant an esophago-gastrostomy and pyloroplasty are performed.

POSTOPERATIVE MANAGEMENT

Immunosuppression – Although CYA based immunosuppression is still used in some centers, it appears that Tacrolimus (FK 506,

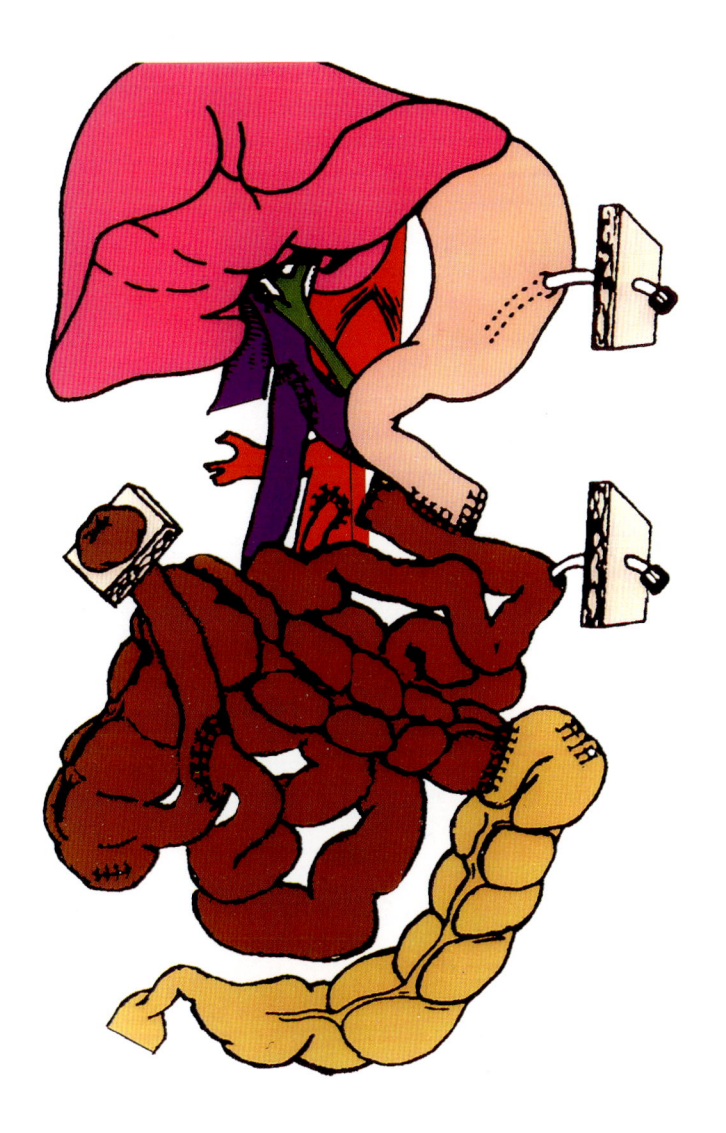

Figure 33.4 – *Isolated intestinal transplantation.*

(Reproduced with permission of Waverly, Williams and Wilkins from Intestinal Transplantation in Composite Visceral Grafts or Alone. Annals of Surgery Vol 216, No 3, September 1992.)

Prograf® based immunosuppression is more potent and is the current treatment choice. Currently, a new immunosuppressive agent, MMF, is being used in combination with Prograf® (1 gram enterally b.i.d in adults or 30 mg/kg/day in 2 divided doses in children). Use of Tacrolimus (FK506, Prograf®) 18 in the intestinal transplantation has significantly reduced the incidence of rejection episodes. Tacrolimus is initiated perioperatively and is given intravenously 0.02-0.03 mg/kg/day, and an oral dose of 0.05 mg/kg/day. The dose adjustment of Tacrolimus is based on the quality of graft function, evidence of graft rejection, and renal dysfunction and daily whole blood levels of Tacrolimus. Desirable 12 hour serum trough levels are 15 to 20 ng/ml for the first 3 to 6 months after transplantation. Intravenous steroid therapy is initiated perioperatively with a 1 gram bolus and is tapered in decrements of 40mg over the first 5 days in adults. Maintenance steroid therapy consists of an oral dose of prednisone, usually 20mg daily. Children smaller than 10kg receive a bolus of hydrocortisone (1 gram) and prednisone 100mg on the first postoperative day, tapered to 10mg per day over 5 days. Supplemental Azathioprine or Cyclophosphamide has been added to the immunosuppressive regimen in the presence of renal toxicity, persistent or recurrent episodes of rejection.

Unmodified bone marrow infusions from the same donor are given in some centers, including those in Pittsburgh and Miami, in an attempt to enhance chimerism and induce tolerance. Bone marrow cells are isolated from the vertebral bodies of the same cadaveric donor.

Intensive Care Unit – The patient is likely to require large volume fluid replacement during the first postoperative day because of sequestration in the intestinal wall and lumen. This fluid is expected to be mobilized during the subsequent postoperative days. Gastric decompression is continued until gastric emptying is normal at which time the patient is started on an oral diet.

A sudden increase in enteric output can signal

an early rejection episode. Intestinal graft rejection may cause a loss of absorptive capacity and an increase in secretory activity of the intestinal lumen. Intestinal rejection can also cause cessation of intestinal function. Observations of losses from the abdominal drains and abdominal dressings can also account for substantial fluid volume deficits in the unstable patient. Hypernatremia, hypokalemia, and metabolic acidosis may occur secondary to hypovolemia, therefore frequent biochemical monitoring is recommended.

Attempts are made to wean the patients from ventilatory support within 48 hours of the operation. Extubation of the patient is based on established respiratory, hemodynamic and neurologic guidelines for the critically ill patient. A patient receiving an isolated intestine transplant is usually transferred out of the intensive care unit to the surgical floor within two to three days postoperatively. The liver- intestine transplant recipient usually requires an extended period in the intensive care unit (days to weeks) due to the more lengthy and traumatic operative experience.

Graft motility recovery is determined by the presence of bowel sounds, the absence of abdominal distention, and the quality and quantity of ileal output. Nutritional considerations for these patients, as well as fluid balance remains extremely important particularly in the early (3 to 4 week) postoperative period. Patients have a relatively high stomal output due to graft adaptation that may necessitate intravenous or enteral fluid replacement.

The potential for alteration in skin integrity around the stoma site due to high ostomy output and diarrhea is a major concern. Postoperative pain management can become a difficult problem leading to alterations in sleep patterns, alterations in thought processes, potential narcotic addiction, and behavioral changes. Most intestinal recipients have a low pain tolerance. This is most likely due to their chronic illness, previous multiple surgical procedures, postoperative incisional pain, and difficult narcotic withdrawal. Liberal administration of opiates can, in turn, result in intestinal dysmotility and graft dysfunction. Some intestinal transplant patients will require larger doses of pain medication over a longer duration of time as compared with other surgical patients.

Nutritional Management – Enteral feeding is started in the form of an elemental diet through a feeding tube and increased as tolerated. TPN is continued until the patient is tolerating enteral and/or oral feeding in terms of caloric intake and protein. The requirement for adults is 1.5 gm protein/ kg/day and 30-35 kcal/kg/day, and up to 100 kcal/kg in children. The absorption of carbohydrates seems to recover early in the postoperative course in comparison with that of amino and fatty acids. Fat malabsorption during the early postoperative course is most likely related to lymphatic interruption at the time of transplantation. For this reason, intralipid administration is favorably recommended during the early postoperative period. A fat free diet is also advised during the early postoperative period.

Monitoring of Graft Function – The early clinical signs of graft dysfunction, whether due to preservation injury or graft rejection are high stomal output along with sluggish or even absent intestinal motility. With intestinal allograft rejection, physical examination reveals abdominal distention with diffuse abdominal pain, infrequent or absent bowel sounds, and edematous or dusky stomal mucosa. Complete recovery of graft function generally occurs 4 to 6 weeks after transplantation, with significant reduction in stomal output.

Radiologic monitoring of graft function is performed by measuring the rate of gastric emptying and the intestinal transit time. A prolonged emptying time or rapid transit time indicate poor functional ability of the transplanted intestine.

An upper endoscopy can provide access to the stomach, duodenum and jejunum. Key emphasis is placed on immediate graft biopsy, when rejection is suspected clinically to make an early diagnosis.

Post-operative complications

The most common complications encountered in the postoperative course are related to technical problems, preservation injury, rejection, graft versus host disease, infections, motility disorders and diarrhea.

Technical Complications – The potential for technical complications involves the vascular and intestinal anastomoses. Vascular complications include stenosis or thrombosis of the arterial or venous vascular systems or both. This can present as an acute or chronic episode. Surgical intervention is usually necessary to re-establish vascularization of the graft. If unsuccessful, retransplantation may be necessary. Intestinal anastomotic leakage is another postoperative complication that may occur during the first postoperative week.

Symptoms and signs of an anastomotic leak include abdominal pain, fever abdominal distention with tenderness. Urgent surgical intervention is necessary to correct this complication.

Preservation Injury – Initial graft dysfunction can occur due to preservation injury. The severity of this phenomenon ranges from mild to severe and is identified endoscopically and histologically by mucosal ulcerations or a sloughing of the entire intestinal mucosa. This is a serious complication because it can result in bacterial translocation. The intestinal mucosa has the ability to regenerate even after severe preservation injury.

Rejection – The appearance of the intestinal mucosa and the detection of mucosal ulcers are important indices of graft rejection. Endoscopy of a dysfunctional graft due to either preservation injury or a rejection episode may show an edematous flat mucosa, multiple ulcerative areas, and even complete sloughing of the intestinal mucosa. There is also a loss of peristalsis.

Rejection is segmental and can be missed even by a complete endoscopy. In mild to moderate rejection the biopsy reveals a mixed infiltrate with villous blunting, cryptitis and depletion of mucus cells. In severe rejection, loss of mucosal pattern, hemorrhage and sloughing can be observed. Biopsy specimens are obtained postoperatively when clinically indicated. Augmentation of maintenance immunosuppression will suffice for treatment of mild rejection, but steroid bolus and the addition of OKT3 may be needed in severe rejection.

Graft Versus Host Disease – Graft versus host disease occurs in the transplanted immunosuppressed patient when donor T cells react against recipient tissue antigens. The intestinal recipient is at high risk due to the abundant amount of lymphoid tissue in the intestine. In intestinal transplant recipients migration of donor lymphocytes from the intestinal graft occurs during the first 5 to 6 weeks after transplantation, with total replacement of the graft with the recipient lymphocytes.[6] GVHD is suspected to occur frequently after intestinal transplantation. GVHD may be diagnosed with skin biopsy of the rash, with chimeric levels in peripheral blood by in situ PCR (polymerase chain reaction) Clinically significant GVHD is uncommon in recipients on FK506 based immunosuppressive regimen.

Infection with or without translocation – Immunosuppressive therapy significantly increases the vulnerability of the patient to common pathogens as well as to opportunistic infections. Patients usually undergo bowel decontamination either orally or by nasogastric tube for 4 to 6 weeks postoperatively and this is restarted if sepsis, persistent rejection or the detection of pathogenic organisms in high concentrations (>106) occurs.[14] Particular attention is given to stool cultures if rejection is suspected, because bacteria and other microorganisms may translocate from the bowel lumen through the damaged mucosa to the blood. Stool microorganisms more than 106 and accompanied by fever are treated with appropriate antibiotic therapy. Blood cultures may become positive within 48 hours after the onset of fever. Immunosuppressive therapy is usually augmented when concomitant rejection is suspected clinically and documented histologically.

The most common viral infection is cytomegalovirus (CMV) and the virus can invade both the recipient tissues and intestinal allograft. Prophylactic therapy for the intestinal recipient consists of Gancyclovir for CMV, Trimethoprim Sulfamethoxazole to prevent Pneumocystic carinii pneumonia, Penicillin VK for Pneumococcus and clarithromycin to prevent atypical Mycobacterium.

Diarrhea – Diarrhea may occur after small intestinal transplantation and may be attributable to a hypersecretory phase, fat malabsorption, rapid transit time or a gut hormonal imbalance. A low fat diet may be effective particularly in patients with fat malabsorption. Surveillance stool cultures, endoscopy, and biopsy are recommended to determine the cause of diarrhea. Administration of Loperamide hydrochloride is effective in most patients to decrease the bowel transit time.

Gastrointestinal Motility Disorders – Abnormal motility of the patient's native gastrointestinal tract and intestinal allograft may occur in the early postoperative period. Disorders such as reflux esophagitis, gastric hypomotility, and pyloric spasm are frequently documented by imaging techniques. Spontaneous resolution of these disorders generally occur 4 to 8 weeks after transplantation.

Outpatient Care – Upon discharge from the hospital, patients are required to remain in the vicinity of the transplant center to be followed biweekly in the transplant clinic. Nutritional, metabolic, and biochemical assessments are performed at each visit. Medication, fluid, and dietary adjustments are instituted as needed. The patients are instructed to notify the transplant center immediately if they experi-

		CLINICAL SMALL BOWEL TRANSPLANTATION			
Pt	Age	Treatment	Diagnosis	Graft	Survival
1	5	OKT3 induction	Intestinal atresia	Liver/SB	>717
2	2	OKT3 induction	NEC	Liver/SB	39
3	0.5	OKT3 induction	Congenital abnormality of the muscularis propria	Multivisceral	44
4	32	OKT3 induction+ MMF Rescue	Crohn's disease	SB**	>578
5	33	OKT3 induction	Venous mesenteric occlusion	Multivisceral	20
6	7	OKT3 induction	Mid-gut volvulus	Liver/SB	63
7	2	Cytoxan+MMF Rescue	Hirsch sprungs disease	SB	>463
8	1	Cytoxan	NEC	Liver/SB	>457
9	2	Cytoxan+MMF Rescue	NEC	Liver/SB	>422
10	28	MMF	Gardner syndrome	Multivisceral	>383
11	34	MMF	Short Bowel 2nd to volvulus	Liver/SB	>368
12	25	MMF	Desmoid tumor	SB/LB	>231
13	47	MMF*	Crohn's disease	Liver/SB	6
14	0.5	MMF*	NEC	Multivisceral	4
15	35	MMF	Mid-gut volvulus	Liver/SB	76
16	39	MMF	Crohn's disease	Liver/SB	>140
17	16	MMF	Intestinal Pseudo-obstruction	Multivisceral	32
18	8	MMF	Megacystic microcolon	Multivisceral	>106
19	4	MMF	NEC	Multivisceral	>15

* Pts who did not receive MMF, or only on for 3 days
** Graft removed at 9.5 months for recurrent Crohn's

Table 33.2 – *Clinical small bowel transplantation at the University of Miami/Jackson Memorial Hospital (Aug 1994 to Aug 1996).*

(Ref. 22, reproduced with permission granted by Blackwell Science, Table 15.2 Transplantation, eds Ginns, Cosmi and Morris)

ence a sudden increase in stoma output, dusky stomal mucosa, abdominal pain, nausea, vomiting, or fever. Prompt evaluation of these signs and symptoms is necessary to determine the presence or absence of rejection or infection. Sepsis and rejection are the major causes of morbidity and mortality in these patients and need to be diagnosed and treated aggressively.

The University of Miami Experience

At the University of Miami Liver and GI Transplantation Program between August 1994 to August 1996, three isolated small bowel, nine combined liver-intestinal and seven multivisceral transplantations were performed. Three of the latter patients received one (n=1) or two kidneys (n=2) with the graft. The recipients were 11 children and 8 adults. The underlying disease, type of operation and outcome are shown in **Table 33.2**. Median length of follow-up was 106 days (4-717). Follow-up is provided through July 1996. All recipients of isolated grafts, five of the combined liver-intestinal recipients and three of the multivisceral recipients are alive.[10,21]

Management – All patients received or were intended to receive unmodified bone marrow infusions from the same donor. Immunosuppression was based on Tacrolimus

(FK506, Prograf) and adjunctive therapy.

Bone marrow cells were isolated from the vertebral bodies of the same cadaveric donor. Infusions of 10×10^8 cells/kg were given in either 2 or 5 divided doses.[10] Three adjunctive agents were tested: OKT3, Cyclophosphamide and MMF. OKT3 was given in the first six patients immediately post-operatively and continued for 10 days at a dose of 2.5 mg/d intravenously for the children and 5.0 mg/d intravenously in the adult patients, although in one patient it was stopped after day 6 due to fever, leukocytosis, and an infection found in the explanted liver and intestine. Patient survival was 33.3% (2/6). Mortalities were due to infectious complications: aorto-intestinal fistula (n=1), intestinal perforation and MSOF (1), pancreatitis, intra-abdominal sepsis and MSOF (1), and disseminated aspergillosis (1). OKT3 induction was discontinued. Of the surviving patients one was converted to MMF therapy, and later had her intestinal graft removed due to an apparent recurrence of Crohn's disease.

In the next 3 patients Cyclophosphamide (1 mg/kg/d IV for 10d) was used (in place of OKT3). In one patient Cyclophosphamide was stopped after 12 days due to rejection requiring OKT3 treatment. The patient was later treated with MMF due to persistent rejection. A second patient received Cyclophosphamide for 8 days. Cyclophosphamide was then discontinued due to fever and leukocytopenia. The third patient received Cyclophosphamide for approximately 3 months, received OKT3 treatment for severe rejection, and was eventually converted to MMF. All patients are alive. The last 10 patients received MMF at the time of transplant in addition to Tacrolimus and steroids. Two of the patients, on life support at the time of transplantation, died within 1 week post transplant. One did not receive MMF at all, the other received it for only 3 days. Both patients died of MSOF, in one case due to deterioration of the general condition, and in the second due to diffuse abdominal sepsis which originated from an enterococcal infection in her native spleen.

Of the remaining 8 patients 6 patients are alive and 2 died. Patient survival was 75% (6/8). The 2 mortalities resulted from a failure in the immunosuppressive regimen, which led to severe rejection in both patients. One patient was treated with multiple boluses of Solumedrol, the other patient received OKT3 and was converted to Cyclophos-phamide. This aggressive treatment caused fatal infections leading to sepsis and MSOF in both patients (POD# 76 & 32). The remaining six patients are currently maintained on MMF. 3 patients were treated with MMF as a rescue agent. One patient who had received OKT3 induction, and 2 patients received Cyclophosphamide.

All patients are alive and have not experienced rejections or viral infections since being placed on MMF. The incidence of rejection was lower in the OKT3 induction patients, however it was also associated with a higher mortality rate. All patients who are alive have well functioning grafts except one whose graft was removed. All 10 are maintained solely on enteral nutrition and receive no parenteral treatment whatsoever. Seven have resumed normal daily activities and three are in the process of complete rehabilitation. OKT3 induction and addition of Cyclophosphamide did not appear to be beneficial in our experience. MMF appears to be an effective adjunct immunosuppressive agent. Due to short follow up and small number of cases our results should not be considered conclusive. The combination of MMF with steroids and Tacrolimus (FK 506) for synergistic effect should be used with caution.[1]

In conclusion, intestinal transplantation can serve as a life saving procedure in the treatment of intestinal failure. The successful patients have undergone excellent rehabilitation. Rejection remains a serious problem. Improvements in immunosuppression with combination of new immunosuppressive agents are under investigation.

ACKNOWLEDGEMENT

We would like to thank the following people for their help in the preparation of this paper: Jennie Benson, Pauline Bethel and Joshua Phipps.

REFERENCES

1. Lillehei RC, Goat B, Miller FA. The physiologic response of the small bowel of the dog to ischemia including prolonged in-vitro preservation of the bowel with successful replacement and survival. *Ann Surg* 1959; **850:**543-560.
2. Cohen Z, Wassef R. In: *Surgery of the Small Intestine*. Nelson, R., Nyhus, L., (eds). Appleton-Century-Crofts, East Norwalk, 1985.
3. Todo S, Tzakis AG, Abu-Elmagd K, Reyes J, Furukawa H., Casavilla A., Selby R, Nour BM, Wright H, Fung JJ, *et al.,* Intestinal transplantation in composite visceral grafts or alone. *Ann Surg* 1992; **216(3):** 223-23.

4. Starzl TE, Todo S, Tzakis A.. Multivisceral and intestinal transplantation. *Trans Proc* 1992; **24(3):** 1217-1223.
5. Goulet O, Revillon D, Jan D, Brousse JN, DePotter S, Cerf-Bensussan N, Rambaud C, Buisson C, Perllerin D, Mougenot JF, *et al.* Small bowel transplantation in children. *Trans Proc* 1990; **22(6):**2499-2500.
6. Deltz E., Schroeder P, Gebhardt H, Gundlach, M., Timmermann, W., Engemann R, Leimenstoll G, Hansman ML, Westphal E, Hammellman H. Successful clinical small bowel transplantation: Report of a case. *Clin Trans* 1989; **3:**89-91.
7. Margreiter R, Konigsrainer A., Schmid T, Koller J, Kornberger R, Oberhuber G, and Furtwangler W. Successful multivisceral transplantation. *Trans Proc* 1992;**24:**1226-1227.
8. Starzl TE, Rowe M, Todo S, Tzakis A. Transplantation of multiple abdominal viscera. *JAMA* 1989; **261:** 1449-1457.
9. Grant D, Wall W, Mimeanlt R. Successful small bowel/liver transplantation. *Lancet* 1990; **335:**181-184.
10. Ingham Clark CL, Wood S, Lennard-Jones JE, Lear PA, Wood RFM. Small bowel transplantation candidates in the United Kingdom. *Trans Proc* 1992; **24(3):**1060-1061.
11. Dudrick SJ, Wilmore DW, Vars HM. Long term total parenteral nutrition with growth, development and positive nitrogen balance. *Surgery* 1968; **169:**134-142.
12. Edes T. Clinical management of short bowel syndrome. *Post Grad Med* **88:** 4, 1990.
13. Grosfeld V, Rescorla F, West K. Short bowel syndrome in infancy and childhood. *Am J Surg* 1986;**151:** 41-46.
14. Lennard-Jones JE. Indications and need for long-term parenteral nutrition: Implications for intestinal transplantation. *Trans Proc* 1990; **22:6:** 2427-2429.
15. Wood R. International symposium on small bowel transplantation. *Trans Proc* 1990; **22:6:** 2423-2426.
16. Starzl TE, Todo, S, Tzakis A. The many faces of multivisceral transplantation. *Surg Gyn Obst* 1991;**172:** 335-344.
17. Starzl TE, Miller C, Broznick B, Makowka, L. An improved technique for multiple organ harvesting. *Surg Gyn & Obst* 1987;**165:**343-348.
18. Staschak-Chicko S, Zamberlan K, Thomson AW. An overview of FK-506 in transplantation and autoimmune disease. *Dialysis and Transplant* 1992; **21:**8.
19. Grant D, Garcia B, Wall W. *et al*. Graft-versus-host disease after clinical small bowel/liver transplantation. *Trans Proc* 1990; **22:**2464.
20. Reyes J, Abu-Elmagd K, Tzakis A *et al*. Infectious complications after human small bowel transplantation. *Trans Proc* 1992;**26:**3.
21. Tzakis A.,Webb M., Nery J *et al*. Experience with clinical intestinal transplantation at the University of Miami. *Trans Proc* 1996; **28:** 2748-2749.
22. Khan FA, Thompson J, Webb M, Nery JR, Olson L, Viciana *et al*. Intestinal and multivisceral transplantation. In: Transplantation. Boston: Blackwell Science (In press)

TECHNIQUES IN
LIVER SURGERY

APPENDIX

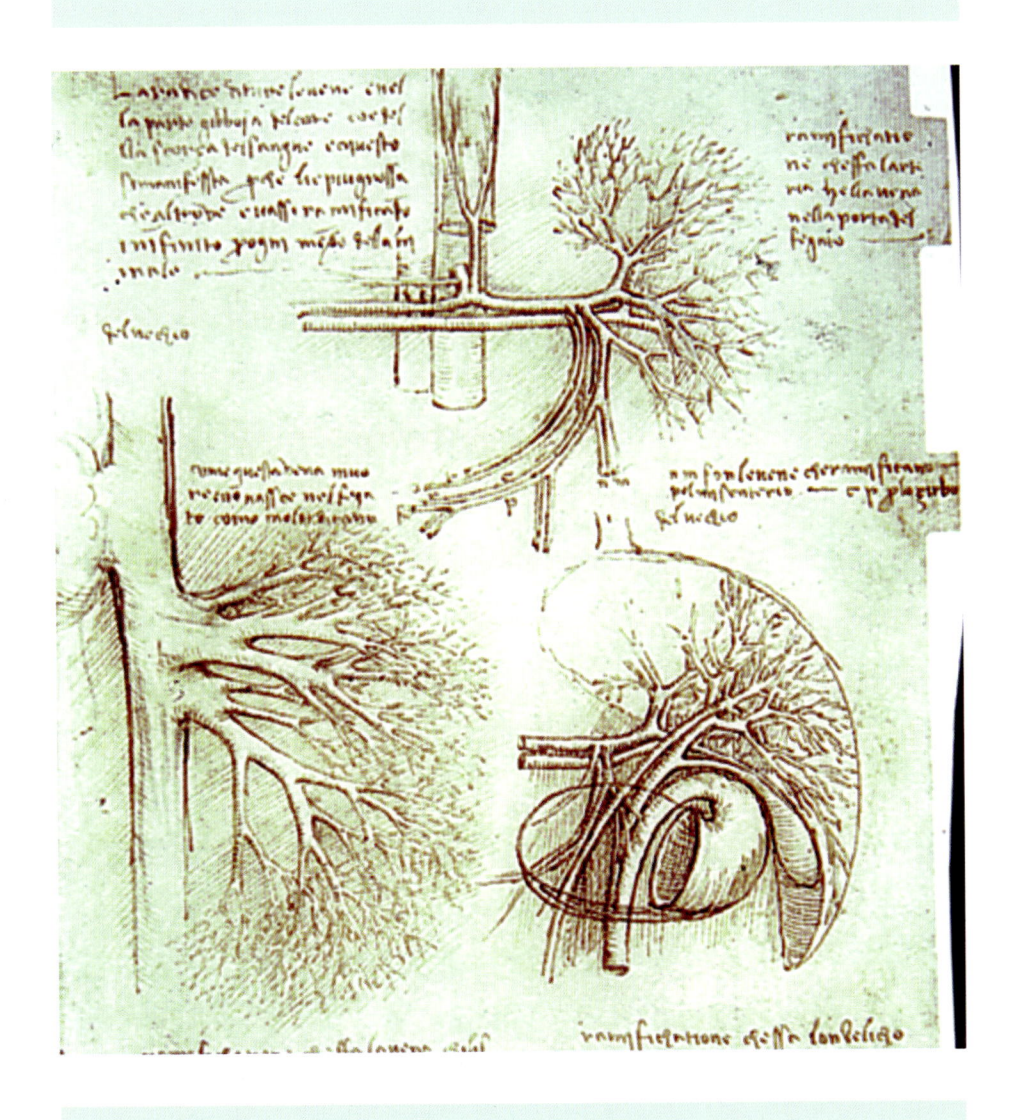

A Delayed Revolution: A History of Liver Surgery

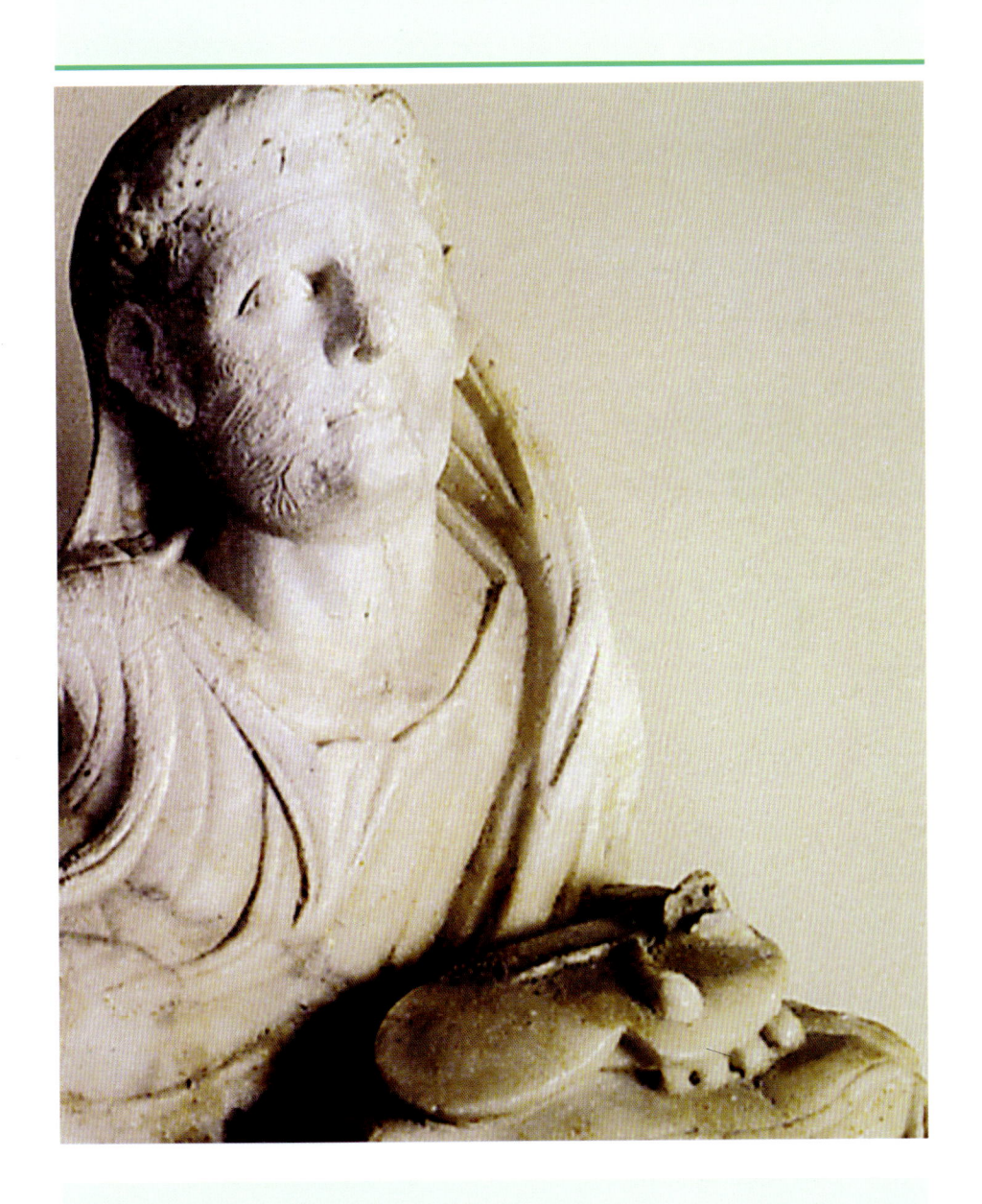

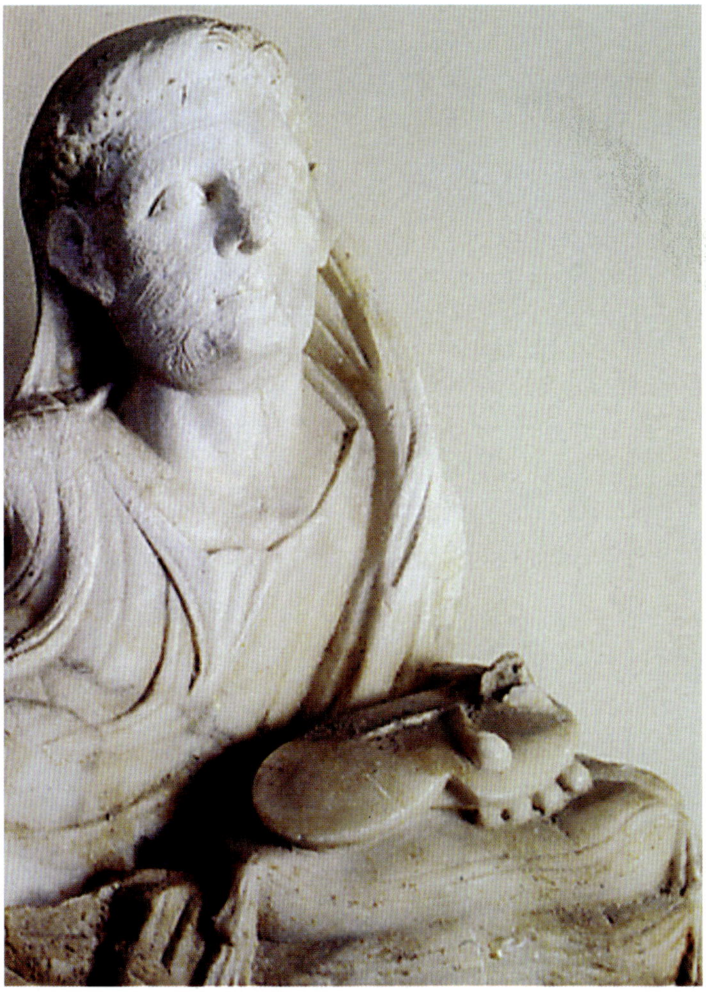

A DELAYED REVOLUTION: A HISTORY OF LIVER SURGERY

Figure A.1 – *An Etruscan funerary urn of a soothsayer holding a liver in his left hand – second century B.C. (Guarnacci Museum, Volterra.)*

Modern liver surgery has a very recent history compared to other branches of surgery which have evolved gradually, achieving technical standardisation and worldwide adoption many decades earlier. The modern era of liver surgery dates back just 40 years, when intra-hepatic segmentary anatomy was classified. Progress from pioneer to the routine surgery is even more recent, corresponding to the advent of ultrasound and the perfection of radiological diagnostics at the beginning of the 1980s. Since then, the increasing number of liver transplants performed has led to an evolution in the expertise of surgical and anesthesiological teams. This, in turn, has had a noticeable effect on resective liver surgery with improvements in intra- and post-operative techniques and care. Resective surgery and transplantation are closely linked, and generally practised by the same teams and liver units which have come into being to provide high quality outcomes in an increasingly complex branch of surgery. Today, specific problems connected with liver surgery in the broadest sense of the term (including major surgery of the biliary system and pancreas) require surgeons to update their knowledge continually, to the point where, we believe, it should be considered a new speciality.

Yet, looking back at the history of surgery, the low level of understanding of the liver lasted for a surprising length of time in relation to other organs or systems, such as the heart, urinary and gastroenteric tracts and lungs.

In ancient times, the liver aroused the curiosity of doctors, philosophers and even poets, but for centuries the perception of the liver in the history of medicine was confined to myth. Its central position in the body, its size and richness of blood, led to the liver being considered a noble organ, used in animal sacrifices to predict the future by the Assyrians, Babylonians, Greeks and the Etruscans (***Figure. A.1***). Several centuries before Roman

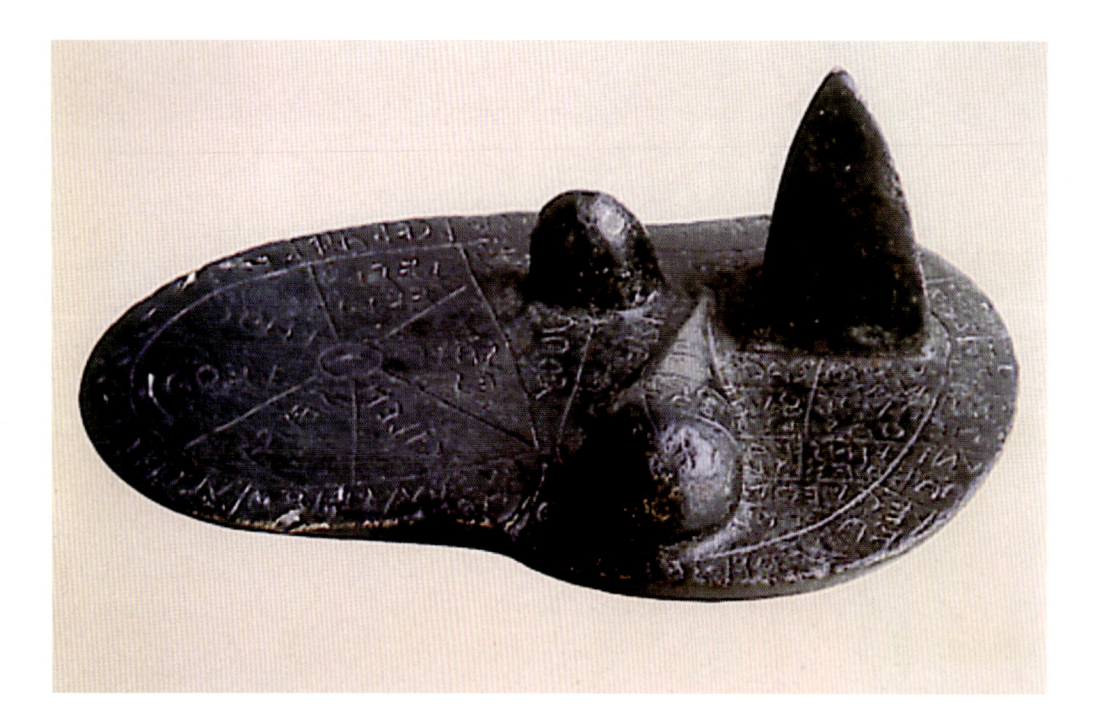

Figure A.2 – *Etruscan liver of Piacenza (Civic Museum, Piacenza).*

civilization, the Etruscans classified the macroscopic anatomy of a lamb's liver, which is very similar to that of man. The mysterious inscriptions on the famous Piacenza Liver (**Figure. A.2**) were a kind of manual for 'trainee' soothsayers.

At this time the legend of Prometheus was born. He dared to steal fire from the forge of Hephaestus to give to man and the merciless Zeus decided to make an example of him. He was bound to a rock in the Caucasus mountains, where every day an eagle came to devour his liver, which then regrew during the night.

The gods also punished other mortals by decreeing that their liver be devoured during the day by eagles or vultures, certain that it would regenerate during the night.

From the age of myths to early medicine in Greece, Hippocrates and Galen had guessed the importance of the liver in digestion and the relationship between liver disease and neuro-psychical manifestations. Hippocrates describes the incision of abscesses on the liver (gallbladder empyema, amebic abscesses?) with cautery or knife, and Galen's extensive description of the anatomy of the human and animal liver dominated medical thought without opposition for 14 centuries afterwards.

In the 1st century A.D. the Alessandrian school handed down, through the books of Celsus, the descriptions of a number of attempts to treat penetrating wounds of the liver, a common occurence given the hand-to-hand combat of the time. Almost all these wounds then proved fatal, giving the liver an age-old reputation as an untouchable organ.

Little progress was made in medicine during the Dark Ages but with the dawning of the Middle Ages around the year 1000, a revival of interest was characterised on a cultural level by the birth of the first free universities, Bologna in 1088 followed by Pavia, Montpellier and Paris. It was in Bologna that anatomical studies began to flourish again at this time thanks to Mondino dei Liuzzi, who repudiated many of the assertions handed down by Galen. But Mondino never mentions the liver in his work. since progress in surgery was still restricted by ecclesiastical dogma and prejudice. Under the papacy of Alexander III, the Council of Tours in 1169 definitively condemned surgical practices with the famous edict "Ecclesia aborret a sanguine" declaring that the Church restricted the performance of any type of surgical practice. Surgeons were almost rejected by official medicine and treated as inferior to practitioners of general medicine. Surgery was

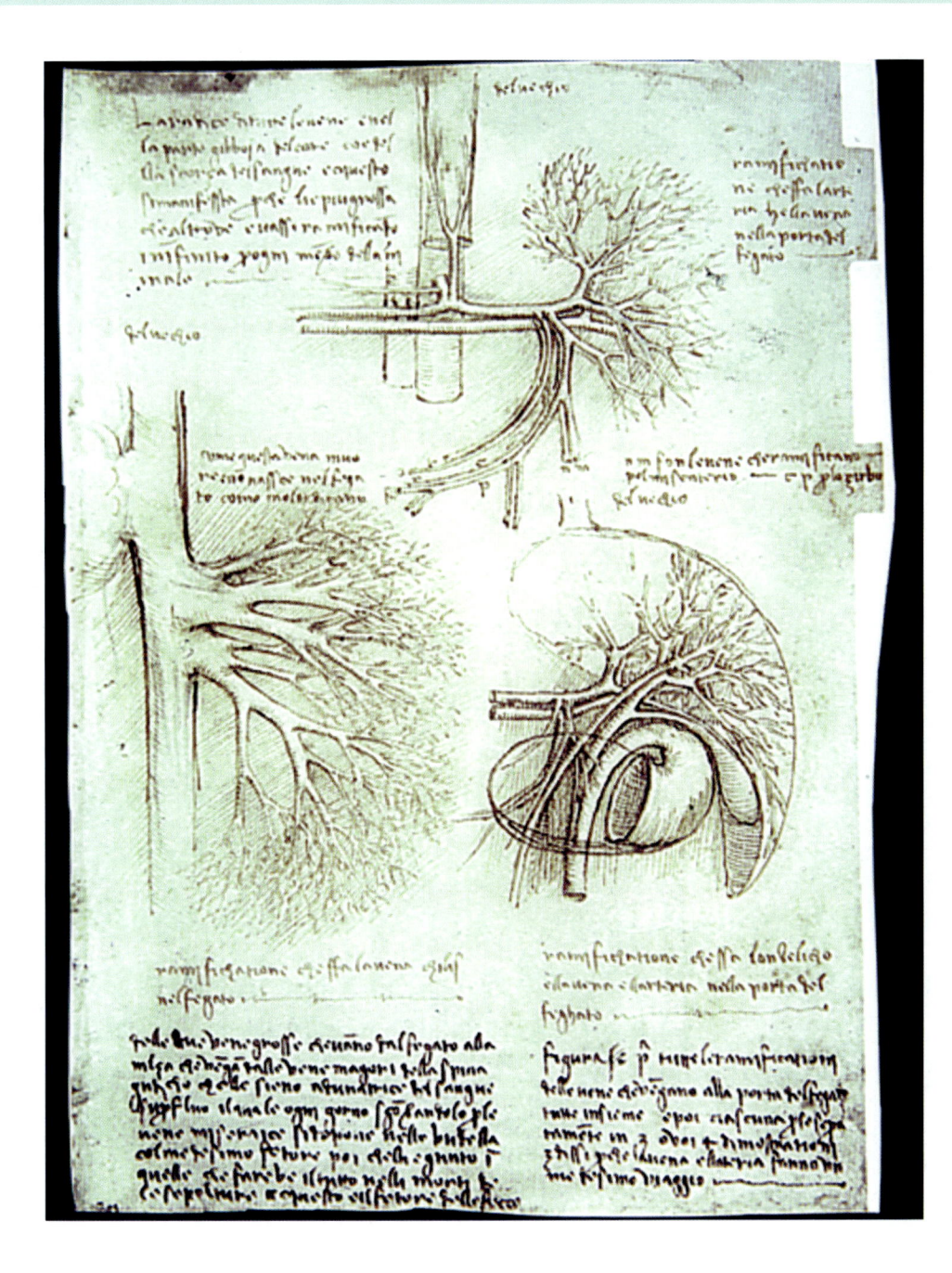

Figure A.3 –
Liver anatomy by Leonardo (from "Quaderni di Anatomia", 1517).

neglected in universities and for centuries it was left to esteemed barbers to incise abscesses and amputate limbs, the only practicable surgical gestures. It was probably a barber who in 1474 performed what the French claim as the first operation for gallstones, in the cloisters of the church of St. Séverin in Paris. Louis XI offered to spare the life of an archer condemned to death if he agreed to be operated on and survived – as indeed he seems to have done.

The flowering of the arts in the Renaissance was accompanied by an awakening of interest in surgery, associated with fundamental changes in the study of human anatomy. At the end of the 15th century, Pope Clement VII finally approved the right to study the human body, removing all hindrances to dissections or autopsies. The first to take advantage of this was that restless genius who had already explored so many other sectors of knowledge, Leonardo da Vinci, who left us with the most artistic images of human and comparative anatomy ever produced, in the Hammer Codex and his Treatise on Anatomy. Many centuries after Galen, Leonardo turned his interest to the liver. The acute observation of his work is illustrated, (**Figure A.3**) in which you can see the division of the afferent pedicles in the two hemilivers, the arrangement of the bile ducts which run together to the portal and arterial pedicles, and the system of hepatic veins. Unfortunately, as he tells us, after having dissected "more than 100 corpses" with

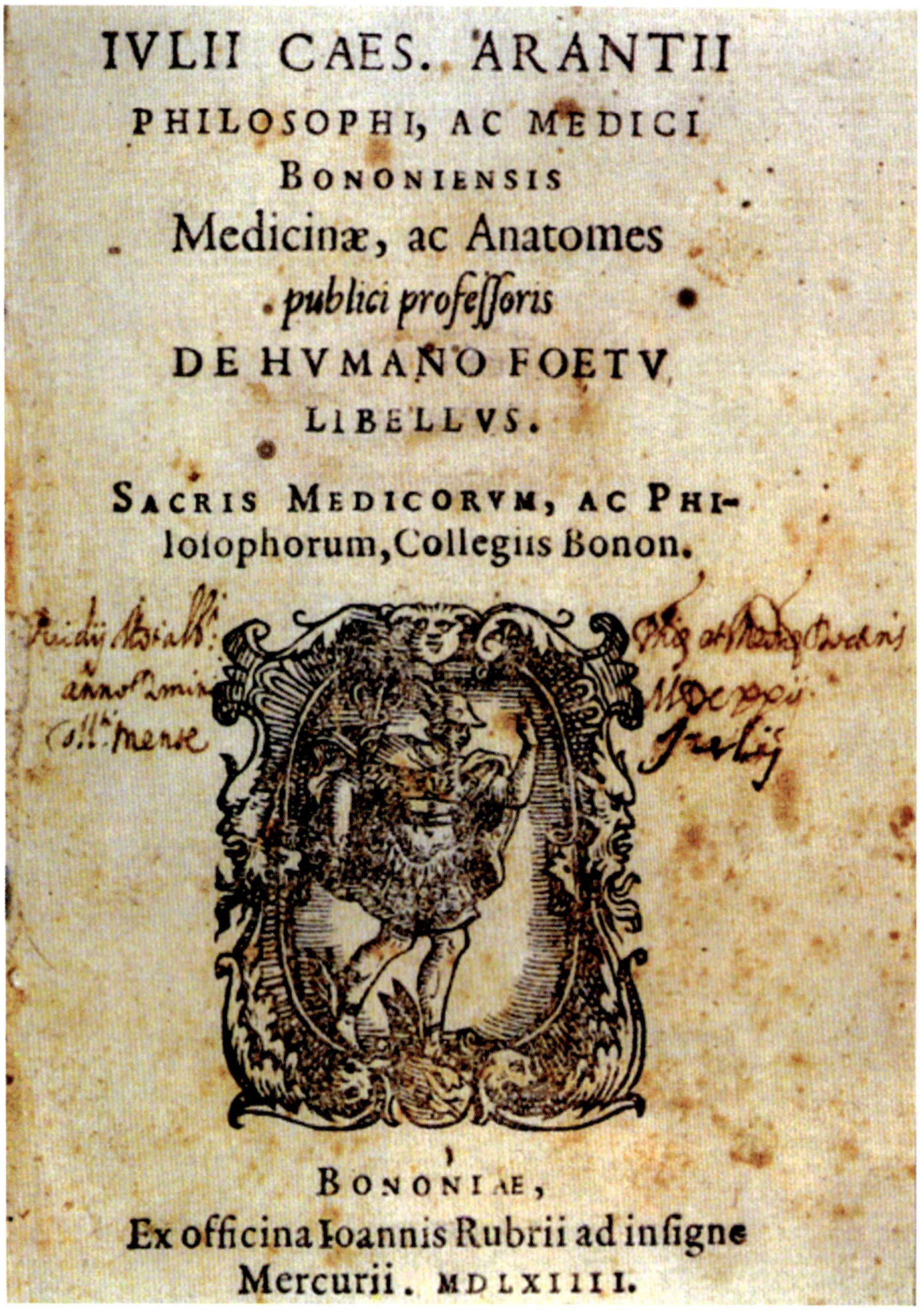
IVLII CAES. ARANTII
PHILOSOPHI, AC MEDICI
BONONIENSIS
Medicinæ, ac Anatomes
publici profeſſoris
DE HVMANO FOETV
LIBELLVS.
SACRIS MEDICORVM, AC PHI-
loſophorum, Collegiis Bonon.
BONONIAE,
Ex officina Ioannis Rubrii ad inſigne
Mercurii. MDLXIIII.

Figure A.4 – *Frontispieces of the book "De Humano Foetu" by Aranzio, published in Bologna in 1564.*

a tenacity worthy of a modern investigator, Leonardo was distracted by other interests. Another more systematic and persistent figure was Andreas Vesalio. A young wanderer (born in Brussels, a student in Montpellier and Paris, professor of anatomy in Padua, and finally, court doctor in Madrid to the melancholy of Carlos V and Felipe II), Vesalio definitively refuted Galen's errors and can be considered as the father of modern anatomy.

More practical and pragmatic than Vesalio, his contemporary, Ambroise Paré was the first to treat liver injury. Paré, inspired by his motto *"I treated him, God cured him"*, had a reputation for competance and self-belief that made him famous throughout Europe, even though it was not enough to heal his king, Henri II d'Orleans, who summoned him to his bedside after being fatally wounded during a tournament. In the mid 16th century Bologna, Giulio Cesare Aranzio studied the anatomy of the human fetus (***Figure A.4***), linking his name to Arantius's duct and the venous ligament which runs from the left branch of the portal vein to the vena cava. At the beginning of the 17th century Adrian van der Spieghel, also known as Spigelius, born in Brussels and professor at Padua, described the anatomy of the caudate lobe, 'lobus exiguus', subsequently also known as the Spigel lobe.

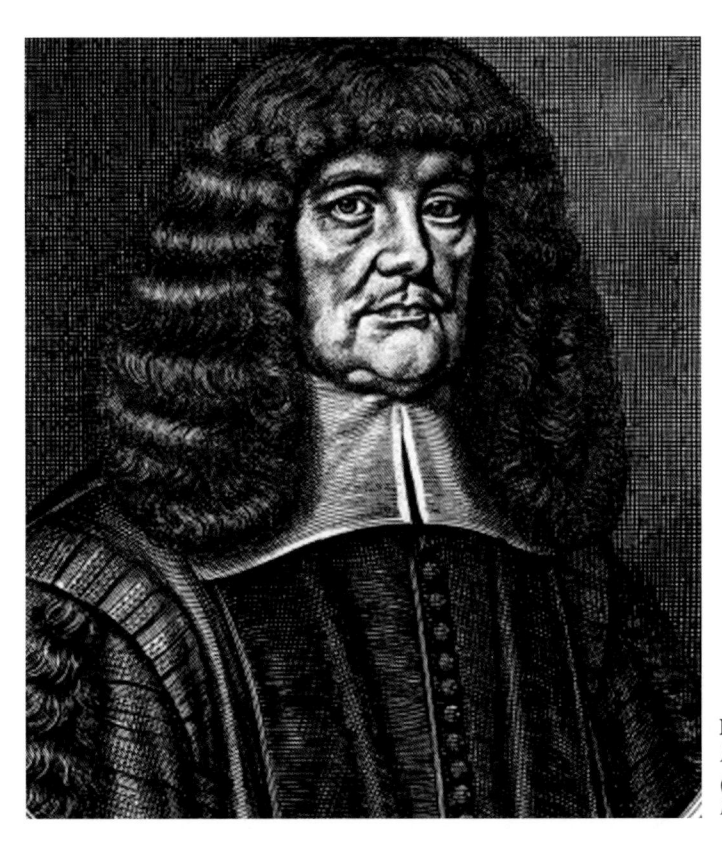

Figure A.5 – *Francis Glisson (Courtesy of the Wellcome Institute Library, London).*

Quod mihi argumento eſt, vaſa fellea nonnunquam alium humorem (ſi forte obvenerit) præter bilem, in inteſtina deferre: arbitrorque, læſo ex contuſione aliqua hepate, ſequi poſſe, per vomitum aut alvum, ſanguinis ejectionem; quod nimirum porus bilarius (magno ægri commodo) partem aliquam ſanguinis hepar opprimentis in ſe recipiat, & ad inteſtina deducat; unde vel motu periſtatico inverſo, ſurſum; vel eodem regulariter ſe habente, deorſum feratur.

Figure A.6 – *Description of post-traumatic hemobilia from "Anatomia Hepatis" by Glisson*

Not until a century later, however, do we find the anatomy of the liver and many aspects of hepatic disease described on a systematic basis, by that most fortunate of classical anatomists, still frequently quoted to this day by all liver surgeons, Francis Glisson of Cambridge (***Figure A.5***). Effectively, Glisson's *Anatomia Hepatis*, published in 1654, laid the foundations for modern liver surgery. Glisson studied the liver and intra-hepatic circulation for many years. He, quite literally 'cooked' several human livers, enabling him to patiently remove the parenchyma from the vessels which he injected with coloured fluid to study the flow of blood. Anatomy provided him with an explanation for a number of physiopathological events, as can be seen from this extract, excellent for its precision, referring to the pathogenesis of post-traumatic hemobilia (***Figure A.6***). Although the writer's knowledge of Latin is somewhat scanty, the translations read roughly as follows, '*I believe that if the liver is injured by a contusion, it may lead to blood leaving the body by way of vomit or the stool; for there is no doubt that the biliary duct takes unto itself (to the great good of the patient) some of the blood issuing into the liver and leads it down to the intestines; from there it is either impelled upwards through reverse peristalsis or downwards the usual way*'.

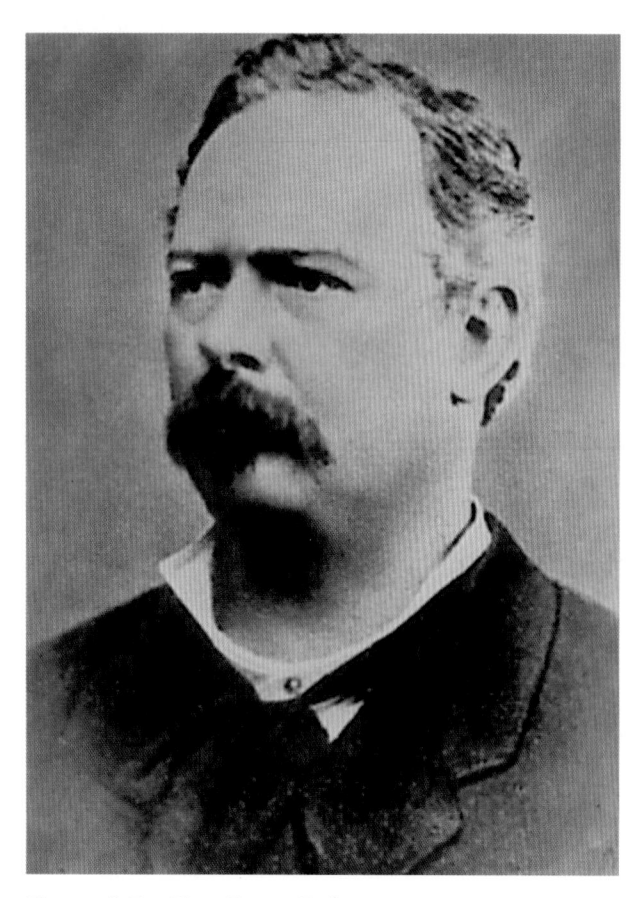

Figure A.7 – *Pietro Loreta. Professor of Surgery at the University of Bologna*

ECHINOCOCCO DEL FEGATO

RESEZIONE DEL FEGATO

ESCISIONE DELLA CISTI

GUARIGIONE

MEMORIA

DEL PROFESSOR PIETRO LORETA

BOLOGNA

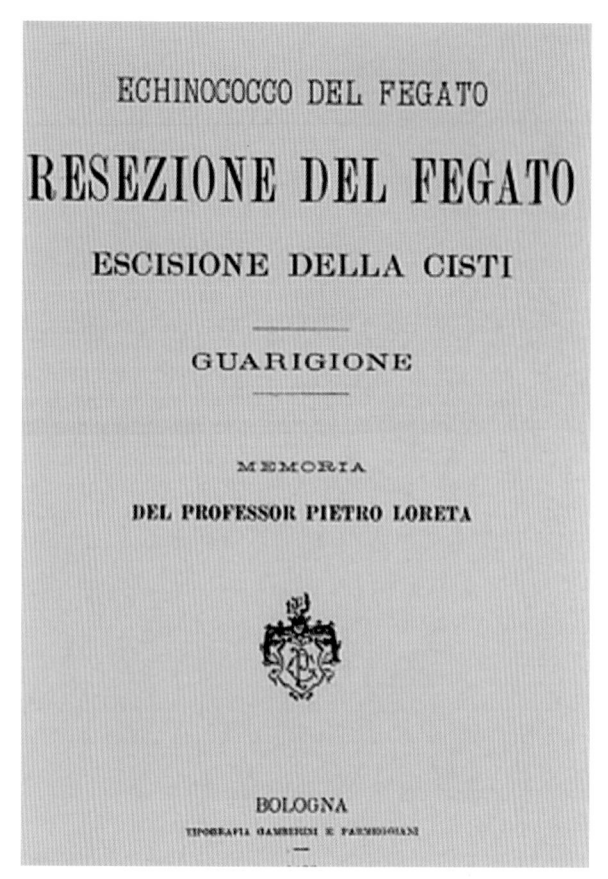

Figure A.8 – *First description of a left lobectomy for a hydatid cyst by Loreta in 1888*

From the two centuries which followed, we have only occasional descriptions of operations carried out for traumatic lesions of the liver, almost always with fatal results. But with every war the level of expertise increased, and in the Franco-Prussian war of 1870, a soldier was operated on for a liver wound by Victor von Bruns, and acutually survived.

The last two decades of the 19th century made a great contribution to the history of liver surgery. In 1888 Langenbuch, 6 years after having completed the first operation for removal of the gallbladder, described the resection of a liver tumor. In the same year, in Bologna, Loreta (***Figure A.7***) operated successfully on a hydatid cyst of the liver, removing part of the left lobe (***Figure A.8***), and Codivilla performed the first duodenopancreatectomy. Other resections were carried out by Postemsky, again in Italy, Burkardt and Vollbrecht in Germany, and in the United States by Keen, who was the first to talk of the finger fracture technique. The introduction of anaesthesia (1846) and antisepsis (1865) laid the foundations for this first revolution in the history of liver surgery. At the same time, the first experimental studies began into liver regeneration and the role of portal blood. Finally, the ancient myth of Prometheus was, in one sense at least, substantiated when Ponfick and later Tillmanns demonstrated that in experimental animals the liver regrew after resection. In Russia in 1877 Nicolai Vladimirovich Eck carried out portacaval anastomosis on 8 dogs. Although 7 of these died, and only 1 survived more than 7 days, (this dog did however manage to escape from the laboratory, so avoiding follow-up). Eck's fistula provided the foundation for physiopathological studies of the portal system and surgery of portal hypertension. At the end of the 19th century, thanks to Rex in Germany and Cantlie in England, there was another resurgence of anatomical studies, which had become completely neglected after the work of Glisson. The former gave his name to the recess in the left branch of the portal vein, and the latter established that the division of the two hemilivers was different from that of the two hepatic lobes and occurred along a constant gallbladder – vena cava plane, which became known as the Cantlie line.

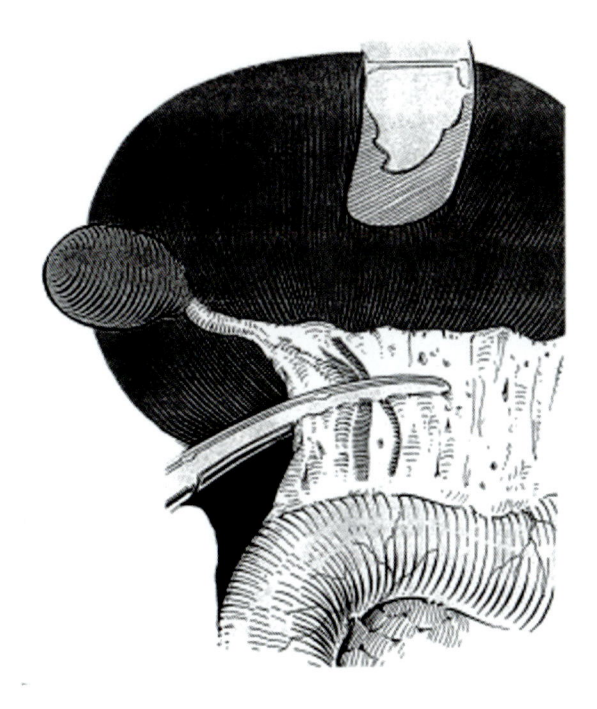

Figure A.9 –
Pringle maneuver

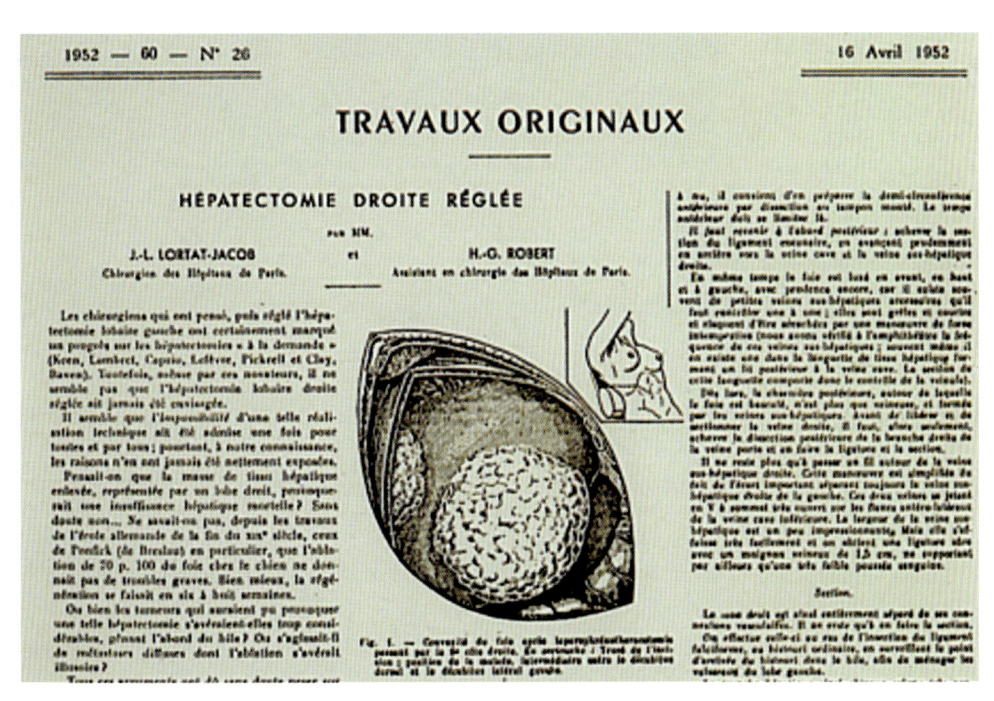

Figure A.10 –
Lortat-Jacob's first paper on right hepatectomy 'reglée' in 1952

At this time the inevitability of parenchymal hemorrhage prevented surgeons from successfully removing liver tumors or treating traumatic wounds of the liver. It was precisely to arrest hemorrhage that the Glaswegian, Hogarth Pringle at the beginning of the 1900s closed the hepatic pedicle by squeezing it between the finger and thumb, the '*Pringle pinch*'. Pringle's patients were unlucky (all 8 bled to death), but Pringle entered triumphantly into the history of surgery and his maneuver, (**Figure A.9**), is carried out every day by at least one surgeon somewhere in the world.

The modern era of liver surgery began in the 1950s, preceded by Couinaud's fundamental anatomical studies, classifying liver segmentation. In 1952, Lortat-Jacob in Paris carried out the first right 'reglée' hepatectomy (**Figure A.10**). The same type of operation with preliminary ligature of the vascular pedicles was carried out on the left lobe by Caprio in Spain, Pettinari in Italy, Honjo in Japan and Quattlebaum (father and son) in the USA. Lin in Taiwan and Longmire in the USA proposed use of special clamps to stop hemorrhage during resection. Until the 1970s, however,

Figure A.11 – *Thomas Starzl*

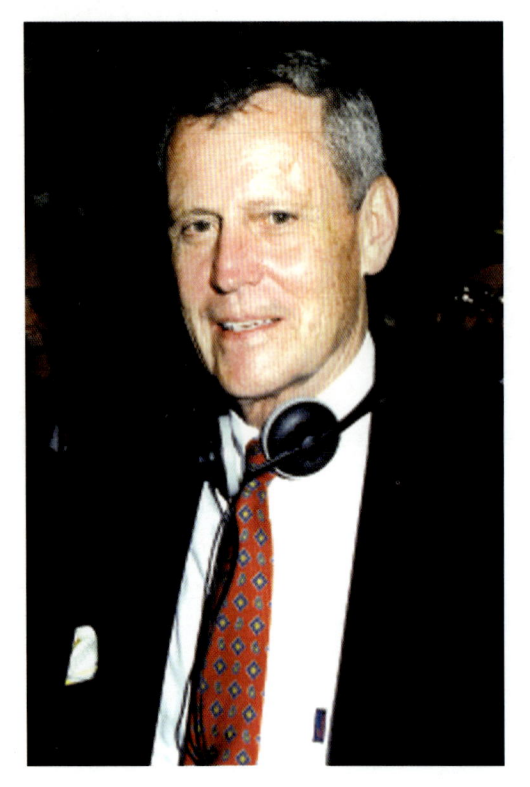

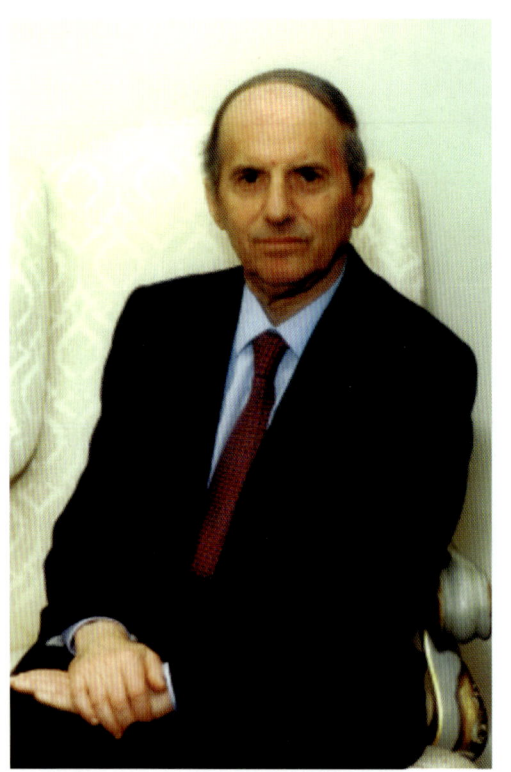

Figure A.12 – *Giuseppe Gozzetti*

liver surgery was restricted to very few centres and each operation was a challenge to the surgeon and a serious threat to the life of the patient, since post-operative mortality following liver resection was over 20%.

Liver surgery really came into its own in the early 1980s, after the introduction of ultrasound and other methods of radiographic diagnosis. Thanks to ultrasound, sub-clinical lesions readily susceptible to surgery could be detected, and this greatly increased the demand for liver surgery. The development of X-ray diagnostics, leading to ever more precise indications, also made a major contribution to improving the long term results of a type of surgery previously considered dangerous, problematical and largely disappointing. Operations on the liver multiplied, first in the East through the impetus of Tôn Thât Tùng, and then throughout the Western world. In Europe, the great impetus in liver surgery came from Stig Bengmark, Leslie Blumgart and Henri Bismuth, who were the first to stress that the results of this type of surgery were better when performed in liver units. An important contribution came from the studies of Huguet who demonstrated the liver's tolerance to ischemia and standardised the procedure for total vascular exclusion of the liver. On a technical level, we also owe a great deal to Japanese surgeons who were responsible for standardising segmentectomies, the use of ultrasound during operations, (Makuuchi) and the introduction of pre-operative portal embolisation.

Again at the beginning of the eighties, a decisive step forward came from the development of liver transplants, thanks to the introduction of cyclosporin (Calne) and other anti-reject agents. Stimulated by the results of Starzl in Pittsburgh (**Figure A.11**), may transplant centres were set up throughout the developed world. The work of Starzl in this field continues to be decisive. After dealing with all the technical problems, Starzl turned his attention to immune tolerance, xenografts and chimerism, laying the foundations for new lines of research. Many surgeons from around the world have spent time in his department before starting their own activities, including the present author, and all scientific papers on transplants refer to at least one of his publications.

Resection and transplantation are inextricably bound together, one contributing to the experience of the other. Transplants improve the skills of the surgical and anaesthesiology teams in areas such as vascular exclusion of the liver , intra- and post-operative care and ex-vivo surgical techniques Resection techniques have become part of the transplantation technique with the procedures of reduced size livers (Bismuth and Houssin), split livers (Pichlmayr and Bismuth) and transplants from living donors (Broelsch). Today, there is an increasing tendency to carry out both types, liver resection and transplantation, with their similar bases and common problems, in the same center and at the same time, to concentrate on surgery involving structures which for anatomical, technical and physiopathological reasons are closely associated with the liver, bile ducts and pancreas. The expertise gained in this type of surgery brings with it a host of problems which now make liver surgery a specialty in its own right. Hepato-Bilio-Pancreatic surgery, should now be considered on a par with other established surgical specialties, such as urology and thoracic, cardio-vascular and plastic surgery, to mention just a few, with its own rules which evolve and oblige surgeons to continually update their knowledge. As well as having demonstrated his skills in all fields of general surgery, Professor Gozzetti of Bologna *(Figure A12)* was one of the first champions of the need for this transformation in liver surgery, a transformation which he was deeply involved in over the last 20 years, making a contribution through his own work. Today the hepato-biliary surgeon must work in tandem with the imaging radiologist, the operating-room radiologist and endoscopist, the oncologist and the gastroenterologist. He must represent a meeting and coordination point for the various disciplines to ensure the rational and coherent treatment of patients.

Index

A

Aberrant arteries, 207, 273

Abscesses, 30, 66, 138-139, 185, 188, 235, 299, 303, 354-355

Accessory artery, 207, 260

Accessory hepatic vein, 29

Adenomas, 114, 160, 108, 242, 259, 265, 331

Albendazole, 179, 189

ALT, 327, 330, 334

Aminopyrine breath test, 143

Anatomical;
  anomalies, 310, 313
  variations, 25, 49, 56, 63, 66, 87, 105-106, 206-208, 253, 260, 289, 309-310, 313
  of the hepatic artery, 206-208, 253, 310

Angiomas, 160

Antifibrinolytic, 289

Aprotinin, 138, 246

Arantius;
  duct, 103, 356
  ligament, 90, 320

Argon;
  beam, 28, 138, 140, 194, 316

Arterial;
  anastomosis, 151, 270, 272, 289, 291, 303
  branches, 5, 52, 56-57, 62, 74, 87, 108, 198, 231, 312, 321, 324
  graft, 273, 290, 304
  hypoplasia, 289

Ascites, 72, 76, 139, 144, 174-175, 299, 330

Ascitic fistulae, 139-140

Auxiliary liver transplantation, 325, 327, 329-336

Axillary vein, 132, 263, 267

Azathioprine, 323, 334, 343

B

Back table procedure, 259

Bare area, 20, 63, 108, 267, 331

Bench reconstruction, 259,

Benign tumors, 50, 114, 160-161, 339

Bilateral subcostal incision, 35, 73, 263-264, 331

Bile ducts, 5, 8, 25, 41, 56, 61, 68, 106-107, 137, 161-162, 173, 179-180, 183, 188-189, 198, 205, 210, 217-219, 222, 233, 313, 355, 361

Biliary;
  complications, 30, 303-304, 315
  confluence, 106-108, 196, 213, 220, 223, 225-226, 228, 232-233
  decompression, 219
  drainage, 106, 139-140, 219-221, 227, 229, 330
  fistulae, 28, 30, 41, 138-140, 179, 185, 187-189, 194, 304
  leakage, 30-31, 66, 76, 84, 108, 139, 183, 198, 220, 299, 303, 332
  reconstruction in liver transplantation, 273

Bilio-enteric anastomosis, 166, 189, 289

Biliostasis, 28, 99, 138-139, 185

Bio-pump, 121, 263, 267, 299

Biological glues, 138, 310, 316

Bone marrow infusions, 339, 343, 346

Budd-Chiari syndrome, 106

Bypass circuit, 263

C

Calot's triangle, 22

Cantlie line, 5, 38, 50, 107, 196, 227, 311, 358

Capsular rupture of the graft, 296

Carcino Embryogenic Antigen, 205

Carcinoma of the biliary tract, 217, 233

Carrel's patch, 259-260, 265, 270, 273, 341

Caudate;
  lobe, 5, 8, 22, 25, 29-30, 35-38, 41, 87, 90, 99, 101, 103-109, 111, 113-115, 119-120, 127, 161, 166, 185, 267, 279-280, 284, 286, 311, 313, 315, 321, 331-333, 356
  lobe vascularization, 105
  process, 20, 87, 103, 105, 114-115

Caustic sclerosing cholangitis, 189

Cavoportal transposition, 299

CEA, 205

Central;
  liver resection, 93, 95-97, 99
  venous pressure, 29, 31, 66, 74, 270, 328

Child-Pugh, 72, 143, 246
  classification, 72, 143

Cholangiocarcinoma, 106-108, 115, 161-162, 166-167, 215, 217, 219, 221, 223, 225, 227, 229, 231-233, 235

Cholangiography, 28, 30, 37, 41, 66, 84, 90, 99, 139, 156, 183, 188, 220-222, 225, 232, 273, 302-303, 313, 321

Cholangiojejunal anastomosis, 227

Cirrhosis, 20, 30, 50, 56, 68, 71-72, 77, 95, 114, 143, 147, 153-155, 159, 161, 165, 246, 299, 323, 327, 335

Clamping;
  of the hepatic pedicle, 29-30, 39, 50, 74, 89, 108, 115, 119, 144, 147, 195, 197, 332
  of the vena cava, 29, 127, 289, 321
  test, 121, 123, 208, 244, 284

Compensatory hypertrophy, 50, 81, 106, 165

Confluence of the bile ducts, 217-219, 222, 233

Couinaud's classification, 6, 8, 19, 45, 49

Cyanocrylate, 138, 165

Cyclophosphamide, 343, 347

Cyclosporin, 323, 360

Cysts, 12-13, 45, 137, 139, 161, 169, 171, 173-176, 179, 181-182, 185-190

D

Dacron mesh, 297

Damage to the biliary tract, 30

Diabetes mellitus, 72

Diaphragm, 13-14, 19, 21, 119-120, 174, 180, 182, 187, 193, 208, 241-242, 244, 253-256, 259, 265, 267, 299, 309, 332-333, 341

Diaphragmatic resection, 13

Dislocation of TIPS, 297

Donor iliac artery conduit, 289

Doppler, 30, 76, 151, 246, 292-294, 303, 321, 323-324, 334

Dorsal ligament, 12, 20-22, 25, 29, 103-104, 107-108, 114, 122, 278

Drainage, 14, 30, 51, 56, 66, 76, 106, 138-140, 174, 179, 183, 185, 187-190, 194-197, 199, 218-222, 227, 229, 232, 234-235, 244-245, 256, 259, 274, 299, 313, 328-330, 342

E

Echinococcus granulosus, 179, 190

Embolization, 71, 81, 163, 165-167, 198, 209, 299
  of a portal branch, 165

Emergency;
  resections, 194
  surgery, 14, 193

Endoprosthesis, 30

Ex situ, 241, 244-245 247
  in vivo, 241, 244-245, 247
  in vivo surgery, 241

Ex vivo, 147, 244
  extracorporeal surgery, 241
  surgery, 241

Extended;
  left hepatectomy, 85, 87-89
  right hepatectomy, 79, 81-84, 132, 144, 166, 197

Extreme liver surgery, 241, 263

F

Falciform ligament, 5-6, 8, 19-20, 26, 35, 45, 50, 53-54, 81-82, 87, 95-96, 107-108, 129, 194, 196, 253, 264, 313-314, 331, 333

Fenestration, 174-176

Fibrin glue, 76, 138, 140, 244, 296, 331-333

Fissure of the right hepatic vein, 56, 59-60, 63, 87, 97, 99

5-Fluorouracil, 205, 211

Focal nodular hyperplasia, 160-161

Fogarty catheter, 293

Fresh frozen plasma, 72, 246, 289, 323

FUDR, 205, 210

Fulminant hepatitis, 144, 285-286

Functional reserve of the liver, 72, 241

G

Galactose test, 143

Ganz's incisure, 50, 56, 61, 66, 87, 99

Gastroduodenal, 207-211, 224, 242, 254-255, 258, 260, 265, 270, 272, 310, 314
  artery, 207-210, 224, 242, 254-255, 258, 260, 265, 270, 272, 310, 314

Gelfoam, 165-166

Glisson's;
  capsule, 26, 28, 37, 41, 45, 50, 54, 56, 75, 81, 83, 95-96, 129, 137, 151, 180, 194, 224, 289, 310, 313
  pedicle, 5-7, 19, 22, 25-26, 29, 45-46, 50, 53-54, 56, 59, 61, 64, 66, 83-84, 87-88, 90, 95, 97, 99, 103, 105, 107-108, 115, 119, 129, 131, 137, 147, 160, 183, 194, 310, 313-315

Glucose tolerance test, 72

Gore-Tex®, 13, 130-132, 290, 316
  prosthesis, 131, 290

Graft Versus Host Disease, 344-345

Green clearance test, 143

Griffith circuit, 267

Growth factor, 270, 274, 323

H

Healey and Schroy's classification, 6, 49

Hemihepatic vascular occlusion, 147-148

Hemiliver, 5, 8, 19, 25-26, 35-38, 41, 50, 81, 87, 90, 104, 106, 108, 113, 128-129, 131, 147, 160, 165, 175, 179, 184, 193-194, 196, 207, 264, 309-315

Hemobilia, 193-194, 197-199, 220, 357

Hepatectomy, 5, 8, 11, 14, 17, 19-21, 23, 25, 27-31, 33, 35, 37, 39, 41, 50, 59, 74, 79, 81-84, 85, 87-89, 105-108, 110-111, 113, 115, 119-121, 128-129, 132, 137, 140, 144, 147, 155, 160, 165-167, 181, 185, 194, 196-197, 199, 245-246, 267-268, 270, 286, 289, 296-298, 300, 312, 319, 321, 324, 327, 330-333, 335, 358-359

Hepatic;
  artery, 19, 22-23, 35, 51, 56, 81-82, 87, 96-97, 106, 108, 110-111, 120, 152, 206-211, 217-219, 224, 228, 231, 233, 242, 253-254, 257-260, 264-265, 270, 272-274, 277, 289-291, 293, 296, 298-300, 302-303, 310-312, 314-315, 320-321, 323-324, 330-332
  hilum, 30, 41, 49, 95, 106, 115, 159, 166, 218, 227-229, 294, 297, 309, 320-321
  hydatidosis, 179, 189-190
  insufficiency, 30, 81, 139, 144, 147, 165-166, 197, 205, 234, 246-247
  metastases, 154, 156, 159, 161-162, 166, 205, 207, 210-211
  segments, 5, 12, 19, 49, 68, 219, 316
  vascular exclusion, 121, 241-244, 246-247
  veins, 6, 19, 21, 30, 35, 38, 40, 56, 59, 63, 66, 68, 74, 90, 103, 105-106, 108, 111, 114, 120, 127, 131, 137, 153, 187, 219, 227, 241, 243-245, 267-268, 277-280, 282, 284-285, 289, 296, 299-300, 310-313, 315, 319-322, 324, 330-333, 355

Hepatocellular carcinoma, (HCC), 14, 50-51, 55, 68, 71, 77, 95, 106, 114-115, 127-128, 140, 143-144, 154-155, 159, 161-162, 166, 205, 211, 292, 323

Hiatus of Wislow, 39

Hilar;
  cholangiocarcinoma, 106, 108, 115, 167, 215, 217,

219, 221, 223, 225, 227, 229, 231, 233, 235
plate, 6, 54, 56, 83, 95, 332
Hilum, 5-6, 22-23, 27, 30, 41, 46, 49-50, 54, 56, 59, 66, 84, 90, 95, 97, 99, 103, 106, 108-109, 114-115, 119, 129, 131, 147, 159, 161, 166, 179, 185, 188-189, 193-194, 196, 218, 227-229, 242, 244, 294, 297, 309, 311, 320-321, 329-331
HTK Breitschneider solution, 241, 244
Hydatid cyst, 12-13, 30, 45, 139, 185, 161, 179, 185-190, 358-359
Hydatidosis, 30, 177, 179, 181, 183, 185, 187, 189-190
Hyperosmolar coma, 180, 189
Hypoplastic portal vein, 294

I

Immunosuppressive treatment, 323
In situ, 241, 243-247, 315-316, 321, 327, 345
Indocyanine, 72, 143, 247
  green clearance, 72, 143, 247
Inferior mesenteric vein, 254-257, 259-260, 289
Intermittent clamping, 74, 89-90, 147, 320
Interposition graft of donor iliac artery, 273
Intestinal transplantation, 339-343, 345, 347-348
Intimal dissection, 289
Intra-arterial chemotherapy, 201, 205, 207, 210
Intra-operative, 14, 19, 30, 49, 71, 73-75, 77, 120, 115, 127, 132, 144, 149, 151-156, 159, 183-184, 188, 190, 198, 209, 246, 289, 292, 295-297, 303, 324, 314, 333-334
  ultrasound, 19, 49, 73-75, 115, 127, 149, 151, 153, 156, 159, 183-184, 190, 303
  Dopppler, 334
Intrabiliary rupture, 189
Intrahepatic hematoma, 193, 198

J

J incision, 11-13, 35, 73, 108, 263-264

Jumping graft, 290, 292, 294-295

K

Kaliaemia, 270
Kehr tube, 189, 196, 273, 303
Kent retractor, 11, 20, 263
Klatskin tumors, 108, 110, 160-161, 166

L

Laparoscopic fenestration, 174, 176
Left;
  hemihepatectomy, 217, 319-321, 323
  hepatectomy, 5, 11, 33, 35, 37, 39, 41, 50, 85, 87-89, 105-108, 194, 196, 331, 333
  hepatic artery, 35, 120, 206-207, 219, 224, 231, 242, 253-254, 264, 312, 314
  hepatic duct, 36-37, 39, 41, 51, 54, 83-84, 87, 95, 99, 107-108, 110-111, 113, 196, 224, 228-229, 231, 312, 321, 331
  hepatic vein, 6, 35, 41, 46, 83, 90, 97, 103-104, 109, 114, 131, 227, 281, 321, 331, 333
  lobectomy, 8, 12, 43, 45-46, 185, 196, 229, 314, 359
  triangular ligaments, 19, 107-108, 129, 242, 333
Left-sided liver graft from a living donor, 320
Lesser omentum, 35, 45, 104-105, 107-108, 242, 253-254, 264
Lesser sac, 39, 108
Lidocaine test, 30, 143-144
Lidocaine-MEGX test, 143
Liver;
  procurement, 251, 253, 255, 257, 259-260
  transplantation, 30, 71, 77, 143-144, 151-152, 174, 176, 197, 199, 241, 247, 249, 260, 263, 273-274, 277, 286, 287, 289, 291, 293, 295, 297, 299, 301, 303-304, 305, 307, 309-313, 315-316, 319, 323-324, 325, 327, 329-336, 348
  volume ratios, 323

Living related liver transplantation, (LRLT), 319-321, 323-324
Lobe, 5-6, 8, 11-12, 14, 19-20, 22, 25, 29-30, 35-38, 41, 45, 49-51, 61, 66, 68, 73, 81, 83-84, 87, 90, 99, 101, 103-109, 111, 113-115, 119-120, 127, 161, 165-166, 173-174, 179-180, 182, 185, 188, 193-197, 218-220, 223-224, 227-229, 232, 235, 242, 246, 254, 267, 279-280, 284, 286, 311-315, 321, 331-333, 356, 358-359
Lobectomy, 8, 12, 43, 45-46, 107, 111, 113, 115, 132, 185, 196, 228-229, 231, 235, 314, 359

M

MEGX, 30, 143-144
Mercedes incision, 11-12, 263
Mesocaval graft, 297
Mesohepatectomy, 95
Metal coils, 165-166
Metastases, 50, 62, 72, 81, 107, 128, 151, 154-156, 159-162, 166, 205, 207, 210-211, 223
Methylene blue, 28, 30, 66, 73, 75-76, 84, 99, 108, 139, 155, 181, 183, 187, 189, 198, 208, 273, 332-333
Middle;
  hepatic artery, 51, 224, 228, 231, 320-321
  hepatic vein, 27, 50-51, 53-54, 81, 83, 87, 97-99, 108, 184, 227, 280, 312-313, 319, 321, 331
Mobilization of the liver, 29, 115, 160, 253, 265
Mycophenolate Mofetil, 339

N

Nasobiliary tube, 30
Normothermic ischemia, 121, 147-148, 189, 241, 246-247

O

Oversized grafts, 296

P

Packing, 193-194, 196-197, 199, 260
Pancreas procurement, 259

Papaverin, 292

Partial pericystectomy, 185-187

PDS®;
   5-0, 274
   6-0, 273

PEEP, 39, 196

Percutaneous drainage, 66, 174, 179, 188, 299

Perendoscopic intubation, 303

Pericystium, 137, 139, 179-188

Piggy-back, 263, 275, 277, 279, 281, 283-286, 296-298, 315, 341-342
   technique, 263, 275, 277, 279, 281, 283-286, 296-298, 315, 342

Pleural effusion, 263

Polycystic liver disease, 173-174, 176

Port, 174, 208, 210

Portacaval anastomosis, 286, 289, 296-297, 335, 358

Portal;
   anastomosis, 270-271, 282, 294
   pedicles, 5, 49, 63, 95, 105, 127
   thrombectomy, 292
   vein, right branch, 23
   vein thrombosis, 72, 76, 246, 292, 294-295, 303-304, 315, 330

Porto-spienic-mesenteric thrombosis, 299

Ports, 205

Positive End Expiratory Pressure, 29, 196

Post-operative liver failure, 71-72, 76

Posterior diaphragmatic vein, 121-123

Pre-operative embolization, 81

Previous portosystemic anastomosis, 297

Pringle's maneuver, 147

Prolene®, 23, 26, 28-29, 38, 46, 66, 76, 90, 108, 127-128, 131, 258, 268, 270, 273, 279-280, 282, 289, 310-312, 316
   Prolene® 3-0, 26, 28-29, 38, 46, 90, 131, 268, 282
   Prolene® 4-0, 108, 127-128, 268, 279-280, 311
   Prolene® 5-0, 29, 258, 270, 289, 311
   Prolene® 6-0, 258, 27

Prolene Mesh®, 316

Proligerous membrane, 179

Pump, 207-210, 244

R

Rapid;
   procurement technique, 259
   technique, 253

Re-transplant, 285-286, 303

Redox;
   tolerance index, 72
   tolerance test, 143

Reduced size;
   grafts, 277, 309, 316
   livers, 286, 316, 315, 324, 361

Rejection, 315, 327-330, 334-335, 339, 343-347

Resection of;
   segment 4, 50-51, 95, 314
   segment 8, 54, 56-57, 59

Retransplantation, 289, 319, 344

Retrograde cholangiography, 30, 302

Rex's recess, 50-51, 54-55, 95, 165, 229, 231

Right;
   adrenal gland, 108, 242, 259, 265, 331
   adrenal vein, 74, 121, 242, 264-265, 278, 300
   branch of the portal vein, 23-24, 29, 56, 61, 87, 105, 111, 166, 194, 277, 280, 311, 313, 332
   hepatectomy, 8, 14, 17, 19-21, 23, 25, 27, 29-31, 35, 37, 39, 79, 81-84, 105, 108, 110-111, 113, 128-129, 132, 144, 165-166, 197, 245, 312, 358
   hepatic artery, 9, 87, 206-207, 224, 228, 253-254, 257-260, 273, 289, 310-312, 314, 332
   hepatic duct, 23, 25, 81, 83-84, 108, 224, 227-229, 311, 332
   hepatic vein, 6, 12-13, 20-22, 25-29, 50-51, 56, 59-60, 63-65, 68, 73, 81-82, 87, 90, 97, 99, 103-104, 108, 111, 120, 131, 183-184, 229, 278, 280-281, 285, 296, 311, 313, 321, 331-333
   inferior hepatic vein, 63, 104
   triangular ligament, 19, 50, 61, 64, 81, 87, 194, 196, 259-260, 278, 331

Round ligament, 8, 19, 53-54, 193-194, 229

Roux-en-Y
   hepaticojejunostomy 315
   loop, 30, 113, 161, 189, 220, 224, 226, 228-230, 235, 274, 302-303, 323, 342

Ruptured sub-capsular hematoma, 194

S

Sagittal fissure, 5, 50, 56, 196

Saphenous vein, 128, 132, 263, 267, 299

Sclerosing cholangitis, 189, 205, 210, 274

Segment 1-, 5-6, 49, 103-104, 107, 114, 217, 219, 224, 227-229, 231-232, 235, 331, 333

Segment 4-, 6, 8, 23, 38, 49-51, 53-55, 66, 81, 83-84, 95, 99, 161, 166, 219, 229, 231, 312-315, 320

Segment 5-, 6, 8, 50, 56, 59, 66, 87, 229

Segment 6-, 8, 61, 63, 66, 120, 127, 186, 198, 229

Segment 7-, 2, 13, 22, 30, 61-64, 66-67, 284

Segment 8-, 6, 27, 54, 56-57, 59-61, 66, 87, 131, 229

Segment 9, 103

Segmentary;
   anatomy, 5, 8, 309, 353
   branches, 49, 56, 61, 220, 224, 229-231

Segmentation, 5, 359

Segmentectomies, 8, 47, 49-51, 53, 55-57, 59, 61, 63, 65-68, 74-75, 137-138, 147, 160, 360,

Segmentectomy, 49-50, 66, 68, 155, 186, 199, 235, 319-321, 323-324

Segments, 5-6, 8, 12, 19, 21, 35, 45, 49-50, 60-61, 64-66, 68, 72, 74, 81, 87, 95, 99, 103, 106, 115, 127-128, 137, 147, 165-166, 174-175, 185, 187, 194, 199, 217-219, 224, 227-232, 235, 246, 259, 296, 309-310, 313-316, 330-331, 333

Selective vascular occlusion, 320

Serous cysts, 173-174

Spigelian;
   lobe, 6, 8, 103, 106, 161, 356
   veins, 107-109, 114, 244-245

Splenic artery, 208-210, 254, 258-260, 272, 289, 291, 310, 330, 333

Split liver, 307, 309, 311-313, 315-316, 330, 361
   transplantation, 307, 309, 311-313, 315-316

Spontaneous spleno-renal shunt, 296

Staining, 49-50, 73

Stenosis of the anastomosis, 303
Sub-total pericystectomy, 182, 184
Subphrenic abscesses, 30, 139, 188, 299
Subsegments, 8, 49, 219
Super-rapid technique, 253
Superior mesenteric vein, 257, 294-295, 303
Swan Ganz catheter, 72

T

Tacrolimus, 323, 339, 342-343, 347
Technetium 99, 208
Technical complications, 289, 344
Temporary porto-caval anastomosis, 277, 285
Thoracophrenolaparotomy, 12
Thrombosis;
   of arterial anastomosis, 303
   of the hepatic artery, 210, 302-303, 315
   of the portal vein, 159, 184, 292
   of the vena cava, 127
Total:
   pericystectomy, 179-181, 186

vascular exclusion, 114, 117, 121-123, 127-128, 130-131, 196, 247, 360
vascular exclusion of the liver, 121-123, 127, 130, 360
vascular occlusion, 74
Transanastomotic drainages, 220
Transjugular intrahepatic portosystemic shunts, (TIPS), 297-299, 303
Traumatic lesions of the liver, 193, 358
Triangular ligaments, 19, 107-108, 129, 193, 242, 265, 320, 333
Tumors of the bile duct, 217

U

Ultrasound dissector, 75, 137, 331-333
Umbilical;
   fissure, 49-50, 333
   ligament, 6, 45-46, 50, 81, 83, 95, 253, 264
University of Wisconsin (UW) solution, 241, 243 245, 257, 259-260, 313, 321, 331, 341

V

Vascular;
   exclusion, 114, 117, 119-121, 127-132, 196, 241-244, 246-247, 360-361
   involvement, 123, 218, 234
   occlusion, 74, 95, 121, 147-148, 320
   TEA, 297
Venous bypass, 263, 267, 270, 274, 277, 286, 289, 321
   ligament, 356
Vicryl®, 13-14, 21, 27, 30, 53-54, 66, 99, 137-139, 181, 183, 187-189, 194, 196, 274, 296, 310
   Vicryl® 3-0, 53, 137, 139, 181, 183, 188, 274
   Vicryl® 4-0, 30, 138, 310
   Vicryl® mesh, 194, 196, 296

W

Wall-stent, 218, 221, 222, 233-236
Warren's operation, 297
Waterjet dissector, 137
Witzel, 274

Acknowledgements

This book is published thanks to the contributions of
– Associazione Trapiantati di Fegato 'G Gozzetti'
– *Bancapulia*, San Severo, Foggia
– Regione Emilia Romagna
– Tito Fugazza, Piacenza